AMA
AMERICAN MEDICAL
ASSOCIATION

MW00993154

HCPCS Level II
Professional 2024

2024 HCPCS LEVEL II, PROFESSIONAL EDITION   ISBN: 978-1-64016-294-5

Notice

Practitioners and researchers must always rely on their own experience and knowledge in evaluating and using any information, methods, compounds or experiments described herein. Because of rapid advances in the medical sciences, in particular, independent verification of diagnoses and drug dosages should be made. To the fullest extent of the law, no responsibility is assumed by Elsevier, authors, editors or contributors for any injury and/or damage to persons or property as a matter of products liability, negligence or otherwise, or from any use or operation of any methods, products, instructions, or ideas contained in the material herein.

Previous editions copyrighted 2023, 2022, 2021, 2020, 2019, 2018, 2017, 2016, 2015, 2014, 2013, 2012, 2011, 2010, 2009, 2008, 2007, 2006, 2005, 2004, 2003, 2002, 2001, 2000

International Standard Book Number: 978-1-64016-294-5

Our Commitment to Accuracy
The American Medical Association (AMA) is committed to producing accurate and reliable materials. To report corrections, please call the AMA Unified Service Center at (800) 621-8335. AMA publication and product updates, errata, and addenda can be found at amaproductupdates.org. The AMA shall not be responsible for, and expressly disclaims liability for, damages of any kind arising out of the use of, reference to, or reliance on, the content of this publication. This publication is for informational purposes only.

To purchase additional copies, contact the AMA at (800) 621-8335 or visit the AMA store at amastore.com. Refer to item number **OP231524**.

Content Strategist: Laura Klein
Content Development Manager: Danielle Frazier
Senior Content Development Specialist: Joshua S. Rapplean
Publishing Services Manager: Deepthi Unni
Project Manager: Nayagi Anandan
Senior Book Designer: Maggie Reid

Printed in Canada

Last digit is the print number: 9   8   7   6   5   4   3   2   1

DEVELOPMENT OF THIS EDITION

Lead Technical Collaborator

Jackie L. Koesterman, CPC
Coding and Reimbursement Specialist
JDK Medical Coding EDU
Grand Forks, North Dakota

CONTENTS

Updates will be posted on codingupdates.com when available.

Check codingupdates.com for Practitioner and Facility Medically Unlikely Edits (MUEs) and Column 1 and Column 2 Edits.

Check the Centers for Medicare & Medicaid Services (www.cms.gov/Manuals/IOM/list.asp) website and codingupdates.com for full and select IOMs.

Notice: 2024 DMEPOS updates were unavailable at the time of printing. Check codingupdates.com for updates and DMEPOS Modifiers in January.

INTRODUCTION

2024 HCPCS quarterly updates available on the companion website at: www.codingupdates.com

The Centers for Medicare & Medicaid Services (CMS) (formerly Health Care Financing Administration [HCFA]) Healthcare Common Procedure Coding System (HCPCS) is a collection of codes and descriptors that represent procedures, supplies, products, and services that may be provided to Medicare beneficiaries and to individuals enrolled in private health insurance programs. The codes are divided as follows:

Level I: Codes and descriptors copyrighted by the American Medical Association's (AMA's) Current Procedural Terminology, ed. 4 (CPT-4). These are five-digit numeric codes representing physician and nonphysician services.

Level II: Includes codes and descriptors copyrighted by the American Dental Association's current dental terminology, seventh edition (CDT-7/8). These are five-digit alphanumeric codes comprising the D series. All other Level II codes and descriptors are alphanumeric and approved and maintained jointly by the editorial panel (consisting of CMS, the Health Insurance Association of America, and the Blue Cross Blue Shield Association). These are five-digit alphanumeric codes representing primarily items and nonphysician services that are not represented in the Level I codes.

Level III: The CMS eliminated Level III local codes. See Program Memorandum AB-02-113.

Headings are provided as a means of grouping similar or closely related items. The placement of a code under a heading does not indicate additional means of classification, nor does it relate to any health insurance coverage categories.

HCPCS also contains modifiers, which are two-digit codes and descriptors used to indicate that a service or procedure that has been performed has been altered by some specific circumstance but unchanged in its definition or code. Modifiers are grouped by levels. Level I modifiers and descriptors are copyrighted by the AMA. Level II modifiers are HCPCS modifiers. Modifiers in the D series are copyrighted by the ADA.

HCPCS is designed to promote uniform reporting and statistical data collection of medical procedures, supplies, products, and services.

HCPCS Disclaimer

Inclusion or exclusion of a procedure, supply, product, or service does not imply any health insurance coverage or reimbursement policy.

HCPCS makes as much use as possible of generic descriptions, but the inclusion of brand names to describe devices or drugs is intended only for indexing purposes; it is not meant to convey endorsement of any particular product or drug.

Updating HCPCS

The primary updates are made annually. Quarterly updates are also issued by CMS.

Medical coding has long been a part of the health care profession. Through the years medical coding systems have become more complex and extensive. Today, medical coding is an intricate and immense process that is present in every health care setting. The increased use of electronic submissions for health care services only increases the need for coders who understand the coding process.

2024 HCPCS Level II was developed to help meet the needs of today's coder.

All material adheres to the latest government versions available at the time of printing.

Annotated

Throughout this text, revisions and additions are indicated by the following symbols:

▶ **New:** Additions to the previous edition are indicated by the color triangle.

⮌ **Revised:** Revisions within the line or code from the previous edition are indicated by the color arrow.

✔ **Reinstated** indicates a code that was previously deleted and has now been reactivated.

✖ ~~Deleted~~ words have been removed from this year's edition.

HCPCS Symbols

✪ **Special coverage instructions** apply to these codes. Usually these special coverage instructions are included in the Internet Only Manuals (IOM). References to the IOM locations are given in the form of Medicare Pub. 100 reference numbers listed below the code. IOM select references are located at codingupdates.com.

⊘ **Not covered or valid by Medicare** is indicated by the "No" symbol. Usually the reason for the exclusion is included in the Internet Only Manuals (IOM) select references at codingupdates.com.

* **Carrier discretion** is an indication that you must contact the individual third-party payers to find out the coverage available for codes identified by this symbol.

Other Drugs approved for Medicare Part B and other FDA-approved drugs are listed as Other.

A2-Z3 **ASC Payment Indicators** identify the 2019 final payment for the code. A list of Payment Indicators is listed in the front matter of this text.

A-Y **OPPS Status Indicators** identify the 2019 final status assigned to the code. A list of Status Indicators is listed in the front matter of this text.

Ⓑ Bill Part B MAC.

Ⓓ Bill DME MAC.

Coding Clinic Indicates the American Hospital Association *Coding Clinic®* for HCPCS references by year, quarter, and page number.

♿ DMEPOS identifies durable medical equipment, prosthetics, orthotics, and supplies that may be eligible for payment from CMS.

♀ Indicates a code for female only.

♂ Indicates a code for male only.

Ⓐ Indicates a code with an indication of age.

🖐 Indicates a code included in the MIPS Quality Measure Specifications.

Qp Indicates there is a maximum allowable number of units of service, per day, per patient for physician/provider services (*see* codingupdates.com for Practitioner Medically Unlikely Edits).

Qh Indicates there is a maximum allowable number of units of service, per day, per patient in the outpatient hospital setting (*see* codingupdates.com for Hospital Medically Unlikely Edits).

Red, green, and blue typeface terms within the Table of Drugs and tabular section are terms added by the publisher and do not appear in the official code set. Information supplementing the official HCPCS Index produced by CMS is *italicized*.

SYMBOLS AND CONVENTIONS

HCPCS Symbols

Special coverage instructions apply to these codes. Usually these instructions are included in the Internet Only Manuals (IOM). References to the IOM locations are given in the form of Medicare Pub. 100 reference numbers listed below the code. IOM select references are located at codingupdates.com.

⊛ **L3540** Miscellaneous shoe additions, sole, full
IOM: 100-2, 15, 290

The Internet Only Manuals (IOM) give instructions regarding use of the code. IOM select references are located at codingupdates.com.

Not covered or valid by Medicare is indicated by the "No" symbol. Usually the reason for the exclusion is included in the IOM references located at codingupdates.com.

⊘ **A65331** Gradient compression stocking, thigh length, 18–30 mm Hg, each
IOM: 100-02, 15, 130; 100-03, 4, 280.1

Carrier discretion is an indication that you must contact the individual third-party payers for the coverage for these codes.

✳ **A6154** Wound pouch, each

A9541 Technetium Tc-99m sulfur colloid, diagnostic, per study dose, up to 20 millicuries

N1 ASC Payment Indicators **A2-Z3** identify the Final OPPS payment for the code.

A0180 Non-emergency transportation: ancillary: lodging-recipient

E ASC Status Indicators **A-Y** identify the Final OPPS status assigned to the code.

A4650 Implantable radiation dosimeter; each ⑧

Bill Part B MAC.

A4606 Oxygen probe for use with oximeter device; replacement ⑧

Bill DME MAC.

Coding Clinic indicates the American Hospital Association *Coding Clinic®* for HCPCS references by year, quarter, and page number.

A4543 Imagining, e.g., gadoteridol injection
Coding Clinic: 2001, Q3, P13-14

Codes shown are for illustration purposes only and may not be current codes.

DMEPOS symbol identifies durable medical equipment, prosthetics, orthotics, and supplies that may be eligible for payment from CMS.

E2210   Wheelchair accessory, bearings, any type, replacement only, each ♿

* **A4233**   Replacement battery, alkaline (other than J cell), for use with medically necessary home blood glucose monitor owned by patient, each ♿

If "incident to" physician service, do not bill; otherwise bill DME MAC

On DMEPOS Fee Schedule.

⊕ **B9000**   Enteral nutrition infusion pump - without alarm [Qp]   γ

Pump will be denied as not medically necessary if medical necessity of pump is not documented

IOM: 100-02, 15, 120; 100-03, 3, 180.2; 100-04, 20, 100.2.2

PEN: On Fee Schedule

On the Parenteral and Enteral Nutrition Items or Services (PEN) with modifier(s) from current PEN Fee Schedule.

A4261   Cervical cap for contraceptive use ♀

Indicates for female only.

A4267   Contraceptive supply, condom, male, each ♂

Indicates for male only.

Indicates a **reinstated** code.

✔ **D2970**   Temporary crown (fractured tooth)

Indicates **new** information or a new code.

▶ **A4614**   Peak expiratory flow rate meter, hand-held

Indicates a **revision** within the line or code.

↩ **J0270**   Injection alprostadil, per 1.25 mcg

Codes shown are for illustration purposes only and may not be current codes.

The strike-through indicates **deleted** information.

→ J1015   Injection, adenosine, 90 mg (not to be used to report any adenosine, phosphate compounds, instead use A9270)   ✖

The "✖" appears in the right margin to indicate deleted information.

Drugs approved for Medicare Part B and other FDA-approved drugs are listed as **Other**. This list may not be all inclusive.

✳ **J0135**   Injection, adalimumab, 20 mg
Other: Adalimumab

Italic typeface indicates publisher-added index items.

Ambulation device, E0100–E0159
AMI, documentation, *G8006–G8011*
Amikacin Sulfate, J0278

D0145   Oral evaluation for a patient under three years of age counseling with primary care giver **A** ◄

Indicates code with age indication.

Indicates the code is included in the MIPS Quality Measure Specifications.

→   **G0101**   Cervical or vaginal cancer screening pelvic and clinical breast examination

G0104   Colorectal cancer screening; flexible sigmoidoscopy **Qp** ◄

Indicates there is a maximum allowable number of units of service, per day, per patient for the **physician/provider** (*see* codingupdates.com, Medically Unlikely Edits).

G0104   Colorectal cancer screening; flexible sigmoidoscopy **Qh** ◄

Indicates there is a maximum allowable number of units of service, per day, per patient for the **hospital outpatient** (*see* codingupdates.com, Medically Unlikely Edits).

Codes shown are for illustration purposes only and may not be current codes.

A2-Z3 ASC Payment Indicators

Final ASC Payment Indicators for CY 2024	
Payment Indicator	**Payment Indicator Definition**
A2	Surgical procedure on ASC list in CY 2007; payment based on OPPS relative payment weight.
B5	Alternative code may be available; no payment made.
D1	Ancillary dental service/item; no separate payment made.
D2	Non office-based dental procedure added in CY 2024 or later.
D5	Deleted/discontinued code; no payment made.
F4	Corneal tissue acquisition, hepatitis B vaccine; paid at reasonable cost.
G2	Non-office-based surgical procedure added in CY 2008 or later; payment based on OPPS relative payment weight.
H2	Brachytherapy source paid separately when provided integral to a surgical procedure on ASC list; payment OPPS rate.
J7	OPPS pass-through device paid separately when provided integral to a surgical procedure on ASC list; payment contractor-priced.
J8	Device-intensive procedure; paid at adjusted rate.
K2	Drugs and biologicals paid separately when provided integral to a surgical procedure on ASC list; payment based on OPPS rate.
K5	Drugs and biologicals for which pricing information is not yet available.
K7	Unclassified drugs and biologicals; payment contractor-priced.
L1	Influenza vaccine; pneumococcal vaccine. Packaged item/service; no separate payment made.
L6	New Technology Intraocular Lens (NTIOL); special payment.
N1	Packaged service/item; no separate payment made.
P2	Office-based surgical procedure added to ASC list in CY 2008 or later with MPFS nonfacility PE RVUs; payment based on OPPS relative payment weight.
P3	Office-based surgical procedure added to ASC list in CY 2008 or later with MPFS nonfacility PE RVUs; payment based on MPFS nonfacility PE RVUs.
R2	Office-based surgical procedure added to ASC list in CY 2008 or later without MPFS nonfacility PE RVUs; payment based on OPPS relative payment weight.
Z2	Radiology or diagnostic service paid separately when provided integral to a surgical procedure on ASC list; payment based on OPPS relative payment weight.
Z3	Radiology or diagnostic service paid separately when provided integral to a surgical procedure on ASC list; payment based on MPFS nonfacility PE RVUs.

CMS-1772-FC, Final Changes to the ASC Payment System and CY 2024 Payment Rates, http://www.cms.gov/Medicare/Medicare-Fee-for-Service-Payment/ASCPayment/ASC-Regulations-and-Notices.html.

A-Y OPPS Status Indicators

	Final OPPS Payment Status Indicators for CY 2024	
Indicator	**Item/Code/Service**	**OPPS Payment Status**
A	Services furnished to a hospital outpatient that are paid under a fee schedule or payment system other than OPPS,* for example:	Not paid under OPPS. Paid by MACs under a fee schedule or payment system other than OPPS. Services are subject to deductible or coinsurance unless indicated otherwise.
	• Ambulance Services	
	• Separately Payable Clinical Diagnostic Laboratory Services	Not subject to deductible or coinsurance.
	• Separately Payable Non-Implantable Prosthetics and Orthotics	
	• Physical, Occupational, and Speech Therapy	
	• Diagnostic Mammography	
	• Screening Mammography	Not subject to deductible or coinsurance.
	Unclassified drugs and biologicals reportable under HCPCS code C9399	Contractor priced at 95 percent of drug or biological's average wholesale price (AWP) using Red Book or an equivalent recognized compendium and paid under OPPS.
B	Codes that are not recognized by OPPS when submitted on an outpatient hospital Part B bill type (12x and 13x)	Not paid under OPPS. • May be paid by MACs when submitted on a different bill type, for example, 75x (CORF), but not paid under OPPS. • An alternate code that is recognized by OPPS when submitted on an outpatient hospital Part B bill type (12x and 13x) may be available.
C	Inpatient Procedures	Not paid under OPPS. Admit patient. Bill as inpatient.
D	Discontinued Codes	Not paid under OPPS or any other Medicare payment system.
E1	Items, Codes and Services: • Not covered by any Medicare outpatient benefit category • Statutorily excluded by Medicare • Not reasonable and necessary	Not paid by Medicare when submitted on outpatient claims (any outpatient bill type).
E2	Items, Codes and Services: For which pricing information and claims data are not available	Not paid by Medicare when submitted on outpatient claims (any outpatient bill type).
F	Corneal Tissue Acquisition; Certain CRNA Services	Not paid under OPPS. Paid at reasonable cost.
G	Pass-Through Drugs and Biologicals	Paid under OPPS; separate APC payment.
H	Pass-Through Device Categories	Separate cost-based pass-through payment; not subject to copayment.
J1	Hospital Part B services paid through a comprehensive APC	Paid under OPPS; all covered Part B services on the claim are packaged with the primary "J1" service for the claim, except services with OPPS status indicator of "F," "G," "H," "L," and "U"; ambulance services; diagnostic and screening mammography; all preventive services; and certain Part B inpatient services.
J2	Hospital Part B Services That May Be Paid Through a Comprehensive APC	Paid under OPPS; Addendum B displays APC assignments when services are separately payable. (1) Comprehensive APC payment based on OPPS comprehensive-specific payment criteria. Payment for all covered Part B services on the claim is packaged into a single payment for specific combinations of services, except services with OPPS status indicator of "F," "G," "H," "L" and "U"; ambulance services; diagnostic and screening mammography; all preventive services; and certain Part B inpatient services. (2) Packaged APC payment if billed on the same claim as a HCPCS code assigned status indicator "J1." (3) In other circumstances, payment is made through a separate APC payment or packaged into payment for other services.

A-Y OPPS Status Indicators—cont'd

	Final OPPS Payment Status Indicators for CY 2024		
Indicator	**Item/Code/Service**	**OPPS Payment Status**	
K	Non-Pass-Through Drugs and Non-Implantable Biologicals, including Therapeutic Radiopharmaceuticals	Paid under OPPS: separate APC payment.	
L	Influenza Vaccine; Pneumococcal Pneumonia Vaccine; Hepatitis B Vaccines; Covid-19 Vaccine; Monoclonal Antibody Therapy Product	Not paid under OPPS. Paid at reasonable cost; not subject to deductible or coinsurance.	
M	Items and Services Not Billable to the MAC	Not paid under OPPS.	
N	Items and Services Packaged into APC Rates	Paid under OPPS; payment is packaged into payment for other services. Therefore, there is no separate APC payment.	
P	Partial Hospitalization	Paid under OPPS; per diem APC payment.	
Q1	STV-Packaged Codes	Paid under OPPS; Addendum B displays APC assignments when services are separately payable. (1) Packaged APC payment if billed on the same claim as a HCPCS code assigned status indicator "S," "T," or "V." (2) Composite APC payment if billed with specific combinations of services based on OPPS composite-specific payment criteria. Payment is packaged into a single payment for specific combinations of services. (3) In other circumstances, payment is made through a separate APC payment.	
Q2	T-Packaged Codes	Paid under OPPS; Addendum B displays APC assignments when services are separately payable. (1) Packaged APC payment if billed on the same claim as a HCPCS code assigned status indicator "T." (2) In other circumstances, payment is made through a separate APC payment.	
Q3	Codes That May Be Paid Through a Composite APC	Paid under OPPS; Addendum B displays APC assignments when services are separately payable. Addendum M displays composite APC assignments when codes are paid through a composite APC. (1) Composite APC payment based on OPPS composite-specific payment criteria. Payment is packaged into a single payment for specific combinations of service. (2) In other circumstances, payment is made through a separate APC payment or packaged into payment for other services.	
Q4	Conditionally packaged laboratory tests	Paid under OPPS or CLFS. (1) Packaged APC payment if billed on the same claim as a HCPCS code assigned published status indicator "J1," "J2," "S," "T," "V," "Q1," "Q2," or "Q3." (2) In other circumstances, laboratory tests should have an SI=A and payment is made under the CLFS.	
R	Blood and Blood Products	Paid under OPPS; separate APC payment.	
S	Procedure or Service, Not Discounted when Multiple	Paid under OPPS; separate APC payment.	
T	Procedure or Service, Multiple Procedure Reduction Applies	Paid under OPPS; separate APC payment.	
U	Brachytherapy Sources	Paid under OPPS; separate APC payment.	
V	Clinic or Emergency Department Visit	Paid under OPPS; separate APC payment.	
Y	Non-Implantable Durable Medical Equipment	Not paid under OPPS. All institutional providers other than home health agencies bill to a DME MAC.	

* Note — Payments "under a fee schedule or payment system other than OPPS" may be contractor priced.

CMS-1772-FC, Final Changes to the ASC Payment System and CY 2024 Payment Rates, http://www.cms.gov/Medicare/Medicare-Fee-for-Service-Payment/HospitalOutpatientPPS/Hospital-Outpatient-Regulations-and-Notices.html.

2024 HCPCS UPDATES

2024 HCPCS New/Revised/Deleted Codes and Modifiers

HCPCS quarterly updates are posted on the companion website (www.codingupdates.com) when available.

NEW CODES/MODIFIERS

JK	C9149	J0137	J1813	J9056	Q4268
JL	C9150	J0174	J1814	J9058	Q4269
A2019	C9151	J0206	J1836	J9059	Q4270
A2020	C9152	J0208	J1920	J9063	Q4271
A2022	C9153	J0216	J1921	J9064	Q4272
A2023	C9154	J0218	J1941	J9196	Q4273
A2024	C9155	J0349	J1961	J9259	Q4274
A2025	C9156	J0457	J2249	J9294	Q4275
A4341	C9157	J0612	J2305	J9296	Q4276
A4342	C9158	J0613	J2329	J9297	Q4277
A4560	C9784	J0665	J2359	J9322	Q4278
A6590	C9785	J0736	J2371	J9323	Q4280
A6591	C9786	J0737	J2372	J9345	Q4281
A7049	C9787	J0801	J2427	J9347	Q4282
A9156	C9788	J0802	J2403	J9350	Q4283
A9268	C9789	J0874	J2561	J9380	Q4284
A9269	C9790	J0889	J2598	J9381	Q4285
A9292	C9791	J1411	J2599	K1035	Q4286
A9573	C9792	J1440	J2781	K1036	Q5127
A9603	E0490	J1449	J2806	L1681	Q5128
A9697	E0491	J1576	J7213	L5991	Q5129
B4148	E0677	J1747	J7214	L8678	Q5130
C9145	E0711	J1805	J7353	M0010	Q5131
C9146	E1905	J1806	J7519	Q4265	S9563
C9147	H2040	J1811	J9029	Q4266	V2526
C9148	H2041	J1812	J9051	Q4267	

REVISED CODES/MODIFIERS

LU	G0460	J1954	K1019	Q5111	S9562
A4344	G0465	J2426	K1028	Q5120	
A4628	J1921	K1004	Q5108	Q5122	

DELETED CODES/MODIFIERS

C1834	C9149	J0610	S0020	U0003
C9146	C9151	J0611	S0030	U0004
C9147	G2023	J0800	S0073	U0005
C9148	G2024	J2370	S0077	

NEW, REVISED, AND DELETED DENTAL CODES

New	D2976	D6089	D9938	D9955	**Revised**
D0396	D2989	D7284	D9939	D9956	D2335
D1301	D2991	D7939	D9954	D9957	D5876

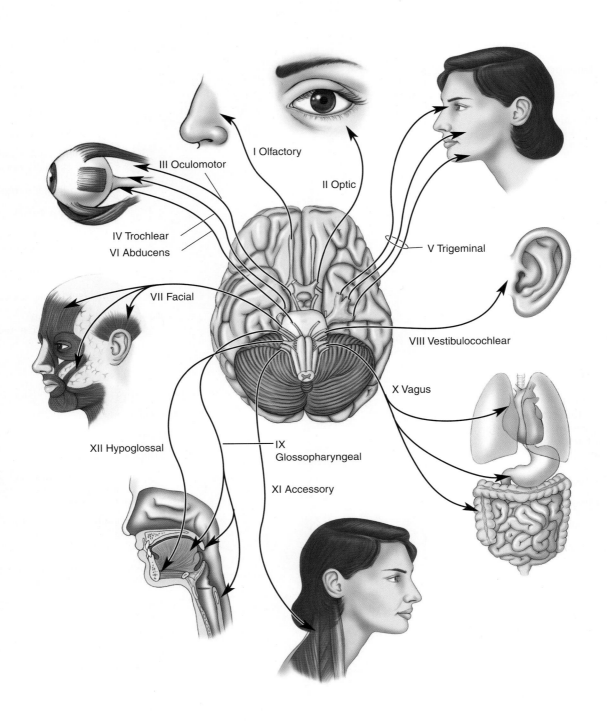

I Olfactory

II Optic

III Oculomotor

IV Trochlear
VI Abducens

V Trigeminal

VII Facial

VIII Vestibulocochlear

XII Hypoglossal

IX Glossopharyngeal

XI Accessory

X Vagus

Plate 1 Cranial Nerves (12 pairs) are known by their numbers (Roman numerals) and names. (Herlihy BL: The Human Body in Health and Illness, ed 6, St. Louis, 2018, Elsevier.)

ANATOMY ILLUSTRATIONS

Superior view

- Supratrochlear nerve
- Medial rectus muscle
- Superior oblique muscle
- Infratrochlear nerve
- Nasociliary nerve
- Trochlear nerve (IV)
- Common tendinous ring
- Ophthalmic nerve (V₁)
- Optic nerve (II)
- Internal carotid artery and nerve plexus
- Oculomotor nerve (III)
- Trochlear nerve (IV)
- Abducent nerve (VI)
- Tentorium cerebelli

- Medial branch } Supraorbital nerve
- Lateral branch
- Levator palpebrae superioris muscle
- Superior rectus muscle
- Lacrimal gland
- Lacrimal nerve
- Lateral rectus muscle
- Frontal nerve
- Maxillary nerve (V₂)
- Meningeal branch of maxillary nerve
- Mandibular nerve (V₃)
- Lesser petrosal nerve
- Meningeal branch of mandibular nerve
- Greater petrosal nerve
- Trigeminal (semilunar) ganglion
- Tentorial (meningeal) branch of ophthalmic nerve

Superior view:
levator palpebrae superioris, superior rectus, and superior oblique muscles partially cut away

- Supratrochlear nerve (cut)
- Supraorbital nerve branches (cut)
- Infratrochlear nerve
- Anterior ethmoidal nerve
- Optic nerve (II)
- Posterior ethmoidal nerve
- Superior branch of oculomotor nerve (III) (cut)
- Nasociliary nerve
- Internal carotid plexus
- Trochlear nerve (IV) (cut)
- Oculomotor nerve (III)
- Abducent nerve (VI)

- Long ciliary nerves
- Short ciliary nerves
- Lacrimal nerve
- Ciliary ganglion
- Parasympathetic root of ciliary ganglion (from inferior branch of oculomotor nerve)
- Sympathetic root of ciliary ganglion (from internal carotid plexus)
- Sensory root of ciliary ganglion (from nasociliary nerve)
- Branches to inferior and medial rectus muscles
- Abducent nerve (VI)
- Inferior branch of oculomotor nerve (III)
- Lacrimal nerve
- Frontal nerve (cut)
- Ophthalmic nerve (V₁)

Proper palmar digital nerves (median nerve)

Medial two lumbricals
innervated by ulnar nerve

Cutaneous innervation
of the median nerve in the hand

Cutaneous innervation
of the dorsal branch of
the ulnar nerve

Cutaneous innervation
of the palmar branch of
the median nerve

Palmar view

Lateral two lumbricals
innervated by median nerve

Dorsal view

Proper palmar
digital nerve
(ulnar nerve)

Intrinsic muscles
innervated by
ulnar nerve except
the thenar muscles
and the two lateral
lumbricals

Common palmar
digital nerve

Hypothenar
muscles
innervated by
ulnar nerve

Common palmar digital nerves
(median nerve)

Cutaneous innervation
of the superficial branch of
the ulnar nerve in
the hand

Thenar muscles
innervated by median nerve

Recurrent branch of median nerve

Palmaris brevis

Deep branch of the
ulnar nerve

Superficial branch of the
ulnar nerve

Palmar branch of the
ulnar nerve

Ulnar nerve

Ulna

Palmar branch of the
median nerve

Median nerve

Radius

Cutaneous innervation
of the palmar branch of
the ulnar nerve

Palmar view

Cutaneous innervation
of the median nerve in the hand

Innervation of the hand, median and ulnar nerves
(palmar view)

Dorsal view

Plate 3 Innervation of the Hand: Median and Ulnar Nerves (From Drake RL, Vogl AW, Mitchell AWM, Tibbitts RM, Richardson PE: Gray's Atlas of Anatomy, ed 2, Philadelphia, 2015, Churchill Livingstone.)

Biceps brachii

Posterior cutaneous nerve of forearm (cut) (from radial nerve)

Lateral cutaneous nerve of forearm (cut) (from musculocutaneous nerve)

Biceps brachii tendon

Radial artery

Brachioradialis

Radial artery

Palmaris longus tendon

Median nerve

Thenar muscles

Palmar branch of median nerve

Palmar aponeurosis

Ulnar nerve

Medial cutaneous nerve of forearm (from medial cord of brachial plexus)

Median nerve

Brachial artery

Medial epicondyle

Bicipital aponeurosis

Ulnar artery

Ulnar nerve

Palmar branch of ulnar nerve

Hypothenar muscles

Radial nerve

Brachial artery

Lateral epicondyle

Radial recurrent artery

Deep branch radial nerve

Radial artery

Supinator

Superficial branch radial nerve

Common interosseous artery

Posterior interosseous artery

Interosseous membrane

Pronator teres (cut)

Perforating branches of anterior interosseous artery

Brachioradialis tendon (cut)

Palmar branch of ulnar nerve

Median nerve

Flexor carpi radialis tendon (cut)

Flexor retinaculum

Superficial palmar branch of radial artery

Palmar branch of median nerve

Median nerve

Recurrent interosseous artery

Ulnar nerve

Humeral head of pronator teres (cut)

Posterior interosseous artery

Anterior ulnar recurrent artery

Humeral head of flexor carpi ulnaris

Posterior ulnar recurrent artery

Ulnar head of pronator teres

Ulnar artery

Anterior interosseous nerve

Anterior interosseous artery

Flexor digitorum superficialis (cut)

Flexor digitorum profundus

Flexor carpi ulnaris tendon (cut)

Ulnar nerve

Palmar branch of ulnar nerve

Deep palmar branch of ulnar artery

Deep palmar arch

Superficial palmar arch

Superior ulnar collateral artery

Inferior ulnar collateral artery

Radial collateral artery

Brachial artery

Radial recurrent artery

Anterior ulnar recurrent artery

Posterior ulnar recurrent artery

Common interosseous artery

Anterior interosseous artery

Ulnar artery

Radial artery

Interosseous membrane

Radius

Ulna

Superficial palmar branch of radial artery

Pisiform

Dorsal branch of ulnar nerve

Superficial palmar arch

Deep palmar arch

Arteries and nerves of forearm (anterior view)

Plate 4 Arteries and Nerves of the Forearm (Anterior View) (From Drake RL, Vogl AW, Mitchell AWM, Tibbitts RM, Richardson PE: Gray's Atlas of Anatomy, ed 2, Philadelphia, 2015, Churchill Livingstone.)

ANATOMY ILLUSTRATIONS

Lateral cutaneous branch of subcostal nerve

Inguinal ligament (Poupart's)

Superficial circumflex iliac vein

Femoral branches of genitofemoral nerve

Lateral femoral cutaneous nerve

Saphenous opening (fossa ovalis)

Fascia lata

Anterior cutaneous branches of femoral nerve

Patellar nerve plexus

Branches of lateral sural cutaneous nerve (from common fibular [peroneal] nerve)

Deep fascia of leg (crural fascia)

Superficial fibular (peroneal) nerve
Medial dorsal cutaneous branch

Intermediate dorsal cutaneous branch

Small saphenous vein and lateral dorsal cutaneous nerve (from sural nerve)

Lateral dorsal digital nerve and vein of 5th toe

Dorsal metatarsal veins

Dorsal digital nerves and veins

Superficial epigastric vein

Ilioinguinal nerve (scrotal branch) (usually passes through superficial inguinal ring)

Genital branch of genitofemoral nerve

Femoral vein

Superficial external pudendal vein

Accessory saphenous vein

Great saphenous vein

Cutaneous branches of obturator nerve

Infrapatellar branch of saphenous nerve

Saphenous nerve (terminal branch of femoral nerve)

Great saphenous vein

Dorsal digital nerves

Dorsal venous arch

Dorsal digital nerve and vein of medial side of great toe

Dorsal digital branch of deep fibular (peroneal) nerve

ANATOMY ILLUSTRATIONS

Plate 5 Superficial Nerves and Veins of Lower Limb: Anterior View. (Copyright 2023 Elsevier Inc. All rights reserved. www. netterimages.com. Image ID: 4846.)

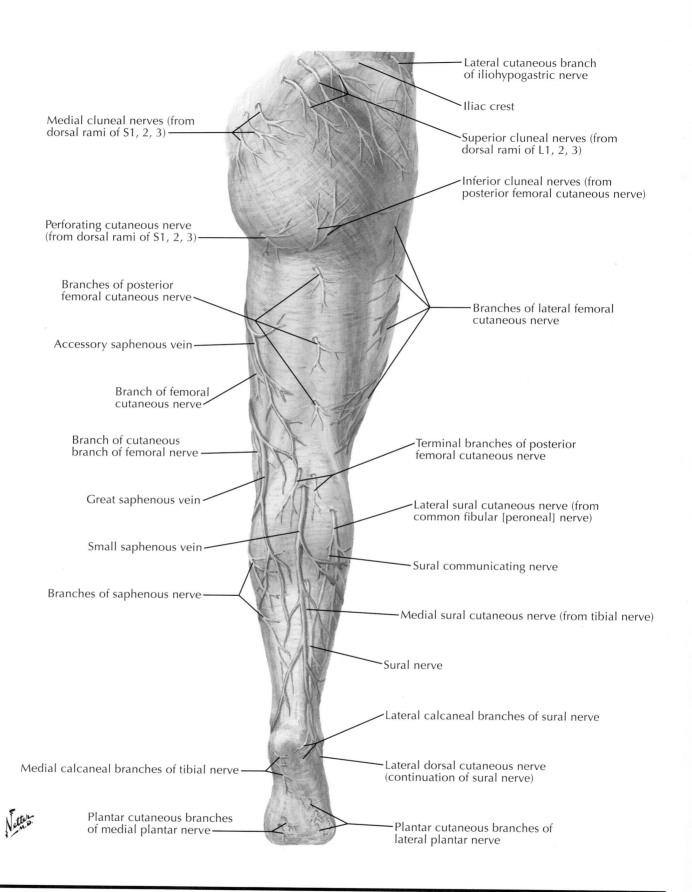

Lateral cutaneous branch of iliohypogastric nerve

Iliac crest

Medial cluneal nerves (from dorsal rami of S1, 2, 3)

Superior cluneal nerves (from dorsal rami of L1, 2, 3)

Inferior cluneal nerves (from posterior femoral cutaneous nerve)

Perforating cutaneous nerve (from dorsal rami of S1, 2, 3)

Branches of posterior femoral cutaneous nerve

Branches of lateral femoral cutaneous nerve

Accessory saphenous vein

Branch of femoral cutaneous nerve

Branch of cutaneous branch of femoral nerve

Terminal branches of posterior femoral cutaneous nerve

Great saphenous vein

Lateral sural cutaneous nerve (from common fibular [peroneal] nerve)

Small saphenous vein

Sural communicating nerve

Branches of saphenous nerve

Medial sural cutaneous nerve (from tibial nerve)

Sural nerve

Lateral calcaneal branches of sural nerve

Medial calcaneal branches of tibial nerve

Lateral dorsal cutaneous nerve (continuation of sural nerve)

Plantar cutaneous branches of medial plantar nerve

Plantar cutaneous branches of lateral plantar nerve

Plate 6 Superficial Nerves and Veins of Lower Limb: Posterior View. (Copyright 2023 Elsevier Inc. All rights reserved. www.netterimages.com. Image ID: 4669.)

ANATOMY ILLUSTRATIONS

Superficial dissections

Anterior superior iliac spine
Lateral femoral cutaneous nerve
Inguinal ligament
Iliopsoas muscle
Superficial circumflex iliac vessels
Superficial epigastric vessels
Superficial and Deep external pudendal vessels

Tensor fasciae latae muscle (*retracted*)
Gluteus minimus and medius muscles
Lateral circumflex femoral artery
Rectus femoris muscle
Vastus lateralis muscle
Vastus medialis muscle
Femoral sheath
Femoral nerve, artery, and vein
Pectineus muscle
Profunda femoris (deep femoral) artery
Gracilis muscle
Adductor longus muscle
Sartorius muscle
Vastus medialis muscle
Fascia lata (*cut*)
Rectus femoris muscle
Vastus lateralis muscle
Tensor fasciae latae muscle

Lateral femoral cutaneous nerve (*cut*)
Sartorius muscle (*cut*)
Iliopsoas muscle
Femoral nerve, artery, and vein
Pectineus muscle
Profunda femoris (deep femoral) artery
Adductor longus muscle
Adductor canal (opened by removal of sartorius muscle)
Saphenous nerve
Nerve to vastus medialis muscle
Adductor magnus muscle
Anteromedial intermuscular septum covers entrance of femoral vessels to popliteal fossa (adductor hiatus)
Sartorius muscle (*cut*)
Superior medial genicular artery (from popliteal artery)
Inferior medial genicular artery (from popliteal artery)

Saphenous nerve and saphenous branch of descending genicular artery
Articular branch of descending genicular artery (emerges from vastus medialis muscle)
Patellar anastomosis
Infrapatellar branch of Saphenous nerve

f. Netter, m.d.

Plate 7 Arteries and Nerves of Thigh: Anterior Views. (Copyright 2023 Elsevier Inc. All rights reserved. www.netterimages.com. Image ID: 4475.)

Deep dissection

Deep circumflex iliac artery

Lateral femoral cutaneous nerve

Sartorius muscle (cut)

Iliopsoas muscle

Tensor fasciae latae muscle (retracted)

Gluteus medius and minimus muscles

Femoral nerve

Rectus femoris muscle (cut)

Ascending, transverse and descending branches of lateral circumflex femoral artery

Lateral circumflex femoral artery

Medial circumflex femoral artery

Pectineus muscle (cut)

Profunda femoris (deep femoral) artery

Perforating branches

Adductor longus muscle (cut)

Vastus lateralis muscle

Vastus intermedius muscle

Rectus femoris muscle (cut)

Saphenous nerve

Anteromedial intermuscular septum (opened)

Vastus medialis muscle

Quadriceps femoris tendon

Patella and patellar anastomosis

Medial patellar retinaculum

Patellar ligament

External iliac artery and vein

Inguinal ligament (Poupart's)

Femoral artery and vein (cut)

Pectineus muscle (cut)

Obturator canal

Obturator externus muscle

Adductor longus muscle (cut)

Anterior branch and Posterior branch of obturator nerve

Quadratus femoris muscle

Adductor brevis muscle

Branches of posterior branch of obturator nerve

Adductor magnus muscle

Gracilis muscle

Cutaneous branch of obturator nerve

Femoral artery and vein (cut)

Descending genicular artery

Articular branch

Saphenous branch

Adductor hiatus

Sartorius muscle (cut)

Adductor magnus tendon

Adductor tubercle on medial epicondyle of femur

Superior medial genicular artery (from popliteal artery)

Infrapatellar branch of Saphenous nerve

Inferior medial genicular artery (from popliteal artery)

Deep dissection

Superior cluneal nerves

Gluteus maximus muscle (*cut*)

Medial cluneal nerves

Inferior gluteal artery and nerve

Pudendal nerve

Nerve to obturator internus
(and superior gemellus)

Posterior femoral
cutaneous nerve

Sacrotuberous ligament

Ischial tuberosity

Inferior cluneal nerves (*cut*)

Adductor magnus muscle

Gracilis muscle

Sciatic nerve

Muscular branches of sciatic nerve

Semitendinosus muscle (*retracted*)

Semimembranosus muscle

Sciatic nerve

Articular branch

Adductor hiatus

Popliteal vein and artery

Superior medial genicular artery

Medial epicondyle of femur

Tibial nerve

Gastrocnemius muscle (medial head)

Medial sural cutaneous nerve

Small saphenous vein

Iliac crest

Gluteal aponeurosis and
gluteus medius muscle (*cut*)

Superior gluteal artery and nerve

Gluteus minimus muscle

Tensor fasciae latae muscle

Piriformis muscle

Gluteus medius muscle (*cut*)

Superior gemellus muscle

Greater trochanter of femur

Obturator internus muscle

Inferior gemellus muscle

Gluteus maximus muscle (*cut*)

Quadratus femoris muscle

Medial circumflex femoral
artery

Vastus lateralis muscle
and iliotibial tract

Adductor minimus part of
adductor magnus muscle

1st perforating artery (from
profunda femoris artery)

Adductor magnus muscle

2nd and 3rd perforating arteries
(from profunda femoris artery)

4th perforating artery (from
profunda femoris artery)

Long head (*retracted*) ⎫ Biceps femoris
Short head ⎬ muscle

Superior lateral genicular artery

Common fibular (peroneal) nerve

Plantaris muscle

Gastrocnemius muscle (lateral head)

Lateral sural cutaneous nerve

Plate 9 Arteries and Nerves of Thigh: Posterior View. (Copyright 2023 Elsevier Inc. All rights reserved. www.netterimages.com. Image ID: 49317.)

ANATOMY ILLUSTRATIONS

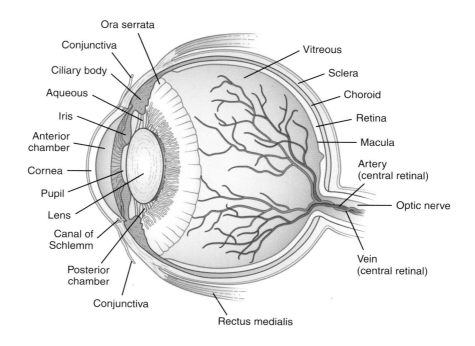

Ora serrata

Conjunctiva

Ciliary body

Aqueous

Iris

Anterior
chamber

Cornea

Pupil

Lens

Canal of
Schlemm

Posterior
chamber

Conjunctiva

Rectus medialis

Vitreous

Sclera

Choroid

Retina

Macula

Artery
(central retinal)

Optic nerve

Vein
(central retinal)

Plate 10   Anatomy of the Eye. (Dehn RW, Asprey DP: Essential Clinical Procedures, ed 3, Philadelphia, 2013, Saunders.)

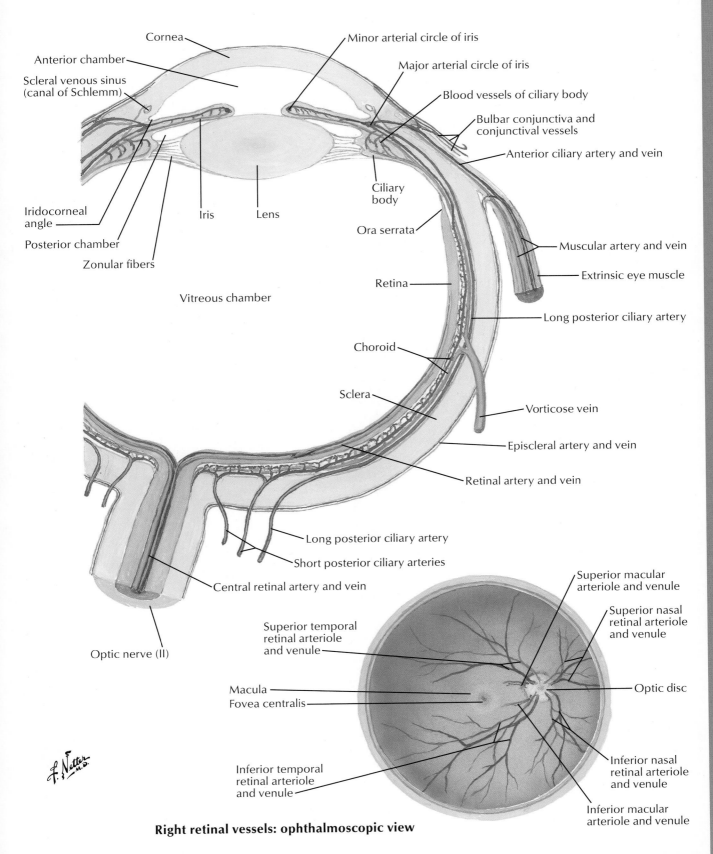

Cornea

Anterior chamber

Scleral venous sinus
(canal of Schlemm)

Minor arterial circle of iris

Major arterial circle of iris

Blood vessels of ciliary body

Bulbar conjunctiva and
conjunctival vessels

Anterior ciliary artery and vein

Ciliary body

Ora serrata

Iridocorneal angle

Posterior chamber

Zonular fibers

Iris

Lens

Muscular artery and vein

Extrinsic eye muscle

Long posterior ciliary artery

Retina

Vitreous chamber

Choroid

Sclera

Vorticose vein

Episcleral artery and vein

Retinal artery and vein

Long posterior ciliary artery

Short posterior ciliary arteries

Central retinal artery and vein

Optic nerve (II)

Superior temporal
retinal arteriole
and venule

Macula

Fovea centralis

Superior macular
arteriole and venule

Superior nasal
retinal arteriole
and venule

Optic disc

Inferior nasal
retinal arteriole
and venule

Inferior temporal
retinal arteriole
and venule

Inferior macular
arteriole and venule

Right retinal vessels: ophthalmoscopic view

f. Netter
M.D.

Plate 11 Intrinsic Arteries and Veins of Eye. (Copyright 2023 Elsevier Inc. All rights reserved. www.netterimages.com. Image ID: 49107.)

ANATOMY ILLUSTRATIONS

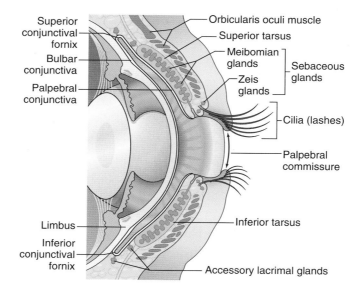

Superior conjunctival fornix
Bulbar conjunctiva
Palpebral conjunctiva
Orbicularis oculi muscle
Superior tarsus
Meibomian glands
Zeis glands
Sebaceous glands
Cilia (lashes)
Palpebral commissure
Limbus
Inferior conjunctival fornix
Inferior tarsus
Accessory lacrimal glands

Plate 12 Anatomy of the Conjunctiva and Eyelids. (Kumar V, Abbas AK, Aster JC: Robbins and Cotran Pathologic Basis of Disease, ed 9, Philadelphia, 2015, Saunders.)

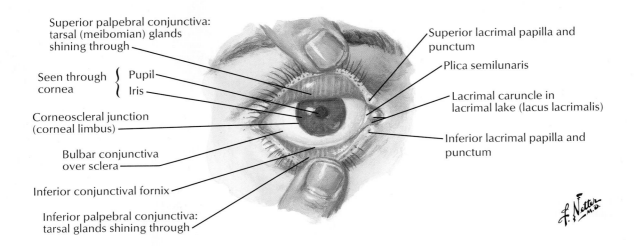

Superior palpebral conjunctiva: tarsal (meibomian) glands shining through

Seen through cornea { Pupil / Iris

Corneoscleral junction (corneal limbus)

Bulbar conjunctiva over sclera

Inferior conjunctival fornix

Inferior palpebral conjunctiva: tarsal glands shining through

Superior lacrimal papilla and punctum

Plica semilunaris

Lacrimal caruncle in lacrimal lake (lacus lacrimalis)

Inferior lacrimal papilla and punctum

ANATOMY ILLUSTRATIONS

Orbital part of lacrimal gland

Palpebral part of lacrimal gland

Excretory ducts of lacrimal gland

Plica semilunaris

Lacrimal caruncle

Inferior lacrimal papilla and punctum

Superior lacrimal papilla and punctum

Lacrimal canaliculi

Lacrimal sac

Nasolacrimal duct

Opening of nasolacrimal duct

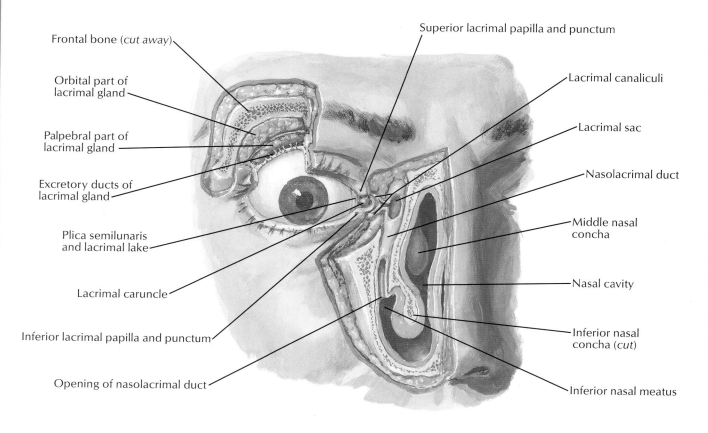

Frontal bone (cut away)

Orbital part of lacrimal gland

Palpebral part of lacrimal gland

Excretory ducts of lacrimal gland

Plica semilunaris and lacrimal lake

Lacrimal caruncle

Inferior lacrimal papilla and punctum

Opening of nasolacrimal duct

Superior lacrimal papilla and punctum

Lacrimal canaliculi

Lacrimal sac

Nasolacrimal duct

Middle nasal concha

Nasal cavity

Inferior nasal concha (cut)

Inferior nasal meatus

Plate 14 Lacrimal Apparatus.

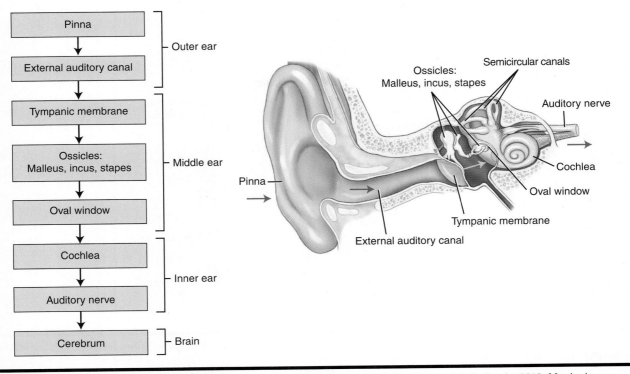

Plate 15 Pathway of Sound. (LaFleur Brooks D, LaFleur Brooks M: Basic Medical Language, ed 4, St. Louis, 2013, Mosby.)

Plate 16 Middle Ear Structures. (©Elsevier Collection.)

RIGHT TYMPANIC MEMBRANE

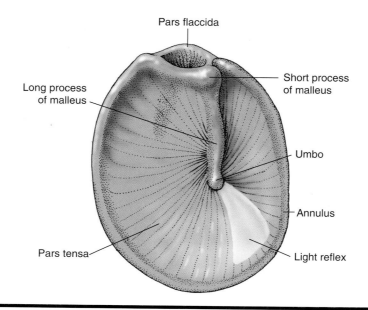

Plate 17 Structural Landmarks of Tympanic Membrane. (Ignatavicius DD, Workman ML: Medical-Surgical Nursing: Patient-Centered Collaborative Care, ed 7, St. Louis, 2013, Saunders.)

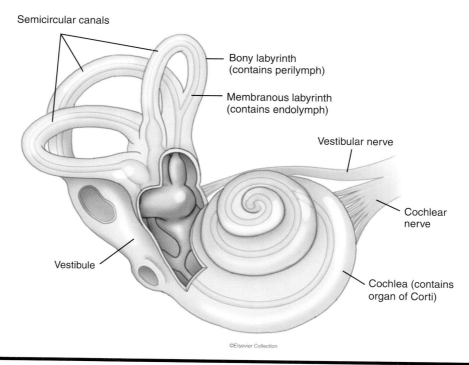

Plate 18 Inner Ear Structures. (©Elsevier Collection.)

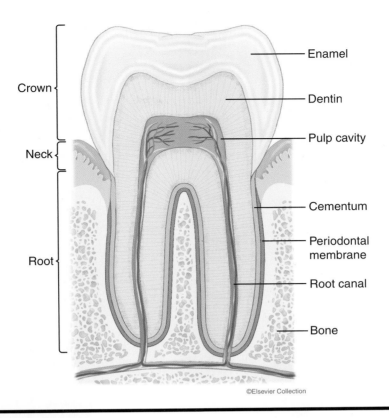

Crown {
Enamel

Dentin

Pulp cavity

Neck {

Root {
Cementum

Periodontal membrane

Root canal

Bone

©Elsevier Collection

Plate 19   The Tooth. (©Elsevier Collection).

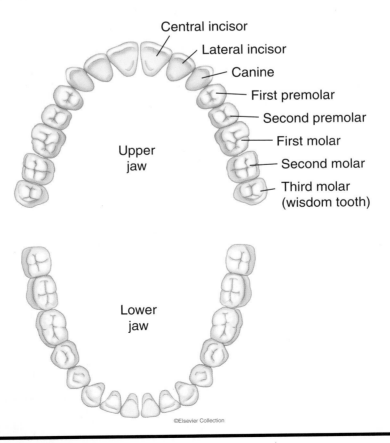

Central incisor

Lateral incisor

Canine

First premolar

Second premolar

First molar

Second molar

Third molar (wisdom tooth)

Upper jaw

Lower jaw

©Elsevier Collection

Plate 20   Adult Teeth. (©Elsevier Collection).

Dorsum of tongue

A, Dorsal view of tongue

- Epiglottis
- Lingual tonsil
- Palatine tonsil
- Foramen cecum
- Vallate papillae
- Fungiform papillae
- Palatoglossal arch
- Filiform papillae
- Foliate papillae

B

- Vallate papillae
- Filiform papillae
- Fungiform papillae
- Lingual tonsil
- Mucous glands
- Intrinsic muscles
- Blood vessels
- Taste buds
- Glands of Von Ebner

© Elsevier Collection

Plate 21 A, Dorsal view of tongue showing the roughened large lingual tonsils on the posterior of the tongue and the foliate papillae on the side. B, Section of dorsal of the tongue showing a cutaway through lingual papillae and showing von Ebner's glands at the base of the vallate papilla. (Brand RW, Isselhard DE: Anatomy of Orofacial Structures: A Comprehensive Approach, ed 8, St. Louis, 2019, Elsevier.)

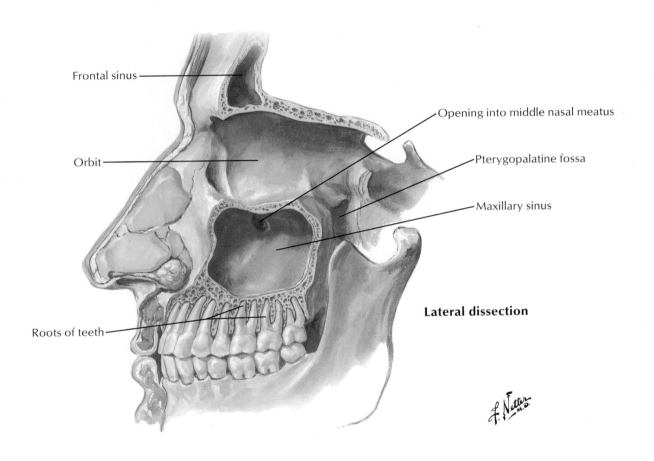

Frontal sinus

Orbit

Roots of teeth

Opening into middle nasal meatus

Pterygopalatine fossa

Maxillary sinus

Lateral dissection

ANATOMY ILLUSTRATIONS

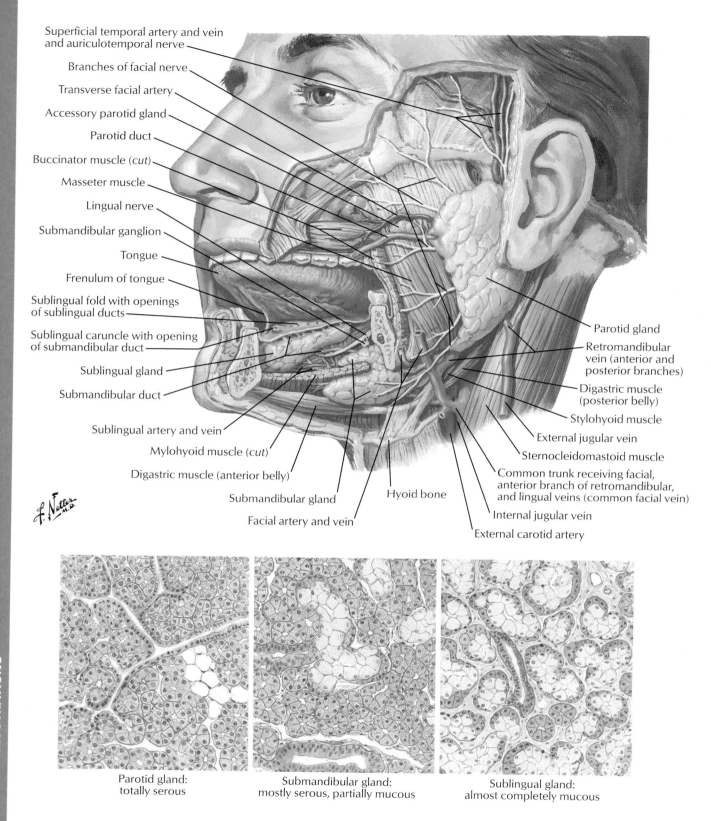

Superficial temporal artery and vein and auriculotemporal nerve

Branches of facial nerve

Transverse facial artery

Accessory parotid gland

Parotid duct

Buccinator muscle (*cut*)

Masseter muscle

Lingual nerve

Submandibular ganglion

Tongue

Frenulum of tongue

Sublingual fold with openings of sublingual ducts

Sublingual caruncle with opening of submandibular duct

Sublingual gland

Submandibular duct

Sublingual artery and vein

Mylohyoid muscle (*cut*)

Digastric muscle (anterior belly)

Submandibular gland

Facial artery and vein

Hyoid bone

Parotid gland

Retromandibular vein (anterior and posterior branches)

Digastric muscle (posterior belly)

Stylohyoid muscle

External jugular vein

Sternocleidomastoid muscle

Common trunk receiving facial, anterior branch of retromandibular, and lingual veins (common facial vein)

Internal jugular vein

External carotid artery

Parotid gland: totally serous

Submandibular gland: mostly serous, partially mucous

Sublingual gland: almost completely mucous

Plate 23 Salivary Glands. (Copyright 2023 Elsevier Inc. All rights reserved. www.netterimages.com. Image ID: 4396.)

Coronary Arteries: Arteriographic Views

Right coronary artery: left anterior oblique view

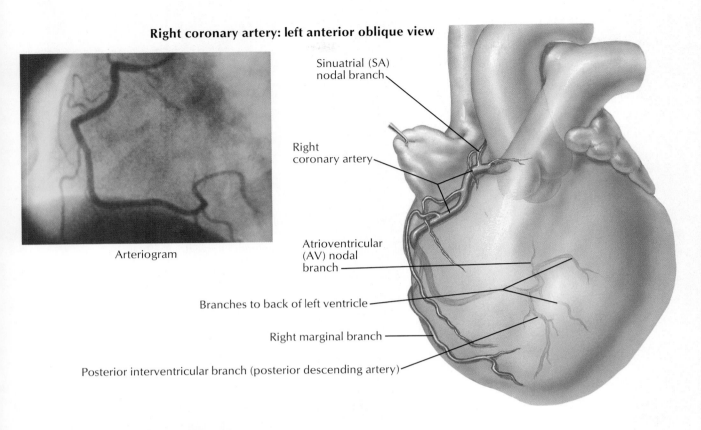

Arteriogram

Sinuatrial (SA) nodal branch

Right coronary artery

Atrioventricular (AV) nodal branch

Branches to back of left ventricle

Right marginal branch

Posterior interventricular branch (posterior descending artery)

Right coronary artery: right anterior oblique view

Sinuatrial (SA) nodal branch

Conus (arteriosus) branch

Right coronary artery

Right marginal branch

Arteriogram

Atrioventricular (AV) nodal branch

Right posterolateral branches (to back of left ventricle)

Posterior interventricular branch (posterior descending artery)

Left coronary artery: left anterior oblique view

Left coronary artery

Circumflex branch

Arteriogram

Anterior interventricular branch (left anterior descending)

Diagonal branches of anterior interventricular branch

Atrioventricular branch of circumflex branch

Left (obtuse) marginal branch

Posterolateral branches

(Perforating) interventricular septal branches

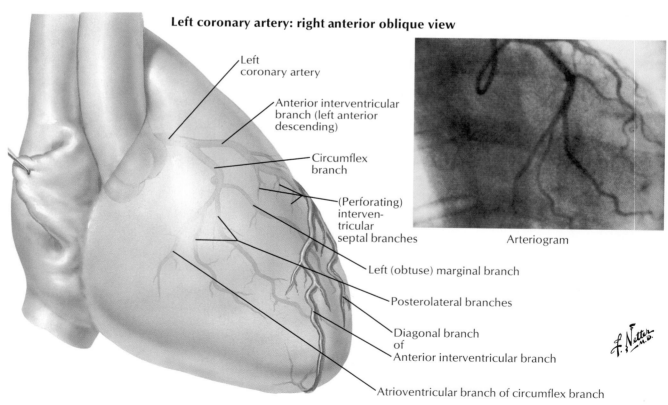

Left coronary artery: right anterior oblique view

Left coronary artery

Anterior interventricular branch (left anterior descending)

Circumflex branch

(Perforating) interventricular septal branches

Arteriogram

Left (obtuse) marginal branch

Posterolateral branches

Diagonal branch of Anterior interventricular branch

Atrioventricular branch of circumflex branch

Plate 25 Coronary Arteries: Arteriographic Views. (Copyright 2023 Elsevier Inc. All rights reserved. www.netterimages.com. Image ID: 4542.)

Corpus callosum

Anterolateral central (lenticulostriate) arteries

Lateral frontobasal (orbitofrontal) artery

Prefrontal artery

Precentral (pre-Rolandic) and central (Rolandic) sulcal arteries

Anterior parietal (postcentral sulcal) artery

Posterior parietal artery

Branch to angular gyrus

Temporal branches (anterior, middle, and posterior)

Middle cerebral artery and branches (deep in lateral cerebral [Sylvian] sulcus)

Anterior communicating artery

Posterior communicating artery

Anterior inferior cerebellar artery (AICA)

Posterior spinal artery

Paracentral artery

Medial frontal branches

Pericallosal artery

Callosomarginal artery

Polar frontal artery

Anterior cerebral arteries

Medial frontobasal (orbitofrontal) artery

Distal medial striate artery (recurrent artery of Heubner)

Internal carotid artery

Anterior choroidal artery

Posterior cerebral artery

Superior cerebellar artery

Basilar and pontine arteries

Labyrinthine (internal acoustic) artery

Vertebral artery

Posterior inferior cerebellar artery (PICA)

Anterior spinal artery

Corpus striatum (caudate and lentiform nuclei)

Anterolateral central (lenticulostriate) arteries

Insula (island of Reil)

Limen of insula

Precentral (pre-Rolandic), central (Rolandic) sulcal, and parietal arteries

Lateral cerebral (Sylvian) sulcus

Temporal branches of middle cerebral artery

Temporal lobe

Middle cerebral artery

Internal carotid artery

Falx cerebri

Callosomarginal arteries and Pericallosal arteries (branches of anterior cerebral arteries)

Trunk of corpus callosum

Internal capsule

Septum pellucidum

Rostrum of corpus callosum

Anterior cerebral arteries

Distal medial striate artery (recurrent artery of Heubner)

Anterior communicating artery

Optic chiasm

f. Netter M.D.

Plate 26 Arteries of Brain: Frontal View and Section. (Copyright 2023 Elsevier Inc. All rights reserved. www.netterimages.com. Image ID: 4588.)

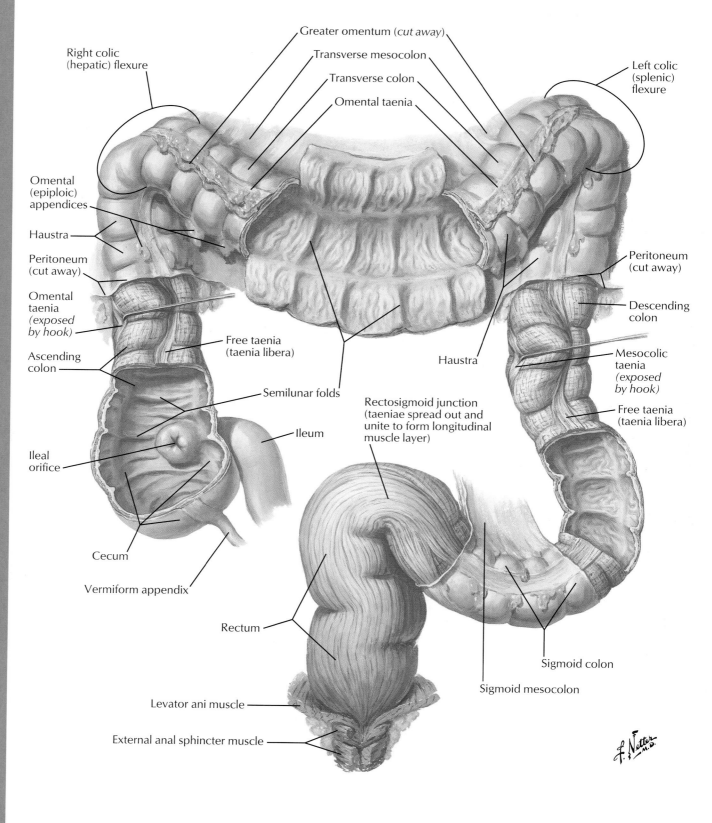

Right colic (hepatic) flexure

Greater omentum (*cut away*)

Transverse mesocolon

Transverse colon

Omental taenia

Left colic (splenic) flexure

Omental (epiploic) appendices

Haustra

Peritoneum (cut away)

Omental taenia *(exposed by hook)*

Ascending colon

Free taenia (taenia libera)

Semilunar folds

Haustra

Peritoneum (cut away)

Descending colon

Mesocolic taenia *(exposed by hook)*

Free taenia (taenia libera)

Ileal orifice

Ileum

Rectosigmoid junction (taeniae spread out and unite to form longitudinal muscle layer)

Cecum

Vermiform appendix

Rectum

Sigmoid colon

Sigmoid mesocolon

Levator ani muscle

External anal sphincter muscle

F. Netter M.D.

ANATOMY ILLUSTRATIONS

Plate 27   Mucosa and Musculature of Large Intestine. (Copyright 2023 Elsevier Inc. All rights reserved. www.netterimages.com. Image ID: 4778.)

xxxviii

Transverse Section: T3–4 Intervertebral Disc, Manubrium

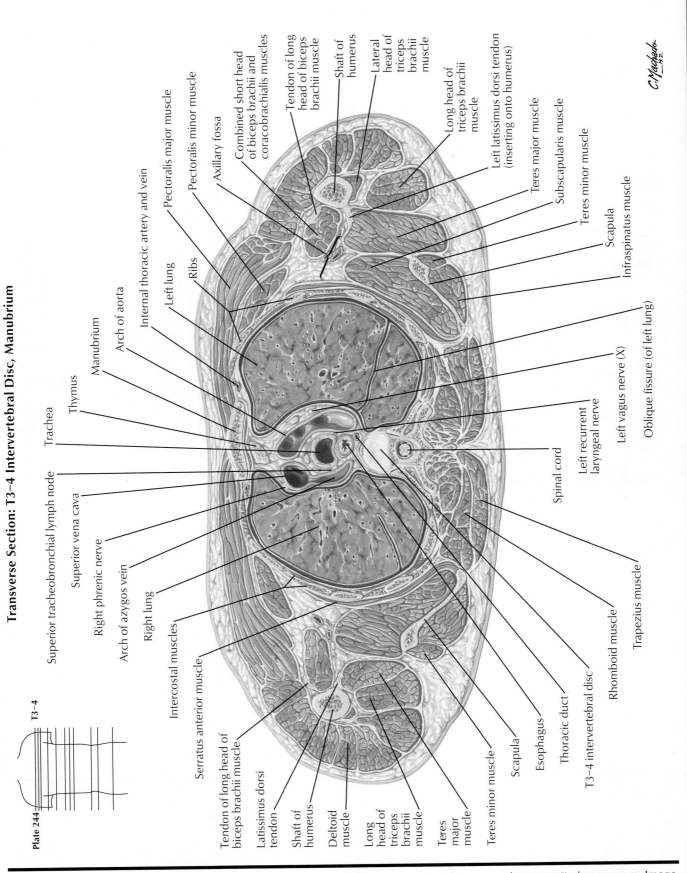

Plate 28 Cross Section of Thorax at T3-4 Disc Level. (Copyright 2023 Elsevier Inc. All rights reserved. www.netterimages.com. Image ID: 4880.)

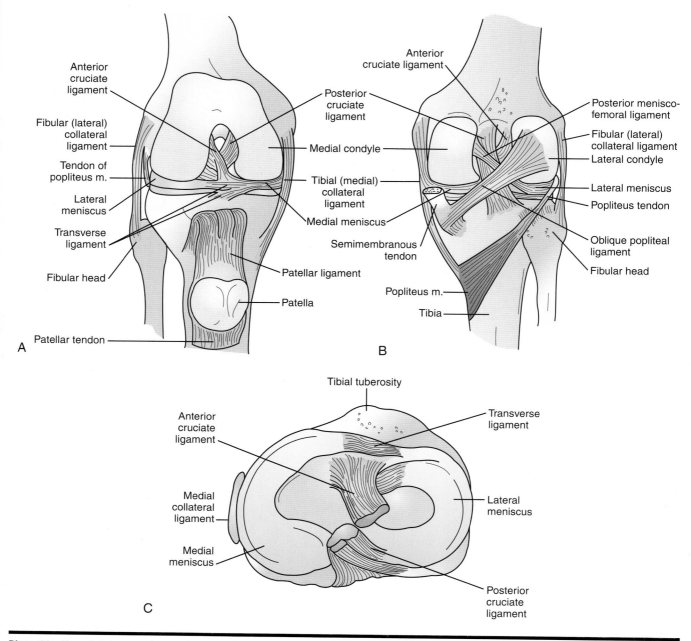

Plate 29 Knee joint opened; anterior, posterior, and proximal views. A, Anterior view of the knee joint, opened by folding the patella and patellar ligament inferiorly. On the lateral side is the fibular collateral ligament, separated by the popliteal tendon from the lateral meniscus. On the medial side, the tibial collateral ligament is attached to the medial meniscus. The anterior and posterior cruciate ligaments are seen between the femoral condyles. B, Posterior view of the opened knee joint with a more complete view of the posterior cruciate ligament. C, The femur is removed, showing the proximal (articular) end of the right tibia. On the medial side is the gently curved medial meniscus; on the lateral side is the more tightly curved lateral meniscus. The anterior end of the medial meniscus is anchored to the surface of the tibia by the transverse ligament. The cut ends of the anterior and posterior cruciate ligaments are shown, as well as the meniscofemoral ligament. (Fritz S: Mosby's Essential Sciences for Therapeutic Massage: Anatomy, Physiology, Biomechanics, and Pathology, ed 5, St. Louis, 2017, Elsevier.)

HCPCS 2024

INDEX

A

Abatacept, J0129
Abciximab, J0130
Abdomen
  dressing holder/binder, A4461, A4463
  pad, low profile, L1270
Abduction control, each, L2624
Abduction restrainer, A4566
Abduction rotation bar, foot, L3140–L3170
  adjustable shoe style positioning device, L3160
  including shoes, L3140
  plastic, heel-stabilizer, off-shelf, L3170
  without shoes, L3150
Abecma, Q2055
AbobotulinumtoxinA, J0586
Absorption dressing, A2001–A2010, A2015–A2021,
  A6251–A6256 ↻
Access, site, occlusive, device, G0269
Access system, A4301
Accessories
  ambulation devices, E0153–E0159
    crutch attachment, walker, E0157
    forearm crutch, platform attachment, E0153
    leg extension, walker, E0158
    replacement, brake attachment, walker, E0159
    seat attachment, walker, E0156
    walker, platform attachment, E0154
    wheel attachment, walker, per pair, E0155
  artificial kidney and machine; (see also ESRD),
    E1510–E1699
    adjustable chair, ESRD patients, E1570
    *automatic peritoneal dialysis system,
      intermittent, E1592*
    bath conductivity meter, hemodialysis, E1550
    *blood leak detector, hemodialysis,
      replacement, E1560*
    blood pump, hemodialysis, replacement, E1620
    cycler dialysis machine, peritoneal, E1594
    deionizer water system, hemodialysis, E1615
    *delivery/installation charges, hemodialysis
      equipment, E1600*
    hemodialysis machine, E1590
    hemostats, E1637
    heparin infusion pump, hemodialysis, E1520
    kidney machine, dialysate delivery system, E1510
    peritoneal dialysis clamps, E1634
    portable travel hemodialyzer, E1635
    reciprocating peritoneal dialysis system, E1630
    replacement, air bubble detector, hemodialysis, E1530
    replacement, pressure alarm, hemodialysis, E1540
    reverse osmosis water system, hemodialysis, E1610
    scale, E1639
    sorbent cartridges, hemodialysis, E1636
    transducer protectors, E1575
    unipuncture control system, E1580
    water softening system, hemodialysis, E1625
    wearable artificial kidney, E1632

Accessories *(Continued)*
  beds, E0271–E0280, E0300–E0326
    bed board, E0273
    bed, board/table, E0315
    bed cradle, E0280
    bed pan, standard, E0275
    bed side rails, E0305–E0310
    bed-pan fracture, E0276
    hospital bed, extra heavy duty, E0302, E0304
    hospital bed, heavy duty, E0301–E0303
    hospital bed, pediatric, electric, E0329
    hospital bed, safety enclosure frame, E0316
    mattress, foam rubber, E0272
    mattress, innerspring, E0271
    over-bed table, E0274
    pediatric crib, E0300
    powered pressure-reducing air mattress, E0277
  wheelchairs, E0950–E1030, E1050–E1298,
    E2300–E2399, K0001–K0109
    accessory tray, E0950
    arm rest, E0994
    back upholstery replacement, E0982
    calf rest/pad, E0995
    commode seat, E0968
    detachable armrest, E0973
    elevating leg rest, E0990
    headrest cushion, E0955
    lateral trunk/hip support, E0956
    loop-holder, E0951–E0952
    manual swingaway, E1028
    manual wheelchair, adapter, amputee, E0959
    manual wheelchair, anti-rollback device, E0974
    manual wheelchair, anti-tipping device, E0971
    *manual wheelchair, hand rim with
      projections, E0967*
    manual wheelchair, headrest extension, E0966
    *manual wheelchair, lever-activated, wheel
      drive, E0988*
    *manual wheelchair, one-arm drive
      attachment, E0958*
    manual wheelchair, power add-on, E0983–E0984
    *manual wheelchair, push activated power
      assist, E0986*
    manual wheelchair, solid seat insert, E0992
    medial thigh support, E0957
    modification, pediatric size, E1011
    narrowing device, E0969
    No. 2 footplates, E0970
    oxygen related accessories, E1352–E1406
    positioning belt/safety belt/pelvic strap, E0978
    power-seating system, E1002–E1010
    *reclining back addition, pediatric size
      wheelchair, E1014*
    residual limb support system, E1020
    safety vest, E0980
    seat lift mechanism, E0985
    seat upholstery replacement, E0981
    shock absorber, E1015–E1018

◄ **New**   ↻ **Revised**   ✔ **Reinstated**   ~~deleted~~ **Deleted**

Accessories *(Continued)*
  wheelchairs *(Continued)*
    shoulder harness strap, E0960
    ventilator tray, E1029–E1030
    wheel lock brake extension, manual, E0961
    wheelchair, amputee, accessories, E1170–E1200
    wheelchair, fully inclining, accessories,
      E1050–E1093
    wheelchair, heavy duty, accessories, E1280–E1298
    wheelchair, lightweight, accessories, E1240–E1270
    wheelchair, semi-reclining, accessories,
      E1100–E1110
    wheelchair, special size, E1220–E1239
    wheelchair, standard, accessories, E1130–E1161
  whirlpool equipment, E1300–E1310
Ace type, elastic bandage, A6448–A6450
Acetaminophen, J0131, J0134, J0136, J0137 ◄
Acetazolamide sodium, J1120
Acetylcysteine
  inhalation solution, J7604, J7608
  injection, J0132
Activity, therapy, G0176
Acyclovir, J0133
Adalimumab, J0135, Q5131 ◄
Additions to
  fracture orthosis, L2180–L2192
    abduction bar, L2300–L2310
    adjustable motion knee joint, L2186
    anterior swing band, L2335
    BK socket, PTB and AFO, L2350
    disk or dial lock, knee flexion, L2425
    dorsiflexion and plantar flexion, L2220
    dorsiflexion assist, L2210
    drop lock, L2405
    drop lock knee joint, L2182
    extended steel shank, L2360
    foot plate, stirrup attachment, L2250
    hip joint, pelvic band, thigh flange, pelvic
      belt, L2192
    integrated release mechanism, L2515
    lacer custom-fabricated, L2320–L2330
    lift loop, drop lock ring, L2492
    limited ankle motion, L2200
    limited motion knee joint, L2184
    long tongue stirrup, L2265
    lower extremity orthrosis, L2200–L2397
    molded inner boot, L2280
    offset knee joint, L2390
    offset knee joint, heavy duty, L2395
    Patten bottom, L2370
    pelvic and thoracic control, L2570–L2680
    plastic shoe insert with ankle joints, L2180
    polycentric knee joint, L2387
    pre-tibial shell, L2340
    quadrilateral, L2188
    ratchet lock knee extension, L2430
    reinforced solid stirrup, L2260
    rocker bottom, custom fabricated, L2232

Additions to *(Continued)*
  fracture orthosis (Continued)
    round caliper/plate attachment, L2240
    split flat caliper stirrups, L2230
    straight knee joint, heavy duty, L2385
    straight knee, or offset knee joints, L2405–L2492
    suspension sleeve, L2397
    thigh/weight bearing, L2500–L2550
    torsion control, ankle joint, L2375
    torsion control, straight knee joint, L2380
    varus/valgus correction, L2270–L2275
    waist belt, L2190
  general additions, orthosis, L2750–L2999
    lower extremity, above knee section, soft
      interface, L2830
    lower extremity, concentric adjustable torsion style
      mechanism, L2861
    lower extremity, drop lock retainer, L2785
    lower extremity, extension, per extension, per
      bar, L2760
    lower extremity, femoral length sock, L2850
    lower extremity, full kneecap, L2795
    lower extremity, high strength, lightweight material,
      hybrid lamination, L2755
    lower extremity, knee control, condylar pad, L2810
    lower extremity, knee control, knee cap, medial or
      lateral, L2800
    lower extremity orthrosis, non-corrosive finish, per
      bar, L2780
    lower extremity orthrosis, NOS, L2999
    lower extremity, plating chrome or nickel, per
      bar, L2750
    lower extremity, soft interface, below knee, L2820
    lower extremity, tibial length sock, L2840
    orthotic side bar, disconnect device, L2768
Adenosine, J0151, J0153
Adhesive, A4364
  bandage, A6413
  disc or foam pad, A5126
  remover, A4455, A4456
  support, breast prosthesis, A4280
  wound, closure, G0168
Adjunctive, dental, D9110–D9999
Administration, chemotherapy, Q0083–Q0085
  both infusion and other technique, Q0085
  infusion technique only, Q0084
  other than infusion technique, Q0083
Administration, Part D
  vaccine, hepatitis B, G0010
  vaccine, influenza, G0008
  vaccine, pneumococcal, G0009
Administrative, Miscellaneous and Investigational,
  A9000–A9999
  alert or alarm device, A9280
  artificial saliva, A9155
  DME delivery set-up, A9901
  exercise equipment, A9300
  external ambulatory insulin delivery system, A9274

◄ **New**   ⊋ **Revised**   ✔ **Reinstated**   ~~deleted~~ **Deleted**

A

3

Administrative, Miscellaneous and Investigational
   (Continued)
   foot pressure off loading/supportive device, A9283
   helmets, A8000–A8004
   home glucose disposable monitor, A9275
   hot-water bottle, ice cap, heat wrap, A9273
   miscellaneous DME, NOS, A9999
   miscellaneous DME supply, A9900
   monitoring feature/device, stand-alone or integrated, A9279
   multiple vitamins, oral, per dose, A9153
   non-covered item, A9270
   non-prescription drugs, A9150
   pediculosis treatment, topical, A9180
   radiopharmaceuticals, A9500–A9700
   reaching grabbing device, A9281
   receiver, external, interstitial glucose monitoring system, A9278
   sensor, invasive, interstitial continuous glucose monitoring, A9276
   single vitamin/mineral trace element, A9152
   spirometer, non-electronic, A9284
   transmitter, interstitial continuous glucose monitoring system, A9277
   wig, any type, A9282
   wound suction, disposable, A9272
Admission, observation, *G0379*
Ado-trastuzumab, J9354
Adrenalin, J0171
Aducanumab-avwa, J0172
Aduhelm, J0172
Advanced life support, *A0390, A0426, A0427, A0433*
   ALS2, A0433
   ALS emergency transport, A0427
   ALS mileage, A0390
   ALS, non-emergency transport, A0426
Aerosol
   compressor, E0571–E0572
   compressor filter, *A7013–A7014,* K0178–K0179
   mask, *A7015,* K0180
Afamelanotide implant, J7352
Aflibercept, J0178
AFO, E1815, E1830, L1900–L1990, L4392, L4396
Afstyla, J7210
Agalsidase beta, J0180
Aggrastat, J3245
A-hydroCort, J1710
Aid, hearing, *V5030–V5263*
Aide, home, health, *G0156, S9122, T1021*
   home health aide/certified nurse assistant, in home, *S9122*
   home health aide/certified nurse assistant, per visit, *T1021*
   home health or hospital setting, *G0156*
Air bubble detector, dialysis, E1530
Air fluidized bed, E0194
Air pressure pad/mattress, E0186, E0197
Air travel and nonemergency transportation, A0140
Alarm
   not otherwise classified, A9280
   pressure, dialysis, E1540
Alatrofloxacin mesylate, J0200

Albumin, human, P9041, P9042
Albuterol
   all formulations, inhalation solution, J7620
   all formulations, inhalation solution, concentrated, J7610, J7611
   all formulations, inhalation solution, unit dose, J7609, J7613
Alcohol, A4244
Alcohol wipes, A4245
Alcohol/substance, assessment, *G0396, G0397, H0001, H0003, H0049*
   alcohol abuse structured assessment, greater than 30 min., G0397
   alcohol abuse structured assessment, 15–30 min., G0396
   alcohol and/or drug assessment, Medicaid, H0001
   alcohol and/or drug screening; laboratory analysis, Medicaid, H0003
   alcohol and/or drug screening, Medicaid, H0049
Aldesleukin (IL2), J9015
Alefacept, J0215
Alemtuzumab, J0202
Alert device, A9280
Alfentanil hydrochloride, J0216 ◀
Alginate dressing, A6196–A6199
   alginate, pad more than 48 sq. cm, A6198
   alginate, pad size 16 sq. cm, A6196
   alginate, pad size more than 16 sq. cm, A6197
   alginate, wound filler, sterile, A6199
Alglucerase, J0205
Alglucosidase, J0220
Alglucosidase alfa, J0221
Allogen, Q4212
Allopurinol sodium, J0206 ◀
Alphanate, J7186
Alpha-1–proteinase inhibitor, human, J0256, J0257
Alprostadil
   injection, J0270
   urethral suppository, J0275
ALS mileage, *A0390*
Alteplase recombinant, J2997
Alternating pressure mattress/pad, A4640, E0180, E0181, E0277
   overlay/pad, alternating, pump, heavy duty, E0181
   powered pressure-reducing air mattress, E0277
   replacement pad, owned by patient, A4640
Alveoloplasty, *D7310–D7321*
   in conjunction with extractions, four or more teeth, D7310
   in conjunction with extractions, one to three teeth, D7311
   not in conjunction with extractions, four or more teeth, D7320
   not in conjunction with extractions, one to three teeth, D7321
Alymsys, Q5126
Amalgam dental restoration, *D2140–D2161*
   four or more surfaces, primary or permanent, D2161
   one surface, primary or permanent, D2140

◀ **New**   ⊃ **Revised**   ✔ **Reinstated**   ~~deleted~~ **Deleted**

Amalgam dental restoration (Continued)
  three surfaces, primary or permanent, D2160
  two surfaces, primary or permanent, D2150
Ambulance, A0021–A0999
  air, A0430, A0431, A0435, A0436
    conventional, transport, one way, fixed wing, A0430
    conventional, transport, one way, rotary wing, A0431
    fixed wing air mileage, A0435
    rotary wing air mileage, A0436
  disposable supplies, A0382–A0398
    ALS routine disposable supplies, A0398
    ALS specialized service disposable supplies, A0394
    ALS specialized service, esophageal intubation, A0396
    BLS routine disposable, A0832
    BLS specialized service disposable supplies, defibrillation, A0384, A0392
  non-emergency transport, fixed wing, S9960
  non-emergency transport, rotary wing, S9961
  oxygen, A0422
Ambulation device, E0100–E0159
  brake attachment, wheeled walker replacement, E0159
  cane, adjustable or fixed, with tip, E0100
  cane, quad or three prong, adjustable or fixed, with tip, E0105
  crutch attachment, walker, E0157
  crutch forearm, each, with tips and handgrips, E0111
  crutch substitute, lower leg platform, with or without wheels, each, E0118
  crutch, underarm, articulating, spring assisted, each, E0117
  crutches forearm, pair, tips and handgrips, E0110
  crutches, underarm, other than wood, pair, with pads, tips and handgrips, E0114
  crutches, underarm, other than wood, with pad, tip, handgrip, with or without shock absorber, each, E0116
  crutches, underarm, wood, each, with pad, tip and handgrip, E0113
  leg extensions, walker, set (4), E0158
  platform attachment, forearm crutch, each, E0153
  platform attachment, walker, E0154
  seat attachment, walker, E0156
  walker, enclosed, four-sided frame, wheeled, posterior seat, E0144
  walker, folding, adjustable or fixed height, E0135
  walker, folding, wheeled, adjustable or fixed height, E0143
  walker, heavy duty, multiple braking system, variable wheel resistance, E0147
  walker, heavy duty, wheeled, rigid or folding, E0149
  walker, heavy duty, without wheels, rigid or folding, E0148
  walker, rigid, adjustable or fixed height, E0130
  walker, rigid, wheeled, adjustable or fixed height, E0141
  walker, with trunk support, adjystable or fixed height, any, E0140
  wheel attachment, rigid, pick up walker, per pair, E0155
Amikacin Sulfate, J0278

Aminolevulinate, J7309
Aminolevulinic acid HCl, J7308
Aminophylline, J0280
Aminolevulinic
  Ameluz, J7345
Amiodarone HCl, J0282, J0283
Amisulpride, C9153 ◀
Amitriptyline HCl, J1320
Ammonia N-13, A9526
Ammonia test paper, A4774
Amnioiwrap2, Q4221
Amnion Bio, Q4211
Amniotic membrane, V2790
Amobarbital, J0300
Amphotericin B, J0285
  Lipid Complex, J0287–J0289
Ampicillin
  sodium, J0290
  sodium/sulbactam sodium, J0295
Amputee
  adapter, wheelchair, E0959
  prosthesis, L5000–L7510, L7520, L7900, L8400–L8465
    above knee, L5200–L5230
    additions to exoskeletal knee-shin systems, L5710–L5782
    additions to lower extremity, L5610–L5617
    additions to socket insert and suspension, L5654–L5699
    additions to socket variations, L5630–L5653
    additions to test sockets, L5618–L5629
    additions/replacements feet-ankle units, L5700–L5707
    ankle, L5050–L5060
    below knee, L5100–L5105
    component modification, L5785–L5795
    endoskeletal, L5810–L5999
    endoskeleton, below knee, L5301–L5312
    endoskeleton, hip disarticulation, L5331–L5341
    fitting endoskeleton, above knee, L5321
    fitting procedures, L5400–L5460
    hemipelvectomy, L5280
    hip disarticulation, L5250–L5270
    initial prosthesis, L5500–L5505
    knee disarticulation, L5150–L5160
    male vacuum erection system, L7900
    partial foot, L5000–L5020
    preparatory prosthesis, L5510–L5600
    prosthetic socks, L8400–L8485
    repair, prosthetic device, L7520
    tension ring, vacuum erection device, L7902
    upper extremity, battery components, L7360–L7368
    upper extremity, other/repair, L7400–L7510
    upper extremity, preparatory, elbow, L6584–L6586
    upper limb, above elbow, L6250
    upper limb, additions, L6600–L6698
    upper limb, below elbow, L6100–L6130
    upper limb, elbow disarticulation, L6200–L6205
    upper limb, endoskeletal, above elbow, L6500
    upper limb, endoskeletal, below elbow, L6400

◀ New ↻ Revised ✓ Reinstated ~~deleted~~ **Deleted**

Amputee *(Continued)*

prosthesis *(Continued)*

    upper limb, endoskeletal, elbow disarticulation, L6450

    upper limb, endoskeletal, interscapular thoracic, L6570

    upper limb, endoskeletal, shoulder disarticulation, L6550

    upper limb, external power, device, L6920–L6975

    upper limb, interscapular thoracic, L6350–L6370

    upper limb, partial hand, L6000–L6025

    upper limb, postsurgical procedures, L6380–L6388

    upper limb, preparatory, shoulder, interscapular, L6588–L6590

    upper limb, preparatory, wrist, L6580–L6582

    upper limb, shoulder disarticulation, L6300–L6320

    upper limb, terminal devices, L6703–L6915, L7007–L7261

    upper limb, wrist disarticulation, L6050–L6055

stump sock, L8470–L8485

    single ply, fitting above knee, L8480

    single ply, fitting, below knee, L8470

    single ply, fitting, upper limb, L8485

wheelchair, E1170–E1190, E1200, K0100

    detachable arms, swing away detachable elevating footrests, E1190

    detachable arms, swing away detachable footrests, E1180

    detachable arms, without footrests or legrest, E1172

    detachable elevating legrest, fixed full length arms, E1170

    fixed full length arms, swing away detachable footrest, E1200

    heavy duty wheelchair, swing away detachable elevating legrests, E1195

    without footrests or legrest, fixed full length arms, E1171

Amygdalin, J3570

Anadulafungin, J0348

Anacaulase-bcdb, J7353 ◀

Analgesia, dental, D9230

Analysis

    saliva, D0418

    semen, G0027

Anaphylaxis, due to vaccine, M1160–M1161, M1163

Angiography, iliac, artery, G0278

Angiography, renal, non-selective, G0275

    non-ophthalmic fluorescent vascular, C9733

    reconstruction, G0288

Angioplasty, C7531–C7535

Anistreplase, J0350

Ankle splint, recumbent, K0126–K0130

Ankle-foot orthosis (AFO), L1900–L1990, L2106–L2116, L4361, L4392, L4396

    ankle gauntlet, custom fabricated, L1904

    ankle gauntlet, prefabricated, off-shelf, L1902

    double upright free plantar dorsiflexion, olid stirrup, calf-band/cuff, custom, L1990

Ankle-foot orthosis *(Continued)*

    fracture orthrosis, tibial fracture, thermoplastic cast material, custom, L2106

    multiligamentus ankle support, prefabricated, off-shelf, L1906

    plastic or other material, custom fabricated, L1940

    plastic or other material, prefabricated, fitting and adjustment, L1932, L1951

    plastic or other material, with ankle joint, prefabricated, fitting and adjustment, L1971

    plastic, rigid anterior tibial section, custom fabricated, L1945

    plastic, with ankle joint, custom, L1970

    posterior, single bar, clasp attachment to shoe, L1910

    posterior, solid ankle, plastic, custom, L1960

    replacement, soft interface material, static AFO, L4392

    single upright free plantar dorsiflection, solid stirrup, calf-band/cuff, custom, L1980

    single upright with static or adjustable stop, custom, L1920

    spiral, plastic, custom fabricated, L1950

    spring wire, dorsiflexion assist calf band, L1900

    static or dynamic AFO, adjustable for fit, minimal ambulation, L4396

    supramalleolar with straps, custom fabricated, L1907

    tibial fracture cast orthrosis, custom, L2108

    tibial fracture orthrosis, rigid, prefabricated, fitting and adjustment, L2116

    tibial fracture orthrosis, semi-rigid, prefabricated, fitting and adjustment, L2114

    tibial fracture orthrosis, soft prefabricated, fitting and adjustment, L2112

    walking boot, prefabricated, off-the-shelf, L4361

Anterior-posterior-lateral orthosis, L0700, L0710

Antibiotic, G8708–G8712

    antibiotic not prescribed or dispensed, G8712

    patient not prescribed or dispensed antibiotic, G8708

    patient prescribed antibiotic, documented condition, G8709

    patient prescribed or dispensed antibiotic, G8710

    prescribed or dispensed antibiotic, G8711

Antidepressant, documentation, G8126–G8128

Anti-emetic, oral, J8498, J8597, Q0163–Q0181

    antiemetic drug, oral NOS, J8597

    antiemetic drug, rectal suppository, NOS, J8498

    diphenhydramine hydrochloride, 50 mg, oral, Q0163

    dolasetron mesylate, 100 mg, oral, Q0180

    dronabinol, 2.5 mg, Q0167

    granisetron hydrochloride, 1 mg, oral, Q0166

    hydroxyzine pomoate, 25 mg, oral, Q0177

    perphenazine, 4 mg, oral, Q0175

    prochlorperazine maleate, 5 mg, oral, Q0164

    promethazine hydrochloride, 12.5 mg, oral, Q0169

    thiethylperazine maleate, 10 mg, oral, Q0174

    trimethobenzamide hydrochloride, 250 mg, oral, Q0173

    unspecified oral dose, Q0181

Anti-hemophilic factor (Factor VIII), J7190–J7192

Anti-inhibitors, per I.U., J7198

◀ **New**   ⏎ **Revised**   ✔ **Reinstated**   ~~deleted~~ **Deleted**

Antimicrobial, prophylaxis, documentation, *D4281, G8201*

Anti-neoplastic drug, NOC, J9999

Antithrombin III, J7197

Antithrombin recombinant, J7196

Antral fistula closure, oral, *D7260*

Apexification, dental, *D3351–D3353*

Apicoectomy, *D3410–D3426*
   anterior, periradicular surgery, D3410
   biscuspid (first root), D3421
   (each additional root), D3426
   molar (first root), D3425

Apomorphine, J0364

Aponvie, C9145 ◀

Appliance
   cleaner, A5131
   pneumatic, E0655–E0673
     non-segmental pneumatic appliance, E0655, E0660, E0665, E0666
     segmental gradient pressure, pneumatic appliance, E0671–E0673
     segmental pneumatic appliance, E0656–E0657, E0667–E0670

Application, heat, cold, *E0200–E0239*
   electric heat pad, moist, E0215
   electric heat pad, standard, E0210
   heat lamp with stand, E0205
   heat lamp without stand, E0200
   hydrocollator unit, pads, E0225
   hydrocollator unit, portable, E0239
   infrared heating pad system, E0221
   non-contact wound warming device, E0231
   paraffin bath unit, E0235
   phototherapy (bilirubin), E0202
   pump for water circulating pad, E0236
   therapeutic lightbox, E0203
   warming card, E0232
   water circulating cold pad with pump, E0218
   water circulating heat pad with pump, E0217

Aprotinin, J0365

Aqueous
   shunt, L8612
   sterile, J7051

ARB/ACE therapy, *G8473–G8475*

Arbutamine HCl, J0395

Arch support, L3040–L3100
   hallus-valgus night dynamic splint, off-shelf, L3100
   intralesional, J3302
   non-removable, attached to shoe, longitudinal, L3070
   non-removable, attached to shoe, longitudinal/ metatarsal, each, L3090
   non-removable, attached to shoe, metatarsal, L3080
   removable, premolded, longitudinal, L3040
   removable, premolded, longitudinal/metatarsal, each, L3060
   removable, premolded, metatarsal, L3050

Arformoterol, J7605

Argatroban, *J0883–J0884, J0891–J0892, J0898–J0899*

Aripiprazole, *C9152, J0400, J0401* ◀

Aripiprazol lauroxil, (aristada), J1944
   aristada initio, H1943

Arm, wheelchair, E0973

Arsenic trioxide, J9017

Artacent cord, Q4216

Arthrography, injection, sacroiliac, joint, *G0259, G0260*

Arthroscopy, knee, surgical, *G0289, S2112*
   chondroplasty, different compartment, knee, G0289
   harvesting of cartilage, knee, S2112

Arthroscopy, shoulder, *C9781* ◀

Artificial
   cornea, L8609
   heart system, miscellaneous component, supply or accessory, L8698
   kidney machines and accessories (see also Dialysis), *E1510–E1699*
   larynx, L8500
   saliva, A9155

Ascent, Q4213

Asparaginase, *J9019–J9021*

Aspirator, VABRA, *A4480*

Assessment
   alcohol/substance (see also Alcohol/substance, assessment), G0396, G0397, H0001, H0003, H0049
   assessment for hearing aid, V5010
   audiologic, V5008–V5020
   cardiac output, M0302
   conformity evaluation, V5020
   fitting/orientation, hearing aid, V5014
   hearing screening, V5008
   itch severity, M1197–M1198, M1205–M1206
   repair/modification hearing aid, V5014
   speech, V5362–V5364

Assistive listening devices and accessories, *V5281–V5290*
   FM/DM system, monaural, V5281

Astramorph, J2275

Atezolizumab, J9022

Atherectomy, PTCA, *C9602, C9603*

Atropine
   inhalation solution, concentrated, J7635
   inhalation solution, unit dose, J7636

Atropine sulfate, J0461

Attachment, walker, *E0154–E0159*
   brake attachment, wheeled walker, replacement, E0159
   crutch attachment, walker, E0157
   leg extension, walker, E0158
   platform attachment, walker, E0154
   seat attachment, walker, E0156
   wheel attachment, rigid pick up walker, E0155

Audiologic assessment, V5008–V5020

Auditory osseointegrated device, L8690–L8694

Auricular prosthesis, *D5914, D5927*

Aurothioglucose, J2910

Avalglucosidase alfa-ngpt, J0219

◀ New   ↻ Revised   ✔ Reinstated   ~~deleted~~ Deleted

Avelumab, J9023
Axobiomembrane, Q4211
Axolotl ambient or axolotl cryo, Q4215
Axolotl graft or axolotl dualgraft, Q4210
Azacitidine, J9025
Azathioprine, J7500, J7501
Azithromycin injection, J0456
Aztreonam, J0457 ◀

B

Back supports, L0621–L0861, L0960
  lumbar orthrosis, L0625–L0627
  lumbar orthrosis, sagittal control, L0641–L0648
  lumbar-sacral orthrosis, L0628–L0640
  lumbar-sacral orthrosis, sagittal-coronal control,
    L0640, L0649–L0651
  sacroiliac orthrosis, L0621–L0624
Baclofen, J0475, J0476
Bacterial sensitivity study, P7001
Bag
  drainage, A4357
  enema, A4458
  irrigation supply, A4398
  urinary, A4358, A5112
Bandage, conforming
  elastic, >5", A6450
  elastic, >3", <5", A6449
  elastic, load resistance 1.25 to 1.34 foot pounds, >3",
    <5", A6451
  elastic, load resistance <1.35 foot pounds, >3",
    <5", A6452
  elastic, <3", A6448
  non-elastic, non-sterile, >5", A6444
  non-elastic, non-sterile, width greater than or equal
    to 3", <5", A6443
  non-elastic, non-sterile, width <3", A6442
  non-elastic, sterile, >5", A6447
  non-elastic, sterile, >3" and <5", A6446
Bamlan and etesev, M0245
Bamlanivimab and etesevima, Q0245
Basiliximab, J0480
Bath, aid, *E0160–E0162, E0235, E0240–E0249*
  bath tub rail, floor base, E0242
  bath tub wall rail, E0241
  bath/shower chair, with/without wheels, E0240
  pad for water circulating heat unit,
    replacement, E0249
  paraffin bath unit, portable, E0235
  raised toilet seat, E0244
  sitz bath chair, E0162
  sitz type bath, portable, with faucet attachment, E0161
  sitz type bath, portable, with/without commode, E0160
  toilet rail, E0243
  transfer bench, tub or toilet, E0248
  transfer tub rail attachment, E0246
  tub stool or bench, E0245

Bathtub
  chair, E0240
  stool or bench, E0245, E0247–E0248
  transfer rail, E0246
  wall rail, E0241–E0242
Battery, L7360, L7364–L7368
  charger, E1066, L7362, L7366
  replacement for blood glucose monitor,
    A4233–A4236
  replacement for cochlear implant device, L8618,
    L8623–L8625
  replacement for TENS, A4630
  ventilator, A4611–A4613
Bebtelovimab, M0222–M0223, Q0222
Beclomethasone inhalation solution, J7622
Bed
  accessories, E0271–E0280, E0300–E0326
    bed board, E0273
    bed cradle, E0280
    bed pan, fracture, metal, E0276
    bed pan, standard, metal, E0275
    mattress, foam rubber, E0272
    mattress innerspring, E0271
    over-bed table, E0274
    power pressure-reducing air mattress, E0277
  air fluidized, E0194
  cradle, any type, E0280
  drainage bag, bottle, A4357, A5102
  hospital, E0250–E0270, E0300–E0329
  pan, E0275, E0276
  rail, E0305, E0310
  safety enclosure frame/canopy, E0316
Behavioral, health, treatment services (Medicaid),
    H0002–H2037
  activity therapy, H2032
  alcohol/drug services, H0001, H0003, H0005–H0016,
    H0020–H0022, H0026–H0029, H0049–H0050,
    H2034–H2036
  assertive community treatment, H0040
  community based wrap-around services, H2021–H2022
  comprehensive community support, H2015–H2016
  comprehensive medication services, H2010
  comprehensive multidisciplinary evaluation, H2000
  crisis intervention, H2011
  day treatment, per diem, H2013
  day treatment, per hour, H2012
  developmental delay prevention activities, dependent
    child of client, H2037
  family assessment, H1011
  foster care, child, H0041–H0042
  health screening, H0002
  hotline service, H0030
  medication training, H0034
  mental health clubhouse services, H2030–H2031
  multisystemic therapy, juveniles, H2033
  non-medical family planning, H1010
  outreach service, H0023
  partial hospitalization, H0035

◀ **New**   ⟳ **Revised**   ✔ **Reinstated**   ~~deleted~~ **Deleted**

◄ **New**   ⊃ **Revised**   ✔ **Reinstated**   ~~deleted~~ **Deleted**

Blood (*Continued*)
  platelets, pheresis, P9034, P9072, P9073, P9100
  platelets, pheresis, irradiated, P9036
  platelets, pheresis, leukocytes reduced, P9035
  platelets, pheresis, leukocytes reduced,
    irradiated, P9037
  pressure monitor, A4660, A4663, A4670
  pump, dialysis, E1620
  red blood cells, deglycerolized, P9039
  red blood cells, irradiated, P9038
  red blood cells, leukocytes reduced, P9016
  red blood cells, leukocytes reduced,
    irradiated, P9040
  red blood cells, washed, P9022
  strips, A4253
  supply, P9010–P9022
  testing supplies, A4770
  tubing, A4750, A4755
Blood collection devices accessory, A4257, E0620
BMI, *G8417–G8422*
Body jacket
  scoliosis, L1300, L1310
Body mass index, *G8417–G8422*
Body sock, L0984
Bond or cement, ostomy skin, A4364
Bone
  density, study, G0130
Boot
  pelvic, E0944
  surgical, ambulatory, L3260
Bortezomib, J9041, J9046, J9048–J9049, J9051 ◀
Brachytherapy radioelements, Q3001
  brachytherapy, LDR, prostate, G0458
  brachytherapy planar source, C2645
  brachytherapy, source, hospital outpatient,
    C1716–C1717, C1719
Breast prosthesis, L8000–L8035, L8600
  adhesive skin support, A4280
  custom breast prosthesis, post mastectomy, L8035
  garment with mastectomy form, post
    mastectomy, L8015
  implantable, silicone or equal, L8600
  mastectomy bra, with integrated breast prosthesis
    form, unilateral, L8001
  mastectomy bra, with prosthesis form, bilateral, L8002
  mastectomy bra, without integrated breast prosthesis
    form, L8000
  mastectomy form, L8020
  mastectomy sleeve, L8010
  nipple prosthesis, L8032
  silicone or equal, with integral adhesive, L8031
  silicone or equal, without integral adhesive, L8030
Breast pump
  accessories, A4281–A4286
    adapter, replacement, A4282
    cap, breast pump bottle, replacement, A4283
    locking ring, replacement, A4286
    polycarbonate bottle, replacement, A4285

Breast pump (*Continued*)
  accessories (*Continued*)
    shield and splash protector, replacement, A4284
    tubing, replacement, A4281
  electric, any type, E0603
  heavy duty, hospital grade, E0604
  manual, any type, E0602
Breathing circuit, A4618
Brentuximab Vedotin, J9042
Brexanolone, J1632
Bridge
  repair, by report, D6980
  replacement, D6930
Bronchoscopy, C7509–C7512
Brolucizumab-dbll, J0179
Brompheniramine maleate, J0945
Budesonide inhalation solution, J7626, J7627,
    J7633, J7634
Bulking agent, L8604, L8607
Bupivacaine, C9144, J0665 ◀
Buprenorphine hydrochlorides, J0592
Buprenorphine/Naloxone, C9154, J0571–J0575 ◀
Burn, compression garment, *A6501–A6513*
  bodysuit, head-foot, A6501
  burn mask, face and/or neck, A6513
  chin strap, A6502
  facial hood, A6503
  foot to knee length, A6507
  foot to thigh length, A6508
  glove to axilla, A6506
  glove to elbow, A6505
  glove to wrist, A6504
  lower trunk, including leg openings, A6511
  trunk, including arms, down to leg openings, A6510
  upper trunk to waist, including arm openings,
    A6509
Bus, nonemergency transportation, A0110
Busulfan, J0594, J8510
Butorphanol tartrate, J0595
Bypass, graft, coronary, artery
  surgery, S2205–S2209

C

C-1 Esterase Inhibitor, J0596–J0598
Cabazitaxel, J9043, J9064 ◀
Cabergoline, oral, J8515
Cabinet/System, ultraviolet, *E0691–E0694*
  multidirectional light system, 6 ft. cabinet, E0694
  timer and eye protection, 4 foot, E0692
  timer and eye protection, 6 foot, E0693
  ultraviolet light therapy system, treatment area
    2 sq ft., E0691
Cabote rilpivir J0741
Cabotegravir, J0739
Caffeine citrate, J0706
Cage, interbody, C1831 ◀
Calaspargase pegol injection-mknl, J9118

◀ **New**   ⤶ **Revised**   ✔ **Reinstated**   ~~deleted~~ **Deleted**

Calcitonin-salmon, J0630
Calcitriol, J0636, *S0169*
Calcium
  disodium edetate, J0600
  gluconate, J0612, J0613 ◀
  glycerophosphate and calcium lactate, J0620
  lactate and calcium glycerophosphate, J0620
  leucovorin, J0640
Calibrator solution, A4256
Camcevi, J1952
Canakinumab, J0638
Cancer, screening
  cervical or vaginal, G0101
  colorectal, G0104–G0106, G0120–G0122, G0328
    alternative to screening colonoscopy, barium enema, G0120
    alternative to screening sigmoidoscopy, barium enema, G0106
    barium enema, G0122
    colonoscopy, high risk, G0105
    colonoscopy, not at high-risk, G0121
    fecal occult blood test, 1-3 simultaneous, G0328
    flexible sigmoidoscopy, G0104
  prostate, G0102, G0103
Cane, E0100, E0105
  accessory, A4636, A4637
Canister
  disposable, used with suction pump, A7000
  non-disposable, used with suction pump, A7001
Cannula, nasal, A4615
Capecitabine, oral, J8520, J8521
Capsaicin patch, J7336
Carbidopa 5 mg/levodopa 20 mg enteral suspension, J7340
Carbon filter, A4680
Carboplatin, J9045
Cardia Event, recorder, implantable, E0616
Cardiokymography, Q0035
Cardiovascular services, M0300–M0301
  Fabric wrapping abdominal aneurysm, M0301
  IV chelation therapy, M0300
Cardioverter-defibrillator, *G0448*
Care
  cancer, M0001
  optimal, M0002–M0003
  supportive, M0004
Care, coordinated, *G9001–G9011, H1002*
  coordinated care fee, home monitoring, G9006
  coordinated care fee, initial rate, G9001
  coordinated care fee, maintenance rate, G9002
  coordinated care fee, physician coordinated care oversight, G9008
  coordinated care fee, risk adjusted high, initial, G9003
  coordinated care fee, risk adjusted low, initial, G9004
  coordinated care fee, risk adjusted maintenance, G9005
  coordinated care fee, risk adjusted maintenance, level 3, G9009

Care, coordinated *(Continued)*
  coordinated care fee, risk adjusted maintenance, level 4, G9010
  coordinated care fee, risk adjusted maintenance, level 5, G9011
  coordinated care fee, scheduled team conference, G9007
  prenatal care, at-risk, enhanced service, care coordination, H1002
Care plan, *G0162*
Carfilzomib, J9047
Caries susceptibility test, *D0425*
Carmustine, J9050
Case management, T1016, T1017
  behavioral health, G0323
  dental, D9991–D9994
Casimersen J1426
Caspofungin acetate, J0637
Cast
  diagnostic, dental, D0470
  hand restoration, L6900–L6915
  materials, special, A4590
  supplies, A4580, A4590, Q4001–Q4051
    body cast, adult, Q4001–Q4002
    cast supplies (e.g., plaster), A4580
    cast supplies, unlisted types, Q4050
    finger splint, static, Q4049
    gauntlet cast, adult, Q4013–Q4014
    gauntlet cast, pediatric, Q4015–Q4016
    hip spica, adult, Q4025–Q4026
    hip spica, pediatric, Q4027–Q4028
    long arm cast, adult, Q4005–Q4006
    long arm cast, pediatric, Q4007–Q4008
    long arm splint, adult, Q4017–Q4018
    long arm splint, pediatric, Q4019–Q4020
    long leg cast, adult, Q4029–Q4030
    long leg cast, pediatric, Q4031–Q4032
    long leg cylinder cast, adult, Q4033–Q4034
    long leg cylinder cast, pediatric, Q4035–Q4036
    long leg splint, adult, Q4041–Q4042
    long leg splint, pediatric, Q4043–Q4044
    short arm cast, adult, Q4009–Q4010
    short arm cast, pediatric, Q4011–Q4012
    short arm splint, adult, Q4021–Q4022
    short arm splint, pediatric, Q4023–Q4024
    short leg cast, adult, Q4037–Q4038
    short leg cast, pediatric, Q4039–Q4040
    short leg splint, adult, Q4045–Q4046
    short leg splint, pediatric, Q4047–Q4048
    shoulder cast, adult, Q4003–Q4004
    special casting material (fiberglass), A4590
    splint supplies, miscellaneous, Q4051
  thermoplastic, L2106, L2126
Caster
  front, for power wheelchair, K0099
  wheelchair, E0997, E0998
Catheter, A4300–A4355
  anchoring device, A4333, A4334, A5200
  cap, disposable (dialysis), A4860
  convert, C7547

◀ New   ⊋ Revised   ✔ Reinstated   ~~deleted~~ **Deleted**

Catheter *(Continued)*
  colorectal *(Continued)*
    coronary artery, C7516–C7529, C7552–C7553
    exchange, C7548
    external collection device, A4327–A4330, A4347–A7048
    female external, A4327–A4328
    indwelling, A4338–A4346
    insertion tray, A4354
    insulin infusion catheter, A4224
    intermittent with insertion supplies, A4353
    irrigation supplies, A4355
    male external, A4324, A4325, *A4326*, A4348
    nephroureteral, C7546
    oropharyngeal suction, A4628
    starter set, A4329
    trachea (suction), A4609, A4610, A4624
    transluminal angioplasty, C2623
    transtracheal oxygen, A4608
    vascular, A4300–A4301
Catheterization, specimen collection, P9612, P9615
CBC, *G0306, G0307*
Cefazolin sodium, J0689, J0690
Cefepime HCl, J0692, J0701, J0703
Cefiderocol, J0699
Cefotaxime sodium, J0698
Ceftaroline fosamil, J0712
Ceftazidime, J0713, J0714
Ceftizoxime sodium, J0715
Ceftolozane 50 mg and tazobactam 25 mg, J0695
Ceftriaxone sodium, J0696
Cefuroxime sodium, J0697
Celera, Q4259
CellCept, K0412
Cellesta cord, Q4214
Cellesta or cellesta duo, Q4184
Cellular therapy, M0075
Cement, ostomy, A4364
Cemiplimab injection-rwlc, J9119
Centrifuge, A4650
Centruroides Immune F(ab), J0716
Cephalin Floculation, blood, P2028
Cephalothin sodium, J1890
Cephapirin sodium, J0710
Certification, physician, home, health (per calendar month), *G0179–G0182*
  Physician certification, home health, G0180
  Physician recertification, home health, G0179
  Physician supervision, home health, complex care, 30 min or more, G0181
  Physician supervision, hospice 30 min or more, G0182
Certolizumab pegol, J0717
Cerumen, removal, *G0268*
Cervical
  cancer, screening, G0101
  cytopathology, G0123, G0124, G0141–G0148
    screening, automated thin layer, manual rescreening, physician supervision, G0145
    screening, automated thin layer preparation, cytotechnologist, physician interpretation, G0143

Cervical *(Continued)*
  cytopathology (Continued)
    screening, automated thin layer preparation, physician supervision, G0144
    screening, by cytotechnologist, physician supervision, G0123
    screening, cytopathology smears, automated system, physician interpretation, G0141
    screening, interpretation by physician, G0124
    screening smears, automated system, manual rescreening, G0148
    screening smears, automated system, physician supervision, G0147
  halo, L0810–L0830
  head harness/halter, E0942
  orthosis, L0100–L0200
    cervical collar molded to patient, L0170
    cervical, flexible collar, L0120–L0130
    cervical, multiple post collar, supports, L0180–L0200
    cervical, semi-rigid collar, L0150–L0160, L0172, L0174
    cranial cervical, L0112–L0113
  traction, E0855, E0856
Cervical cap contraceptive, A4261
Cervical-thoracic-lumbar-sacral orthosis (CTLSO), L0700, L0710
Cetuximab, J9055
Chair
  adjustable, dialysis, E1570
  lift, E0627
  rollabout, E1031
  sitz bath, E0160–E0162
  transport, E1035–E1039
    chair, adult size, heavy duty, greater than 300 pounds, E1039
    chair, adult size, up to 300 pounds, E1038
    chair, pediatric, E1037
    multi-positional patient transfer system, extra-wide, greater than 300 pounds, E1036
    multi-positional patient transfer system, up to 300 pounds, E1035
Change
  ureterostomy tube, C7549
Chaplain Services, Q9001–Q9003
Chelation therapy, M0300
Chemical endarterectomy, M0300
Chemistry and toxicology tests, P2028–P3001
Chemotherapy
  administration (hospital reporting only), Q0083–Q0085
  drug, oral, not otherwise classified, J8999
  drugs; (see also drug by name), J9000–J9999
Chest shell (cuirass), E0457
Chest Wall Oscillation System, E0483
  hose, replacement, A7026
  vest, replacement, A7025
Chest wrap, E0459
Chin cup, cervical, L0150

◄ **New**   ⭮ **Revised**   ✔ **Reinstated**   ~~deleted~~ **Deleted**

Chloramphenicol sodium succinate, J0720
Chlordiazepoxide HCl, J1990
Chloromycetin sodium succinate, J0720
Chloroprocaine HCl, J2401–J2402
Chloroprocaine hcl ophthalmic, J2403
Chloroquine HCl, J0390
Chlorothiazide sodium, J1205
Chlorpromazine HCl, J3230
   Chlorpromazine HCL, 5 mg, oral, Q0161
Chorionic gonadotropin, J0725
Choroid, lesion, destruction, *G0186*
Chromic phosphate P32 suspension, A9564
Chromium CR-51 sodium chromate, A9553
Cidofovir, J0740
Cilastatin sodium, imipenem, J0743
Ciltacabtagene, Q2056
Cinacalcet, J0604
Ciprofloxacin
   for intravenous infusion, J0744
   octic suspension, J7342
Cisplatin, J9060
Cladribine, J9065
Clamp
   dialysis, A4918
   external urethral, A4356
Cleanser, wound, A6260
Cleansing agent, dialysis equipment, A4790
Clindamycin phosphate, J0736, *J0737* ◄
Clofarabine, J9027
Clonidine, J0735
Closure, wound, adhesive, tissue, *G0168*
Clotting time tube, A4771
Clubfoot wedge, L3380
Cocaine, C9143
Cochlear prosthetic implant, L8614
   accessories, L8615–L8617, *L8618*
   batteries, L8621–L8624
   replacement, L8619, L8627–L8629
     external controller component, L8628
     external speech processor and controller, integrated
       system, L8619
     external speech processor, component, L8627
     transmitting coil and cable, integrated, L8629
Cocoon, membrane, Q4264
Codeine phosphate, J0745
Cold/Heat, application, E0200–E0239
   bilirubin light, E0202
   electric heat pad, moist, E0215
   electric heat pad, standard, E0210
   heat lamp with stand, E0205
   heat lamp, without stand, E0200
   hydrocollator unit, E0225
   hydrocollator unit, portable, E0239
   infrared heating pad system, E0221
   non-contact wound warming device, E0231
   paraffin bath unit, E0235
   pump for water circulating pad, E0236
   therapeutic lightbox, E0203

Cold/Heat, application *(Continued)*
   warming card, non-contact wound warming
     device, E0232
   water circulating cold pad, with pump, E0218
   water circulating heat pad, with pump, E0217
Colistimethate sodium, J0770
Collagen
   meniscus implant procedure, G0428
   skin test, G0025
   urinary tract implant, L8603
   wound dressing, A2006–A2014, **A6020–A6024**
Collagenase, Clostridium histolyticum, J0775
Collar, cervical
   multiple post, L0180–L0200
   nonadjust (foam), L0120
Collection and preparation, saliva, *D0417*
Colorectal, screening, cancer, *G0104–G0106,*
   G0120–G0122, G0328
Coly-Mycin M, J0770
Comfort items, A9190
Commode, E0160–E0175
   chair, E0170–E0171
   lift, E0172, E0625
   pail, E0167
   seat, wheelchair, E0968
Complete, blood, count, *G0306, G0307*
Composite dressing, A6200–A6205
Compressed gas system, E0424–E0446
   oximeter device, E0445
   portable gaseous oxygen system, purchase, E0430
   portable gaseous oxygen system, rental, E0431
   portable liquid oxygen, rental, container/supplies,
     E0434
   portable liquid oxygen, rental, home liquefier,
     E0433
   portable liquid oxygen system, purchase, container/
     refill adapter, E0435
   portable oxygen contents, gaseous, 1 month,
     E0443
   portable oxygen contents, liquid, 1 month, E0444
   stationary liquid oxygen system, purchase, use of
     reservoir, E0440
   stationary liquid oxygen system, rental, container/
     supplies, E0439
   stationary oxygen contents, gaseous, 1 month,
     E0441
   stationary oxygen contents, liquid, 1 month, E0442
   stationary purchase, compressed gas system, E0425
   stationary rental, compressed gaseous oxygen
     system, E0424
   topical oxygen delivery system, NOS, E0446
Compression
   bandage, A4460
   burn garment, A6501–A6512
   stockings, A6530–A6549
Compressor, E0565, E0570, E0571, E0572,
   E0650–E0652, K1031–K1033
Conductive gel/paste, *A4558*

Conductivity meter, bath, dialysis, E1550
Conference, team, G0175, G9007, *S0220, S0221*
   coordinate care fee, scheduled team conference, G9007
   medical conference/physician/interdisciplinary team,
     patient present, 30 min, S0220
   medical conference physician/interdisciplinary team,
     patient present, 60 min, S0221
   scheduled interdisciplinary team conference, patient
     present, G0175
Congo red, blood, P2029
Consultation, S0285, S0311, T1040, T1041
   dental, D9311
   Telehealth, G0425–G0427
Contact layer, A6206–A6208
Contact lens, V2500–V2599
Continent device, A5081, A5082, A5083
Continuous glucose monitoring system
   receiver, A9278, E2103, *S1037*
   sensor, A9276, *S1035*
   transmitter, A9277, *S1036*
Continuous passive motion exercise device, E0936
Continuous positive airway pressure
    device(CPAP), E0601
   compressor, K0269
Contraceptive
   cervical cap, A4261
   condoms, A4267, A4268
   diaphragm, A4266
   intratubal occlusion device, A4264
   intrauterine, copper, J7300
   intrauterine, levonorgestrel releasing, J7296–J7298,
     J7301
   patch, J7304
   spermicide, A4269
   supply, A4267–A4269
   vaginal ring, J7303
Contracts, maintenance, ESRD, A4890
Contrast, Q9951–Q9969
   HOCM, Q9958–Q9964
   injection, iron based magnetic resonance, per ml, Q9953
   injection, non-radioactive, non-contrast,
    visualization adjunct, Q9968
   injection, octafluoropropane microspheres,
    per ml, Q9956
   injection, perflexane lipid microspheres, per ml, Q9955
   injection, perflutren lipid microspheres, per ml, Q9957
   LOCM, Q9965–Q9967
   LOCM, 400 or greater mg/ml iodine, per ml, Q9951
   oral magnetic resonance contrast, Q9954
   Tc-99m per study dose, Q9969
Contrast material
   injection during MRI, A4643
   low osmolar, A4644–A4646
Coordinated, care, G9001–G9011
   CORF, registered nurse- face-face, G0128
Corneal tissue processing, V2785
Corset, spinal orthosis, L0970–L0976
   LSO, corset front, L0972
   LSO, full corset, L0976

Corset, spinal orthosis *(Continued)*
   TLSO, corset front, L0970
   TLSO, full corset, L0974
Corticorelin ovine triflutate, J0795
Corticotropin (acthar gel), J0801 ◄
Corticotropin (ani), J0802 ◄
Corvert (see Ibutilide fumarate)
Cosyntropin, J0833, J0834
Cough stimulating device, A7020, E0482
Counseling
   alcohol misuse, G0443
   cardiovascular disease, G0448
   control of dental disease, D1310, D1320
   immunization, G0310–G0315
   obesity, G0447
   sexually transmitted infection, G0445
Count, blood, G0306, G0307
Counterpulsation, external, G0166
Cover, wound
   alginate dressing, A6196–A6198
   foam dressing, A6209–A6214
   hydrogel dressing, A6242–A6248
   non-contact wound warming cover, and accessory,
    A6000, E0231, E0232
   specialty absorptive dressing, A6251–A6256
Covid-19 convalescent plasma, C9507 ◄
Covid test, K1034
CPAP (continuous positive airway pressure)
    device, E0601
   headgear, K0185
   humidifier, A7046
   intermittent assist, E0452
Cradle, bed, E0280
Cranial electrotherapy stimulation (CES), K1002
Crib, E0300
Cromolyn sodium, inhalation solution, unit dose,
   J7631, J7632
Crotalidae polyvalent immune fab, J0840
Crowns, D2710–D2983, D4249, D6720–D6794
   clinical crown lengthening-hard tissue, D4249
   fixed partial denture retainers, crowns, D6710–D6794
   single restoration, D2710–D2983
Crutches, E0110–E0118
   accessories, A4635–A4637, K0102
   crutch substitute, lower leg, E0118
   forearm, E0110–E0111
   underarm, E0112–E0117
Cryoprecipitate, each unit, P9012
CTLSO, L0700, L0710, L1000–L1120
   addition, axilla sling, L1010
   addition, cover for upright, each, L1120
   addition, kyphosis pad, L1020
   addition, kyphosis pad, floating, L1025
   addition, lumbar bolster pad, L1030
   addition, lumbar rib pad, L1040
   addition, lumbar sling, L1090
   addition, outrigger, L1080
   addition, outrigger bilateral, vertical extensions,
    L1085
   addition, ring flange, L1100

◄ **New**   ⊃ **Revised**   ✔ **Reinstated**   ~~deleted~~ **Deleted**

CTLSO *(Continued)*
addition, ring flange, molded to patient model, L1110
addition, sternal pad, L1050
addition, thoracic pad, L1060
addition, trapezius sling, L1070
anterior-posterior-lateral control, molded to patient model (CTLSO), L0710
cervical, thoracic, lumbar, sacral orthrosis (CTLSO), L0700
furnishing initial orthrosis, L1000
immobilizer, infant size, L1001
tension based scoliosis orthosis, fitting, L1005
Cuirass, E0457
Culture sensitivity study, P7001
Cushion, wheelchair, E0977
Cutaquig, J1551
Cyanocobalamin Cobalt C057, A9559
Cycler dialysis machine, E1594
Cyclophosphamide, J9070, J9071
oral, J8530
Cyclosporine, J7502, J7515, J7516
Cygnus matrix, Q4199
Cystourethroscopy, C7550, C7554, C9761 ↻
Cytarabine, J9100
liposome, J9098
Cytomegalovirus immune globulin (human), J0850
Cytopathology, cervical or vaginal, G0123, G0124, G0141–G0148

D

Dacarbazine, J9130
Daclizumab, J7513
Dactinomycin, J9120
Dalalone, J1100
Dalbavancin, 5mg, J0875
Dalteparin sodium, J1645
Daprodustat, oral, J0889 ◄
Daptomycin, J0874, J0877, J0878 ◄
Daratumumab, J9144, J9145
Darbepoetin Alfa, J0881–J0882
Daunorubicin
Citrate, J9151
HCl, J9150
DaunoXome (see Daunorubicin citrate)
Debridement
bone, C7500
Decitabine, J0893, J0894
Decubitus care equipment, E0180–E0199
air fluidized bed, E0194
air pressure mattress, E0186
air pressure pad, standard mattress, E0197
dry pressure mattress, E0184
dry pressure pad, standard mattress, E0199
gel or gel-like pressure pad mattress, standard, E0185
gel pressure mattress, E0196
heel or elbow protector, E0191
positioning cushion, E0190

Decubitus care equipment *(Continued)*
power pressure reducing mattress overlay, with pump, E0181, E0183
powered air flotation bed, E0193
pump, alternating pressure pad, replacement, E0182
synthetic sheepskin pad, E0189
water pressure mattress, E0187
water pressure pad, standard mattress, E0198
Deferoxamine mesylate, J0895
Defibrillator, external, E0617, K0606
battery, K0607
electrode, K0609
garment, K0608
Degarelix, J9155
Deionizer, water purification system, E1615
Delivery/set-up/dispensing, A9901
Denileukin diftitox, J9160
Denosumab, J0897
Density, bone, study, G0130
Dental procedures
adjunctive general services, D9110–D9999
alveoloplasty, D7310–D7321
analgesia, D9230
diagnostic, D0120–D0999
endodontics, D3000–D3999
evaluations, D0120–D0180
implant services, D6000–D6199
implants, D3460, D5925, D6010–D6067, D6075–D6199
laboratory, D0415–D0999
maxillofacial, D5900–D5999
orthodontics, D8000–D8999
periodontics, D4000–D4999
preventive, D1000–D1999
prosthetics, D5911–D5960, D5999
prosthodontics, fixed, D6200–D6999
prosthodontics, removable, D5000–D5999
restorative, D2000–D2999
scaling, D4341–D4346, D6081
Dentures, D5110–D5899
Depo-estradiol cypionate, J1000
Dermacell, dermacell awn or dermacell awn porous, Q4122
Dermal filler injection, G0429
Desmopressin acetate, J2597
Destruction, lesion, choroid, G0186
Detector, blood leak, dialysis, E1560
Developmental testing, G0451
Devices, other orthopedic, E1800–E1841
assistive listening device, V5267–V5290
Dexamethasone
acetate, J1094
inhalation solution, concentrated, J7637
inhalation solution, unit dose, J7638
intravitreal implant, J7312
lacrimal ophthalmic insert, J1096
oral, J8540
sodium phosphate, J1100
Dextran, J7100

◄ **New**   ↻ **Revised**   ✔ **Reinstated**   ~~deleted~~ **Deleted**

Dextrose
  saline (normal), J7042
  water, J7060, J7070
Dextrose, 5% in lactated ringers infusion, J7121
Dextrostick, A4772
Diabetes
  evaluation, G0245, G0246
  shoes (fitting/modifications), A5500–A5508
    deluxe feature, depth-inlay shoe, A5508
    depth inlay shoe, A5500
    molded from cast patient's foot, A5501
    shoe with metatarsal bar, A5505
    shoe with off-set heel(s), A5506
    shoe with rocker or rigid-bottom rocker, A5503
    shoe with wedge(s), A5504
    specified modification NOS, depth-inlay shoe, A5507
  training, outpatient, G0108, G0109
Diagnostic
  dental services, D0100–D0999
  copper, A9592
  florbetaben, Q9983
  flutemetamol F18, Q9982
  mammography, digital image, G9899, G9900
  radiology services, R0070–R0076
Dialysate
  concentrate additives, A4765
  solution, *A4720–A4728*
  testing solution, A4760
Dialysis
  air bubble detector, E1530
  bath conductivity, meter, E1550
  chemicals/antiseptics solution, A4674
  circuit, C7513–C7515, **C7530**
  disposable cycler set, A4671
  emergency, G0257
  equipment, E1510–E1702
  extension line, A4672–A4673
  filter, A4680
  fluid barrier, E1575
  home, S9335, S9339
  kit, A4820
  pressure alarm, E1540
  shunt, A4740
  supplies, A4650–A4927
  tablo hemodialysis system, E1629
  tourniquet, A4929
  unipuncture control system, E1580
  unscheduled, G0257
  venous pressure clamp, A4918
Dialyzer, A4690
Diaper, T1500, T4521–T4540, T4543, T4544
  adult incontinence garment, A4520, A4553
  incontinence supply, rectal insert, any type, each, A4337
  disposable penile wrap, T4545
Diathermy low frequency ultrasonic treatment device for home use, K1004
Diazepam, J3360
Diazoxide, J1730

Diclofenac, J1130
Dicyclomine HCl, J0500
Diethylstilbestrol diphosphate, J9165
Difelikefalin (for ESRD on dialysis), J0879
Digital behavioral therapy, A9291
Digoxin, J1160
Digoxin immune fab (ovine), J1162
Dihydroergotamine mesylate, J1110
Dimenhydrinate, J1240
Dimercaprol, J0470
Dimethyl sulfoxide (DMSO), J1212
Diphenhydramine HCl, J1200
Dipyridamole, J1245
Disarticulation
  lower extremities, prosthesis, L5000–L5999
    above knee, L5200–L5230
    additions exoskeletal-knee-shin system, L5710–L5782
    additions to lower extremities, L5610–L5617
    additions to socket insert, L5654–L5699
    additions to socket variations, L5630–L5653
    additions to test sockets, L5618–L5629
    additions/replacements, feet-ankle units, L5700–L5707
    ankle, L5050–L5060
    below knee, L5100–L5105
    component modification, L5785–L5795
    endoskeletal, L5810–L5999
    endoskeletal, above knee, L5321
    endoskeletal, hip disarticulation, L5331–L5341
    endoskeleton, below knee, L5301–L5312
    hemipelvectomy, L5280
    hip disarticulation, L5250–L5270
    immediate postsurgical fitting, L5400–L5460
    initial prosthesis, L5500–L5505
    knee disarticulation, L5150–L5160
    partial foot, L5000–L5020
    preparatory prosthesis, L5510–L5600
  upper extremities, prosthesis, L6000–L6692
    above elbow, L6250
    additions to upper limb, L6600–L6698
    below elbow, L6100–L6130
    elbow disarticulation, L6200–L6205
    endoskeletal, below elbow, L6400
    endoskeletal, interscapular thoracic, L6570–L6590
    endoskeletal, shoulder disarticulation, L6550
    immediate postsurgical procedures, L6380–L6388
    interscapular/thoracic, L6350–L6370
    partial hand, L6000–L6026
    shoulder disarticulation, L6300–L6320
    wrist disarticulation, L6050–L6055
Disease
  status, oncology, G9063–G9139
Dispensing, fee, pharmacy, *G0333, Q0510–Q0514, S9430*
  dispensing fee inhalation drug(s), 30 days, Q0513
  dispensing fee inhalation drug(s), 90 days, Q0514
  inhalation drugs, 30 days, as a beneficiary, G0333
  initial immunosuppressive drug(s), post transplanr, G0510

Dispensing, fee, pharmacy *(Continued)*
oral anti-cancer, oral anti-emetic,
immunosuppressive, first prescription, Q0511
oral anti-cancer, oral anti-emetic, immunosuppressive,
subsequent preparation, Q0512
Disposable collection and storage bag for breast milk, K1005
Disposable supplies, ambulance, A0382, A0384, A0392–A0398
DME
miscellaneous, A9900–A9999
DME delivery, set up, A9901
DME supple, NOS, A9999
DME supplies, A9900
DMSO, J1212
Dobutamine HCl, J1250
Docetaxel, J9171
Documentation
antidepressant, G8126–G8128
blood pressure, G8476–G8478
bypass, graft, coronary, artery, documentation, G8160–G8163
CABG, G8160–G8163
dysphagia, G8232
dysphagia, screening, G8232, V5364
ECG, 12–lead, G8705, G8706
eye, functions, G8315–G8333
influenza, immunization, G8482–G8484, M1169
kidney health evaluation, M1189–M1190
medical reason, M1178, M1183–M1185, M1194, M1201–M1202
pharmacologic therapy for osteoporosis, G8635
physician for DME, G0454
prophylactic antibiotic, G8702, G8703
prophylactic parenteral antibiotic, G8629–G8632
prophylaxis, DVT, G8218
prophylaxis, thrombosis, deep, vein, G8218
urinary, incontinence, G8063, G8267
vaccine, immunization, M1172
Dolasetron mesylate, J1260
Dome and mouthpiece (for nebulizer), A7016
Dopamine HCl, J1265
Doripenem, J1267
Dornase alpha, inhalation solution, unit dose form, J7639
Dostarlimab-gxly, J9272
Doxercalciferol, J1270
Doxil, J9001
Doxorubicin HCl, J9000, J9002
Drainage
bag, A4357, A4358
board, postural, E0606
bottle, A5102
Dressing
alginate, A6196–A6199
collagen, A6020–A6024
composite, A6200–A6205
contact layer, A6206–A6208
foam, A6209–A6215

Dressing *(Continued)*
gauze, A6216–A6230, A6402–A6406
holder/binder, A4462
hydrocolloid, A6234–A6241
hydrogel, A6242–A6248
specialty absorptive, A6251–A6256
transparent film, A6257–A6259
tubular, A6457
wound, K0744–K0746
Droperidol, J1790
and fentanyl citrate, J1810
Dropper, A4649
Drugs; (see also Table of Drugs)
administered through a metered dose inhaler, J3535
antiemetic, J8498, J8597, Q0163–Q0181
chemotherapy, J8500–J9999
disposable delivery system, 50 ml or greater per hour, A4305
disposable delivery system, 5 ml or less per hour, A4306
immunosuppressive, J7500–J7599
infusion supplies, A4221, A4222, A4230–A4232
inhalation solutions, J7608–J7699
non-prescription, A9150
not otherwise classified, J3490, J7599, J7699, J7799, J7999, J8499, J8999, J9999
oral, NOS, J8499
prescription, oral, J8499, J8999
Dry pressure pad/mattress, E0179, E0184, E0199
Duel layer impax membrane, Q4262
Durable medical equipment (DME), E0100–E1830, K Codes
additional oxygen related equipment, E1352–E1406
arm support, wheelchair, E2626–E2633
artificial kidney machines/accessories, E1500–E1699
attachments, E0156–E0159
bath and toilet aides, E0240–E0249
canes, E0100–E0105
commodes, E0160–E0175
crutches, E0110–E0118
decubitus care equipment, E0181–E0199
DME, respiratory, inexpensive, purchased, A7000–A7509
gait trainer, E8000–E8002
heat/cold application, E0200–E0239
hospital beds and accessories, E0250–E0373
humidifiers/nebulizers/compressors, oxygen IPPB, E0550–E0585
infusion supplies, E0776–E0791
IPPB machines, E0500
jaw motion rehabilitation system, E1700–E1702
miscellaneous, E1902–E2120
monitoring equipment, home glucose, E0607
negative pressure, E2402
non-pneumatic compressor, E0677 ◀
other orthopedic devices, E1800–E1841
oxygen/respiratory equipment, E0424–E0487
pacemaker monitor, E0610–E0620
patient lifts, E0621–E0642
pneumatic compressor, E0650–E0676

Durable medical equipment (DME) *(Continued)*
  rollout chair/transfer system, E1031–E1039
  safety equipment, E0700–E0705
  speech device, E2500–E2599
  suction pump/room vaporizers, E0600–E0606
  temporary DME codes, regional carriers, K0000–K9999
  TENS/stimulation device(s), E0720–E0770
  traction equipment, E0830–E0900
  trapeze equipment, fracture frame, E0910–E0948
  walkers, E0130–E0155
  wheelchair accessories, E2201–E2397
  wheelchair, accessories, E0950–E1030
  wheelchair, amputee, E1170–E1200
  wheelchair cusion/protection, E2601–E2621
  wheelchair, fully reclining, E1050–E1093
  wheelchair, heavy duty, E1280–E1298
  wheelchair, lightweight, E1240–E1270
  wheelchair, semi-reclining, E1100–E1110
  wheelchair, skin protection, E2622–E2625
  wheelchair, special size, E1220–E1239
  wheelchair, standard, E1130–E1161
  whirlpool equipment, E1300–E1310
Duraclon, (see Clonidine)
Dyphylline, J1180
Dysphagia, screening, documentation, G8232, V5364
Dystrophic, nails, trimming, G0127

E

Ear mold, V5264, V5265
Ecallantide, J1290
Echocardiography image, C9786 ◀
Echocardiography injectable contrast material, A9700
  ECG, 12–lead, G8704
Eculizumab, J1300
ED, visit, G0380–G0384
Edetate
  calcium disodium, J0600
  disodium, J3520
Educational Services
  chronic kidney disease, G0420, G0421
Efgartigimod, J9332
Eflapegrastim-xnst, J1449 ◀
Eggcrate dry pressure pad/mattress, E0184, E0199
EKG, G0403–G0405
Elbow
  disarticulation, endoskeletal, L6450
  orthosis (EO), E1800, L3700–L3740, L3760, L3671
    dynamic adjustable elbow flexion device, E1800
    elbow arthrosis, L3702–L3766
  protector, E0191
Electric hand, L7007–L7008
Electric, nerve, stimulator, transcutaneous, A4595, E0720–E0749
  conductive garment, E0731
  electric joint stimulation device, E0762

Electric, nerve, stimulator, transcutaneous *(Continued)*
  electrical stimulator supplies, A4595, A4596
  electromagnetic wound treatment device, E0769
  electronic salivary reflex stimulator, E0755
  EMG, biofeedback device, E0746
  functional electrical stimulator, nerve and/or muscle groups, E0770
  functional stimulator sequential muscle groups, E0764
  incontinence treatment system, E0740
  nerve stimulator (FDA), treatment nausea and vomiting, E0765
  osteogenesis stimulator, electrical, surgically implanted, E0749
  osteogenesis stimulator, low-intensity ultrasound, E0760
  osteogenesis stimulator, non-invasive, not spinal, E0747
  osteogenesis stimulator, non-invasive, spinal, E0748
  radiowaves, non-thermal, high frequency, E0761
  stimulator, electrical shock unit, E0745
  stimulator for scoliosis, E0744
  TENS, four or more leads, E0730
  TENS, two lead, E0720
Electrical stimulation device used for cancer treatment, E0766
Electrical work, dialysis equipment, A4870
Electrodes, per pair, A4555, A4556
Electromagnetic, therapy, G0295, G0329
Electronic medication compliance, T1505
Electronic positional obstructive sleep apnea treatment, K1001
Elevating leg rest, K0195
Elliotts B solution, J9175
Elotuzumab, J9176
Emapalumab injection-lzsg, J9210
Emergency department, visit, G0380–G0384
EMG, E0746
Eminase, J0350
Encephalitis, due to vaccine, M1162
Endarterectomy, chemical, M0300
Endodontic procedures, D3000–D3999
  periapical services, D3410–D3470
  pulp capping, D3110, D3120
  root canal therapy, D3310–D3353
  therapy, D3310–D3330
Endodontics, dental, D3000–D3999
Endoscope sheath, A4270
Endoscopic
  outlet reduction, C9785 ◀
  retrograde cholangiopancreatography, C7541–C7544
  sleeve gastroplasty, C9784 ◀
Endoskeletal system, addition, L5848, L5856–L5857, L5925, L5961, L5969
Enema, bag, A4458
Enfuvirtide, J1324
Enoxaparin sodium, J1650
Enteral
  feeding supply kit (syringe) (pump) (gravity), B4034–B4036, B4148 ◀
  formulae, B4149–B4156, B4157–B4162

◀ **New** ↻ **Revised** ✓ **Reinstated** ~~deleted~~ **Deleted**

Enteral *(Continued)*
nutrition infusion pump (with alarm) (without), B9000, B9002
therapy, supplies, B4000–B9999
enteral and parenteral pumps, B9002–B9999
enteral formula/medical supplies, B0434–B4162
parenteral solutions/supplies, B4164–B5200
Epcoritamab-bysp, C9155 ◀
Epinephrine, J0171, J0173
Epirubicin HCl, J9178
Epoetin alpha, J0885, Q4081
Epoetin alpha-epbx, Retacrit (for ESRD on dialysis), Q5105
Epoetin alpha-epbx, Retacrit (non-ESRD use), Q5106
Epoetin beta, J0887–J0888
Epoprostenol, J1325
Eptinezumab-jjmr, J3032
Equipment
decubitus, E0181–E0199
exercise, A9300, E0935, E0936
orthopedic, E0910–E0948, E1800–E8002
oxygen, E0424–E0486, E1353–E1406
pump, E0781, E0784, E0791
respiratory, E0424–E0601
safety, E0700, E0705
traction, E0830–E0900
transfer, E0705
trapeze, E0910–E0912, E0940
whirlpool, E1300, E1310
Eravacycline injection, J0122
Erection device, tension ring, *L7902*
Ergonovine maleate, J1330
Eribulin mesylate, J9179
Ertapenem sodium, J1335
Erythromycin lactobionate, J1364
Esketamine, nasal spray, S0013
Esmolol hydrochloride, J1805, J1806 ◀
ESRD (End-Stage Renal Disease); (see also Dialysis)
diagnosis of, M1187
machines and accessories, E1500–E1699
adjustable chair, ESRD, E1570
centrifuge, dialysis, E1500
dialysis equipment, NOS, E1699
hemodialysis, air bubble detector, replacement, E1530
hemodialysis, bath conductivity meter, E1550
hemodialysis, blood leak detector, replacement, E1560
hemodialysis, blood pump, replacement, E1620
hemodialysis equipment, delivery/installation charges, E1600
hemodialysis, heparin infusion pump, E1520
hemodialysis machine, E1590
hemodialysis, portable travel hemodialyzer system, E1635
hemodialysis, pressure alarm, E1540
hemodialysis, reverse osmosis water system, E1615
hemodialysis, sorbent cartridges, E1636
hemodialysis, transducer protectors, E1575
hemodialysis, unipuncture control system, E1580

ESRD *(Continued)*
machines and accessories *(Continued)*
hemodialysis, water softening system, E1625
hemostats, E1637
peritoneal dialysis, automatic intermittent system, E1592
peritoneal dialysis clamps, E1634
peritoneal dialysis, cycler dialysis machine, E1594
peritoneal dialysis, reciprocating system, E1630
scale, E1639
wearable artificial kidney, E1632
plumbing, A4870
supplies, A4651–A4929
acetate concentrate solution, hemodialysis, A4708
acid concentrate solution, hemodialysis, A4709
activated carbon filters, hemodialysis, A4680
ammonia test strip, dialysis, A4774
automatic blood pressure monitor, A4670
bicarbonate concentrate, powder, hemodialysis, A4707
bicarbonate concentrate, solution, A4706
blood collection tube, vaccum, dialysis, A4770
blood glucose test strip, dialysis, A4772
blood pressure cuff only, A4663
blood tubing, arterial and venous, hemodialysis, A4755
blood tubing, arterial or venous, hemodialysis, A4750
chemicals/antiseptics solution, clean dialysis equipment, A4674
dialysate solution, non-dextrose, A4728
dialysate solution, peritoneal dialysis, A4720–A4726, A4760–A4766
dialyzers, hemodialysis, A4690
disposable catheter tips, peritoneal dialysis, A4860
disposable cycler set, dialysis machine, A4671
drainage extension line, dialysis, sterile, A4672
extension line easy lock connectors, dialysis, A4673
fistula cannulation set, hemodialysis, A4730
injectable anesthetic, dialysis, A4737
occult blood test strips, dialysis, A4773
peritoneal dialysis, catheter anchoring device, A4653
protamine sulfate, hemodialysis, A4802
serum clotting timetube, dialysis, A4771
shunt accessory, hemodialysis, A4740
sphygmomanometer, cuff and stethoscope, A4660
syringes, A4657
topical anesthetic, dialysis, A4736
treated water, peritoneal dialysis, A4714
"Y set" tubing, peritoneal dialysis, A4719
Estrogen conjugated, J1410
Estrone (5, Aqueous), J1435
Etelcalcetide, J0606
Eteplirsen, J1428
Ethanolamine oleate, J1430
Etidronate disodium, J1436
Etonogestrel implant system, J7307
Etoposide, J9181
oral, J8560

◀ **New** ⊃ **Revised** ✔ **Reinstated** ~~deleted~~ **Deleted**

Etranacogene dezaparvovec-drlb, J1411 ◄
Euflexxa, J7323
Evaluation
  conformity, V5020
  contact lens, S0592
  dental, D0120–D0180
  diabetic, G0245, G0246
  footwear, G8410–G8416
  hearing, S0618, V5008, V5010
  hospice, G0337
  multidisciplinary, H2000
  nursing, T1001
  ocularist, S9150
  performance measurement, S3005
  resident, T2011
  speech, S9152
  team, T1024
Everolimus, J7527
Evinacumab-dgnb J1305
Examination
  gynecological, S0610–S0613
  ophthalmological, S0620, S0621
  oral, D0120–D0160
  pinworm, Q0113
Excision
  cervical nodes, C7503
  neuroma, C7551
Exercise
  class, S9451
  equipment, A9300
External
  ambulatory infusion pump, E0781, E0784
  ambulatory infusion pump continuous glucose
    sensing, E0787
  ambulatory insulin delivery system, A9274
  power, battery components, L7360–L7368
  power, elbow, L7160–L7191
  urinary supplies, A4356–A4359
Extractions; (see also Dental procedures),
  D7111–D7140, D7251
Extremity
  belt/harness, E0945
  traction, E0870–E0880
Eye
  case, V2756
  functions, documentation, G8315–G8333
  lens (contact) (spectacle), V2100–V2615
  pad, patch, A6410–A6412
  prosthetic, V2623, V2629
  service (miscellaneous), V2700–V2799
  stent, S1091

F

Face tent, oxygen, A4619
Faceplate, ostomy, A4361
Facility services, dental, G0330

Factor IX, J7193, J7194, J7195, J7200–J7202,
  J7213 ◄
Factor VIIA coagulation factor, recombinant,
  J7189, J7205, J7212
Factor VIII, anti-hemophilic factor, J7182, J7185,
  J7190–J7192, J7207–J7209, J7214 ◄
Factor X, J7175
Factor XIII, anti-hemophilic factor, J7180, J7188
Factor XIII, A-subunit, J7181
Family Planning Education, H1010
Faricimab-svoa, J2777
Fecal microbiota, J1440 ◄
Fee
  coordinated care, G9001–G9011
  dispensing, pharmacy, G0333, Q0510–Q0514,
    S9430
Fentanyl citrate, J3010
  and droperidol, J1810
Fern test, Q0114
Ferric derisomaltose, J1437
Ferric pyrophosphate citrate powder, J1444
Ferumoxytol, Q0138, Q0139
Filgrastim (G-CSF & TBO), J1442, J1447,
  Q5101
Filler, wound
  alginate dressing, A6199
  foam dressing, A6215
  hydrocolloid dressing, A6240, A6241
  hydrogel dressing, A6248
  not elsewhere classified, A6261, A6262
Film, transparent (for dressing), A6257–A6259
Filter
  aerosol compressor, A7014
  dialysis carbon, A4680
  ostomy, A4368
  tracheostoma, A4481
  ultrasonic generator, A7014
Fistula cannulation set, A4730
Flebogamma, J1572
Florbetapir F18, A9586
Flortaucipir, A9601
Flotufolastat, C9156 ◄
Flowmeter, E0440, E0555, E0580
Floxuridine, J9200
Fluconazole, injection, J1450
Fludarabine phosphate, J8562, J9185
Fluid barrier, dialysis, E1575
Fluid flow, Q4206
Flunisolide inhalation solution, J7641
Fluocinolone, J7311, J7313
  (Yutiq), J7314
Fluoride treatment, D1201–D1205
Fluorodeoxyglucose F-18 FDG, A9552
Fluorodopa, A9602
Fluoroestradiol F 18, A9591
Fluorouracil, J9190
Fluphenazine decanoate, J2680
Foam
  dressing, A6209–A6215
  pad adhesive, A5126

Folding walker, E0135, E0143
Foley catheter, A4312–A4316, A4338–A4346
  indwelling catheter, specialty type, A4340–A4342 ◀
  indwelling catheter, three-way, continuous
    irrigation, A4346
  indwelling catheter, two-way, all silicone, A4344
  indwelling catheter, two-way latex, A4338
  insertion tray with drainage bag, A4312
  insertion tray with drainage bag, three-way,
    continuous irrigation, A4316
  insertion tray with drainage bag, two-way
    latex, A4314
  insertion tray with drainage bag, two-way,
    silicone, A4315
  insertion tray without drainage bag, A4313
Fomepizole, J1451
Fomivirsen sodium intraocular, J1452
Fondaparinux sodium, J1652
Foot care, G0247
Footdrop splint, L4398
Footplate, E0175, E0970, L3031
Footwear, orthopedic, L3201–L3265
  additional charge for split size, L3257
  Benesch boot, pair, child, L3213
  Benesch boot, pair, infant, L3212
  Benesch boot, pair, junior, L3214
  custom molded shoe, prosthetic shoe, L3250
  custom shoe, depth inlay, L3230
  ladies' shoe, depth inlay, L3216
  ladies' shoe, hightop, L3217
  ladies' shoe, oxford, L3215
  ladies' shoe, oxford/brace, L3224
  men's shoe, depth inlay, L3221
  men's shoe, hightop, L3222
  men's shoe, oxford, L3219
  men's shoe, oxford/brace, L3225
  molded shoe, custom fitted, Plastazote, L3253
  non-standard size or length, L3255
  non-standard size or width, L3254
  Plastazote sandal, L3265
  shoe, hightop, child, L3206
  shoe, hightop, infant, L3204
  shoe, hightop, junior, L3207
  shoe molded/patient model, Plastazote, L3252
  shoe, molded/patient model, silicone, L3251
  shoe, oxford, child, L3202
  shoe, oxford, infant, L3201
  shoe, oxford, junior, L3203
  surgical boot, child, L3209
  surgical boot, infant, L3208
  surgical boot, junior, L3211
  surgical boot/shoe, L3260
Forearm crutches, E0110, E0111
Formoterol, J7640
  fumarate, J7606
Fosaprepitant, J1453, J1456
Foscarnet sodium, J1455
Fosphenytoin, Q2009

Fracture
  bedpan, E0276
  frame, E0920, E0930, E0946–E0948
    attached to bed/weights, E0920
    attachments for complex cervical traction,
      E0948
    attachments for complex pelvic traction,
      E0947
    dual, cross bars, attached to bed, E0946
    free standing/weights, E0930
  orthosis, L2106–L2136, L3980–L3984
    ankle/foot orthosis, fracture, L2106–L2128
    KAFO, fracture orthosis, L2132–L2136
    upper extremity, fracture orthosis, L3980–L3984
  orthotic additions, L2180–L2192, L3995
    addition to upper extremity orthosis, sock,
      fracture, L3995
    additions lower extremity fracture, L2180–L2192
Fragmin, (see Dalteparin sodium), *J1645*
Frames (spectacles), V2020, V2025
  deluxe frame, V2025
  purchases, V2020
Fremanezumab-vfrm, J3031
Fulvestrant, J9393–J9395
Furosemide, J1940, J1941 ◀
Fusion
  finger joints, C7506

G

Gadobutrol, A9585
Gadofosveset trisodium, A9583
Gadopiclenol, A9573 ◀
Gadoxetate disodium, A9581
Gait trainer, E8000–E8002
Gallium Ga67, A9556
Gallium illuccix, A9596
Gallium locametz, A9800
Gallium nitrate, J1457
Galsulfase, J1458
Gamma globulin, J1460, J1560
  injection, gamma globulin (IM), 1cc, J1460
  injection, gamma globulin (IM), over 10cc, J1560
Gammagard liquid, J1569
Gammaplex, J1557
Gamunex, J1561
Ganciclovir
  implant, J7310
  sodium, J1570, J1574
Garamycin, J1580
Gas system
  compressed, E0424, E0425
  gaseous, E0430, E0431, E0441, E0443
  liquid, E0434–E0440, E0442, E0444
Gastric electrophysiology mapping, C9787 ◀
Gastric freezing, hypothermia, M0100
Gatifloxacin, J1590

◀ New   ↻ Revised   ✔ Reinstated   ~~deleted~~ Deleted

Gauze
> impregnated, A6222–A6233, A6266
> non-impregnated, A6402–A6404

Gefitinib, J8565

Gel
> conductive, A4558
> pressure pad, E0185, E0196

Gemcitabine HCl, not otherwise specified, J9196, J9201, ◄
> Infugem, J9198

Gemtuzumab ozogamicin, J9203

Generator
> *neurostimulator (implantable), high frequency, C1822*
> *neurostimulator (implantable), non-rechargeable, C1827*
> *neurostimulator (implantable), rechargeable, C1826*
> ultrasonic with nebulizer, E0574–E0575

Gentamicin (Sulfate), J1580

***Gingival procedures,** D4210–D4240*
> *gingival flap procedure, D4240–D4241*
> *gingivectomy or gingivoplasty, D4210–D4212*

Glasses
> air conduction, V5070
> binaural, V5120–V5150
>> *behind the ear, V5140*
>> *body, V5120*
>> *glasses, V5150*
>> *in the ear, V5130*
> bone conduction, V5080
> frames, V2020, V2025
> hearing aid, V5230

Glaucoma
> *screening, G0117, G0118*

Gloves, A4927

Glucagon HCl, J1610, J1611

Glucose
> monitor with integrated lancing/blood sample collection, E2101
> monitor with integrated voice synthesizer, E2100
> test strips, A4253, A4772

Gluteal pad, L2650

Glycopyrrolate, inhalation solution, concentrated, J7642

Glycopyrrolate, inhalation solution, unit dose, J7643

Gold
> *foil dental restoration, D2410–D2430*
>> *gold foil, one surface, D2410*
>> *gold foil, two surfaces, D2420*
>> *gold foil, three surfaces, D2430*
> sodium thiomalate, J1600

Golimumab, J1602

Gomco drain bottle, A4912

Gonadorelin HCl, J1620

Goserelin acetate implant; (see also Implant), J9202

Grab bar, trapeze, E0910, E0940

Grade-aid, wheelchair, E0974

***Gradient, compression stockings,** A6530–A6549*
> *below knee, 18–30 mmHg, A6530*

***Gradient, compression stockings** (Continued)*
> *below knee, 30–40 mmHg, A6531*
> *below knee, thigh length, 18–30 mmHg, A6533*
> *full length/chap style, 18–30 mmHg, A6536*
> *full length/chap style, 30–40 mmHg, A6537*
> *full length/chap style, 40–50 mmHg, A6538*
> *garter belt, A6544*
> *non-elastic below knee, 30–50 mmhg, A6545*
> *sleeve, NOS, A6549*
> *thigh length, 30–40 mmHg, A6534*
> *thigh length, 40–50 mmHg, A6535*
> *waist length, 18–30 mmHg, A6539*
> *waist length, 30–40 mmHg, A6540*
> *waist length, 40–50 mmHg, A6541*

Granisetron HCl, J1626
> XR, J1627

Gravity traction device, E0941

Gravlee jet washer, A4470

***Guidelines, practice, oncology,** G9056–G9062*

H

Habilitation, prevocational, waiver, T2047

Hair analysis (excluding arsenic), P2031
> *Halaven, Injection, eribulin mesylate, 0.1 mg, J9179*

Hallus-Valgus dynamic splint, L3100

Hallux prosthetic implant, L8642

Halo procedures, L0810–L0860
> *addition HALO procedure, MRI compatible systems, L0859*
> *addition HALO procedure, replacement liner, L0861*
> *cervical halo/jacket vest, L0810*
> *cervical halo/Milwaukee type orthosis, L0830*
> *cervical halo/plaster body jacket, L0820*

Haloperidol, J1630
> decanoate, J1631

Halter, cervical head, E0942

Hand finger orthosis, prefabricated, L3923

Hand restoration, L6900–L6915
> orthosis (WHFO), E1805, E1825, L3800–L3805, L3900–L3954
> partial prosthesis, L6000–L6020
>> *partial hand, little and/or ring finger remaining, L6010*
>> *partial hand, no finger, L6020*
>> *partial hand, thumb remaining, L6000*
>> *transcarpal/metacarpal or partial hand disarticulation prosthesis, L6025*
> rims, wheelchair, E0967

Handgrip (cane, crutch, walker), A4636

Harness, E0942, E0944, E0945

Headgear (for positive airway pressure device), K0185

Hearing
> *aid, V5030–V5267, V5298*
>> *aid-body worn, V5100*
>> *assistive listening device, V5268–V5274, V5281–V5290*
>> *battery, use in hearing device, V5266*

◄ **New** ↻ **Revised** ✔ **Reinstated** ~~deleted~~ **Deleted**

Hearing (Continued)
 aid (Continued)
  *contralateral routing, V5171–V5172, V5181,
   V5211–V5115, V5221*
  dispensing fee, binaural, V5160
  dispensing fee, monaural hearing aid, any type, V5241
  dispensing fee, unspecified hearing aid, V5090
  ear impression, each, V5275
  ear mold/insert, disposable, any type, V5265
  ear mold/insert, not disposable, V5264
  glasses, air conduction, V5070
  glasses, bone conduction, V5080
  hearing aid, analog, binaural, CIC, V5248
  hearing aid, analog, binaural, ITC, V5249
  hearing aid, analog, monaural, CIC, V5242
  hearing aid, analog, monaural, ITC, V5243
  hearing aid, BICROS, V5210–V5240
  hearing aid, binaural, V5120–V5150
  hearing aid, CROS, V5170–V5200
  hearing aid, digital, V5254–V5261
  *hearing aid, digitally programmable, V5244–V5247,
   V5250–V5253*
  hearing aid, disposable, any type, binaural, V5263
  hearing aid, disposable, any type, monaural, V5262
  hearing aid, monaural, V5030–V5060
  hearing aid, NOC, V5298
  *hearing aid or assistive listening device/supplies/
   accessories, NOS, V5267*
  hearing service, miscellaneous, V5299
  semi-implantable, middle ear, V5095
 assessment, S0618, V5008, V5010
 devices, L8614, V5000–V5169, V5171–V5179,
  V5181–V5209, V5211–V5219, V5221–V5299
 services, V5000–V5999
Heat
 application, E0200–E0239
 infrared heating pad system, A4639, E0221
 lamp, E0200, E0205
 pad, A9273, E0210, E0215, E0237, E0249
Heater (nebulizer), E1372
***Heavy duty, wheelchair,** E1280–E1298, K0006,
  K0007, K0801–K0886*
 detachable arms, elevating legrests, E1280
 detachable arms, swing away detachable footrest, E1290
 extra heavy duty wheelchair, K0007
 fixed full length arms, elevating legrest, E1295
 *fixed full length arms, swing away detachable
  footrest, E1285*
 heavy duty wheelchair, K0006
 *power mobility device, not coded by DME PDAC or
  no criteria, K0900*
 power operated vehicle, group 2, K0806–K0808
 power operated vehicle, NOC, K0812
 power wheelchair, group 1, K0813–K0816
 power wheelchair, group 2, K0820–K0843
 power wheelchair, group 3, K0848–K0864
 power wheelchair, group 4, K0868–K0886
 power wheelchair, group 5, pediatric, K0890–K0891
 power wheelchair, NOC, K0898

***Heavy duty, wheelchair** (Continued)
 power-operated vehicle, group 1, K0800–K0802
 *special wheelchair seat depth and/or width, by
  construction, E1298*
 special wheelchair seat depth, by upholstery, E1297
 special wheelchair seat height from floor, E1296
Heel
 elevator, air, E0370
 protector, E0191
 shoe, L3430–L3485
 stabilizer, L3170
Helicopter, ambulance; (see also Ambulance)
Helmet
 cervical, L0100, L0110
 head, A8000–A8004
Hemin, J1640
Hemipelvectomy prosthesis, L5280
Hemi-wheelchair, E1083–E1086
Hemodialysis machine, E1590
Hemodialyzer, portable, E1635
Hemofil M, J7190
Hemophilia clotting factor, J7190–J7198
 anti-inhibitor, per IU, J7198
 anti-thrombin III, human, per IU, J7197
 Factor IX, complex, per IU, J7194
 *Factor IX, purified, non-recombinant, per IU,
  J7193*
 Factor IX, recombinant, J7195
 Factor VIII, human, per IU, J7190
 Factor VIII, porcine, per IU, J7191
 Factor VIII, recombinant, per IU, NOS, J7192
 *injection, antithrombin recombinant, 50 i.u.,
  J7196*
 NOC, J7199
Hemostats, A4850, *E1637*
Hemostix, A4773
Hepagam B
 IM, J1571
 IV, J1573
Heparin
 infusion pump, dialysis, E1520
 lock flush, J1642
 sodium, J1643, J1644
***Hepatitis B, vaccine, administration,** G0010*
Hep-Lock (U/P), J1642
Hexalite, A4590
High osmolar contrast material, Q9958–Q9964
 HOCM, 400 or greater mg/ml iodine, Q9964
 HOCM, 150–199 mg/ml iodine, Q9959
 HOCM, 200–249 mg/ml iodine, Q9960
 HOCM, 250–299 mg/ml iodine, Q9961
 HOCM, 300–349 mg/ml iodine, Q9962
 HOCM, 350–399 mg/ml iodine, Q9963
 HOCM, up to 149 mg/ml iodine, Q9958
Hip
 disarticulation prosthesis, L5250, L5270
 orthosis (HO), L1600–L1690
Hip-knee-ankle-foot orthosis (HKAFO), L2040–L2090

◄ New ⊋ Revised ✔ Reinstated ~~deleted~~ Deleted

Histrelin
    acetate, J1675
    implant, J9225
HKAFO, L2040–L2090
Home
    certification, home health, G0180
    glucose, monitor, E0607, E2100, E2101, S1030, S1031
    health, aide, G0156, S9122, T1021
    health, aide, in home, per hour, S9122
    health, aide, per visit, T1021
    health, clinical, social worker, G0155
    health, data collection, G0322
    health, hospice, each 15 min, G0156
    health, occupational, therapist, G0152
    health, physical therapist, G0151
    health, physician, certification, G0179–G0182
    health, respiratory therapy, S5180, S5181
    recertification, home health, G0179
    supervision, home health, G0181
    supervision, hospice, G0182
    therapist, speech, S9128
Home Health Agency Services, T0221, T1022
    care improvement home visit assessment, G9187
Home sleep study test, G0398–G0400
HOPPS, C1000–C9999
Hospice care
    assisted living facility, Q5002
    hospice facility, Q5010
    inpatient hospice facility, Q5006
    inpatient hospital, Q5005
    inpatient psychiatric facility, Q5008
    long-term care facility, Q5007
    nursing long-term facility, Q5003
    patient's home, Q5001
    services, M1154, M1159, M1186
    skilled nursing facility, Q5004
Hospice, evaluation, pre-election, *G0337*
Hospice physician supervision, *G0182*
Hospital
    bed, E0250–E0304, E0328, E0329
    observation, G0378, G0379
    outpatient clinic visit, assessment, G0463
Hospital Outpatient Payment System, C1000–C9999
Hot water bottle, A9273
Human fibrinogen concentrate, J7178
Humidifier, A7046, E0550–E0563
    durable, diring IPPB treatment, E0560
    durable, extensive, IPPB, E0550
    durable glass bottle type, for regulator, E0555
    heated, used with positive airway pressure device, E0562
    non-heated, used with positive airway pressure, E0561
    water chamber, humidifier, replacement, positive airway device, A7046
Hyalgan, J7321
Hyalomatrix, Q4117
Hyaluronan, J7326, J7327
    derivative, J7332
    durolane, J7318

Hyaluronan *(Continued)*
    gel-Syn, J7328
    genvisc, J7320
    hymovis, J7322
    trivisc, J7329
Hyaluronate, sodium, J7317
Hyaluronidase, J3470, J9316
    ovine, J3471–J3473
Hydralazine HCl, J0360
Hydraulic patient lift, E0630
Hydrocollator, E0225, E0239
Hydrocolloid dressing, A6234–A6241
Hydrocortisone
    acetate, J1700
    sodium phosphate, J1710
    sodium succinate, J1720
Hydrogel dressing, A6231–A6233, A6242–A6248
Hydromorphone, J1170
Hydroxyprogesterone caproate, J1725–J1726, J1729
Hydroxyzine HCl, J3410
Hygienic item or device, disposable or non-disposable, any type, each, A9286
Hylan G-F 20, J7322
Hyoscyamine Sulfate, J1980
Hyperbaric oxygen chamber, topical, A4575
Hypertonic saline solution, J7130, *J7131*

I

Ibandronate sodium, J1740
Ibuprofen, J1741
Ibutilide Fumarate, J1742
Icatibant, J1744
Ice
    cap, E0230
    collar, E0230
Idarubicin HCl, J9211
Idursulfase, J1743
Ifosfamide, J9208
Iliac, artery, angiography, G0278
Iloprost, Q4074
Imaging, PET, G0219, G0235
    any site, NOS, G0235
    whole body, melanoma, non-covered indications, G0219
Imiglucerase, J1786
Immune globulin, J1575
    Bivigam, 500 mg, J1556
    Cuvitru, J1555
    Flebogamma, J1572
    Gammagard liquid, J1569
    Gammaplex, J1557
    Gamunex, J1561
    HepaGam B, J1571
    Hizentra, J1559
    Intravenous services, supplies and accessories, Q2052
    NOS, J1566

◄ **New**   ↻ **Revised**   ✔ **Reinstated**   ~~deleted~~ **Deleted**

Immune globulin *(Continued)*
  Octagam, J1568
  Panzyga, J1576 ◀
  Privigen, J1459
  Rho(D), J2788, *J2790, J2791*
  Rhophylac, J2791
  Subcutaneous, J1562
  Xembify, J1558
Immunization counseling, G0310–G0315
Immunosuppressive drug, not otherwise classified, J7599
Implant
  access system, A4301
  aqueous shunt, L8612
  bimatoprost, intracameral implant, J7351
  breast, L8600
  buprenorphine implant, J0570
  cochlear, L8614, L8619
  collagen, urinary tract, L8603
  dental, D3460, D5925, D6010–D6067, D6075–D6199
    crown, provisional, D6085
    endodontic endosseous implant, D3460
    facial augmentation implant prosthesis, D5925
    implant supported prosthetics, D6055–D6067, D6075–D6077
    other implant services, D6080–D6199
    surgical placement, D6010–D6051
  dextranomer/hyaluronic acid copolymer, L8604
  ganciclovir, J7310
  hallux, L8642
  infusion pump, programmable, E0783, E0786
    implantable, programmable, E0783
    implantable, programmable, replacement, E0786
  joint, L8630, L8641, L8658
    interphalangeal joint spacer, silicone or equal, L8658
    metacarpophalangeal joint implant, L8630
    metatarsal joint implant, L8641
  lacrimal duct, A4262, A4263
  maintenance procedures, D6080
  maxillofacial, D5913–D5937
    auricular prosthesis, D5914
    auricular prosthesis, replacement, D5927
    cranial prosthesis, D5924
    facial augmentation implant prosthesis, D5925
    facial prosthesis, D5919
    facial prosthesis, replacement, D5929
    mandibular resection prosthesis, with guide flange, D5934
    mandibular resection prosthesis, without guide flange, D5935
    nasal prosthesis, D5913
    nasal prosthesis, replacement, D5926
    nasal septal prosthesis, D5922
    obturator prosthesis, definitive, D5932
    obturator prosthesis, modification, D5933
    obturator prosthesis, surgical, D5931
    obturator/prosthesis, interim, D5936
    ocular prosthesis, D5916
    ocular prosthesis, interim, D5923
    orbital prosthesis, D5915

Implant *(Continued)*
  maxillofacial (Continued)
    orbital prosthesis, replacement, D5928
    trismus appliance, not for TM treatment, D5937
  metacarpophalangeal joint, L8630
  metatarsal joint, L8641
  neurostimulator pulse generator, L8679, L8681–L8688
  not otherwise specified, L8699
  ocular, L8610
  ossicular, L8613
  osteogenesis stimulator, E0749
  percutaneous access system, A4301
  removal, dental, D6100
  repair, dental, D6090
  replacement implantable intraspinal catheter, E0785
  sinuva, J7402
  synthetic, urinary, L8606
  urinary tract, L8603, L8606
  vascular graft, L8670
Implantable radiation dosimeter, A4650
Impregnated gauze dressing, A6222–A6230, *A6231–A6233*
Inclisiran, J1306
Incobotulinumtoxin a, J0588
Incontinence
  appliances and supplies, A4310, A4331, A4332, A4360, A5071–A5075, *A5081–A5093, A5102–A5114*
  garment, A4520, T4521–T4543
    adult sized disposable incontinence product, T4522–T4528
    any type, e.g. brief, diaper, A4520
    pediatric sized disposable incontinence product, T4529–T4532
    youth sized disposable incontinence product, T4533–T4534
  supply, A4335, A4356–A4360
    bedside drainage bag, A4357
    disposable external urethral clamp/compression device, A4360
    external urethral clamp or compression device, A4356
    incontinence supply, miscellaneous, A4335
    urinary drainage bag, leg or abdomen, A4358
  treatment system, E0740
Indium IN-111
  carpromab pendetide, A9507
  ibritumomab tiuxetan, A9542
  labeled autologous platelets, A9571
  labeled autologous white blood cells, A9570
  oxyquinoline, A9547
  pentetate, A9548
  pentetreotide, A9572
  satumomab, A4642
Index visit, M1196, M1204
Inebilizumab-cdon, J1823
Infliximab injection, J1745
Influenza
  afluria, Q2035
  agriflu, Q2034
  flulaval, Q2036
  fluvirin, Q2037
  fluzone, Q2038

◀ **New**   ↻ **Revised**   ✔ **Reinstated**   ~~deleted~~ **Deleted**

Influenza *(Continued)*
  immunization, documentation, G8482–G8484
  not otherwise specified, Q2039
  vaccine, administration, G0008
  virus vaccine, Q2034–Q2039
Infusion
  covid, M0249, M0250
  pump, ambulatory, with administrative
    equipment, E0781
  pump, continuous glucose sensing supplies for
    maintenance, A4226
  pump, heparin, dialysis, E1520
  pump, implantable, E0782, E0783
  pump, implantable, refill kit, A4220
  pump, insulin, E0784
  pump, mechanical, reusable, E0779, E0780
  pump, uninterrupted infusion of Epiprostenol, K0455
  replacement battery, A4602
  saline, J7030–J7060
  supplies, A4219, A4221, A4222, A4225, A4230–A4232,
    E0776–E0791
  therapy, other than chemotherapeutic drugs,
    Q0081, Q2054
Inhalation solution; (see also drug name),
  J7608–J7699, Q4074
Injection device, needle-free, *A4210*
Injections; (see also drug name), J0120–J2504,
  J0223, J0224, J0591, J0691, J0693, J0699, J0741,
  J0742, J0791, J0896, J1201, J1303, J1305, J1426,
  J1427, J1429, J1445, J1448, J1554, J1823,
  J1942–J1944, J2406, J2506, J2794, J2798, J3031,
  J3399, J7169, J7204, J7208, J7311, J7313, J7314,
  J7320, J7321, J7332, J9032, J9036, J9037,
  J9039, J9057, J9118, J9153, J9173, J9177, J9199,
  J9201, J9210, J9223, J9229, J9247, J9269, J9271,
  J9272, J9299, J9308, J9309, J9313, J9314, J9316,
  J9317, J9348, J9349, J9353, J9355, J9356, Q0244,
  Q0249, Q5112–Q5118, Q5122, Q5123, Q9950,
  Q9991, Q9992
  ado-trastuzumab emtansine, 1 mg, J9354
  aripiprazole, extended release, J0401
  arthrography, sacroiliac, joint, G0259, G0260
  carfilzomib, 1 mg, J9047
  certolizumab pegol, J0717
  dental service, D9610, D9630
    other drugs/medicaments, by report, D9630
    therapeutic parenteral drug, single
      administration, D9610
    therapeutic parenteral drugs, two or more
      administrations, different medications, D9612
  dermal filler (LDS), G0429
  filgrastim, J1442
  interferon beta-1a, IM, Q3027
  interferon beta-1a, SC, Q3028
  omacetaxine mepesuccinate, 0.01 mg, J9262
  pertuzumb, 1 mg, J9306
  sculptra, 0.5 mg, Q2028
  supplies for self-administered, A4211
  vincristine, 1 mg, J9371
  ziv-aflibercept, 1 mg, J9400

Injections *(Continued)*
Inlay/onlay dental restoration, *D2510–D2664*
INR, monitoring, *G0248–G0250*
  demonstration prior to initiation, home INR, G0248
  physician review and interpretation, home INR, G0250
  provision of test materials, home INR, G0249
Insertion tray, A4310–A4316
Instillation, hexaminolevulinate hydrochloride,
  A9589
Insulin, J1811–J1815, J1817, *S5550–S5571* ◀
  ambulatory, external, system, A9274
  treatment, outpatient, G9147
Integra flowable wound matrix, *Q4114*
Interferon
  Alpha, J9212–J9215
  Beta-1a, J1826, Q3027, Q3028
  Beta-1b, J1830
  Gamma, J9216
Intermittent
  assist device with continuous positive airway
    pressure device, E0470–E0472
  limb compression device, E0676
  peritoneal dialysis system, E1592
  positive pressure breathing machine (IPPB), E0500
Interphalangeal joint, prosthetic implant,
  L8658, L8659
Interscapular thoracic prosthesis
  endoskeletal, L6570
  upper limb, L6350–L6370
Intervention, alcohol/substance (not tobacco),
  G0396–G0397
Intervention, tobacco, *G9016*
Intraconazole, J1835
Intraocular
  lenses, V2630–V2632
Intraoral radiographs, dental, *D0210–D0240*
  intraoral-complete series, D0210
  intraoral-occlusal image, D0420
  intraoral-periapical-each additional image, D0230
  intraoral-periapical-first radiographic image, D0220
Intrapulmonary percussive ventilation system, E0481
Intrauterine copper contraceptive, J7300
Inversion/eversion correction device, A9285
Iodine I-123
  iobenguane, A9582
  ioflupane, A9584
  sodium iodide, A9509, A9516
Iodine I-125
  serum albumin, A9532
  sodium iodide, A9527
  sodium iothalamate, A9554
Iodine I-131
  iodinated serum albumin, A9524
  sodium iodide capsule, A9517, A9528
  sodium iodide solution, A9529–A9531
Iodine Iobenguane sulfate I-131, A9508
Iodine swabs/wipes, A4247
IPD
  system, E1592
Ipilimumab, J9228

◀ **New**   ↻ **Revised**   ✔ **Reinstated**   ~~deleted~~ **Deleted**

IPPB machine, E0500
Ipratropium bromide, inhalation solution, unit dose, J7644, J7645
Irinotecan, J9205, J9206
Iron
    Dextran, J1750
    sucrose, J1756
Irrigation solution for bladder calculi, Q2004
Irrigation supplies, A4320–A4322, A4355, A4397–A4400
    irrigation supply, sleeve, each, A4397
    irrigation syringe, bulb, or piston, each, A4320
    irrigation tubing set, bladder irrigation, A4355
    ostomy irrigation set, A4400
    ostomy irrigation supply, bag, A4398
    ostomy irrigation supply, cone/catheter, A4399
Irrigation/evacuation system, bowel
    control unit, E0350
    disposable supplies for, E0352
    manual pump enema, A4459
    tubing, K1013
Isatuximab-irfc, J9227
Isavuconazonium, J1833
Islet, transplant, *G0341–G0343, S2102*
Isoetharine HCl, inhalation solution
    concentrated, J7647, J7648
    unit dose, J7649, J7650
Isolates, B4150, B4152
Isoproterenol HCl, inhalation solution
    concentrated, J7657, J7658
    unit dose, J7659, J7660
Isosulfan blue, Q9968
Item, non-covered, A9270
IUD, *J7300, S4989*
IV pole, each, E0776, K0105
Ixabepilone, J9207

J

Jacket
    scoliosis, L1300, L1310
Jaw, motion, rehabilitation system, *E1700–E1702*
Jemperli, J9272
Jenamicin, J1580
Jetria, (ocriplasmin), *J7316*

K

Kadcyla, ado-trastuzumab emtansine, 1 mg, *J9354*
Kanamycin sulfate, J1840, J1850
Kartop patient lift, toilet or bathroom; (see also Lift), E0625
Keramatrix or kerasorb, J4165
Ketorolac thomethamine, J1885
Kidney
    diagnosis of CKD stage 5, M1188
    ESRD supply, A4650–A4927
    machine, E1500–E1699
    machine, accessories, E1500–E1699

Kidney (*Continued*)
    system, E1510
    wearable artificial, E1632
Kits
    enteral feeding supply (syringe) (pump) (gravity), B4034–B4036
    fistula cannulation (set), A4730
    parenteral nutrition, B4220–B4224
        administration kit, per day, B4224
        supply kit, home mix, per day, B4222
        supply kit, premix, per day, B4220
    surgical dressing (tray), A4550
    tracheostomy, A4625
Knee
    arthroscopy, surgical, G0289, S2112, S2300
        knee, surgical, harvesting cartilage, S2112
        knee, surgical, removal loose body, chondroplasty, different compartment, G0289
        shoulder, surgical, thermally-induced, capsulorraphy, S2300
    disarticulation, prosthesis, L5150, L5160
    joint, miniature, L5826
    orthosis (KO), E1810, L1800–L1885, K1014
        dynamic adjustable elbow entension/flexion device, E1800
        dynamic adjustable knee extension/flexion device, E1810
        static-progressive devices, E1801, E1806, E1811, E1816–E1818, E1831, E1841
Knee-ankle-foot device with microprocessor control, L2006
Knee-ankle-foot orthosis (KAFO), K1007, L2000–L2039, L2126–L2136
    addition, high strength, lightweight material, L2755
    base procedure, used with any knee joint, double upright, double bar, L2020
    base procedure, used with any knee joint, full plastic double upright, L2036
    base procedure, used with any knee joint, single upright, single bar, L2000
    foot orthosis, double upright, double bar, without knee joint, L2030
    foot orthosis, single upright, single bar, without knee joint, L2010
Kovaltry, J7211
Kyphosis pad, L1020, L1025

L

Labetalol hydrochloride, J1920, J1921 ◀
Laboratory
    dental, D0415–D0999
        adjunctive pre-diagnostic tests, mucosal abnormalities, D0431
        analysis saliva sample, D0418
        caries risk assessment, low, D0601
        caries risk assessment, moderate, D0602
        caries susceptibility tests, D0425

◀ **New**   ⏎ **Revised**   ✔ **Reinstated**   ~~deleted~~ **Deleted**

Laboratory (Continued)
  dental (Continued)
    collection and preparation, saliva sample, D0417
    collection of microorganisms for culture and sensitivity, D0415
    diagnostic casts, D0470
    oral pathology laboratory, D0472–D0502
    processing, D0414
    pulp vitality tests, D0460
  services, P0000–P9999
  viral culture, D0416

Laboratory tests
  chemistry, P2028–P2038
    cephalin flocculation, blood, P2028
    congo red, blood, P2029
    hair analysis, excluding arsenic, P2031
    mucoprotein, blood, P2038
    thymol turbidity, blood, P2033
  microbiology, P7001
  miscellaneous, P9010–P9615, Q0111–Q0115
    blood, split unit, P9011
    blood, whole, transfusion, unit, P9010
    catheterization, collection specimen, multiple patients, P9615
    catheterization, collection specimen, single patient, P9612
    cryoprecipitate, each unit, P9012
    fern test, Q0114
    fresh frozen plasma, donor retested, each unit, P9060
    fresh frozen plasma (single donor), frozen within 8 hours, P9017
    fresh frozen plasma, within 8–24 hours of collection, each unit, P9059
    granulocytes, pheresis, each unit, P9050
    infusion, albumin (human), 25%, 20 ml, P9046
    infusion, albumin (human), 25%, 50 ml, P9047
    infusion, albumin (human), 5%, 250 ml, P9045
    infusion, albumin (human), 5%, 50 ml, P9041
    infusion, plasma protein fraction, human, 5%, 250 ml, P9048
    infusion, plasma protein fraction, human, 5%, 50 ml, P9043
    KOH preparation, Q0112
    pinworm examinations, Q0113
    plasma, cryoprecipitate reduced, each unit, P9044
    plasma, pooled, multiple donor, frozen, P9023
    platelet rich plasma, each unit, P9020
    platelets, each unit, P9019
    platelets, HLA-matched leukocytes reduced, apheresis/pheresis, each unit, P9052
    platelets, irradiated, each unit, P9032
    platelets, leukocytes reduced, CMV-neg, aphresis/pheresis, each unit, P9055
    platelets, leukocytes reduced, each unit, P9031
    platelets, leukocytes reduced, irradiated, each unit, P9033
    platelets, pheresis, each unit, P9034
    platelets, pheresis, irradiated, each unit, P9036

Laboratory tests (Continued)
  miscellaneous (Continued)
    platelets, pheresis, leukocytes reduced, CMV-neg, irradiated, each unit, P9053
    platelets, pheresis, leukocytes reduced, each unit, P9035
    platelets, pheresis, leukocytes reduced, irradiated, each unit, P9037
    post-coital, direct qualitative, vaginal or cervical mucous, Q0115
    red blood cells, deglycerolized, each unit, P9039
    red blood cells, each unit, P9021
    red blood cells, frozen/deglycerolized/washed, leukocytes reduced, irradiated, each unit, P9057
    red blood cells, irradiated, each unit, P9038
    red blood cells, leukocytes reduced, CMV-neg, irradiated, each unit, P9058
    red blood cells, leukocytes reduced, each unit, P9016
    red blood cells, leukocytes reduced, irradiated, each unit, P9040
    red blood cells, washed, each unit, P9022
    travel allowance, one way, specimen collection, home/nursing home, P9603, P9604
    wet mounts, vaginal, cervical, or skin, Q0111
    whole blood, leukocytes reduced, irradiated, each unit, P9056
    whole blood or red blood cells, leukocytes reduced, CMV-neg, each unit, P9051
    whole blood or red blood cells, leukocytes reduced, frozen, deglycerol, washed, each unit, P9054
  toxicology, P3000–P3001, Q0091

Lacrimal duct, implant
  permanent, A4263
  temporary, A4262
Lactated Ringer's infusion, J7120
Laetrile, J3570
Lanadelumab-flyo, J0593
Lancet, A4258, A4259
Language, screening, V5363
Lanreotide, J1930, J1932
Laronidase, J1931
Larynx, artificial, L8500
Laser blood collection device and accessory, A4257, E0620
LASIK, S0800
Lead investigation, T1029
Lead wires, per pair, A4557
Lecanemab-irmb, J0174 ◀
Leg
  bag, A4358, A5105, A5112
    leg or abdomen, vinyl, with/without tubes, straps, each, A4358
    urinary drainage bag, leg bag, leg/abdomen, latex, with/without tube, straps, A5112
    urinary suspensory, leg bag, with/without tube, each, A5105

Leg (*Continued*)
  bag (*Continued*)
  extensions for walker, E0158
  rest, elevating, K0195
  rest, wheelchair, E0990
  strap, replacement, A5113–A5114
Legg Perthes orthosis, L1700–L1755
  Newington type, L1710
  Patten bottom type, L1755
  Scottish Rite type, L1730
  Tachdjian type, L1720
  Toronto type, L1700
Lenacapavir, J1961 ◄
Lens
  aniseikonic, V2118, V2318
  contact, V2500–V2599
    gas permeable, V2510–V2513
    hydrophilic, V2520–V2523
    other type, V2599
    PMMA, V2500–V2503
    scleral, gas, V2530–V2531
  eye, V2100–V2615, V2700–V2799
    bifocal, glass or plastic, V2200–V2299
    contact lenses, V2500–V2599
    low vision aids, V2600–V2615
    miscellaneous, V2700–V2799
    single vision, glass or plastic, V2100–V2199
    trifocal, glass or plastic, V2300–V2399
    variable asphericity, V2410–V2499
  intraocular, V2630–V2632
    anterior chamber, V2630
    iris supported, V2631
    new technology, category 4, IOL, Q1004
    new technology, category 5, IOL, Q1005
    posterior chamber, V2632
    telescopic lens, C1840
  low vision, V2600–V2615
    hand held vision aids, V2600
    single lens spectacle mounted, V2610
    telescopic and other compound lens system, V2615
  progressive, V2781
Lepirudin, J1945
Lesion, destruction, choroid, *G0186*
Leucovorin calcium, J0640
Leukocyte poor blood, each unit, P9016
Leuprolide acetate, J1950, J1951, J1954, J9217, J9219 ◄
Leuprolide injectable, camcevi, J1952
Levalbuterol, all formulations, inhalation solution
  concentrated, J7607, J7612
  unit dose, J7614, J7615
Levetiracetam, J1953
Levocarnitine, J1955
Levofloxacin, J1956
Levoleucovorin injection, J0641
Levoleucovorin injection (khapzory), J0642
Levonorgestrel, (contraceptive), implants and supplies, J7306
Levorphanol tartrate, J1960

Lexidronam, A9604
Lidocaine HCl, J2001
Lift
  patient (includes seat lift), E0621–E0635
    bathroom or toilet, E0625
    mechanism incorporated into a combination lift-chair, E0627
    patient lift, electric, E0635
    patient lift, hydraulic or mechanical, E0630
    separate seat lift mechanism, patient owned furniture, non-electric, E0629
    sling or seat, canvas or nylon, E0621
  shoe, L3300–L3334
    lift, elevation, heel, L3334
    lift, elevation, heel and sole, cork, L3320
    lift, elevation, heel and sole, Neoprene, L3310
    lift, elevation, heel, tapered to metatarsals, L3300
    lift, elevation, inside shoe, L3332
    lift, elevation, metal extension, L3330
Lightweight, wheelchair, *E1087–E1090, E1240–E1270*
  detachable arms, swing away detachable, elevating leg rests, E1240
  detachable arms, swing away detachable footrest, E1260
  fixed full length arms, swing away detachable elevating legrests, E1270
  fixed full length arms, swing away detachable footrest, E1250
  high strength, detachable arms desk, E1088
  high strength, detachable arms desk or full length, E1090
  high strength, fixed full length arms, E1087
  high strength, fixed length arms swing away footrest, E1089
Lincomycin HCl, J2010
Linezolid, J2020, J2021
Liquid barrier, ostomy, A4363
Listening devices, assistive, *V5281–V5290*
  personal Bluetooth FM/DM, V5286
  personal FM/DM adapter/boot coupling device for receiver, V5289
  personal FM/DM binaural, 2 receivers, V5282
  personal FM/DM, direct audio input, V5285
  personal FM/DM, ear level receiver, V5284
  personal FM/DM monaural, 1 receiver, V5281
  personal FM/DM neck, loop induction receiver, V5283
  personal FM/DM transmitter assistive listening device, V5288
  transmitter microphone, V5290
Lodging, recipient, escort nonemergency transport, A0180, A0200
LOPS, *G0245–G0247*
  follow-up evaluation and management, G0246
  initial evaluation and management, G0245
  routine foot care, G0247
Lorazepam, J2060
Loss of protective sensation, *G0245–G0247*
Low osmolar contrast material, Q9965–Q9967
Loxapine, for inhalation, J2062
LSO, L0621–L0640
Lubricant, A4332, A4402
Lumbar flexion, L0540

◄ **New**   ⊋ **Revised**   ✔ **Reinstated**   ~~deleted~~ **Deleted**

Lumbar-sacral orthosis (LSO), L0621–L0640
Lutetium, A9607
LVRS, services, G0302–G0305
Lymphocyte immune globulin, J7504, J7511

M

Machine
   IPPB, E0500
   kidney, E1500–E1699
Magnesium sulphate, J3475
Maintenance contract, ESRD, A4890
Mammography, screening, G9899, G9900
Mannitol, J2150, J7665
Marker, tissue, A4648
Mask
   aerosol, K0180
   oxygen, A4620
Mastectomy
   bra, L8000
   form, L8020
   prosthesis, L8030, L8600
   sleeve, L8010
Matristem, Q4118
   micromatrix, 1 mg, Q4118
Mattress
   air pressure, E0186
   alternating pressure, E0277
   dry pressure, E0184
   gel pressure, E0196
   hospital bed, E0271, E0272
   non-powered, pressure reducing, E0373
   overlay, E0371–E0372
   powered, pressure reducing, E0277
   water pressure, E0187
Measurement period
   ace inhibior, M1200, M1203
   anaphylaxis, M1155
   bone marrow transplant, M1157
   chemotherapy, M1156
   dementia, M1164
   herpes zoster, M1174, M1176
   hospice services, M1159, M1165, M1167, M1191
   immunocompromising condition (history of), M1158
   influenza vaccine, M1168, M1170
   left ventricular function testing, G8682
   pneumococcal conjugate, M1179
   td or tdap vaccine, M1171, M1173
Mecasermin, J2170
Mechlorethamine HCl, J9230
Medicaid, codes, T1000–T9999
Medical and surgical supplies, A4206–A8999
Medical nutritional therapy, G0270, G0271
Medical services, other, M0000–M9999
Medications, high-risk, M1209–M1210
Medroxyprogesterone acetate, J1050
Meloxicam, J1738
Melphalan flufenamide J9247
Melphalan NOS, J9245, J9246
Melphalan oral, J8600
Membrane graft/wrap, Q4205

Mental, health, training services, C7900–C7902, G0177
Meperidine, J2175
   and promethazine, J2180
Mepivacaine HCl, J0670
Mepolizumab, J2182
Meropenem, J2184, J2185
Mesna, J9209
Metacarpophalangeal joint, prosthetic implant, L8630, L8631
Metaproterenol sulfate, inhalation solution
   concentrated, J7667, J7668
   unit dose, J7669, J7670
Metaraminol bitartrate, J0380
Metatarsal joint, prosthetic implant, L8641
Meter, bath conductivity, dialysis, E1550
Methacholine chloride, J7674
Methadone HCl, J1230
Methergine, J2210
Methocarbamol, J2800
Methotrexate
   oral, J8610
   sodium, J9250, J9260
Methyldopate HCl, J0210
Methylene blue, Q9968
Methylnaltrexone, J2212
Methylprednisolone
   acetate, J1020–J1040
      injection, 20 mg, J1020
      injection, 40 mg, J1030
      injection, 80 mg, J1040
   oral, J7509
   sodium succinate, J2920, J2930
Metoclopramide HCl, J2765
Metronidazole, J1836 ◀
Micafungin sodium, J2247, J2248
Microbiology test, P7001
Midazolam HCl, J2250, J2251
Mileage
   ALS, A0390
   ambulance, A0380, A0390
Milrinone lactate, J2260
Mini-bus, nonemergency transportation, A0120
Minocycline hydrochloride, J2265
Mirvetuximab soravtansine-gynx, J9063 ◀
Miscellaneous and investigational, A9000–A9999
Mitomycin, J7315, J9280, J9281
Mitoxantrone HCl, J9293
MNT, G0270, G0271
Mobility device, physician, service, G0372
Modalities, with office visit, M0005–M0008
Mogamulizumab injection-kpkc, J9201
Moisture exchanger for use with invasive mechanical ventilation, A4483
Moisturizer, skin, A6250
Molecular diagnostic test reader, K1035 ◀
Molecular pathology procedure, G0452
Monitor
   blood glucose, home, E0607
   blood pressure, A4670
   pacemaker, E0610, E0615
Monitoring feature/device, A9279

◀ New   ↻ Revised   ✔ Reinstated   ~~deleted~~ Deleted

Monitoring, INR, G0248–G0250
  demonstration prior to initiation, G0248
  physician review and interpretation, G0250
  provision of test materials, G0249
Monoclonal antibodies, J7505
Morphine sulfate, J2270, J2272
  epidural or intrathecal use, J2274
Mosunetuzumab-axgb, J9350 ◄
Motion, jaw, rehabilitation system, E1700–E1702
  motion rehabilitation system, E1700
  replacement cushions, E1701
  replacement measuring scales, E1702
Mouthpiece (for respiratory equipment), A4617
Moxetumomab pasudotox-tdfx, J9313
Moxifloxacin, J2280, J2281
Mucoprotein, blood, P2038
Multiaxial ankle, L5986
Multidisciplinary services, H2000–H2001, T1023–T1028
Multiple post collar, cervical, L0180–L0200
  occipital/mandibular supports, adjustable, L0180
  occipital/mandibular supports, adjustable cervical bars, L0200
  SQMI, Guilford, Taylor types, L0190
Multi-Podus type AFO, L4396
Muromonab-CD3, J7505
Mycophenolate mofetil, J7517, J7519 ◄
Mycophenolic acid, J7518
MyOwn skin, Q4226

N

Nabilone, J8650
Nadofaragene firadenovec-vncg, J9029 ◄
Nails, trimming, dystrophic, G0127
Nalbuphine HCl, J2300
Naloxone HCl, J2310, J2311
Naltrexone, J2315
Nandrolone
  decanoate, J2320
Narrowing device, wheelchair, E0969
Nasal
  application device, K0183
  pillows/seals (for nasal application device), K0184
  vaccine inhalation, J3530
Nasogastric tubing, B4081, B4082
Natalizumab, J2323
Nebulizer, E0570–E0585
  aerosol compressor, E0571, *E0572*
  aerosol mask, A7015
  corrugated tubing, disposable, A7010
  filter, disposable, A7013
  filter, non-disposable, A7014
  heater, E1372
  large volume, disposable, prefilled, A7008
  large volume, disposable, unfilled, A7007
  not used with oxygen, durable, glass, A7017
  pneumatic, administration set, A7003, A7005, A7006
  pneumatic, nonfiltered, A7004

Nebulizer (Continued)
  portable, E0570
  small volume, A7003–A7005
  ultrasonic, E0575
  ultrasonic, dome and mouthpiece, A7016
  ultrasonic, reservoir bottle, non-disposable, A7009
  water collection device, large volume nebulizer, A7012
Necitumumab, J9295
Needle, A4215
  bone marrow biopsy, C1830
  non-coring, A4212
  with syringe, A4206–A4209
Negative pressure wound therapy pump, E2402
  accessories, A6550
Nelarabine, J9261
Neonatal transport, ambulance, base rate, A0225
Neostigmine methylsulfate, J2710
Neotrim, Q4265–Q4267 ◄
Nerve, conduction, sensory, test, G0255
Nerve stimulator with batteries, E0765
Nesiritide injection, J2324, *J2325*
Neupogen, injection, filgrastim, 1 mcg, J1442
Neuromuscular stimulator, A4560, E0745 ◄
Neurophysiology, intraoperative, monitoring, G0453
Neurostimulator
  battery recharging system, L8695
  external antenna, L8696
  implantable pulse generator, L8679
  pulse generator, L8681–L8688
    dual array, non-rechargeable, with extension, L8688
    dual array, rechargeable, with extension, L8687
    patient programmer (external), replacement only, L8681
    radiofrequency receiver, L8682
    radiofrequency transmitter (external), sacral root receiver, bowel and bladder management, L8684
    radiofrequency transmitter (external), with implantable receiver, L8683
    single array, rechargeable, with extension, L8686
Nipple prosthesis, custom fabricated, reusable, L8033
Nipple prosthesis, prefabricated, reusable, L8032
Nitrogen N-13 ammonia, A9526
Nivol relatlimab, J9298
NMES, E0720–E0749
Nonchemotherapy drug, oral, NOS, J8499
Noncovered services, A9270
Nonemergency transportation, A0080–A0210
Nonimpregnated gauze dressing, A6216–A6221, A6402–A6404
Nonprescription drug, A9150
Not otherwise classified drug, J3490, J7599, J7699, J7799, J8499, J8999, J9999, Q0181
Novafix, Q4208
NPH, J1820
NPWT, pump, E2402

◄ **New**   ⊃ **Revised**   ✔ **Reinstated**   ~~deleted~~ **Deleted**

NTIOL category 3, Q1003
NTIOL category 4, Q1004
NTIOL category 5, Q1005
Nursing care, T1030–T1031
Nursing service, direct, skilled, outpatient, G0128
Nusinersen, J2326
Nutrition
    counseling, dental, *D1310, D1320*
    enteral infusion pump, B9002
    parenteral infusion pump, B9004, B9006
    parenteral solution, B4164–B5200
    therapy, medical, G0270, G0271

O

O & P supply/accessory/service, L9900
Observation
    admission, *G0379*
    hospital, *G0378*
Obturator prosthesis
    definitive, *D5932*
    interim, *D5936*
    surgical, *D5931*
Occipital/mandibular support, cervical, L0160
Occlusive device, placement, G0269
Occupational, therapy, G0129, S9129
Ocrelizumab, J2350
Ocriplasmin, J7316
Octafluoropropane, Q9956
Octagam, J1568
Octreotide acetate, J2353, J2354
Ocular prosthetic implant, L8610
Ofatumumab, J9302
Olanzapine, J2358–J2359 ◀
Olaratumab, J9285
Oliceridine, C9101
Olipudase alfa-rpcp, J0218 ◀
Omacetaxine Mepesuccinate, J9262
Omadacycline, J0121
Omalizumab, J2357
Omegaven, B4187
OnabotulinumtoxinA, J0585
Oncology
    disease status, *G9063–G9139*
    practice guidelines, *G9056–G9062*
    visit, *G9050–G9055*
Ondansetron HCl, J2405
Ondansetron oral, Q0162
One arm, drive attachment, K0101
Ophthalmological examination, refraction, S0621
Oprelvekin, J2355
Oral and maxillofacial surgery, D7111–D7999
    alveoloplasty, *D7310–D7321*
    complicated suturing, *D7911–D7912*
    excision of bone tissue, *D7471–D7490*
    extractions, local, *D7111–D7140*
    other repair procedures, *D7920–D7999*
    other surgical procedures, *D7260–D7295*

Oral and maxillofacial surgery (Continued)
    reduction of dislocation/TMJ dysfunction, *D7810–D7899*
    repair of traumatic wounds, *D7910*
    surgical excision, intra-osseous lesions, *D7440–D7465*
    surgical excision, soft tissue lesions, *D7410–D7415*
    surgical extractions, *D7210–D7251*
    surgical incision, *D7510–D7560*
    treatment of fractures, compound, *D7710–D7780*
    treatment of fractures, simple, *D7610–D7680*
    vestibuloplasty, *D7340–D7350*
Oral device/appliance, E0485–E0486, E0490–E0491, K1028, K1029 ◀
Oral interface, A7047
Oral mucoadhesive, A9156 ◀
Oral, NOS, drug, J8499
Oral/nasal mask, A7027
    nasal pillows, A7029
    oral cushion, A7028
Oritavancin, J2406, J2407
Oropharyngeal suction catheter, A4628
Orphenadrine, J2360
Orthodontics, D8000–D8999
Orthopedic shoes
    arch support, L3040–L3100
    footwear, *L3000–L3649*, L3201–L3265
    insert, L3000–L3030
    lift, L3300–L3334
    miscellaneous additions, L3500–L3595
    positioning device, K1015, L3140–L3170
    transfer, L3600–L3649
    wedge, L3340–L3420
Orthotic additions
    carbon graphite lamination, L2755
    fracture, L2180–L2192, L3995
    halo, L0860
    lower extremity, L2200–L2999, L4320
    ratchet lock, L2430
    scoliosis, L1010–L1120, L1210–L1290
    shoe, L3300–L3595, L3649
    spinal, L0970–L0984
    upper limb, L3810–L3890, *L3900, L3901,* L3970–L3974, *L3975–L3978,* L3995
Orthotic devices
    ankle-foot (AFO); (see also Orthopedic shoes), E1815, E1816, E1830, L1900–L1990, L2102–L2116, L3160, L4361, *L4397*
    anterior-posterior-lateral, L0700, L0710
    cervical, L0100–L0200
    cervical-thoracic-lumbar-sacral (CTLSO), L0700, L0710
    elbow (EO), E1800, E1801, L3700–L3740, L3760–L3761, *L3762*
    fracture, L2102–L2136, L3980–L3986
    halo, L0810–L0830
    hand, (WHFO), E1805, E1825, L3807, L3900–L3954, *L3956*
    hand, finger, prefabricated, L3923

Orthotic devices (Continued)
　hip (HO), L1600–L1690
　hip-knee-ankle-foot (HKAFO), L2040–L2090
　interface material, E1820
　knee (KO), E1810, E1811, L1800–L1885
　knee-ankle-foot (KAFO); (see also Orthopedic
　　shoes), L2000–L2038, L2126–L2136
　Legg Perthes, L1700–L1755
　lumbar, L0625–L0651
　multiple post collar, L0180–L0200
　not otherwise specified, L0999, L1499, L2999,
　　L3999, L5999, L7499, L8039, L8239
　pneumatic splint, L4350–L4380
　pronation/supination, E1818
　repair or replacement, L4000–L4210
　replace soft interface material, L4390–L4394
　sacroiliac, L0600–L0620, *L0621–L0624*
　scoliosis, L1000–L1499
　shoe, (see Orthopedic shoes)
　shoulder (SO), L1840, L3650, L3674, *L3678*
　shoulder-elbow-wrist-hand (SEWHO), L3960–L3978
　side bar disconnect, L2768
　spinal, cervical, L0100–L0200
　spinal, DME, K0112–K0116
　thoracic, L0210, *L0220*
　thoracic-hip-knee-ankle (THKO), L1500–L1520
　toe, E1830
　wrist-hand-finger (WHFO), E1805, E1806, E1825,
　　L3806–L3809, L3900–L3954, *L3956*
Orthovisc, J7324
Ossicula prosthetic implant, L8613
Osteogenesis stimulator, E0747–E0749, E0760
Osteotomy, segmented or subapical, *D7944*
Ostomy
　accessories, A5093
　belt, A4396
　pouches, A4416–A4435, *A5056, A5057*
　skin barrier, A4401–A4449, *A4462*
　supplies, A4361–A4421, A5051–A5149, *A5200*
Otto Bock, prosthesis, *L7007*
Outpatient payment system, hospital, *C1000–C9999*
Overdoor, traction, *E0860*
Oxacillin sodium, J2700
Oxaliplatin, J9263
Oxygen
　ambulance, A0422
　battery charger, E1357
　battery pack/cartridge, E1356
　catheter, transtracheal, A7018
　chamber, hyperbaric, topical, A4575
　concentrator, E1390–E1391
　DC power adapter, E1358
　delivery system (topical), E0446
　equipment, E0424–E0486, E1353–E1406
　Liquid oxygen system, E0433
　mask, A4620
　medication supplies, A4611–A4627
　rack/stand, E1355

Oxygen (Continued)
　regulator, E1352, E1353
　respiratory equipment/supplies, E0424–E0480,
　　A4611–A4627, *E0481*
　supplies and equipment, E0425–E0444, E0455
　tent, E0455
　tubing, A4616
　water vapor enriching system, E1405, E1406
　wheeled cart, E1354
Oxymorphone HCl, J2410
Oxytetracycline HCl, J2460
Oxytocin, J2590

P

Pacemaker monitor, E0610, E0615
Pacemaker permanent insertion, C7537–C7578
Pacemaker removal, C7540
Paclitaxel, J9267
Paclitaxel protein-bound particles, J9264
Pad
　correction, CTLSO, L1020–L1060
　gel pressure, E0185, E0196
　heat, A9273, E0210, E0215, E0217, E0238, E0249
　　electric heat pad, moist, E0215
　　electric heat pad, standard, E0210
　　*hot water bottle, ice cap or collar, heat and/or cold
　　　wrap, A9273*
　　*pad for water circulating heat unit, replacement
　　　only, E0249*
　　water circulating heat pad with pump, E0217
　orthotic device interface, E1820
　sheepskin, E0188, E0189
　water circulating cold with pump, E0218
　water circulating heat unit, E0249
　water circulating heat with pump, E0217
Pafolacianine, A9603 ◄
Pail, for use with commode chair, E0167
Pain assessment, *G8730–G8732*
Pain management, chronic, G3002–G3003
**Pain measured by the Visual Analog Scale (VAS)
　or Numeric Pain Scale,** G2136–G2141,
　　G2146–G2147 ◄
Palate, prosthetic implant, L8618
Palifermin, J2425
Paliperidone palmitate, J2426–J2427 ◄
Palonosetron, J2469, J8655
Pamidronate disodium, J2430
Pan, for use with commode chair, E0167
Panitumumab, J9303
Papanicolaou screening smear (Pap), P3000,
　　P3001, Q0091
　cervical or vaginal, up to 3 smears, by technician, P3000
　*cervical or vaginal, up to 3 smears, physician
　　interpretation, P3001*
　obtaining, preparing and conveyance, Q0091
Papaverine HCl, J2440

◄ **New**　⤶ **Revised**　✔ **Reinstated**　~~deleted~~ **Deleted**

Paraffin, A4265
 bath unit, E0235
Parenteral nutrition
 administration kit, B4224
 not otherwise specified, B4185
 pump, B9004, B9006
 solution, B4164, B4184, B4186
  compounded amino acid and carbohydrates, with
   electrolytes, B4189–B4199, B5000–B5200
  nutrition additives, homemix, B4216
  nutrition administration kit, B4224
  nutrition solution, amino acid, B4168–B4178
  nutrition solution, carbohydrates, B4164, B4180
  nutrition solution, per 10 grams, liquid, B4185
  nutrition supply kit, homemix, B4222
 supply kit, B4220, B4222
Paricalcitol, J2501
Parking fee, nonemergency transport, A0170
Partial Hospitalization, OT, G0129
Pasireotide long acting, J2502
Paste, conductive, A4558
Pathology and laboratory tests, miscellaneous,
 P9010–P9615
Pathology, surgical, G0416, M1193, M1195
Patient support system, E0636, M1207–M1208
Patient transfer system, E1035–E1036
Patisiran injection, J0222
Pediculosis (lice) treatment, A9180
PEFR, peak expiratory flow rate meter, A4614
Pegademase bovine, J2504
Pegaptanib, J2503
Pegaspargase, J9266
Pegcetacoplan, intravitreal, J2781 ◄
Pegfilgrastim, J2505, Q5111, Q5122, Q5127, Q5130 ◄
Peginesatide, J0890
Pegloticase, J2507
Pelvic
 belt/harness/boot, E0944
 traction, E0890, E0900, E0947
Pemetrexed, J9294, J9296–J9297, J9304–J9305,
 J9322-J9323 ◄
Penicillin
 G benzathine/G benzathine and penicillin G
  procaine, J0558, J0561
 G potassium, J2540
 G procaine, aqueous, J2510
Pentamidine isethionate, J2545, J7676
Pentastarch, 10% solution, J2513
Pentazocine HCl, J3070
Pentobarbital sodium, J2515
Pentostatin, J9268
Peramivir, J2547
Percussor, E0480
Percutaneous
 biliary drainage catheter, C7545
 breast biopsies, C7501–C7502
 vertebral augmentations, C7507–C7508
 vertebroplasties, C7504–C7505
Percutaneous access system, A4301

Perflexane lipid microspheres, Q9955
Perflutren lipid microspheres, Q9957
Periapical service, D3410–D3470
 apicoectomy, bicuspid, first root, D3421
 apicoectomy, each additional root, D3426
 apicoectomy, molar, first root, D3425
 apicoectomy/periradicular surgery-anterior, D3410
 biological materials, aid soft and osseous tissue
  regeneration/periradicular surgery, D3431
 bone graft, per tooth, periradicular surgery, D3429
 endodonic endosseous implant, D3460
 guided tissue regeneration/periradicular surgery, D3432
 intentional replantation, D3470
 periradicular surgery without apicoectomy, D3427
 retrograde filling, per root, D3430
 root amputation, D3450
Periodontal procedures, D4000–D4999
Periodontics, dental, D4000–D4999
Peroneal strap, L0980
Peroxide, A4244
Perphenazine, J3310
Personal care services, T1019–T1021
 home health aide or CAN, per visit, T1021
 per diem, T1020
 provided by home health aide or CAN, per
  15 minutes, T1019
Pertuzumab, J9306, J9316
Pessary, A4561, A4562
PET, G0219, G0235, G0252
Pharmacologic therapy, G8633
Pharmacy, fee, G0333
Phenobarbital sodium, J2560–J2561 ◄
Phentolamine mesylate, J2760
~~Phenylephrine HCl, J2370~~
Phenylephrine hydrochloride, J2371–J2372 ◄
Phenylephrine/ketorolac ophthalmic solution, J1097
Phenytoin sodium, J1165
Phisohex solution, A4246
Photofrin, (see Porfimer sodium)
Photorefraction keratectomy, (PRK), S0810
Phototherapeutic keratectomy, (PTK), S0812
Phototherapy light, E0202
Phytonadione, J3430
Pillow, cervical, E0943
Pin retention (per tooth), D2951
Pinworm examination, Q0113
Plasma
 multiple donor, pooled, frozen, P9023, P9070
 single donor, fresh frozen, P9017, P9071
Plasminogen, J2998
Plastazote, L3002, L3252, L3253, L3265,
 L5654–L5658
 addition to lower extremity socket insert, L5654
 addition to lower extremity socket insert, above
  knee, L5658
 addition to lower extremity socket insert, below
  knee, L5655
 addition to lower extremity socket insert, knee
  disarticulation, L5656

◄ **New**   ↄ **Revised**   ✔ **Reinstated**   ~~deleted~~ **Deleted**

Plastazote *(Continued)*
 foot insert, removable, plastazote, L3002
 foot, molded shoe, custom fitted, plastazote, L3253
 foot, shoe molded to patient model, plastazote, L3252
 plastazote sandal, L3265
Platelet, P9073, P9100
 concentrate, each unit, P9019
 rich plasma, each unit, P9020
Platelets, *P9031–P9037, P9052–P9053, P9055*
Platform attachment
 forearm crutch, E0153
 walker, E0154
Plazomicin injection, J0291
Plerixafor, J2562
Plicamycin, J9270
Plumbing, for home ESRD equipment, A4870
Pneumatic
 appliance, E0655–E0673, L4350–L4380
 compressor, E0650–E0652
 splint, L4350–L4380
 ventricular assist device, Q0477, Q0480–Q0505
Pneumatic nebulizer
 administration set, small volume, filtered, A7006
 administration set, small volume, nonfiltered, A7003
 administration set, small volume, nonfiltered, nondisposable, A7005
 small volume, disposable, A7004
Pneumococcal
 vaccine, administration, G0009
Polatuzumab vedotin-piiq, J9309
Pontics, *D6210–D6252*
Porfimer sodium, J9600
Portable
 equipment transfer, R0070–R0076
 gaseous oxygen, K0741, K0742
 hemodialyzer system, E1635
 liquid oxygen system, E0433
 x-ray equipment, Q0092
Positioning seat, T5001
Positive airway pressure device, accessories, A7030–A7039, E0561–E0562
Positive expiratory pressure device, E0484
Post-coital examination, Q0115
Postural drainage board, E0606
Potassium
 chloride, J3480
 hydroxide preparation(KOH), Q0112
Pouch
 fecal collection, A4330
 ostomy, A4375–A4378, A5051–A5054, A5061–A5065
 urinary, A4379–A4383, A5071–A5075
Practice, guidelines, oncology, *G9056–G9062*
Pralatrexate, J9307
Pralidoxime chloride, J2730
Prednisolone
 acetate, J2650
 oral, J7510

Prednisone, J7512
Prefabricated crown, *D2930–D2933*
Preparation kits, dialysis, A4914
Preparatory prosthesis, L5510–L5595
 chemotherapy, J8999
 nonchemotherapy, J8499
Prescription digital behavioral therapy, A9291–A9292 ◀
Pressure
 alarm, dialysis, E1540
 pad, A4640, E0180–E0199
 ~~Pressure sensor system, C1834~~
Preventive dental procedures, *D1000–D1999*
Privigen, J1459
Procainamide HCl, J2690
Procedure
 HALO, L0810–L0861
 noncovered, G0293, G0294
 scoliosis, L1000–L1499
Prochlorperazine, J0780
Progenamatrix, Q4222
Programmer/Programable, A9268–A9269 ◀
Prolonged Service
 home or residence, G0318
 hospital inpatient/observation, G0316
 nursing facility, G0317
Prolotherapy, M0076
Promazine HCl, J2950
Promethazine
 and meperdine, J2180
 HCl, J2550
Propranolol HCl, J1800
Prostate, cancer, screening, *G0102, G0103*
Prosthesis
 artificial larynx battery/accessory, L8505
 auricular, D5914
 breast, L8000–L8035, L8600
 dental, D5911–D5960, D5999
 eye, L8610, L8611, V2623–V2629
 fitting, L5400–L5460, L6380–L6388
 foot/ankle one piece system, L5979
 hand, L6000–L6020, L6026
 implants, L8600–L8690
 larynx, L8500
 lower extremity, L5700–L5999, L8640–L8642
 mandible, L8617
 maxilla, L8616
 maxillofacial, provided by a non-physician, L8040–L8048
 miscellaneous service, L8499
 obturator, D5931–D5933, D5936
 ocular, V2623–V2629
 repair of, L7520, L8049
 socks (shrinker, sheath, stump sock), L8400–L8485
 taxes, orthotic/prosthetic/other, L9999
 tracheo-esophageal, L8507–L8509
 upper extremity, L6000–L6999
 vacuum erection system, L7900

◀ **New** ⤶ **Revised** ✔ **Reinstated** ~~deleted~~ **Deleted**

Prosthetic additions
 lower extremity, L5610–L5999
 powered upper extremity range of motion assist
  device, L8701–L8702
 upper extremity, L6600–L7405
Prosthetic, eye, V2623
Prosthodontic procedure
 fixed, D6200–D6999
 removable, D5000–D5899
Prosthodontics, removable, *D5110–D5899*
Protamine sulfate, J2720
Protectant, skin, A6250
Protector, heel or elbow, E0191
Protein C Concentrate, J2724
Protirelin, J2725
Psychotherapy, group, partial hospitalization,
 G0410–G0411
Pulp capping, D3110, D3120
Pulpotomy, D3220
 partial, D3222
 vitality test, D0460
Pulse generator, E2120
Pump
 alternating pressure pad, E0182
 ambulatory infusion, E0781, E0787
 ambulatory insulin, E0784
 blood, dialysis, E1620
 breast, E0602–E0604
 enteral infusion, B9000, B9002
 external infusion, E0779
 heparin infusion, E1520
 implantable infusion, E0782, E0783
 implantable infusion, refill kit, A4220
 infusion, supplies, A4226, A4230, A4232
 negative pressure wound therapy, E2402
 parenteral infusion, B9004, B9006
 suction, portable, E0600
 water circulating pad, E0236
 wound, negative, pressure, E2402
Purification system, E1610, E1615
Pyridoxine HCl, J3415

Q

Quad cane, E0105
Quinupristin/dalfopristin, J2770

R

Rack/stand, oxygen, E1355
Radiesse, Q2026
Radioelements for brachytherapy, Q3001
Radiograph, dental, D0210–D0340
Radiological, supplies, A4641, A4642
Radiology service, R0070–R0076
Radiopharmaceutical diagnostic and
 therapeutic imaging agent, A4641, A4642,
 A9500–A9699

Radiosurgery, robotic, G0339–G0340
Radiosurgery, stereotactic, G0339, G0340
Rail
 bathtub, E0241, E0242, E0246
 bed, E0305, E0310
 toilet, E0243
Ranibizumab, J2778, Q5128 ◀
Rasburicase, J2783
Ravulizumab injection-cwvz, J1303
Reaching/grabbing device, A9281
Reagent strip, A4252
Re-cement
 crown, D2920
 inlay, D2910
Reciprocating peritoneal dialysis
 system, E1630
Reclast, J3488, *J3489*
Reclining, wheelchair, E1014, E1050–E1070,
 E1100–E1110
Reconstruction, angiography, G0288
Rectal Control System for Vaginal insertion,
 A4563
Red blood cells, P9021, P9022
Regadenoson, J2785
Regular insulin, *J1815,* J1820
Regulator, oxygen, E1353
Rehabilitation
 cardiac, S9472
 program, H2001
 psychosocial, H2017, H2018
 pulmonary, S9473
 system, jaw, motion, E1700–E1702
 vestibular, S9476
Releuko, Q5125
Remdesivir, J0248
Remimazolam, J2249 ◀
Removal, cerumen, G0268
Repair
 contract, ESRD, A4890
 durable medical equipment, E1340
 maxillofacial prosthesis, L8049
 orthosis, L4000–L4130
 prosthetic, L7500, L7510
Replacement
 battery, A4630
 pad (alternating pressure), A4640
 tanks, dialysis, A4880
 tip for cane, crutches, walker, A4637
 underarm pad for crutches, A4635
Resin dental restoration, D2330–D2394
Reslizumab, J2786
Respiratory
 DME, A7000–A7527
 equipment, E0424–E0601
 function, therapeutic, procedure, G0237–G0239,
 S5180–S5181
 supplies, A4604–A4629, A7049 ◀
Restorative dental procedure, D2000–D2999
Restraint, any type, E0710–E0711 ◀
Reteplase, *J2993*

◀ New   ↻ Revised   ✔ Reinstated   ~~deleted~~ **Deleted**

Retifanlimab-dlwr, J9345 ◀
Revascularization, C9603–C9608
Revefenacin inhalation solution, J7677
Rezafungin, J0349 ◀
Rho(D) immune globulin, human, J2788, J2790, J2792
Rib belt, thoracic, A4572, L0220
Rilanocept, J2793
RimabotulinumtoxinB, J0587
Ring, ostomy, A4404
Ringers lactate infusion, J7120
Risankizumab, J2327
Risk-adjusted functional status
  elbow, wrist or hand, G8667–G8670
  hip, G8651–G8654
  lower leg, foot or ankle, G8655–G8658
  lumbar spine, G8659–G8662
  neck, cranium, mandible, thoracic spine, ribs, or other, G8671–G8674
  shoulder, G8663–G8666
Risperidone (risperdal consta), J2794
  (perseris), J2798
  (uzedy), C9158 ◀
Rituximab, J9312
  abbs (Truxina), Q5115
Robin-Aids, L6000, L6010, L6020, L6855, L6860
Rocking bed, E0462
Rolapitant, J8670
Rollabout chair, E1031
Romidepsin, J9315
Romiplostim, J2796
Romosozumab injection-aqqg, J3111
Root canal therapy, D3310–D3353
Ropivacaine HCl, J2795
Rubidium Rb-82, A9555
Rybrevant, J9061
Rylaze, J9021

S

Sacituzumab govitecan-hziy, J9317
Sacral nerve stimulation test lead, A4290
Safety equipment, E0700
  vest, wheelchair, E0980
Saline
  hypertonic, J7130, *J7131*
  infusion, J7030–J7060
  solution, A4216–A4218, J7030–J7050
Saliva
  artificial, A9155
  collection and preparation, D0417
Samarium SM 153 Lexidronamm, A9605
Sargramostim (GM-CSF), J2820
Scale, E1639
Scoliosis, L1000–L1499
  additions, L1010–L1120, L1210–L1290
Screening
  alcohol misuse, G0442
  cancer, cervical or vaginal, G0101

Screening (Continued)
  colorectal, cancer, G0104–G0106, G0120–G0122, G0328
  cytopathology cervical or vaginal, G0123, G0124, G0141–G0148
  depression, G0444
  dysphagia, documentation, V5364
  enzyme immunoassay, G0432
  glaucoma, G0117, G0118
  infectious agent antibody detection, G0433, G0435
  language, V5363
  mammography, digital image, G9899, G9900
  prostate, cancer, G0102, G0103
  speech, V5362
  TB, M1003 ◀
Sculptra, Q2028
Sealant
  skin, A6250
  tooth, D1351
Seat
  attachment, walker, E0156
  insert, wheelchair, E0992
  lift (patient), E0621, E0627–E0629
  upholstery, wheelchair, E0975, *E0981*
Sebelipase alfa , J2840
Secretin, J2850
Semi-reclining, wheelchair, E1100, E1110
Sensitivity study, P7001
Sensory nerve conduction test, G0255
Sermorelin acetate, Q0515
Serum clotting time tube, A4771
Service
  Allied Health, home health, hospice, G0151–G0161
  behavioral health and/or substance abuse, H0001–H9999
  doula birth worker, T1032–T1033
  hearing, V5000–V5999
  laboratory, P0000–P9999
  mental, health, training, G0177
  non-covered, A9270
  oncology, M0010 ◀
  physician, for mobility device, G0372
  pulmonary, for LVRS, G0302–G0305
  skilled, RN/LPN, home health, hospice, G0162
  social, psychological, G0409–G0411
  speech-language, V5336–V5364
  therapeutic, C9784–C9792 ◀
  vision, V2020–V2799
SEWHO, L3960–L3974, L3975–L3978
SEXA, G0130
Sheepskin pad, E0188, E0189
Shoes
  arch support, L3040–L3100
  for diabetics, A5500–A5514
  insert, L3000–L3030, *L3031*
  lift, L3300–L3334
  miscellaneous additions, L3500–L3595
  orthopedic, L3201–L3265

Shoes *(Continued)*
  positioning device, L3140–L3170
  transfer, L3600–L3649
  wedge, L3340–L3485
Shoulder
  disarticulation, prosthetic, L6300–L6320, L6550
  orthosis (SO), L3650–L3674
  spinal, cervical, L0100–L0200
Shoulder sling, A4566
Shoulder-elbow-wrist-hand orthosis (SEWHO),
  L3960–L3969, *L3971–L3978*
Shunt accessory for dialysis, A4740
  aqueous, L8612
Sigmoidoscopy, cancer screening, G0104, G0106
Siltuximab, J2860
Sincalide, J2805–J2806 ◀
Sipuleucel-T, Q2043
Sirolimus, J7520, J9331
Sitz bath, E0160–E0162
Skin
  barrier, ostomy, A4362, A4363, A4369–A4373,
   A4385, A5120
  bond or cement, ostomy, A4364
  sealant, protectant, moisturizer, A6250
  substitute, Q4100–Q4258, Q4265–Q4286 ◀
Sling, A4565
  patient lift, E0621, E0630, E0635
Smear, Papanicolaou, screening, *P3000, P3001, Q0091*
SNCT, *G0255*
Social worker, clinical, home, health, *G0155*
Social worker, nonemergency transport, A0160
Social work/psychological services, CORF, *G0409*
Sock
  body sock, L0984
  prosthetic sock, *L8417,* L8420–L8435, L8470,
   L8480, L8485
  stump sock, L8470–L8485
Sodium
  chloride injection, J2912
  ferric gluconate complex in sucrose, J2916
  fluoride F-18, A9580
  hyaluronate
   Euflexxa, J7323
   GELSYN-3, J7328
   Hyalgan, J7321
   Orthovisc, J7324
   Supartz, J7321
   Synvisc and Synvisc-One, J7325
   Visco-3, J7321
  phosphate P32, A9563
  pyrophosphate, J1443
  succinate, J1720
  thiosulfate, J0208 ◀
Solution
  calibrator, A4256
  dialysate, A4760
  elliotts b, J9175
  enteral formulae, B4149–B4156, *B4157–B4162*
  parenteral nutrition, B4164–B5200

Solvent, adhesive remover, *A4455*
Somatrem, J2940
Somatropin, J2941
Sorbent cartridge, ESRD, E1636
Special size, wheelchair, *E1220–E1239*
Specialty absorptive dressing, A6251–A6256
Specialty care, H2040–H2041 ◀
Spectacle lenses, *V2100–V2199*
Spectinomycin HCl, J3320
Speech assessment, V5362–V5364
Speech generating device, E2500–E2599, K1009
Speech, pathologist, *G0153*
Speech-Language pathology, services, *V5336–V5364*
Spesolimab-sbzo, J1747 ◀
Spherocylinder, single vision, *V2100–V2114*
  bifocal, V2203–V2214
  trifocal, V2303–V2314
Spinal orthosis
  cervical, L0100–L0200
  cervical-thoracic-lumbar-sacral (CTLSO),
   L0700, L0710
  DME, K0112–K0116
  halo, L0810–L0830
  multiple post collar, L0180–L0200
  scoliosis, L1000–L1499
  torso supports, L0960
Splint, A4570, L3100, L4350–L4380
  ankle, L4390–L4398
  dynamic, E1800, E1805, E1810, E1815, E1825,
   E1830, E1840
  footdrop, L4398
  supplies, miscellaneous, Q4051
Standard, wheelchair, *E1130, K0001*
Static progressive stretch, E1801, E1806, E1811,
  E1816, E1818, E1821
Status
  disease, oncology, G9063–G9139
STELARA, ustekinumab, 1 mg, J3357
Stent, transcatheter, placement, *C9600, C9601*
Stereotactic, radiosurgery, *G0339, G0340*
Sterile cefuroxime sodium, J0697
Sterile water, A4216–A4217
Stimulation, electrical, non-attended, *G0281–G0283*
Stimulators
  neuromuscular, E0744, E0745
  osteogenesis, electrical, E0747–E0749
  salivary reflex, E0755
  stoma absorptive cover, A5083
  transcutaneous, electric, nerve, A4595–A4596,
   E0720–E0749
  ultrasound, E0760
Stockings
  gradient, compression, A6530–A6549
  surgical, A4490–A4510
Stoma, plug or seal, A5081
Stomach tube, B4083
Streptokinase, J2995
Streptomycin, J3000

◀ New ↻ Revised ✔ Reinstated ~~deleted~~ Deleted

Streptozocin, J9320

Strip, blood glucose test, A4253–A4772
  urine reagent, A4250

Strontium-89 chloride, supply of, A9600

Study, bone density, G0130

Stump sock, L8470–L8485

Stylet, A4212

Substance/Alcohol, assessment, G0396, G0397, *H0001, H0003, H0049*

Succinylcholine chloride, J0330

Suction pump
  gastric, home model, E2000
  portable, E0600
  respiratory, home model, E0600

Sumatriptan succinate, J3030

Supartz, J7321

Supplies
  battery, A4233–A4236, A4601, A4611–A4613, A4638
  cast, A4580, A4590, Q4001–Q4051
  catheters, A4300–A4306
  continuous glucose monitor, A4238, A4239
  contraceptive, A4267–A4269
  diabetic shoes, A5500–A5513
  dialysis, A4653–A4928
  DME, other, A4630–A4640
  dressings, A6000–A6513
  electrical stimulator (external), L8678 ◀
  enteral, therapy, B4000–B9999
  hip orthosis, L1681 ◀
  incontinence, A4310–A4355, A5102–A5200
  infusion, A4221, A4222, A4230–A4232, E0776–E0791
  needle, A4212, A4215
  needle-free device, A4210
  ostomy, A4361–A4434, A5051–A5093, A5120–A5200
  parenteral, therapy, B4000–B9999
  radiological, A4641, A4642
  refill kit, infusion pump, A4220
  respiratory, A4604–A4629
  self-administered injections, A4211
  splint, Q4051
  sterile water/saline and/or dextrose, A4216–A4218
  surgical, miscellaneous, A4649
  syringe, A4206–A4209, A4213, A4232
  syringe with needle, A4206–A4209
  ultrasonic diathermy treatment, K1036 ◀
  urinary, external, A4356–A4360

Supply/accessory/service, A9900

Support
  arch, L3040–L3090
  cervical, L0100–L0200
  spinal, L0960
  stockings, L8100–L8239

Surederm, Q4220

Surgery, oral, D7000–D7999

Surgical
  arthroscopy, knee, G0289, S2112
  boot, L3208–L3211
  dressing, A6196–A6406

Surgical *(Continued)*
  procedure, noncovered, G0293, G0294
  stocking, A4490–A4510
  supplies, A4649
  tray, A4550

Surgicord, Q4218–Q4219

Surgraft, Q4209, Q4263, Q4268–Q4269 ◀

Susvimo, J2779

Sutimlimab-jome, J1302

Swabs, betadine or iodine, A4247

Synojoynt, J7331

Synvisc and Synvisc-One, J7325

Syringe, A4213
  with needle, A4206–A4209

System
  external, ambulatory insulin, A9274
  rehabilitation, jaw, motion, E1700–E1702
  transport, E1035–E1039

T

Tables, bed, E0274, E0315

Tacrolimus
  oral, J7503, J7507, J7508
  parenteral, J7525

Tagraxofusp injections-erzs, J9269

Taliglucerase, J3060

Talimogene laheroareovec, J9325

Tape, A4450–A4452

Taxi, non-emergency transportation, A0100

Team, conference, G0175, G9007, S0220, S0221

Tebentafusp-tebn, J9274

Technetium TC 99M
  Arcitumomab, A9568
  Bicisate, A9557
  Depreotide, A9536
  Disofenin, A9510
  Exametazine, A9521
  Exametazine labeled autologous white blood cells, A9569
  Fanolesomab, A9566
  Glucepatate, A9550
  Labeled red blood cells, A9560
  Macroaggregated albumin, A9540
  Mebrofenin, A9537
  Mertiatide, A9562
  Oxidronate, A9561
  Pentetate, A9539, A9567
  Pertechnetate, A9512
  Pyrophosphate, A9538
  Sestamibi, A9500
  Succimer, A9551
  Sulfur colloid, A9541
  Teboroxime, A9501
  Tetrofosmin, A9502
  Tilmanocept, A9520

Teclistamab-cqyv, J9380 ◀

◀ New   ⊃ Revised   ✔ Reinstated   ~~deleted~~ Deleted

Tedizolid phosphate, J3090
TEEV, J0900
Telavancin, J3095
Telehealth, Q3014, G0320–G0321
Telehealth transmission, T1014
Temozolomide
    injection, J9328
    oral, J8700
Temporary codes, Q0000–Q9999, S0009–S9999
Temporomandibular joint, D0320, D0321
Temsirolimus, J9330
Tenecteplase, J3101
Teniposide, Q2017
TENS, A4595–A4596, E0720–E0749
Tent, oxygen, E0455
Teplizumab-mzwv, J9381 ◄
Teprotumumab-trbw, J3241
Terbutaline sulfate, J3105
    inhalation solution, concentrated, J7680
    inhalation solution, unit dose, J7681
Teriparatide, J3110
Terminal devices, L6700–L6895
Test
    sensory, nerve, conduction, G0255
Testosterone
    cypionate and estradiol cypionate, J1071
    enanthate, J3121
    undecanoate, J3145
Tetanus immune globulin, human, J1670
Tetracycline, J0120
Tezepelumab, J2356
Thallous Chloride TL 201, A9505
Theophylline, J2810
Therapeutic lightbox, A4634, E0203
Therapy
    activity, G0176
    electromagnetic, G0295, G0329
    endodontic, D3222–D3330
    enteral, supplies, B4000–B9999
    immune checkpoint inhibitor, M1180
    medical, nutritional, G0270, G0271
    occupational, *G0129, H5300, S9129*
    occupational, health, G0152
    parenteral, supplies, B4000–B9999
    respiratory, function, procedure, G0237–S0239,
        S5180, S5181
    speech, home, G0153, S9128
    wound, negative, pressure, pump, E2402
Theraskin, Q4121
Thermometer, A4931–A4932
    dialysis, A4910
Thiamine HCl, J3411
Thiethylperazine maleate, J3280
Thiotepa, J9340
Thoracic orthosis, L0210
Thoracic-hip-knee-ankle (THKAO), L1500–L1520

Thoracic-lumbar-sacral orthosis (TLSO)
    scoliosis, L1200–L1290
    spinal, L0450–L0492
Thymol turbidity, blood, P2033
Thyroidectomy, C7555
Thyrotropin Alfa, J3240
Tigecycline, J3243, J3244
Tinzarparin sodium, J1655
Tip (cane, crutch, walker) replacement, A4637
Tire, wheelchair, E2211–E2225, E2381–E2395
Tirofiban, J3246
Tisagenlecleucel, Q2040
Tisotumab vedotin-TFTV, J9273
Tissue marker, A4648
Tixagev and cilgav, Q0221
TLSO, L0450–L0492, L1200–L1290
Tobacco
    intervention, G9016, G0029–G0030 ↻
Tobramycin
    inhalation solution, unit dose, J7682, J7685
    sulfate, J3260
Tocilizumab, J2362
Toe device, E1831
Tofersen, C9157 ◄
Toilet accessories, E0167–E0179, E0243, E0244, E0625
Tolazoline HCl, J2670
Toll, non emergency transport, A0170
Tomographic radiograph, dental, D0322
Topical hyperbaric oxygen chamber, A4575
Topotecan, J8705, J9351
Torsemide, J3265
Trabectedin, J9352
Tracheostoma heat moisture exchange system,
    A7501–A7509
Tracheostomy
    care kit, A4629
    filter, A4481
    speaking valve, L8501
    supplies, A4623, A4629, A7523–A7524
    tube, A7520–A7522
Tracheotomy mask or collar, A7525–A7526
Traction
    cervical, E0855, E0856
    device, ambulatory, E0830
    equipment, E0840–E0948
    extremity, E0870–E0880
    pelvic, E0890, E0900, E0947
Training
    diabetes, outpatient, G0108, G0109
    home health or hospice, G0162
    services, mental, health, G0177
Transcutaneous electrical nerve stimulator
    (TENS), E0720–E0770, K1016–K1020
Transducer protector, dialysis, E1575
Transfer (shoe orthosis), L3600–L3640
Transfer system with seat, E1035

◄ New   ↻ Revised   ✔ Reinstated   ~~deleted~~ Deleted

Transparent film (for dressing), A6257–A6259

Transplant
heart (history of), M1151–M1152
islet, G0341–G0343, S2102

Transport
chair, E1035–E1039
system, E1035–E1039
x-ray, R0070–R0076

Transportation
ambulance, A0021–A0999, Q3019, Q3020
corneal tissue, V2785
EKG (portable), R0076
handicapped, A0130
non-emergency, A0080–A0210, T2001–T2005
service, including ambulance, A0021, A0999, T2006
taxi, non-emergency, A0100
toll, non-emergency, A0170
volunteer, non-emergency, A0080, A0090
x-ray (portable), R0070, R0075, R0076

Transportation services
air services, A0430, A0431, A0435, A0436
ALS disposable supplies, A0398
ALS mileage, A0390
ALS specialized service, A0392, A0394, A0396
ambulance, ALS, A0426, A0427, A0433
ambulance, outside state, Medicaid, A0021
ambulance oxygen, A0422
ambulance, waiting time, A0420
ancillary, lodging, escort, A0200
ancillary, lodging, recipient, A0180
ancillary, meals, escort, A0210
ancillary, meals, recipient, A0190
ancillary, parking fees, tolls, A0170
BLS disposable supplies, A0382
BLS mileage, A0380
BLS specialized service, A0384
emergency, neonatal, one-way, A0225
extra ambulance attendant, A0424
ground mileage, A0425
non-emergency, air travel, A0140
non-emergency, bus, A0110
non-emergency, case worker, A0160
non-emergency, mini-bus, A0120
non-emergency, no vested interest, A0080
non-emergency, taxi, A0100
non-emergency, wheelchair van, A0130
non-emergency, with vested interest, A0090
paramedic intercept, A0432
response and treat, no transport, A0998
specialty transport, A0434

Transtracheal oxygen catheter, A7018
Trapeze bar, E0910–E0912, E0940
Trauma, response, team, G0390
Tray
insertion, A4310–A4316
irrigation, A4320

Tray *(Continued)*
surgical; (see also kits), A4550
wheelchair, E0950

Trastuzumab injection excludes biosimilar, J9316, J9355
anns (kanjinti), Q5117
dkst (Ogivri), Q5114
dttb (Ontruzant), Q5112
fam-trastuzumab deruxtecan-nxki, J9358
pkrb (Herzuma), Q5113
qyyp (trazimera), Q5116

Trastuzumab and Hyaluronidase-oysk, J9356

Treatment
bone, G0412–G0415
pediculosis (lice), A9180
services, behavioral health, H0002–H2037

Tremelimumab-actl, J9347 ◄
Treprostinil, J3285
Triamcinolone, J3301–J3303
acetonide, J3300, J3301
diacetate, J3302
hexacetonide, J3303
inhalation solution, concentrated, J7683
inhalation solution, unit dose, J7684

Triferic avnu J1445
Triflupromazine HCl, J3400
Trifocal, glass or plastic, V2300–V2399
aniseikonic, V2318
lenticular, V2315, V2321
specialty trifocal, by report, V2399
sphere, plus or minus, V2300–V2302
spherocylinder, V2303–V2314
trifocal add-over 3.25d, V2320
trifocal, seg width over 28 mm, V2319

Trigeminal division block anesthesia, D9212
Trilaciclib J1448
Triluron intraarticular injection, J7332
Trimethobenzamide HCl, J3250
Trimetrexate glucuoronate, J3305
Trimming, nails, dystrophic, G0127
Triptorelin pamoate, J3315
Trismus appliance, D5937
Truss, L8300–L8330
addition to standard pad, scrotal pad, L8330
addition to standard pad, water pad, L8320
double, standard pads, L8310
single, standard pad, L8300
Tube/Tubing
anchoring device, A5200
blood, A4750, A4755
corrugated tubing, non-disposable, used with large volume nebulizer,10 feet, A4337
drainage extension, A4331
gastrostomy, B4087, B4088
irrigation, A4355
larynectomy, A4622
nasogastric, B4081, B4082

◄ **New** ⤺ **Revised** ✔ **Reinstated** ~~deleted~~ **Deleted**

Tube/Tubing (Continued)
oxygen, A4616
serum clotting time, A4771
stomach, B4083
suction pump, each, A7002
tire, K0091, K0093, K0095, K0097
tracheostomy, A4622
urinary drainage, K0280

U

Ublituximab-xiiy, J2329 ◀
Ultrasonic nebulizer, E0575
Ultrasound, S8055, S9024
paranasal sinus ultrasound, S9024
ultrasound guidance, multifetal pregnancy reduction, technical component, S8055
Ultraviolet, cabinet/system, E0691, E0694
Ultraviolet light therapy system, A4633, E0691–E0694
light therapy system in 6 foot cabinet, E0694
replacement bulb/lamp, A4633
therapy system panel, 4 foot, E0692
therapy system panel, 6 foot, E0693
treatment area 2 sq feet or less, E0691
Unclassified drug, J3490
Underpads, disposable, A4554
Unipuncture control system, dialysis, E1580
Upper extremity addition, locking elbow, L6693
Upper extremity fracture orthosis, L3980–L3999
Upper limb prosthesis, L6000–L7499
Urea, J3350
Ureterostomy supplies, A4454–A4590
Urethral suppository, Alprostadil, J0275
Urinal, E0325, E0326
Urinary
catheter, A4338–A4346, A4351–A4353
indwelling catheter, A4338–A4346
intermittent urinary catheter, A4351–A4353
male external catheter, A4349
collection and retention (supplies), A4310–A4360
bedside drainage bag, A4357
disposable external urethral clamp, A4360
external urethral clamp, A4356
female external urinary collection device, A4328
insertion trays, A4310–A4316, A4354–A4355
irrigation syringe, A4322
irrigation tray, A4320
male external catheter/integral collection chamber, A4326
perianal fecal collection pouch, A4330
therapeutic agent urinary catheter irrigation, A4321
urinary drainage bag, leg/abdomen, A4358
supplies, external, A4335, A4356–A4358
bedside drainage bag, A4357
external urethral clamp/compression device, A4356
incontinence supply, A4335
urinary drainage bag, leg or abdomen, A4358

Urinary (Continued)
supplies, external (Continued)
tract endoscope, C1747
tract implant, collagen, L8603
tract implant, synthetic, L8606
Urine
sensitivity study, P7001
system, K1006
tests, A4250
Urofollitropin, J3355
Urokinase, J3364, J3365
Ustekinumab, J3357, J3758
U-V lens, V2755

V

Vabra aspirator, A4480
Vaccination, administration
flublok, Q2033
hepatitis B, G0010
influenza virus, G0008
pneumococcal, G0009
Vaccine
administration, influenza, G0008
administration, pneumococcal, G0009
hepatitis B, administration, G0010
Vaginal
cancer, screening, G0101
cytopathologist, G0123
cytopathology, G0123, G0124, G0141–G0148
screening, cervical/vaginal, thin-layer, cytopathologist, G0123
screening, cervical/vaginal, thin-layer, physician interpretation, G0124
screening cytopathology smears, automated, G0141–G0148
Vancomycin HCl, J3370–J3372
Vaporizer, E0605
Vascular
catheter (appliances and supplies), A4300–A4306
disposable drug delivery system, >50 ml/hr, A4305
disposable drug delivery system, <50 ml/hr, A4306
implantable access catheter, external, A4300
implantable access total, catheter, A4301
graft material, synthetic, L8670
Vasopressin, J2598–J2599 ◀
Vasoxyl, J3390
Vedolizumab, J3380
Vehicle, power-operated, K0800–K0899
Velaglucerase alfa, J3385
Venous pressure clamp, dialysis, A4918
Ventilator
battery, A4611–A4613
home ventilator, any type, E0465, E0466
used with invasive interface (e.g., tracheostomy tube), E0465

Ventilator *(Continued)*
home ventilator, any type *(Continued)*
used with non-invasive interface (e.g., mask, chest shell), E0466
moisture exchanger, disposable, A4483
Ventricular assist device, Q0478–Q0504, Q0506–Q0509
battery clips, electric or electric/pneumatic, replacement, Q0497
battery, lithium-ion, electric or electric/pneumatic, replacement, Q0506
battery, other than lithium-ion, electric or electric/ pneumatic, replacement, Q0496
battery, pneumatic, replacement, Q0503
battery/power-pack charger, electric or electric/ pneumatic, replacement, Q0495
belt/vest/bag, carry external components, replacement, Q0499
driver, replacement, Q0480
ejection, fraction, left, M1150
emergency hand pump, electric or electric/pneumatic, replacement, Q0494
emergency power source, electric, replacement, Q0490
emergency power source, electric/pneumatic, replacement, Q0491
emergency power supply cable, electric, replacement, Q0492
emergency power supply cable, electric/pneumatic, replacement, Q0493
filters, electric or electric/pneumatic, replacement, Q0500
holster, electric or electric/pneumatic, replacement, Q0498
leads (pneumatic/electrical), replacement, Q0487
microprocessor control unit, electric/pneumatic combination, replacement, Q0482
microprocessor control unit, pneumatic, replacement, Q0481
miscellaneous supply, external VAD, Q0507
miscellaneous supply, implanted device, Q0508
miscellaneous supply, implanted device, payment not made under Medicare Part A, Q0509
mobility cart, replacement, Q0502
monitor control cable, electric, replacement, Q0485
monitor control cable, electric/pneumatic, Q0486
monitor/display module, electric, replacement, Q0483
monitor/display module, electric/electric pneumatic, replacement, Q0484
power adapter, pneumatic, replacement, vehicle type, Q0504
power adapter, vehicle type, Q0478
power module, replacement, Q0479
power-pack base, electric, replacement, Q0488
power-pack base, electric/pneumatic, replacement, Q0489

Ventricular assist device *(Continued)*
shower cover, electric or electric/pneumatic, replacement, Q0501
Verteporfin, J3396
Vest, safety, wheelchair, E0980
Vinblastine sulfate, J9360
Vincristine sulfate, J9370, J9371
Vinorelbine tartrate, J9390
Vision service, V2020–V2799
bifocal, glass or plastic, V2200–V2299
contact lenses, V2500–V2599
frames, V2020–V2025
intraocular lenses, V2630–V2632
low-vision aids, V2600–V2615
miscellaneous, V2700–V2799
prosthetic eye, V2623–V2629
spectacle lenses, V2100–V2199
trifocal, glass or plastic, V2300–V2399
variable asphericity, V2410–V2499
Visit, emergency department, G0380–G0384
Visual, function, postoperative cataract surgery, G0915–G0918
Vitamin B-12 cyanocobalamin, J3420
Vitamin K, J3430
Voice
amplifier, L8510
prosthesis, L8511–L8514
Von Willebrand Factor Complex, human, J7179, J7183, J7187
Voriconazole, J3465
Vutrisiran, J0225

W

Waiver, T2012–T2050
assessment/plan of care development, T2024
case management, per month, T2022
day habilitation, per 15 minutes, T2021
day habilitation, per diem, T2020
habilitation, educational, per diem, T2012
habilitation, educational, per hour, T2013
habilitation, prevocational, per diem, T2014
habilitation, prevocational, per hour, T2015
habilitation, residential, 15 minutes, T2017
habilitation, residential, per diem, T2016
habilitation, supported employment, 15 minutes, T2019
habilitation, supported employment, per diem, T2018
targeted case management, per month, T2023
waiver services NOS, T2025
Walker, E0130–E0149
accessories, A4636, A4637
attachments, E0153–E0159
enclosed, four-sided frame, E0144
folding (pickup), E0135
folding, wheeled, E0143
heavy duty, multiple braking system, E0147
heavy duty, wheeled, rigid or folding, E0149

◄ **New** ⟳ **Revised** ✔ **Reinstated** ~~deleted~~ **Deleted**

Walker (*Continued*)
  heavy duty, without wheels, E0148
  rigid (pickup), E0130
  rigid, wheeled, E0141
  with trunk support, E0140
Walking splint, L4386
Washer, Gravlee jet, *A4470*
Water
  dextrose, J7042, J7060, J7070
  distilled (for nebulizer), A7018
  pressure pad/mattress, E0187, E0198
  purification system (ESRD), E1610, E1615
  softening system (ESRD), E1625
  sterile, A4714
WBC/CBC, *G0306*
Wedges, shoe, L3340–L3420
Wellness, promoting, M0005
Wellness visit; annual, *G0438*, *G0439*
Wet mount, Q0111
Wheel attachment, rigid pickup walker, E0155
Wheelchair, E0950–E1298, K0001–K0108,
  K0801–K0899
  accessories, E0192, E0950–E1030, E1065–E1069,
    E2211–E2230, E2300–E2399, *E2626–E2633*
  amputee, E1170–E1200
  back, fully reclining, manual, E1226
  component or accessory, not otherwise
    specified, K0108
  cushions, E2601–E2625
  custom manual wheelchair base, K0008
  custom motorized/power base, K0013
  dynamic positioning hardware for back, E2398
  foot box, E0954
  heavy duty, E1280–E1298, K0006, K0007,
    K0801–K0886
  lateral thigh or knee support, E0953
  lightweight, E1087–E1090, E1240–E1270
  narrowing device, E0969
  power add-on, E0983–E0984
  reclining, fully, E1014, E1050–E1070,
    E1100–E1110
  semi-reclining, E1100–E1110
  shock absorber, E1015–E1018
  specially sized, E1220, E1230
  standard, E1130, K0001
  stump support system, K0551
  tire, E0999
  transfer board or device, E0705
  tray, K0107
  van, non-emergency, A0130
  youth, E1091
WHFO with inflatable air chamber, L3807
Whirlpool equipment, E1300–E1310
Whirlpool tub, walk-in, portable, K1003
WHO, wrist extension, L3914
Wig, A9282
Wipes, A4245, A4247
Wound
  cleanser, A6260

Wound (*Continued*)
  closure, adhesive, G0168
  cover
    alginate dressing, A6196–A6198
    collagen dressing, A6020–A6024
    foam dressing, A6209–A6214
    hydrocolloid dressing, A6234–A6239
    hydrogel dressing, A6242–A6247
    non-contact wound warming cover, and
      accessory, E0231–E0232
    specialty absorptive dressing, A2001–A2010,
      A2015–A2025, A6251–A6256
  filler
    alginate dressing, A6199
    collagen based, A6010
    foam dressing, A6215
    hydrocolloid dressing, A6240–A6241
    hydrogel dressing, A6248
    not elsewhere classified, A6261–A6262
Woundfix, Woundfix Plus, Q4217
  matrix, Q4114
  pouch, A6154
  therapy, negative, pressure, pump, E2402
  wound suction, A9272, K0743
Wrapping, fabric, abdominal aneurysm, *M0301*
Wrist
  disarticulation prosthesis, L6050, L6055
  electronic wrist rotator, L7259
  hand/finger orthosis (WHFO), E1805, E1825,
    L3800–L3954

X

Xenon Xe 133, A9558
Xenon Xe 129, C9150 ◀
Xipere, J3299
X-ray
  equipment, portable, Q0092, R0070, R0075
  single, energy, absorptiometry (SEXA), G0130
  transport, R0070–R0076
Xylocaine HCl, J2000

Y

Yttrium Y-90 ibritumomab, A9543

Z

Ziconotide, J2278
Zidovudine, J3485
Ziprasidone mesylate, J3486
Zoledronic acid, J3489
Zynlonta, J9359

TABLE OF DRUGS

IA	Intra-arterial administration
IU	International unit
IV	Intravenous administration
IM	Intramuscular administration
IT	Intrathecal
SC	Subcutaneous administration
INH	Administration by inhaled solution
VAR	Various routes of administration
OTH	Other routes of administration
ORAL	Administered orally

Intravenous administration includes all methods, such as gravity infusion, injections, and timed pushes. The "VAR" posting denotes various routes of administration and is used for drugs that are commonly administered into joints, cavities, tissues, or topical applications, in addition to other parenteral administrations. Listings posted with "OTH" indicate other administration methods, such as suppositories or catheter injections.

Blue typeface terms are added by publisher.

DRUG NAME	DOSAGE	METHOD OF ADMINISTRATION	HCPCS CODE	
A				
Abatacept	10 mg	IV	**J0129**	
Abbokinase	5,000 IU vial	IV	J3364	
	250,000 IU vial	IV	J3365	
Abbokinase, Open Cath	5,000 IU vial	IV	J3364	
Abciximab	10 mg	IV	**J0130**	
Abelcet	10 mg	IV	J0289	
Abilify Maintena	1 mg		J0401	
ABLC	50 mg	IV	J0285	
AbobotulinumtoxinA	5 units	IM	**J0586**	
Abraxane	1 mg		J9264	
Accuneb	1 mg		J7613	
Acetadote	100 mg		J0132	
Acetaminophen	10 mg	IV	**J0131, J0136-J0137**	◀
Acetazolamide sodium	up to 500 mg	IM, IV	**J1120**	
Acetylcysteine				
injection	100 mg	IV	**J0132**	
unit dose form	per gram	INH	**J7604, J7608**	
Achromycin	up to 250 mg	IM, IV	J0120	
Actemra	1 mg		J3262	
~~ACTH~~	~~up to 40 units~~	~~IV, IM, SC~~	~~J0800~~	
~~Acthar~~	~~up to 40 units~~	~~IV, IM, SC~~	~~J0800~~	
Acthib			J3490	
Acthrel	1 mcg		J0795	
Actimmune	3 million units	SC	J9216	
Activase	1 mg	IV	J2997	
Acyclovir	5 mg		**J0133**	
			J8499	
Adagen	25 IU		J2504	
Adalimumab	20 mg	SC, IM	**J0135 , Q5131**	◀
Adcetris	1 mg	IV	J9042	
~~Adenocard~~	~~1 mg~~	~~IV~~	~~J0153~~	
~~Adenoscan~~	~~1 mg~~	~~IV~~	~~J0153~~	

◀ **New**   ↻ **Revised**   ✔ **Reinstated**   ~~deleted~~ **Deleted**

DRUG NAME	DOSAGE	METHOD OF ADMINISTRATION	HCPCS CODE
Adenosine	1 mg	IV	J0153
Ado-trastuzumab Emtansine	1 mg	IV	J9354
Adrenalin Chloride	up to 1 ml ampule	SC, IM	J0171
Adrenalin, epinephrine	0.1 mg	SC, IM	J0171
Adriamycin, PFS, RDF	10 mg	IV	J9000
Adrucil	500 mg	IV	J9190
Aduhelm	2 mg	IV	J0172
Advate	per IU		J7192
Afamelanotide implant	1 mg	IV	J7352
Aflibercept	1 mg	OTH	J0178
Agalsidase beta	1 mg	IV	J0180
Aggrastat	0.25 mg	IM, IV	J3246
A-hydrocort	up to 50 mg	IV, IM, SC	J1710
	up to 100 mg		J1720
Akineton	per 5 mg	IM, IV	J0190
Akynzeo	300 mg and 0.5 mg		J8655
Alatrofloxacin mesylate, injection	100 mg	IV	J0200
Albumin			P9041, P9045, P9046, P9047
Albuterol	0.5 mg	INH	J7620
concentrated form	1 mg	INH	J7610, J7611
unit dose form	1 mg	INH	J7609, J7613
Aldesleukin	per single use vial	IM, IV	J9015
Aldomet	up to 250 mg	IV	J0210
Aldurazyme	0.1 mg		J1931
Alefacept	0.5 mg	IM, IV	J0215
Alemtuzumab	1 mg		J0202
Alfentanil hydrochloride	500 mcg	IM	J0216 ◄
Alferon N	250,000 IU	IM	J9215
Alglucerase	per 10 units	IV	J0205
Alglucosidase alfa	10 mg	IV	J0220, J0221
Alimta	10 mg		J9305
Alkaban-AQ	1 mg	IV	J9360
Alkeran	2 mg	ORAL	J8600
	50 mg	IV	J9245
AlloDerm	per square centimeter		Q4116
AlloSkin	per square centimeter		Q4115
Allopurinol sodium	1 mg	IM	J0206 ◄
Aloxi	25 mcg		J2469
Alpha 1-proteinase inhibitor, human	10 mg	IV	J0256, J0257
Alphanate			J7186
AlphaNine SD	per IU		J7193
Alprolix	per IU		J7201
Alprostadil			
injection	1.25 mcg	OTH	J0270
urethral suppository	each	OTH	J0275
Alteplase recombinant	1 mg	IV	J2997

◄ **New** ↻ **Revised** ✓ **Reinstated** ~~deleted~~ **Deleted**

DRUG NAME	DOSAGE	METHOD OF ADMINISTRATION	HCPCS CODE
Alupent	per 10 mg	INH	**J7667, J7668**
noncompounded, unit dose	10 mg	INH	J7669
unit dose	10 mg	INH	J7670
AmBisome	10 mg	IV	J0289
Amcort	per 5 mg	IM	J3302
A-methaPred	up to 40 mg	IM, IV	J2920
	up to 125 mg	IM, IV	J2930
Amgen	1 mcg	SC	J9212
Amifostine	500 mg	IV	**J0207**
Amikacin sulfate	100 mg	IM, IV	**J0278**
Aminocaproic Acid			J3490
Aminolevulinic acid HCl	unit dose (354 mg)	OTH	**J7308**
Aminolevulinic acid HCl 10% Gel	10 mg	OTH	**J7345**
Aminolevulinate	1 g	OTH	**J7309**
Aminophylline/Aminophyllin	up to 250 mg	IV	**J0280**
Amiodarone HCl	30 mg	IV	**J0282-J0283** ◄
Amitriptyline HCl	up to 20 mg	IM	**J1320**
Amobarbital	up to 125 mg	IM, IV	**J0300**
Amphadase	1 ml		J3470
Amphocin	50 mg	IV	J0285
Amphotericin B	50 mg	IV	**J0285**
Amphotericin B, lipid complex	10 mg	IV	**J0287-J0289**
Ampicillin			
sodium	up to 500 mg	IM, IV	**J0290**
sodium/sulbactam sodium	per 1.5 g	IM, IV	**J0295**
Amvuttra	1 mg	IM	J0225 ◄
Amygdalin			J3570
Amytal	up to 125 mg	IM, IV	J0300
Anabolin LA 100	up to 50 mg	IM	J2320
Anadulafungin	1 mg	IV	**J0348**
Anascorp	up to 120 mg	IV	J0716
Anastrozole	1 mg		J8999
Ancef	500 mg	IV, IM	J0690
Andrest 90-4	1 mg	IM	J3121
Andro-Cyp	1 mg		J1071
Andro-Cyp 200	1 mg		J1071
Andro L.A. 200	1 mg	IM	J3121
Andro-Estro 90-4	1 mg	IM	J3121
Andro/Fem	1 mg		J1071
Androgyn L.A.	1 mg	IM	J3121
Androlone-50	up to 50 mg		J2320
Androlone-D 100	up to 50 mg	IM	J2320
Andronaq-50	up to 50 mg	IM	J3140
Andronaq-LA	1 mg		J1071
Andronate-100	1 mg		J1071
Andronate-200	1 mg		J1071
Andropository 100	1 mg	IM	J3121
Andryl 200	1 mg	IM	J3121
Anectine	up to 20 mg	IM, IV	J0330

◄ New   ↻ Revised   ✔ Reinstated   ~~deleted~~ Deleted

DRUG NAME	DOSAGE	METHOD OF ADMINISTRATION	HCPCS CODE
Anergan 25	up to 50 mg	IM, IV	J2550
	12.5 mg	ORAL	Q0169
Anergan 50	up to 50 mg	IM, IV	J2550
	12.5 mg	ORAL	Q0169
Angiomax	1 mg		J0583
Anidulafungin	1 mg	IV	J0348
Anistreplase	30 units	IV	**J0350**
Antiflex	up to 60 mg	IM, IV	J2360
Anti-Inhibitor	per IU	IV	**J7198**
Antispas	up to 20 mg	IM	J0500
Antithrombin III (human)	per IU	IV	**J7197**
Antithrombin recombinant	50 IU	IV	**J7196**
Anzemet	10 mg	IV	J1260
	50 mg	ORAL	S0174
	100 mg	ORAL	Q0180
Apidra Solostar	per 50 units		J1817
A.P.L.	per 1,000 USP units	IM	J0725
Apligraf	per square centimeter		Q4101
Apomorphine Hydrochloride	1 mg	SC	**J0364**
Aprepitant	1 mg	IV	**J0185**
Aprepitant	5 mg	ORAL	J8501
Apresoline	up to 20 mg	IV, IM	J0360
Aprotinin	10,000 kiu		**J0365**
AquaMEPHYTON	per 1 mg	IM, SC, IV	J3430
Aralast	10 mg	IV	J0256
Aralen	up to 250 mg	IM	J0390
Aramine	per 10 mg	IV, IM, SC	J0380
Aranesp			
ESRD use	1 mcg		J0882
Non-ESRD use	1 mcg		J0881
Arbutamine	1 mg	IV	**J0395**
Arcalyst	1 mg		J2793
Aredia	per 30 mg	IV	J2430
Arfonad, *see* Trimethaphan camsylate			
Arformoterol tartrate	15 mcg	INH	**J7605**
Argatroban			
(for ESRD use)	1 mg	IV	**J0884, J0892, J0899**
(for non-ESRD use)	1 mg	IV	**J0883, J0891, J0898**
Aridol	25% in 50 ml	IV	J2150
	5 mg	INH	J7665
			J8999
Arimidex			
Aripiprazole	0.25 mg	IM	**J0400**
Aripiprazole, extended release	1 mg	IV	**J0401**
Aripiprazole lauroxil	1 mg	IV	**J1942**
Aripiprazole lauroxil (aristada)	1 mg	IV	**J1944**
Aripiprazole lauroxil (aristada initio)	1 mg	IV	**J1943**
Aristocort Forte	per 5 mg	IM	J3302

◄ **New**   ↺ **Revised**   ✓ **Reinstated**   ~~deleted~~ **Deleted**

DRUG NAME	DOSAGE	METHOD OF ADMINISTRATION	HCPCS CODE
Aristocort Intralesional	per 5 mg	IM	J3302
Aristospan Intra-Articular	per 5 mg	VAR	J3303
Aristospan Intralesional	per 5 mg	VAR	J3303
Arixtra	per 0.5 m		J1652
Aromasin			J8999
Arranon	50 mg		J9261
Arrestin	up to 200 mg	IM	J3250
	250 mg	ORAL	Q0173
Arsenic trioxide	1 mg	IV	**J9017**
Arzerra	10 mg		J9302
Asparaginase	1,000 units	IV, IM	**J9019**
	10,000 units	IV, IM	**J9020**
Astagraf XL	0.1 mg		J7508
Astramorph PF	up to 10 mg	IM, IV, SC	J2270
Atezolizumab	10 mg	IV	**J9022**
Atgam	250 mg	IV	J7504
Ativan	2 mg	IM, IV	J2060
Atropine			
concentrated form	per mg	INH	**J7635**
unit dose form	per mg	INH	**J7636**
sulfate	0.01 mg	IV, IM, SC	**J0461**, J7636
Atrovent, unit dose form	per mg	INH	J7644, J7645
ATryn	50 IU	IV	J7196
Aurothioglucose	up to 50 mg	IM	**J2910**
Autologous cultured chondrocytes implant		OTH	**J7330**
Autoplex T	per IU	IV	J7198, J7199
AUVI-Q	0.15 mg		J0171
Avastin	10 mg		J9035
Avelox	100 mg		J2280
Avelumab	10 mg	IV	**J9023**
Avonex	30 mcg	IM	J1826
	1 mcg	IM	Q3027
	1 mcg	SC	Q3028
Azacitidine	1 mg	SC	**J9025**
Azasan	50 mg		J7500
Azathioprine	50 mg	ORAL	**J7500**
Azathioprine, parenteral	100 mg	IV	**J7501**
Azithromycin, dihydrate	1 gram	ORAL	**Q0144**
Azithromycin, injection	500 mg	IV	**J0456**
Aztreonam	100 mg	IM	**J0457**
B			
Baciim			J3490
Bacitracin			J3490
Baclofen	10 mg	IT	**J0475**
Baclofen for intrathecal trial	50 mcg	OTH	**J0476**
Bactocill	up to 250 mg	IM, IV	J2700
BAL in oil	per 100 mg	IM	J0470

◀ New   ↻ Revised   ✔ Reinstated   deleted **Deleted**

DRUG NAME	DOSAGE	METHOD OF ADMINISTRATION	HCPCS CODE	
Bamlan and etesev		IV	**M0245**	
Bamlanivimab and etesevima	2100 mg	IV	**Q0245**	
Banflex	up to 60 mg	IV, IM	J2360	
Basiliximab	20 mg		**J0480**	
BCG live intravesical instillation	1 mg	OTH	**J9030**	
Bebulin	per IU		J7194	
Beclomethasone inhalation solution, unit dose form	per mg	INH	**J7622**	
Belantamab mafodotin-blmf	0.5 mg	IV	**J9037**	
Belatacept	1 mg	IV	**J0485**	
Beleodaq	10 mg		J9032	
Belimumab	10 mg	IV	**J0490**	
Belinostat	10 mg	IV	**J9032**	
Bena-D 10	up to 50 mg	IV, IM	J1200	
Bena-D 50	up to 50 mg	IV, IM	J1200	
Benadryl	up to 50 mg	IV, IM	J1200	
Benahist 10	up to 50 mg	IV, IM	J1200	
Benahist 50	up to 50 mg	IV, IM	J1200	
Ben-Allergin-50	up to 50 mg	IV, IM	J1200	
	50 mg	ORAL	Q0163	
Bendamustine HCl				
Apotex	1 mg	IV	J9058	◄
Baxter	1 mg	IV	J9059	◄
Bendeka	1 mg	IV	**J9034**	
Treanda	1 mg	IV	**J9033**	
Vivimusta	1 mg	IV	J9056	◄
Bendamustine HCl (Belrapzo/bendamustine)	1 mg	IV	**J9036**	
Benefix	per IU	IV	J7195	
Benlysta	10 mg		J0490	
Benoject-10	up to 50 mg	IV, IM	J1200	
Benoject-50	up to 50 mg	IV, IM	J1200	
Benralizumab	1 mg	IV	**J0517**	
Bentyl	up to 20 mg	IM	J0500	
Benzocaine			J3490	
Benztropine mesylate	per 1 mg	IM, IV	**J0515**	
Berinert	10 units		J0597	
Berubigen	up to 1,000 mcg	IM, SC	J3420	
Beta amyloid	per study dose	OTH	**A9599**	
Betalin 12	up to 1,000 mcg	IM, SC	J3420	
Betameth	per 3 mg	IM, IV	J0702	
Betamethasone Acetate			J3490	

◄ **New**   ↻ **Revised**   ✔ **Reinstated**   ~~deleted~~ **Deleted**

DRUG NAME	DOSAGE	METHOD OF ADMINISTRATION	HCPCS CODE
Betamethasone Acetate & Betamethasone Sodium Phosphate	per 3 mg	IM	**J0702**
Betamethasone inhalation solution, unit dose form	per mg	INH	**J7624**
Betaseron	0.25 mg	SC	J1830
Bethanechol chloride	up to 5 mg	SC	**J0520**
Bethkis	300 mg		J7682
Bevacizumab	10 mg	IV	**J9035**
Bevacizumab-adcd	10 mg	IM	**Q5129**
Bevacizumab-awwb	10 mg	IV	**Q5107**
Bevacizumab-bvzr (Zirabev)	10 mg	IV	**Q5118**
Bezlotoxumab	10 mg	IV	**J0565**
Bicillin C-R	100,000 units		J0558
Bicillin C-R 900/300	100,000 units	IM	J0558, J0561
Bicillin L-A	100,000 units	IM	J0561
BiCNU	100 mg	IV	J9050
Biperiden lactate	per 5 mg	IM, IV	**J0190**
Bitolterol mesylate			
concentrated form	per mg	INH	**J7628**
unit dose form	per mg	INH	**J7629**
Bivalirudin	1 mg	IV	**J0583**
Blenoxane	15 units	IM, IV, SC	J9040
Bleomycin sulfate	15 units	IM, IV, SC	**J9040**
Blinatumomab	1 microgram	IV	**J9039**
Blincyto	1 mcg		J9039
Boniva	1 mg		J1740
Bortezomib	0.1 mg	IV	**J9041**
Bortezomib	0.1 mg		**J9046, J9049, J9051**
Botox	1 unit		J0585
Bravelle	75 IU		J3355
Brentuximab Vedotin	1 mg	IV	**J9042**
Brethine			
concentrated form	per 1 mg	INH	J7680
unit dose	per 1 mg	INH	J7681
	up to 1 mg	SC, IV	J3105
Bricanyl Subcutaneous	up to 1 mg	SC, IV	J3105
Brompheniramine maleate	per 10 mg	IM, SC, IV	**J0945**
Bronkephrine, *see* Ethylnorepinephrine HCl			

◄ **New**   ↵ **Revised**   ✔ **Reinstated**   ~~deleted~~ **Deleted**

DRUG NAME	DOSAGE	METHOD OF ADMINISTRATION	HCPCS CODE
Bronkosol			
concentrated form	per mg	INH	J7647, J7648
unit dose form	per mg	INH	J7649, J7650
Brovana			J7605
Budesonide inhalation solution			
concentrated form	0.25 mg	INH	J7633, J7634
unit dose form	0.5 mg	INH	J7626, J7627
Bumetanide			J3490
Bupivacaine	0.5 mg	IM	J0655, J3490 ◄
Buprenex	0.3 mg		J0592
Buprenorphine Hydrochloride	0.1 mg	IM	J0592
Buprenorphine/Naloxone	1 mg	ORAL	J0571
	< = 3 mg	ORAL	J0572
	> 3 mg but < = 6 mg	ORAL	J0573
	> 6 mg but < = 10 mg	ORAL	J0574
	> 10 mg	ORAL	J0575
Buprenorphine extended release	< = 100 mg	ORAL	Q9991
	> 100 mg	ORAL	Q9992
Burosumab-twza	1 mg	IV	J05894
Busulfan	1 mg	IV	J0594
	2 mg	ORAL	J8510
Butorphanol tartrate	1 mg		J0595
C			
C1 Esterase Inhibitor	10 units	IV	J0596-J0599
Cabazitaxel	1 mg	IV	J9043, J9064 ◄
Cabergoline	0.25 mg	ORAL	J8515
Cabote Rilpivir	2 mg/3 mg	IV	J0741
Cabotegravir	1 mg	IM	J0739
Cafcit	5 mg	IV	J0706
Caffeine citrate	5 mg	IV	J0706
Caine-1	10 mg	IV	J2001
Caine-2	10 mg	IV	J2001
Calaspargase pegol-mknl	10 units	IV	J9118
Calcijex	0.1 mcg	IM	J0636
Calcimar	up to 400 units	SC, IM	J0630
Calcitonin-salmon	up to 400 units	SC, IM	J0630
Calcitriol	0.1 mcg	IM	J0636
Calcitrol			J8499
~~Calcium Disodium Versenate~~	~~up to 1,000 mg~~	~~IV, SC, IM~~	~~J0600~~

◄ **New**   ↻ **Revised**   ✔ **Reinstated**   ~~deleted~~ **Deleted**

DRUG NAME	DOSAGE	METHOD OF ADMINISTRATION	HCPCS CODE	
Calcium gluconate	10 mg	IM	**J0611-J0613**	◄
Calcium glycerophosphate and calcium lactate	per 10 ml	IM, SC	**J0620**	
Caldolor	100 mg	IV	J1741	
Calphosan	per 10 ml	IM, SC	J0620	
Camcevi	1 mg	IV	**J1952**	
Camptosar	20 mg	IV	J9206	
Canakinumab	1 mg	SC	**J0638**	
Cancidas	5 mg		J0637	
Capecitabine	150 mg	ORAL	**J8520**	
	500 mg	ORAL	**J8521**	
Capsaicin patch	per sq cm	OTH	**J7336**	
Carbidopa 5 mg/levodopa 20 mg enteral suspension		IV	**J7340**	
Carbocaine	per 10 ml	VAR	J0670	
Carbocaine with Neo-Cobefrin	per 10 ml	VAR	J0670	
Carboplatin	50 mg	IV	**J9045**	
Carfilzomib	1 mg	IV	**J9047**	
Carimune	500 mg		J1566	
Carmustine	100 mg	IV	**J9050**	
Carnitor	per 1 g	IV	J1955	
Carticel			J7330	
Casimersen	10 mg	IV	**J1426**	
Caspofungin acetate	5 mg	IV	**J0637**	
Cathflo Activase	1 mg		J2997	
Caverject	per 1.25 mcg		J0270	
~~Cayston~~	~~500 mg~~		~~S0073~~	
Cefadyl	up to 1 g	IV, IM	J0710	
Cefazolin sodium	500 mg	IV, IM	**J0889-J0690**	◄
Cefepime hydrochloride	500 mg	IV	**J0692, J0701, J0703**	◄
Cefiderocol	10 mg	IV	J0699	
Cefizox	per 500 mg	IM, IV	J0715	
Cefotaxime sodium	per 1 g	IV, IM	**J0698**	
Cefotetan			J3490	
Cefoxitin sodium	1 g	IV, IM	**J0694**	
Ceftaroline fosamil	1 mg	IV	**J0712**	
Ceftazidime	per 500 mg	IM, IV	**J0713**	
Ceftazidime and avibactam	0.5 g/0.125 g	IV	**J0714**	
Ceftizoxime sodium	per 500 mg	IV, IM	**J0715**	
Ceftolozane 50 mg and Tazobactam 25 mg		IV	**J0695**	

◄ **New**   ↻ **Revised**   ✔ **Reinstated**   ~~deleted~~ **Deleted**

DRUG NAME	DOSAGE	METHOD OF ADMINISTRATION	HCPCS CODE
Ceftriaxone sodium	per 250 mg	IV, IM	J0696
Cefuroxime sodium, sterile	per 750 mg	IM, IV	J0697
Celestone Soluspan	per 3 mg	IM	J0702
CellCept	250 mg	ORAL	J7517
Cel-U-Jec	per 4 mg	IM, IV	Q0511
Cenacort A-40	1 mg		J3300
	per 10 mg	IM	J3301
Cenacort Forte	per 5 mg	IM	J3302
Centruroides Immune F(ab)	up to 120 mg	IV	J0716
Cephalothin sodium	up to 1 g	IM, IV	J1890
Cephapirin sodium	up to 1 g	IV, IM	J0710
Ceprotin	10 IU		J2724
Ceredase	per 10 units	IV	J0205
Cerezyme	10 units		J1786
Cerliponase alfa	1 mg	IV	J0567
Certolizumab pegol	1 mg	SC	J0717
Cerubidine	10 mg	IV	J9150
Cetirizine hydrochloride	0.5 mg	IM	J1201
Cetuximab	10 mg	IV	J9055
Chealamide	per 150 mg	IV	J3520
Chirhostim	1 mcg	IV	J2850
Chloramphenicol Sodium Succinate	up to 1 g	IV	J0720
Chlordiazepoxide HCl	up to 100 mg	IM, IV	J1990
Chloromycetin Sodium Succinate	up to 1 g	IV	J0720
Chloroprocaine	1mg		J2401-J2403 ◄
Chloroquine HCl	up to 250 mg	IM	J0390
Chlorothiazide sodium	per 500 mg	IV	J1205
Chlorpromazine	5 mg	ORAL	Q0161
Chlorpromazine HCl	up to 50 mg	IM, IV	J3230
Cholografin Meglumine	per ml		Q9961
Chorex-5	per 1,000 USP units	IM	J0725
Chorex-10	per 1,000 USP units	IM	J0725
Chorignon	per 1,000 USP units	IM	J0725
Chorionic Gonadotropin	per 1,000 USP units	IM	J0725
Choron 10	per 1,000 USP units	IM	J0725
Cidofovir	375 mg	IV	J0740
Cilastatin sodium, imipenem	per 250 mg	IV, IM	J0743
Cimzia	1 mg	SC	J0717
Cinacalcet	1 mg	ORAL	J0604

◄ **New** ↻ **Revised** ✓ **Reinstated** ~~deleted~~ **Deleted**

DRUG NAME	DOSAGE	METHOD OF ADMINISTRATION	HCPCS CODE
Cinryze	10 units		J0598
Cipro IV	200 mg	IV	J0706
Ciprofloxacin	200 mg	IV	**J0706**
otic suspension	6 mg	OTH	**J7342**
			J3490
Cisplatin, powder or solution	per 10 mg	IV	**J9060**
Cladribine	per mg	IV	**J9065**
Claforan	per 1 gm	IM, IV	J0698
Cleocin Phosphate			J3490
Clindamycin			J3490
Clindamycin phosphate	300 mg	IM	**J0736, J0737**
Clofarabine	1 mg	IV	**J9027**
Clolar	1 mg		J9027
Clonidine Hydrochloride	1 mg	Epidural	**J0735**
Coagulation factor Xa (recombinant), inactivated-zhzo (Andexxa)	10 mg		J7169
Cobex	up to 1,000 mcg	IM, SC	J3420
Codeine phosphate	per 30 mg	IM, IV, SC	**J0745**
Codimal-A	per 10 mg	IM, SC, IV	J0945
Cogentin	per 1 mg	IM, IV	J0515
Colistimethate sodium	up to 150 mg	IM, IV	**J0770**
Collagenase, Clostridium Histolyticum	0.01 mg	OTH	**J0775**
Coly-Mycin M	up to 150 mg	IM, IV	J0770
Compa-Z	up to 10 mg	IM, IV	J0780
Copanlisib	1 mg	IV	**J9057**
Compazine	up to 10 mg	IM, IV	J0780
	5 mg	ORAL	Q0164
			J8498
Compounded drug, not otherwise classified			**J7999**
Compro			J8498
Conray	per ml		Q9961
Conray 30	per ml		Q9958
Conray 43	per ml		Q9960
Copaxone	20 mg		J1595
Cophene-B	per 10 mg	IM, SC, IV	J0945
Copper contraceptive, intrauterine		OTH	**J7300**
Cordarone	30 mg	IV	J0282
Corgonject-5	per 1,000 USP units	IM	J0725
Corifact	1 IU		J7180
Corticorelin ovine triflutate	1 mcg		**J0795**

◄ **New**   ↻ **Revised**   ✔ **Reinstated**   ~~deleted~~ **Deleted**

DRUG NAME	DOSAGE	METHOD OF ADMINISTRATION	HCPCS CODE
Corticotropin	up to 40 units	IV, IM, SC	J0801-J0802 ◄
Cortisone Acetate Micronized			J3490
Cortrosyn	per 0.25 mg	IM, IV	J0835
Corvert	1 mg		J1742
Cosmegen	0.5 mg	IV	J9120
Cosyntropin	per 0.25 mg	IM, IV	J0833, J0834
Cotranzine	up to 10 mg	IM, IV	J0780
Crizanlizumab-tmca		IV	J0791
Crofab	up to 1 gram		J0840
Cromolyn Sodium			J8499
Cromolyn sodium, unit dose form	per 10 mg	INH	J7631, J7632
Crotalidae immune f(ab')2 (equine)	120 mg	IV	J0841
Crotalidae Polyvalent Immune Fab	up to 1 gram	IV	J0840
Crysticillin 600 A.S.	up to 600,000 units	IM, IV	J2510
Cubicin	1 mg		J0878
Cutaquig	100 mg	IM	J1551
Cuvitru			J7799
Cyclophosphamide	100 mg	IV	J9070
oral	25 mg	ORAL	J8530
Cyclosporine	25 mg	ORAL	J7515
	100 mg	ORAL	J7502
parenteral	250 mg	IV	J7516
Cymetra	1 cc		Q4112
Cyramza	5 mg		J9308
Cysto-Conray II	per ml		Q9958
Cystografin	per ml		Q9958
Cytarabine	100 mg	SC, IV	J9100
Cytarabine liposome	10 mg	IT	J9098
CytoGam	per vial		J0850
Cytomegalovirus immune globulin intravenous (human)	per vial	IV	J0850
Cytosar-U	100 mg	SC, IV	J9100
Cytovene	500 mg	IV	J1570
Cytoxan	100 mg	IV	J8530, J9070
D			
D-5-W, infusion	1000 cc	IV	J7070
Dacarbazine	100 mg	IV	J9130
Daclizumab	25 mg	IV	J7513
Dacogen	1 mg		J0894
Dactinomycin	0.5 mg	IV	J9120

◄ **New** ↻ **Revised** ✔ **Reinstated** ~~deleted~~ **Deleted**

DRUG NAME	DOSAGE	METHOD OF ADMINISTRATION	HCPCS CODE
Dalalone	1 mg	IM, IV, OTH	J1100
Dalalone L.A.	1 mg	IM	J1094
Dalbavancin	5 mg	IV	**J0875**
Dalteparin sodium	per 2500 IU	SC	**J1645**
Daprodustat	1 mg	oral	**J0889**
Daptomycin	1 mg	IV	**J0874, J0877, J0878**
Daratumumab	10 mg	IV	**J9145**
Darbepoetin Alfa	1 mcg	IV, SC	**J0881, J0882**
Darzalex	10 mg		J9145
Daunorubicin citrate, liposomal formulation	10 mg	IV	**J9151**
Daunorubicin HCl	10 mg	IV	**J9150**
Daunoxome	10 mg	IV	J9151
DDAVP	1 mcg	IV, SC	J2597
Decadron	1 mg	IM, IV, OTH	J1100
	0.25 mg		J8540
Decadron Phosphate	1 mg	IM, IV, OTH	J1100
Decadron-LA	1 mg	IM	J1094
Deca-Durabolin	up to 50 mg	IM	J2320
Decaject	1 mg	IM, IV, OTH	J1100
Decaject-L.A.	1 mg	IM	J1094
Decitabine	1 mg	IV	**J0893, J0894**
Decolone-50	up to 50 mg	IM	J2320
Decolone-100	up to 50 mg	IM	J2320
De-Comberol	1 mg		J1071
Deferoxamine mesylate	500 mg	IM, SC, IV	**J0895**
Definity	per ml		J3490, Q9957
Degarelix	1 mg	SC	**J9155**
Dehist	per 10 mg	IM, SC, IV	J0945
Deladumone	1 mg	IM	J3121
Deladumone OB	1 mg	IM	J3121
Delatest	1 mg	IM	J3121
Delatestadiol	1 mg	IM	J3121
Delatestryl	1 mg	IM	J3121
Delestrogen	up to 10 mg	IM	J1380
Delta-Cortef	5 mg	ORAL	J7510
Demadex	10 mg/ml	IV	J3265
Demerol HCl	per 100 mg	IM, IV, SC	J2175
Denileukin diftitox	300 mcg	IV	**J9160**

◄ **New**   ↻ **Revised**   ✔ **Reinstated**   ~~deleted~~ **Deleted**

DRUG NAME	DOSAGE	METHOD OF ADMINISTRATION	HCPCS CODE
Denosumab	1 mg	SC	**J0897**
Deoxycholic acid	1 mg	IM	J0591
DepAndro 100	1 mg		J1071
DepAndro 200	1 mg		J1071
DepAndrogyn	1 mg		J1071
DepGynogen	up to 5 mg	IM	J1000
DepMedalone 40	20 mg	IM	J1020
	40 mg	IM	J1030
	80 mg	IM	J1040
DepMedalone 80	20 mg	IM	J1020
	40 mg	IM	J1030
	80 mg	IM	J1040
DepoCyt	10 mg		J9098
Depo-estradiol cypionate	up to 5 mg	IM	**J1000**
Depogen	up to 5 mg	IM	J1000
Depoject	20 mg	IM	J1020
	40 mg	IM	J1030
	80 mg	IM	J1040
Depo-Medrol	20 mg	IM	J1020
	40 mg	IM	J1030
	80 mg	IM	J1040
Depopred-40	20 mg	IM	J1020
	40 mg	IM	J1030
	80 mg	IM	J1040
Depopred-80	20 mg	IM	J1020
	40 mg	IM	J1030
	80 mg	IM	J1040
Depo-Provera Contraceptive	1 mg		J1050
Depotest	1 mg		J1071
Depo-Testadiol	1 mg		J1071
Depo-Testosterone	1 mg		J1071
Depotestrogen	1 mg		J1071
Dermagraft	per square centimeter		Q4106
Desferal Mesylate	500 mg	IM, SC, IV	J0895
Desmopressin acetate	1 mcg	IV, SC	**J2597**
Dexacen-4	1 mg	IM, IV, OTH	J1100
Dexacen LA-8	1 mg	IM	J1094

◀ **New**   ⟲ **Revised**   ✓ **Reinstated**   ~~deleted~~ **Deleted**

DRUG NAME	DOSAGE	METHOD OF ADMINISTRATION	HCPCS CODE
Dexamethasone			
concentrated form	per mg	INH	J7637
intravitreal implant	0.1 mg	OTH	J7312
lacrimal ophthalmic insert	0.1 mg	OTH	J1096
unit form	per mg	INH	J7638
oral	0.25 mg	ORAL	J8540
acetate	1 mg	IM	J1094
sodium phosphate	1 mg	IM, IV, OTH	J1100
Dexasone	1 mg	IM, IV, OTH	J1100
Dexasone L.A.	1 mg	IM	J1094
Dexferrum	50 mg		J1750
Dexone	0.25 mg	ORAL	J8540
	1 mg	IM, IV, OTH	J1100
Dexone LA	1 mg	IM	J1094
Dexpak	0.25 mg	ORAL	J8540
Dexrazoxane hydrochloride	250 mg	IV	J1190
Dextran 40	500 ml	IV	J7100
Dextran 75	500 ml	IV	J7110
Dextrose 5%/normal saline solution	500 ml = 1 unit	IV	J7042
Dextrose/water (5%)	500 ml = 1 unit	IV	J7060
D.H.E. 45	per 1 mg		J1110
Diamox	up to 500 mg	IM, IV	J1120
Diazepam	up to 5 mg	IM, IV	J3360
Diazoxide	up to 300 mg	IV	J1730
Dibent	up to 20 mg	IM	J0500
Diclofenac sodium	37.5	IV	J1130
Dicyclomine HCl	up to 20 mg	IM	J0500
Didronel	per 300 mg	IV	J1436
Diethylstilbestrol diphosphate	250 mg	IV	J9165
Diflucan	200 mg	IV	J1450
DigiFab	per vial		J1162
Digoxin	up to 0.5 mg	IM, IV	J1160
Digoxin immune fab (ovine)	per vial		J1162
Dihydrex	up to 50 mg	IV, IM	J1200
	50 mg	ORAL	Q0163
Dihydroergotamine mesylate	per 1 mg	IM, IV	J1110
Dilantin	per 50 mg	IM, IV	J1165
Dilaudid	up to 4 mg	SC, IM, IV	J1170
	250 mg	OTH	S0092

◄ New   ↻ Revised   ✔ Reinstated   ~~deleted~~ **Deleted**

DRUG NAME	DOSAGE	METHOD OF ADMINISTRATION	HCPCS CODE
Dilocaine	10 mg	IV	J2001
Dilomine	up to 20 mg	IM	J0500
Dilor	up to 500 mg	IM	J1180
Dimenhydrinate	up to 50 mg	IM, IV	**J1240**
Dimercaprol	per 100 mg	IM	**J0470**
Dimethyl sulfoxide	50%, 50 ml	OTH	J1212
Dinate	up to 50 mg	IM, IV	J1240
Dioval	up to 10 mg	IM	J1380
Dioval 40	up to 10 mg	IM	J1380
Dioval XX	up to 10 mg	IM	J1380
Diphenacen-50	up to 50 mg	IV, IM	J1200
	50 mg	ORAL	Q0163
Diphenhydramine HCl			
IV	up to 50 mg	IV, IM	**J1200**
oral	50 mg	ORAL	**Q0163**
Diprivan	10 mg		J2704
			J3490
Dipyridamole	per 10 mg	IV	**J1245**
Disotate	per 150 mg	IV	J3520
Di-Spaz	up to 20 mg	IM	J0500
Ditate-DS	1 mg	IM	J3121
Diuril Sodium	per 500 mg	IV	J1205
D-Med 80	20 mg	IM	J1020
	40 mg	IM	J1030
	80 mg	IM	J1040
DMSO, Dimethyl sulfoxide 50%	50 ml	OTH	**J1212**
Dobutamine HCl	per 250 mg	IV	**J1250**
Dobutrex	per 250 mg	IV	J1250
Docefrez	1 mg		J9171
Docetaxel	20 mg	IV	**J9170**
Dolasetron mesylate			
injection	10 mg	IV	**J1260**
tablets	100 mg	ORAL	**Q0180**
Dolophine HCl	up to 10 mg	IM, SC	J1230
Dommanate	up to 50 mg	IM, IV	J1240
Donbax	10 mg		J1267
Dopamine	40 mg		**J1265**
Dopamine HCl	40 mg		**J1265**
Doribax	10 mg		J1267
Doripenem	10 mg	IV	**J1267**

◀ **New**   ↻ **Revised**   ✔ **Reinstated**   ~~deleted~~ **Deleted**

DRUG NAME	DOSAGE	METHOD OF ADMINISTRATION	HCPCS CODE
Dornase alpha, unit dose form	per mg	INH	J7639
Dotarem	0.1 ml		A9575
Doxercalciferol	1 mcg	IV	J1270
Doxil	10 mg	IV	J9000, Q2050
Doxorubicin HCL	10 mg	IV	J9000
Doxy	100 mg		J3490
Dramamine	up to 50 mg	IM, IV	J1240
Dramanate	up to 50 mg	IM, IV	J1240
Dramilin	up to 50 mg	IM, IV	J1240
Dramocen	up to 50 mg	IM, IV	J1240
Dramoject	up to 50 mg	IM, IV	J1240
Dronabinol	2.5 mg	ORAL	Q0167
Droperidol	up to 5 mg	IM, IV	J1790
Droperidol and fentanyl citrate	up to 2 ml ampule	IM, IV	J1810
Droxia		ORAL	J8999
Drug administered through a metered dose inhaler		INH	J3535
DTIC-Dome	100 mg	IV	J9130
Dua-Gen L.A.	1 mg	IM	J3121
DuoNeb	up to 2.5 mg		J7620
Duopa	20 ml		J7340
Duoval P.A.	1 mg	IM	J3121
Durabolin	up to 50 mg	IM	J2320
Duracillin A.S.	up to 600,000 units	IM, IV	J2510
Duraclon	1 mg	Epidural	J0735
Dura-Estrin	up to 5 mg	IM	J1000
Duragen-10	up to 10 mg	IM	J1380
Duragen-20	up to 10 mg	IM	J1380
Duragen-40	up to 10 mg	IM	J1380
Duralone-40	20 mg	IM	J1020
	40 mg	IM	J1030
	80 mg	IM	J1040
Duralone-80	20 mg	IM	J1020
	40 mg	IM	J1030
	80 mg	IM	J1040
Duralutin, *see* Hydroxyprogesterone Caproate			
Duramorph	up to 10 mg	IM, IV, SC	J2270, J2274
Duratest-100	1 mg		J1071
Duratest-200	1 mg		J1071
Duratestrin	1 mg		J1071
Durathate-200	1 mg	IM	J3121

◄ **New**   ⟲ **Revised**   ✔ **Reinstated**   ~~deleted~~ **Deleted**

DRUG NAME	DOSAGE	METHOD OF ADMINISTRATION	HCPCS CODE
Durvalumab	10 mg	IV	J9173
Dymenate	up to 50 mg	IM, IV	J1240
Dyphylline	up to 500 mg	IM	J1180
Dysport	5 units		J0586
Dalvance	5 mg		J0875
E			
Ecallantide	1 mg	SC	J1290
Eculizumab	10 mg	IV	J1300
Edaravone	1 mg	IV	J1301
Edetate calcium disodium	up to 1,000 mg	IV, SC, IM	J0600
Edetate disodium	per 150 mg	IV	J3520
Efgartigimod	2 mg	IM	J9332
Eflapegrastim-xnst	0.1 mg	IM	J1449 ◄
Elaprase	1 mg		J1743
Elavil	up to 20 mg	IM	J1320
Elelyso	10 units		J3060
Eligard	7.5 mg		J9217
Elitek	0.5 mg		J2783
Ellence	2 mg		J9178
Elliotts B solution	1 ml	OTH	J9175
Eloctate	per IU		J7205
Elosulfase alfa	1 mg	IV	J1322
Elotuzumab	1 mg	IV	J9176
Eloxatin	0.5 mg		J9263
Elspar	10,000 units	IV, IM	J9020
Emapalunab-lzsg	1 mg	IV	J9210
Emend			J1453, J8501
Emete-Con, *see* Benzquinamide			
Eminase	30 units	IV	J0350
Empliciti	1 mg		J9176
Enbrel	25 mg	IM, IV	J1438
Endrate ethylenediamine-tetra-acetic acid	per 150 mg	IV	J3520
Enfortumab vedotin-ejfv	0.25 mg	IM	J9177
Enfuvirtide	1 mg	SC	J1324
Engerix-B			J3490
Enovil	up to 20 mg	IM	J1320
Enoxaparin sodium	10 mg	SC	J1650
Entyvio			J3380
Eovist	1 ml		A9581
Epinephrine			J0173, J7799 ◄

◄ New   ⮌ Revised   ✔ Reinstated   ~~deleted~~ **Deleted**

DRUG NAME	DOSAGE	METHOD OF ADMINISTRATION	HCPCS CODE
Epinephrine, adrenalin	0.1 mg	SC, IM	J0171
Epirubicin hydrochloride	2 mg		J9178
Epoetin alfa, ESRD use	100 units	IV, SC	Q4081
Epoetin alfa, non-ESRD use	1000 units	IV	J0885
Epoetin alfa-epbx (Retacrit) ESRD use	100 units	IV	Q5105
Epoetin alfa-epbx (Retacrit) non-ESRD use	1000 units	IV	Q5106
Epoetin beta, ESRD use	1 mcg	IV	J0887
Epoetin beta, non-ESRD use	1 mcg	IV	J0888
Epogen	1,000 units		J0885
			Q4081
Epoprostenol	0.5 mg	IV	J1325
Eptifibatide, injection	5 mg	IM, IV	J1327
Eravacycline	1 mg	IV	J0122
Eraxis	1 mg	IV	J0348
Erbitux	10 mg		J9055
Ergonovine maleate	up to 0.2 mg	IM, IV	J1330
Eribulin mesylate	0.1 mg	IV	J9179
Erivedge	150 mg		J8999
Ertapenem sodium	500 mg	IM, IV	J1335
Erwinase	1,000 units	IV, IM	J9019
	10,000 units	IV, IM	J9020
Erythromycin lactobionate	500 mg	IV	J1364
Esmolol hydrochloride	10 mg	IM	J1805, J1806
Estra-D	up to 5 mg	IM	J1000
Estradiol			
L.A.	up to 10 mg	IM	J1380
L.A. 20	up to 10 mg	IM	J1380
L.A. 40	up to 10 mg	IM	J1380
Estradiol cypionate	up to 5 mg	IM	J1000
Estradiol valerate	up to 10 mg	IM	J1380
Estra-L 20	up to 10 mg	IM	J1380
Estra-L 40	up to 10 mg	IM	J1380
Estra-Testrin	1 mg	IM	J3121
Estro-Cyp	up to 5 mg	IM	J1000
Estrogen, conjugated	per 25 mg	IV, IM	J1410
Estroject L.A.	up to 5 mg	IM	J1000
Estrone	per 1 mg	IM	J1435
Estrone 5	per 1 mg	IM	J1435
Estrone Aqueous	per 1 mg	IM	J1435
Estronol	per 1 mg	IM	J1435

◄ **New**　↻ **Revised**　✓ **Reinstated**　deleted **Deleted**

DRUG NAME	DOSAGE	METHOD OF ADMINISTRATION	HCPCS CODE
Estronol-L.A.	up to 5 mg	IM	J1000
Etanercept, injection	25 mg	IM, IV	J1438
Etelcalcetide	0.1 mg	IV	Q4078
Eteplirsen	10 mg	IV	J1428
Ethamolin	100 mg		J1430
Ethanolamine	100 mg		J1430, J3490
Ethyol	500 mg	IV	J0207
Etidronate disodium	per 300 mg	IV	J1436
Etonogestrel implant			J7307
Etopophos	10 mg	IV	J9181
Etoposide	10 mg	IV	J9181
oral	50 mg	ORAL	J8560
Etranacogene dezaparvovec-drlb	per dose	IM	J1411 ◄
Euflexxa	per dose	OTH	J7323
Everolimus	0.25 mg	ORAL	J7527
Everone	1 mg	IM	J3121
Evinacumab-dgnb	5 mg	IV	J1305
Evomela	50 mg		J9245
Eylea	1 mg	OTH	J0178
F			
Fabrazyme	1 mg	IV	J0180
Factor IX			
anti-hemophilic factor, purified, non-recombinant	per IU	IV	J7193
anti-hemophilic factor, recombinant	per IU	IV	J7195, J7200-J7202
complex	per IU	IV	J7194
coagulation (recombinant)	1 IU	IV	J7213 ◄
Factor VIIa (coagulation factor, recombinant)	1 mcg	IV	J7189
Factor VIII (anti-hemophilic factor)	per IU	IV	J7208
human	per IU	IV	J7190
porcine	per IU	IV	J7191
recombinant	per IU	IV	J7182, J7185, J7192, J7188
Factor VIII (anti-hemophilic factor, recombinant)			
(Afstyla)	per IU	IV	J7210
Esperoct	per IU	IV	J7204
Jivi	per IU	IV	J7208
(Kovaltry)	per IU	IV	J7211
Novoeight	per IU	IV	J7182
Obizur	per IU	IV	J7188
Xyntha	per IU	IV	J7185

◄ New   ↻ Revised   ✔ Reinstated   ~~deleted~~ Deleted

DRUG NAME	DOSAGE	METHOD OF ADMINISTRATION	HCPCS CODE
Factor VIII, anti-hemophilic factor (recombinant)(esperoct)	per IU	IV	J7204
Factor VIII (recombinant)	per IU	IV	J7205, J7207, J7209, J7214 ◄
Factor X (human)	per IU	IV	J7175
Factor XIII A-subunit (recombinant)	per IU	IV	J7181
Factors, other hemophilia clotting	per IU	IV	J7196
Factrel	per 100 mcg	SC, IV	J1620
Fam-trastuzumab deruxtecan-nxki	1 mg	IM	J9358
Famotidine			J3490
Faricimab-svoa	0.1 mg	IM	J2777
Faslodex	25 mg		J9395
Fecal microbiota	1 ml		J1440 ◄
Feiba NF			J7198
Feiba VH Immuno	per IU	IV	J7196
Fentanyl citrate	0.1 mg	IM, IV	J3010
Feraheme	1 mg		Q0138, Q0139
Ferric carboxymaltose	1 mg	IV	J1439
Ferric pyrophosphate citrate powder	0.1 mg of iron	IV	J1444
Ferric pyrophosphate citrate solution (triferic)	0.1 mg of iron	IV	J1443
Ferric pyrophosphate citrate solution (triferic avnu)	0.1 mg of iron	IV	J1445
Ferrlecit	12.5 mg		J2916
Ferumoxytol	1 mg		Q0138, Q0139
Filgrastim-aafi	1 mcg	IV	Q5110
Filgrastim			
(G-CSF)	1 mcg	SC, IV	J1442, Q5101
(TBO)	1 mcg	IV	J1447
Firazyr	1 mg	SC	J1744
Firmagon	1 mg		J9155
Flebogamma	500 mg	IV	J1572
	1 cc		J1460
Flexoject	up to 60 mg	IV, IM	J2360
Flexon	up to 60 mg	IV, IM	J2360
Flolan	0.5 mg	IV	J1325
Flo-Pred	5 mg		J7510
Florbetaben f18, diagnostic	per study dose	IV	Q9983
Floxuridine	500 mg	IV	J9200
Fluconazole	200 mg	IV	J1450
Fludara	1 mg	ORAL	J8562
	50 mg	IV	J9185
Fludarabine phosphate	1 mg	ORAL	J8562
	50 mg	IV	J9185

◄ New   ↪ Revised   ✔ Reinstated   ~~deleted~~ Deleted

DRUG NAME	DOSAGE	METHOD OF ADMINISTRATION	HCPCS CODE
Flunisolide inhalation solution, unit dose form	per mg	INH	J7641
Fluocinolone		OTH	J7311, J7313
Fluocinolone acetonide (Yutiq)	0.01 mg	OTH	J7314
Fluorouracil	500 mg	IV	J9190
Fluphenazine decanoate	up to 25 mg		J2680
Flutamide			J8999
Flutemetamol f18, diagnostic	per study dose	IV	Q9982
Folex	5 mg	IA, IM, IT, IV	J9250
	50 mg	IA, IM, IT, IV	J9260
Folex PFS	5 mg	IA, IM, IT, IV	J9250
	50 mg	IA, IM, IT, IV	J9260
Follutein	per 1,000 USP units	IM	J0725
Folotyn	1 mg		J9307
Fomepizole	15 mg		J1451
Fomivirsen sodium	1.65 mg	Intraocular	J1452
Fondaparinux sodium	0.5 mg	SC	J1652
Formoterol	12 mcg	INH	J7640
Formoterol fumarate	20 mcg	INH	J7606
Fortaz	per 500 mg	IM, IV	J0713
Fosaprepitant	1 mg	IV	J1453, J1456
Foscarnet sodium	per 1,000 mg	IV	J1455
Foscavir	per 1,000 mg	IV	J1455
Fosnetupitant 235 mg and palonosetron 0.25 mg		IV	J1454
Fosphenytoin	50 mg	IV	Q2009
Fragmin	per 2,500 IU		J1645
Fremanezumab-vfrm	1 mg	IV	J3031
FUDR	500 mg	IV	J9200
Fulvestrant	25 mg	IM	J9393, J9394, J9395
Fungizone intravenous	50 mg	IV	J0285
Furomide M.D.	up to 20 mg	IM, IV	J1940
Furosemide	up to 20 mg	IM, IV	J1940, J1941 ◄
G			
Gablofen	10 mg		J0475
	50 mcg		J0476
Gadavist	0.1 ml		A9585
Gadopiclenol	1 ml	IM	A9573 ◄
Gadoxetate disodium	1 ml	IV	A9581
Gallium nitrate	1 mg	IV	J1457
Galsulfase	1 mg	IV	J1458

◄ New   ⮌ Revised   ✔ Reinstated   ~~deleted~~ Deleted

DRUG NAME	DOSAGE	METHOD OF ADMINISTRATION	HCPCS CODE
Gamastan	1 cc	IM	J1460
	over 10 cc	IM	J1560
Gamma globulin	1 cc	IM	J1460
	over 10 cc	IM	J1560
Gammagard Liquid	500 mg	IV	J1569
Gammagard S/D			J1566
GammaGraft	per square centimeter		Q4111
Gammaplex	500 mg	IV	J1557
Gammar	1 cc	IM	J1460
	over 10 cc	IM	J1560
Gammar-IV, *see* Immune globin intravenous (human)			
Gamulin RH			
immune globulin, human	100 IU		J2791
	1 dose package, 300 mcg	IM	J2790
immune globulin, human, solvent detergent	100 IU	IV	J2792
Gamunex	500 mg	IV	J1561
Ganciclovir, implant	4.5 mg	OTH	J7310
Ganciclovir sodium	500 mg	IV	J1570, J1574
Ganirelix			J3490
Garamycin, gentamicin	up to 80 mg	IM, IV	J1580
Gastrografin	per ml		Q9963
Gatifloxacin	10 mg	IV	J1590
Gazyva	10 mg		J9301
Gefitinib	250 mg	ORAL	J8565
Gel-One	per dose	OTH	J7326
Gemcitabine HCl	200 mg	IV	J9201, J9196
Gemcitabine HCl, not otherwise specified	200 mg	IV	J9201
Gemcitabine HCl (Infugem)	100 mg	IV	J9198
Gemsar	200 mg	IV	J9201
Gemtuzumab ozogamicin	5 mg	IV	J9300
Gengraf	100 mg		J7502
	25 mg	ORAL	J7515
Genotropin	1 mg		J2941
Gentamicin Sulfate	up to 80 mg	IM, IV	J1580, J7699
Gentran	500 ml	IV	J7100
Gentran 75	500 ml	IV	J7110
Geodon	10 mg		J3486
Gesterol 50	per 50 mg		J2675
Givosiran	0.5 mg	IM	J0223
Glassia	10 mg	IV	J0257

◄ **New**   ↺ **Revised**   ✔ **Reinstated**   ~~deleted~~ **Deleted**

DRUG NAME	DOSAGE	METHOD OF ADMINISTRATION	HCPCS CODE
Glatiramer Acetate	20 mg	SC	J1595
Gleevec (Film-Coated)	400 mg		J8999
GlucaGen	per 1 mg		J1610
Glucagon HCl	per 1 mg	SC, IM, IV	J1610, J1611
Glukor	per 1,000 USP units	IM	J0725
Glycopyrrolate			
concentrated form	per 1 mg	INH	J7642
unit dose form	per 1 mg	INH	J7643
Gold sodium thiomalate	up to 50 mg	IM	J1600
Golimumab	1 mg	IV	J1602
Golodirsen	10 mg	IM	J1429
Gonadorelin HCl	per 100 mcg	SC, IV	J1620
Gonal-F			J3490
Gonic	per 1,000 USP units	IM	J0725
Goserelin acetate implant	per 3.6 mg	SC	J9202
Graftjacket	per square centimeter		Q4107
Graftjacket Xpress	1 cc		Q4113
Granisetron HCl			
extended release	0.1 mg	IV	J1627
injection	100 mcg	IV	J1626
oral	1 mg	ORAL	Q0166
Guselkumab	1 mg	IV	J1628
Gynogen L.A. A10	up to 10 mg	IM	J1380
Gynogen L.A. A20	up to 10 mg	IM	J1380
Gynogen L.A. A40	up to 10 mg	IM	J1380
H			
Halaven	0.1 mg		J9179
Haldol	up to 5 mg	IM, IV	J1630
Haloperidol	up to 5 mg	IM, IV	J1630
Haloperidol decanoate	per 50 mg	IM	J1631
Haloperidol Lactate	up to 5 mg		J1630
Hectoral	1 mcg	IV	J1270
Helixate FS	per IU		J7192
Hemin	1 mg		J1640
Hemofil M	per IU	IV	J7190
Hemophilia clotting factors (e.g., anti-inhibitors)	per IU	IV	J7198
NOC	per IU	IV	J7199
Hepagam B	0.5 ml	IM	J1571
	0.5 ml	IV	J1573
Heparin sodium	1,000 units	IV, SC	J1643, J1644

◀ **New**   ↪ **Revised**   ✔ **Reinstated**   ~~deleted~~ **Deleted**

DRUG NAME	DOSAGE	METHOD OF ADMINISTRATION	HCPCS CODE
Heparin sodium (heparin lock flush)	10 units	IV	J1642
Heparin Sodium (Procine)	per 1,000 units		J1644
Hep-Lock	10 units	IV	J1642
Hep-Lock U/P	10 units	IV	J1642
Herceptin	10 mg	IV	J9355
Hexabrix 320	per ml		Q9967
Hexadrol Phosphate	1 mg	IM, IV, OTH	J1100
Hexaminolevulinate hydrochloride	100 mg	IV	A9589
Histaject	per 10 mg	IM, SC, IV	J0945
Histerone 50	up to 50 mg	IM	J3140
Histerone 100	up to 50 mg	IM	J3140
Histrelin			
acetate	10 mcg		J1675
implant	50 mg	OTH	J9225, J9226
Hizentra, *see* Immune globulin			
Humalog	per 5 units		J1815
	per 50 units		J1817
Human fibrinogen concentrate	100 mg	IV	J7178
Human fibrinogen concentrate (fibryga)	1 mg	IV	J7177
Humate-P	per IU		J7187
Humatrope	1 mg		J2941
Humira	20 mg		J0135
Humulin	per 5 units		J1815
	per 50 units		J1817
Hyalgan, Spurtaz or VISCO-3	per dose	IA	J7321
Hyaluronan or derivative	per dose	IV	J7327
Durolane	1 mg	IA	J7318
Gel-Syn	0.1 mg	IA	J7328
Gelsyn-3	0.1 mg	IV	J7328
Gen Visc 850	1 mg	IA	J7320
Hyalgan or supartz	per dose	IA	J7321
Hymovis	1 mg	IA	J7322
Synojoynt	1 mg	VAR	J7331
Triluron	1 mg	IV	J7332
Trivisc	1 mg	IV	J7329
Hyaluronic Acid			J3490
Hyaluronidase	up to 150 units	SC, IV	J3470
Hyaluronidase			
ovine	up to 999 units	VAR	J3471
ovine	per 1000 units	VAR	J3472
recombinant	1 usp	SC	J3473

◀ **New**   ↻ **Revised**   ✔ **Reinstated**   deleted **Deleted**

DRUG NAME	DOSAGE	METHOD OF ADMINISTRATION	HCPCS CODE
Hyate:C	per IU	IV	J7191
Hybolin Decanoate	up to 50 mg	IM	J2320
Hycamtin	0.25 mg	ORAL	J8705
	4 mg	IV	J9351
Hydralazine HCl	up to 20 mg	IV, IM	J0360
Hydrate	up to 50 mg	IM, IV	J1240
Hydrea			J8999
Hydrocortisone acetate	up to 25 mg	IV, IM, SC	J1700
Hydrocortisone sodium phosphate	up to 50 mg	IV, IM, SC	J1710
Hydrocortisone succinate sodium	up to 100 mg	IV, IM, SC	J1720
Hydrocortone Acetate	up to 25 mg	IV, IM, SC	J1700
Hydrocortone Phosphate	up to 50 mg	IM, IV, SC	J1710
Hydromorphone HCl	up to 4 mg	SC, IM, IV	J1170
Hydroxyprogesterone Caproate	1 mg	IM	J1725
(Makena)	10 mg	IV	J1726
NOS	10 mg	IV	J1729
Hydroxyurea			J8999
Hydroxyzine HCl	up to 25 mg	IM	J3410
Hydroxyzine Pamoate	25 mg	ORAL	Q0177
Hylan G-F 20		OTH	J7322
Hylenex	1 USP unit		J3473
Hyoscyamine sulfate	up to 0.25 mg	SC, IM, IV	J1980
Hyperrho S/D	300 mcg		J2790
	100 IU		J2792
Hyperstat IV	up to 300 mg	IV	J1730
Hyper-Tet	up to 250 units	IM	J1670
HypRho-D	300 mcg	IM	J2790
			J2791
	50 mcg		J2788
Hyrexin-50	up to 50 mg	IV, IM	J1200
Hyzine-50	up to 25 mg	IM	J3410
I			
Ibalizumab-uiyk	10 mg	IV	J1746
Ibandronate sodium	1 mg	IV	J1740
Ibuprofen	100 mg	IV	J1741
Ibutilide fumarate	1 mg	IV	J1742
Icatibant	1 mg	SC	J1744
Idamycin	5 mg	IV	J9211
Idarubicin HCl	5 mg	IV	J9211
Idursulfase	1 mg	IV	J1743

◄ **New**   ↻ **Revised**   ✔ **Reinstated**   ~~deleted~~ **Deleted**

DRUG NAME	DOSAGE	METHOD OF ADMINISTRATION	HCPCS CODE
Ifex	1 g	IV	J9208
Ifosfamide	1 g	IV	J9208
Ilaris	1 mg		J0638
Iloprost	20 mcg	INH	Q4074
Ilotycin, *see* Erythromycin lactobionate			
Iluvien	0.01 mg		J7313
Imferon	50 mg		J1750
Imiglucerase	10 units	IV	J1786
Imipenem 4 mg, cilistatin 4 mg, relebactam 2 mg			J0742
Imitrex	6 mg	SC	J3030
Imlygic	per 1 million plaque forming units		J9325, J9999
Immune globulin			
Asceniv	500 mg	IV	J1554
Bivigam	500 mg	IV	J1556
Cuvitru	100 mg	IV	J1555
Flebogamma	500 mg	IV	J1572
Gammagard Liquid	500 mg	IV	J1569
Gammaplex	500 mg	IV	J1557
Gamunex	500 mg	IV	J1561
HepaGam B	0.5 ml	IM	J1571
	0.5 ml	IV	J1573
Hizentra	100 mg	SC	J1559
Hyaluronidase, (HYQVIA)	100 mg	IV	J1575
NOS	500 mg	IV	J1566, J1599
Octagam	500 mg	IV	J1568
Panzyga	500 mg	IV	J1576
Privigen	500 mg	IV	J1459
Rhophylac	100 IU	IM	J2791
Subcutaneous	100 mg	SC	J1562
Xembify	100 mg	IM	J1558
Immunosuppressive drug, not otherwise classified			J7599
Imuran	50 mg	ORAL	J7500
	100 mg	IV	J7501
Inapsine	up to 5 mg	IM, IV	J1790
Inclisiran	1 mg	IM	J1306
Incobotulinumtoxin type A	1 unit	IM	J0588
Increlex	1 mg		J2170
Inderal	up to 1 mg	IV	J1800
Inebilizumab-cdon	1 mg	IV	J1823

◀ **New**   ↻ **Revised**   ✔ **Reinstated**   ~~deleted~~ **Deleted**

DRUG NAME	DOSAGE	METHOD OF ADMINISTRATION	HCPCS CODE
Infed	50 mg		J1750
Infergen	1 mcg	SC	J9212
Inflectra			Q5102
Infliximab			
dyyb	10 mg	IM, IV	Q5103
abda	10 mg	IM, IV	Q5104
axxq, biosimilar, (AVSOLA)	10 mg	IM, IV	Q5121
qbtx	10 mg	IM, IV	Q5109
Infumorph	10 mg		J2274
Injectafer	1 mg		J1439
Injection factor XL, glycopegylated	1 IU	IV	J7203
Injection sulfur hexafluoride lipid microspheres	per ml	IV	Q9950
Innohep	1,000 iu	SC	J1655
Innovar	up to 2 ml ampule	IM, IV	J1810
Inotuzumab orogamicin	0.1 mg	IV	J9229
Insulin	5 units, 50 units	SC	J1811–J1815 ◄
Insulin-Humalog	per 50 units		J1817
Insulin lispro	50 units	SC	J1817
Intal, unit dose form	per 10 mg	INH	J7631, J7632
Integra			
Bilayer Matrix Wound Dressing (BMWD)	per square centimeter		Q4104
Dermal Regeneration Template (DRT)	per square centimeter		Q4105
Flowable Wound Matrix	1 cc		Q4114
Matrix	per square centimeter		Q4108
Integrilin IV injection	5 mg	IM, IV	J1327
Interferon alfa-2a, recombinant	3 million units	SC, IM	J9213
Interferon alfa-2b, recombinant	1 million units	SC, IM	J9214
Interferon alfa-n3 (human leukocyte derived)	250,000 IU	IM	J9215
Interferon alphacon-1, recombinant	1 mcg	SC	J9212
Interferon beta-1a	30 mcg	IM	J1826
	1 mcg	IM	Q3027
	1 mcg	SC	Q3028
Interferon beta-1b	0.25 mg	SC	J1830
Interferon gamma-1b	3 million units	SC	J9216
Intrauterine copper contraceptive		OTH	J7300
Intron-A	1 million units		J9214
Invanz	500 mg		J1335
Invega Sustenna	1 mg		J2426
Ipilimumab	1 mg	IV	J9228

◄ **New**   ⊃ **Revised**   ✔ **Reinstated**   ~~deleted~~ **Deleted**

DRUG NAME	DOSAGE	METHOD OF ADMINISTRATION	HCPCS CODE
Ipratropium bromide, unit dose form	per mg	INH	J3535, J7620, J7644, J7645
Irinotecan	20 mg	IV	J9206, J9205
Iron dextran	50 mg	IV, IM	J1750
Iron oxide, superparamagnetic	per study dose		A9697
Iron sucrose	1 mg	IV	J1756
Irrigation solution for Tx of bladder calculi	per 50 ml	OTH	Q2004
Isatuximab-irfc	10 mg	IV	J9227
Isavuconazonium	1 mg	IV	J1833
Isocaine HCl	per 10 ml	VAR	J0670
Isoetharine HCl			
concentrated form	per mg	INH	J7647, J7648
unit dose form	per mg	INH	J7649, J7650
Isoproterenol HCl			
concentrated form	per mg	INH	J7657, J7658
unit dose form	per mg	INH	J7659, J7660
Isovue	per ml		Q9966, Q9967
Isuprel			
concentrated form	per mg	INH	J7657, J7658
unit dose form	per mg	INH	J7659, J7660
Itraconazole	50 mg	IV	J1835
Ixabepilone	1 mg	IV	J9207
Ixempra	1 mg		J9207
J			
Jemperli	10 mg	IV	J9272
Jenamicin	up to 80 mg	IM, IV	J1580
Jetrea	0.125 mg		J7316
Jevtana	1 mg		J9043
K			
Kabikinase	per 250,000 IU	IV	J2995
Kadcyla	1 mg		J9354
Kalbitor	1 mg		J1290
~~Kaleinate~~	~~per 10 ml~~	~~IV~~	~~J0610~~
Kanamycin sulfate	up to 75 mg	IM, IV	J1850
	up to 500 mg	IM, IV	J1840
Kantrex	up to 75 mg	IM, IV	J1850
	up to 500 mg	IM, IV	J1840
Keflin	up to 1 g	IM, IV	J1890
Kefurox	per 750 mg		J0697
Kefzol	500 mg	IV, IM	J0690

◀ **New**   ↩ **Revised**   ✔ **Reinstated**   ~~deleted~~ **Deleted**

DRUG NAME	DOSAGE	METHOD OF ADMINISTRATION	HCPCS CODE
Kenaject-40	1 mg		J3300
	per 10 mg	IM	J3301
Kenalog-10	1 mg		J3300
	per 10 mg	IM	J3301
Kenalog-40	1 mg		J3300
	per 10 mg	IM	J3301
Kepivance	50 mcg		J2425
Keppra	10 mg		J1953
Keroxx	1 cc	IV	Q4202
Kestrone 5	per 1 mg	IM	J1435
Ketorolac tromethamine	per 15 mg	IM, IV	J1885
Key-Pred 25	up to 1 ml	IM	J2650
Key-Pred 50	up to 1 ml	IM	J2650
Key-Pred-SP, see Prednisolone sodium phosphate			
Keytruda	1 mg		J9271
K-Flex	up to 60 mg	IV, IM	J2360
Khapzory	0.5 mg	IV	J0642
Kinevac	5 mcg	IV	J2805
Kitabis PAK	per 300 mg		J7682
Klebcil	up to 75 mg	IM, IV	J1850
	up to 500 mg	IM, IV	J1840
Koate-HP (anti-hemophilic factor)			
human	per IU	IV	J7190
porcine	per IU	IV	J7191
recombinant	per IU	IV	J7192
Kogenate			
human	per IU	IV	J7190
porcine	per IU	IV	J7191
recombinant	per IU	IV	J7192
Konakion	per 1 mg	IM, SC, IV	J3430
Konyne-80	per IU	IV	J7194
Krystexxa	1 mg		J2507
Kyleena	19.5 mg	OTH	J7296
Kyprolis	1 mg		J9047
Kytril	1 mg	ORAL	Q0166
	1 mg	IV	S0091
	100 mcg	IV	J1626
L			
L.A.E. 20	up to 10 mg	IM	J1380
Labetalol hydrochloride	5 mg	IM	J1920, J1921

◀ **New**   ↺ **Revised**   ✓ **Reinstated**   ~~deleted~~ **Deleted**

DRUG NAME	DOSAGE	METHOD OF ADMINISTRATION	HCPCS CODE
Laetrile, Amygdalin, vitamin B-17			**J3570**
Lanadelumab-flyo	1 mg	IV	**J0593**
Lanoxin	up to 0.5 mg	IM, IV	J1160
Lanreotide	1 mg	SC	**J1930, J1932**
Lantus	per 5 units		J1815
Largon, *see* Propiomazine HCl			
Laronidase	0.1 mg	IV	**J1931**
Lasix	up to 20 mg	IM, IV	J1940
L-Caine	10 mg	IV	J2001
Lecanemab-irmb	1 mg	IM	**J0174** ◀
Lefamulin	1 mg		**J0691**
Lemtrada	1 mg		J0202
Lenacapavir	1 mg	IM	**J1961** ◀
Lepirudin	50 mg		**J1945**
Leucovorin calcium	per 50 mg	IM, IV	**J0640**
Leukeran			J8999
Leukine	50 mcg	IV	J2820
Leuprolide acetate	per 1 mg	IM	**J9218**
Leuprolide acetate (for depot suspension)	per 3.75 mg	IM	**J1950**
	7.5 mg	IM	**J1954, J9217** ◀
Leuprolide acetate (for depot suspension) (fensolvi)	0.25 mg	IV	**J1951**
Leuprolide acetate implant	65 mg	OTH	**J9219**
Leustatin	per mg	IV	J9065
Levalbuterol HCl			
concentrated form	0.5 mg	INH	**J7607, J7612**
unit dose form	0.5 mg	INH	**J7614, J7615**
Levaquin I.U.	250 mg	IV	J1956
Levetiracetam	10 mg	IV	**J1953**
Levocarnitine	per 1 gm	IV	**J1955**
Levo-Dromoran	up to 2 mg	SC, IV	J1960
Levofloxacin	250 mg	IV	**J1956**
Levoleucovorin NOS	0.5 mg	IV	**J0641**
Levonorgestrel implant		OTH	**J7306**
Levonorgestrel-releasing intrauterine contraceptive system	52 mg	OTH	**J7297, J7298**
Kyleena	19.5 mg	OTH	**J7296**
Levorphanol tartrate	up to 2 mg	SC, IV	**J1960**
Levsin	up to 0.25 mg	SC, IM, IV	J1980
Levulan Kerastick	unit dose (354 mg)	OTH	J7308
Lexiscan	0.1 mg		J2785
Librium	up to 100 mg	IM, IV	J1990

◀ **New**   ↩ **Revised**   ✔ **Reinstated**   ~~deleted~~ **Deleted**

DRUG NAME	DOSAGE	METHOD OF ADMINISTRATION	HCPCS CODE
Lidocaine HCl	10 mg	IV	**J2001**
Lidoject-1	10 mg	IV	J2001
Lidoject-2	10 mg	IV	J2001
Liletta	52 mg	OTH	J7297
Lincocin	up to 300 mg	IV	J2010
Lincomycin HCl	up to 300 mg	IV	**J2010**
Linezolid	200 mg	IV	**J2020, J2021**
Lioresal	10 mg	IT	J0475
			J0476
Liposomal			
Cytarabine	2.27 mg	IV	**J9153**
Daunorubicin	1 mg	IV	**J9153**
Liquaemin Sodium	1,000 units	IV, SC	J1644
LMD (10%)	500 ml	IV	J7100
Locort	1.5 mg		J8540
Lorazepam	2 mg	IM, IV	**J2060**
Lovenox	10 mg	SC	J1650
Loxapine	1 mg	OTH	**J2062**
Lucentis	0.1 mg		J2778
Lufyllin	up to 500 mg	IM	J1180
Lumasiran	0.5 mg	IV	**J0224**
Lumason	per ml		Q9950
Luminal Sodium	up to 120 mg	IM, IV	J2560
Lumizyme	10 mg		J0221
Lupon Depot	7.5 mg		J9217
	3.75 mg		J1950
Lupron	per 1 mg	IM	J9218
	per 3.75 mg	IM	J1950
	7.5 mg	IM	J9217
Lurbinectedin	0.1 mg	IV	J9223
Luspatercept-aamt	0.25 mg	IM	J0896
Lyophilized, *see* Cyclophosphamide, lyophilized			
M			
Macugen	0.3 mg		J2503
Magnesium sulfate	500 mg		**J3475**
Magnevist	per ml		A9579
Makena	1 mg		J1725
Mannitol	25% in 50 ml	IV	**J2150**
	5 mg	INH	**J7665**
Marcaine			J3490

◀ **New** ↻ **Revised** ✔ **Reinstated** ~~deleted~~ **Deleted**

DRUG NAME	DOSAGE	METHOD OF ADMINISTRATION	HCPCS CODE
Margetuximab-cmkb	5 mg	IV	J9353
Marinol	2.5 mg	ORAL	Q0167
Marmine	up to 50 mg	IM, IV	J1240
Matulane	50 mg		J8999
Maxipime	500 mg	IV	J0692
MD-76R	per ml		Q9963
MD Gastroview	per ml		Q9963
Mecasermin	1 mg	SC	J2170
Mechlorethamine HCl (nitrogen mustard), HN2	10 mg	IV	J9230
Medralone 40	20 mg	IM	J1020
	40 mg	IM	J1030
	80 mg	IM	J1040
Medralone 80	20 mg	IM	J1020
	40 mg	IM	J1030
	80 mg	IM	J1040
Medrol	per 4 mg	ORAL	J7509
Medroxyprogesterone acetate	1 mg	IM	J1050
Mefoxin	1 g	IV, IM	J0694
Megestrol Acetate			J8999
Meloxicam	1 mg	IV	J1738
Melphalan (evomela)	1 mg	IV	J9246
Melphanlan flufenamide	1 mg	IV	J9247
Melphalan HCl	50 mg	IV	J9245
Melphalan, oral	2 mg	ORAL	J8600
Menoject LA	1 mg		J1071
Mepergan injection	up to 50 mg	IM, IV	J2180
Meperidine and promethazine HCl	up to 50 mg	IM, IV	J2180
Meperidine HCl	per 100 mg	IM, IV, SC	J2175
Mepivacaine HCl	per 10 ml	VAR	J0670
Mepolizumab	1 mg	IV	J2182
Mercaptopurine			J8999
Meropenem	100 mg	IV	J2184, J2185
Merrem	100 mg		J2185
Mesna	200 mg	IV	J9209
Mesnex	200 mg	IV	J9209
Metaprel			
concentrated form	per 10 mg	INH	J7667, J7668
unit dose form	per 10 mg	INH	J7669, J7670

◄ New   ↻ Revised   ✔ Reinstated   ~~deleted~~ Deleted

2024 TABLE OF DRUGS M

DRUG NAME	DOSAGE	METHOD OF ADMINISTRATION	HCPCS CODE
Metaproterenol sulfate			
concentrated form	per 10 mg	INH	**J7667, J7668**
unit dose form	per 10 mg	INH	**J7669, J7670**
Metaraminol bitartrate	per 10 mg	IV, IM, SC	**J0380**
Metastron	per millicurie		A9600
Methacholine chloride	1 mg	INH	**J7674**
Methadone HCl	up to 10 mg	IM, SC	**J1230**
Methergine	up to 0.2 mg		J2210
Methocarbamol	up to 10 ml	IV, IM	**J2800**
Methotrexate LPF	5 mg	IV, IM, IT, IA	J9250
	50 mg	IV, IM, IT, IA	J9260
Methotrexate, oral	2.5 mg	ORAL	**J8610**
Methotrexate sodium	5 mg	IV, IM, IT, IA	**J9250**
	50 mg	IV, IM, IT, IA	**J9260**
Methyldopate HCl	up to 250 mg	IV	**J0210**
Methylergonovine maleate	up to 0.2 mg		J2210
Methylnaltrexone	0.1 mg	SC	**J2212**
Methylprednisolone acetate	20 mg	IM	**J1020**
	40 mg	IM	**J1030**
	80 mg	IM	**J1040**
Methylprednisolone, oral	per 4 mg	ORAL	**J7509**
Methylprednisolone sodium succinate	up to 40 mg	IM, IV	**J2920**
	up to 125 mg	IM, IV	**J2930**
Metoclopramide HCl	up to 10 mg	IV	**J2765**
Metrodin	75 IU		J3355
Metronidazole	10 mg	IM	**J1836**, J3490 ◄
Metvixia	1 g	OTH	J7309
Miacalcin	up to 400 units	SC, IM	J0630
Micafungin sodium	1 mg		**J2247, J2248**
MicRhoGAM	50 mcg		J2788
Midazolam HCl	per 1 mg	IM, IV	**J2250, J2251**
Milrinone lactate	5 mg	IV	**J2260**
Minocine	1 mg		J2265
Minocycline Hydrochloride	1 mg	IV	**J2265**
Mircera	1 mcg		J0887, J0888
Mirena	52 mg	OTH	J7297, J7298
Mirvetuximab soravtansine-gynx	1 mg	IM	**J9063** ◄
Mithracin	2,500 mcg	IV	J9270
Mitomycin	0.2 mg	Ophthalmic	**J7315**
	5 mg	IV	**J9280**

◄ **New**　⤾ **Revised**　✔ **Reinstated**　~~deleted~~ **Deleted**

DRUG NAME	DOSAGE	METHOD OF ADMINISTRATION	HCPCS CODE
Mitosol	0.2 mg	Ophthalmic	J7315
	5 mg	IV	J9280
Mitoxantrone HCl	per 5 mg	IV	J9293
Mogamulizumab-kpkc	1 mg	IV	J9204
Mometasone furoate sinus implant, (sinuva)	10 mcg	OTH	J7402
Monocid, *see* Cefonicic sodium			
Monoclate-P			
human	per IU	IV	J7190
porcine	per IU	IV	J7191
Monoclonal antibodies, parenteral	5 mg	IV	J7505
Mononine	per IU	IV	J7193
Monovisc			J7327
Morphine sulfate	up to 10 mg	IM, IV, SC	J2270, J2272
preservative-free	10 mg	SC, IM, IV	J2274
Mosunetuzumab-axgb	1 mg	IM	J9350
Moxetumomab Pasudotox-tdfk	0.01 mg	IV	J9313
Moxifloxacin	100 mg	IV	J2280, J2281
Mozobil	1 mg		J2562
M-Prednisol-40	20 mg	IM	J1020
	40 mg	IM	J1030
	80 mg	IM	J1040
M-Prednisol-80	20 mg	IM	J1020
	40 mg	IM	J1030
	80 mg	IM	J1040
Mucomyst			
unit dose form	per gram	INH	J7604, J7608
Mucosol			
injection	100 mg	IV	J0132
unit dose	per gram	INH	J7604, J7608
MultiHance	per ml		A9577
MultiHance Multipack	per ml		A9578
Muromonab-CD3	5 mg	IV	J7505
Muse		OTH	J0275
	1.25 mcg	OTH	J0270
Mustargen	10 mg	IV	J9230
Mutamycin			
	0.2 mg	Ophthalmic	J7315
	5 mg	IV	J9280
Mycamine	1 mg		J2248
Mycophenolate Mofetil	250 mg	ORAL	J7517, J7519

◀ **New** ↻ **Revised** ✔ **Reinstated** ~~deleted~~ **Deleted**

DRUG NAME	DOSAGE	METHOD OF ADMINISTRATION	HCPCS CODE
Mycophenolic acid	180 mg	ORAL	**J7518**
Myfortic	180 mg		J7518
Myleran	1 mg		J0594
	2 mg	ORAL	J8510
Mylotarg	5 mg	IV	J9300
Myobloc	per 100 units	IM	J0587
Myochrysine	up to 50 mg	IM	J1600
Myolin	up to 60 mg	IV, IM	J2360
N			
Nabilone	1 mg	ORAL	**J8650**
Nadofaragene firadenovec-vncg	per therapeutic dose	IM	**J9029** ◄
Nafcillin			J3490
Naglazyme	1 mg		J1458
Nalbuphine HCl	per 10 mg	IM, IV, SC	**J2300**
Naloxone HCl	per 1 mg	IM, IV, SC	**J2310, J2311, J3490**
Naltrexone			J3490
Naltrexone, depot form	1 mg	IM	**J2315**
Nandrobolic L.A.	up to 50 mg	IM	J2320
Nandrolone decanoate	up to 50 mg	IM	**J2320**
Narcan	1 mg	IM, IV, SC	J2310
Naropin	1 mg		J2795
Nasahist B	per 10 mg	IM, SC, IV	J0945
Nasal vaccine inhalation		INH	**J3530**
Natalizumab	1 mg	IV	**J2323**
Natrecor	0.1 mg		J2325
Navane, *see* Thiothixene			
Navelbine	per 10 mg	IV	J9390
Naxitamab-gqgk	1 mg	IV	**J9348**
ND Stat	per 10 mg	IM, SC, IV	J0945
Nebcin	up to 80 mg	IM, IV	J3260
NebuPent	per 300 mg	INH	J2545, J7676
Necitumumab	1 mg	IV	**J9295**
Nelarabine	50 mg	IV	**J9261**
Nembutal Sodium Solution	per 50 mg	IM, IV, OTH	J2515
Neocyten	up to 60 mg	IV, IM	J2360
Neo-Durabolic	up to 50 mg	IM	J2320
Neoquess	up to 20 mg	IM	J0500
Neoral	100 mg		J7502
	25 mg		J7515

◄ **New**   ↻ **Revised**   ✔ **Reinstated**   ~~deleted~~ **Deleted**

DRUG NAME	DOSAGE	METHOD OF ADMINISTRATION	HCPCS CODE
Neosar	100 mg	IV	J9070
Neostigmine methylsulfate	up to 0.5 mg	IM, IV, SC	J2710
~~Neo-Synephrine~~	~~up to 1 ml~~	~~SC, IM, IV~~	~~J2370~~
Nervocaine 1%	10 mg	IV	J2001
Nervocaine 2%	10 mg	IV	J2001
Nesiritide	0.1 mg	IV	J2325
Netupitant 300 mg and palonosetron 0.5 mg		ORAL	J8655
Neumega	5 mg	SC	J2355
Neupogen			
(G-CSF)	1 mcg	SC, IV	J1442
Neutrexin	per 25 mg	IV	J3305
Nipent	per 10 mg	IV	J9268
Nitroglycerin	5 mg	IM	J2305
Nivol relatlimab	3mg/1mg	IM	J9298
Nivolumab	1 mg	IV	J9299
Nolvadex			J8999
Nordryl	up to 50 mg	IV, IM	J1200
	50 mg	ORAL	Q0163
Norflex	up to 60 mg	IV, IM	J2360
Norzine	up to 10 mg	IM	J3280
Not otherwise classified drugs			J3490
other than inhalation solution administered through DME			J7799
inhalation solution administered through DME			J7699
anti-neoplastic			J9999
chemotherapeutic		ORAL	J8999
immunosuppressive			J7599
nonchemotherapeutic		ORAL	J8499
Novantrone	per 5 mg	IV	J9293
Novarel	per 1,000 USP Units		J0725
Novolin	per 5 units		J1815
	per 50 units		J1817
Novolog	per 5 units		J1815
	per 50 units		J1817
Novo Seven	1 mcg	IV	J7189
Novoeight			J7182
NPH	5 units	SC	J1815
Nplate	100 units		J0587
	10 mcg		J2796
Nubain	per 10 mg	IM, IV, SC	J2300
Nulecit	12.5 mg		J2916

◀ **New**   ↩ **Revised**   ✔ **Reinstated**   ~~deleted~~ **Deleted**

DRUG NAME	DOSAGE	METHOD OF ADMINISTRATION	HCPCS CODE
Nulicaine	10 mg	IV	J2001
Nulojix	1 mg	IV	J0485
Numorphan	up to 1 mg	IV, SC, IM	J2410
Numorphan H.P.	up to 1 mg	IV, SC, IM	J2410
Nusinersen	0.1 mg	IV	J2326
Nutropin	1 mg		J2941
O			
Oasis Burn Matrix	per square centimeter		Q4103
Oasis Wound Matrix	per square centimeter		Q4102
Obinutuzumab	10 mg		J9301
Ocriplasmin	0.125 mg	IV	J7316
Ocrelizumab	1 mg	IV	J2350
Octagam	500 mg	IV	J1568
Octreotide Acetate, injection	1 mg	IM	J2353
	25 mcg	IV, SQ	J2354
Oculinum	per unit	IM	J0585
Ofatumumab	10 mg	IV	J9302
Ofev			J8499
Ofirmev	10 mg	IV	J0131
O-Flex	up to 60 mg	IV, IM	J2360
Oforta	10 mg		J8562
Olanzapine	1 mg, 0.5 mg	IM	J2358-J2359 ◄
Olaratumab	10 mg	IV	J9285
Olipudase alfa-rpcp	1 mg	IM	J0218 ◄
Omadacycline	1 mg	IV	J0121
Omacetaxine Mepesuccinate	0.01 mg	IV	J9262
Omalizumab	5 mg	SC	J2357
Omnipaque	per ml		Q9965, Q9966, Q9967
Omnipen-N	up to 500 mg	IM, IV	J0290
	per 1.5 gm	IM, IV	J0295
Omniscan	per ml		A9579
Omnitrope	1 mg		J2941
Omontys	0.1 mg	IV, SC	J0890
OnabotulinumtoxinA	1 unit	IM	J0585
Onasemnogene abeparvovec-xioi, per treatment, vector genomes	up to 5x10 15	IM	J3399
Oncaspar	per single dose vial	IM, IV	J9266
Oncovin	1 mg	IV	J9370
Ondansetron HCl	1 mg	IV	J2405
	1 mg	ORAL	Q0162
Onivyde	1 mg		J9205

◄ New   ↻ Revised   ✔ Reinstated   ~~deleted~~ Deleted

DRUG NAME	DOSAGE	METHOD OF ADMINISTRATION	HCPCS CODE	
Opana	up to 1 mg		J2410	
Opdivo	1 mg		J9299	
Oprelvekin	5 mg	SC	**J2355**	
Optimark	per ml		A9579	
Optiray	per ml		Q9966, Q9967	
Optison	per ml		Q9956	
Oraminic II	per 10 mg	IM, SC, IV	J0945	
Orapred	per 5 mg	ORAL	J7510	
Orbactiv	10 mg		J2407	
Orencia	10 mg		J0129	
Oritavancin (kimyrsa)	10 mg	IV	**J2406**	
Oritavancin (orbactiv)	10 mg	IV	**J2407**	
Ormazine	up to 50 mg	IM, IV	J3230	
Orphenadrine citrate	up to 60 mg	IV, IM	**J2360**	
Orphenate	up to 60 mg	IV, IM	J2360	
Orthovisc		OTH	**J7324**	
Or-Tyl	up to 20 mg	IM	**J0500**	
Osmitrol			J7799	
Ovidrel			J3490	
Oxacillin sodium	up to 250 mg	IM, IV	**J2700**	
Oxaliplatin	0.5 mg	IV	**J9263**	
Oxilan	per ml		Q9967	
Oxlumo	0.5 mg	IV	J0224	◄
Oxymorphone HCl	up to 1 mg	IV, SC, IM	**J2410**	
Oxytetracycline HCl	up to 50 mg	IM	**J2460**	
Oxytocin	up to 10 units	IV, IM	**J2590**	
Ozurdex	0.1 mg		J7312	
P				
Paclitaxel	1 mg	IV	**J9267**	
Paclitaxel protein-bound particles	1 mg	IV	**J9259, J9264**	◄
Pafolacianine	0.1 mg	IM	**J9603**	◄
Palifermin	50 mcg	IV	**J2425**	
Paliperidone palmitate	1 mg	IM	**J2426-J2427**	◄
Palonosetron HCl	25 mcg	IV	**J2469**	
Netupitant 300 mg and palonosetron 0.5 mg		ORAL	**J8655**	
Pamidronate disodium	per 30 mg	IV	**J2430**	
Panhematin	1 mg		J1640	
Panitumumab	10 mg	IV	**J9303**	
Papaverine HCl	up to 60 mg	IV, IM	**J2440**	

◄ **New**   ↻ **Revised**   ✔ **Reinstated**   ~~deleted~~ **Deleted**

DRUG NAME	DOSAGE	METHOD OF ADMINISTRATION	HCPCS CODE	
Paragard T 380 A		OTH	J7300	
Paraplatin	50 mg	IV	J9045	
Paricalcitol, injection	1 mcg	IV, IM	J2501	
Pasireotide, long acting	1 mg	IV	J2502	
Pathogen(s) test for platelets		OTH	P9100	
Patisiran	0.1 mg	IV	J0222	
Peforomist	20 mcg		J7606	
Pegademase bovine	25 IU		J2504	
Pegaptinib	0.3 mg	OTH	J2503	
Pegaspargase	per single dose vial	IM, IV	J9266	
Pegasys			J3490	
Pegcetacoplan	1 mg	IVT	J2781	◄
Pegfilgrastim-bmez, biosimilar, (ziextenzo)	0.5 mg	IM	Q5120	
Pegfilgrastim-cbqv	0.5 mg	IM	Q5111	◄
Pegfilgrastim-fpgk	0.5 mg	IM	Q5127	◄
Pegfilgrastim-jmdb	0.5 mg	SC	Q5108	
Pegfilgrastim-pbbk	0.5 mg	IM	Q5130	◄
Peginesatide	0.1 mg	IV, SC	J0890	
Peg-Intron			J3490	
Pegloticase	1 mg	IV	J2507	
Pembrolizumab	1 mg	IV	J9271	
Pemetrexed	10 mg	IV	J9294, J9296-J9297, J9305, J9314, J9322-J9323	◄
Pemetrexed (Pemfexy)	10 mg	IV	J9304	
Penicillin G Benzathine	100,000 units	IM	J0561	
Penicillin G Benzathine and Penicillin G Procaine	100,000 units	IM	J0558	
Penicillin G potassium	up to 600,000 units	IM, IV	J2540	
Penicillin G procaine, aqueous	up to 600,000 units	IM, IV	J2510	
Penicillin G Sodium			J3490	
Pentam	per 300 mg		J7676	
Pentamidine isethionate	per 300 mg	INH, IM	J2545, J7676	
Pentastarch, 10%	100 ml		J2513	
Pentazocine HCl	30 mg	IM, SC, IV	J3070	
Pentobarbital sodium	per 50 mg	IM, IV, OTH	J2515	
Pentostatin	per 10 mg	IV	J9268	
Peramivir	1 mg	IV	J2547	
Perjeta	1 mg		J9306	
Permapen	up to 600,000	IM	J0561	

◄ New   ↻ Revised   ✔ Reinstated   ~~deleted~~ Deleted

DRUG NAME	DOSAGE	METHOD OF ADMINISTRATION	HCPCS CODE	
Perphenazine				
injection	up to 5 mg	IM, IV	**J3310**	
tablets	4 mg	ORAL	**Q0175**	
Persantine IV	per 10 mg	IV	J1245	
Pertuzumab	1 mg	IV	**J9306**	
Pet Imaging				
Fluciclovine F-18, diagnostic	1 millcurie	IV	**A9588**	
Gallium Ga-68, dotatate, diagnostic	0.1 millicurie	IV	**A9587**	
Gallium ga-68, psma-11, (ucla)	1 millicurie	IV	**A9594**	
Gallium ga-68, psma-11, (ucsf)	1 millicurie	IV	**A9593**	
Pfizerpen	up to 600,000 units	IM, IV	J2540	
Pfizerpen A.S.	up to 600,000 units	IM, IV	J2510	
Phenadoz			J8498	
Phenazine 25	up to 50 mg	IM, IV	J2550	
	12.5 mg	ORAL	Q0169	
Phenazine 50	up to 50 mg	IM, IV	J2550	
	12.5 mg	ORAL	Q0169	
Phenergan	12.5 mg	ORAL	Q0169	
	up to 50 mg	IM, IV	J2550	
			J8498	
Phenobarbital sodium	up to 120 mg	IM, IV	**J2560-J2561**	◀
Phentolamine mesylate	up to 5 mg	IM, IV	**J2760**	
Phenylephrine HCl	up to 1 ml	SC, IM, IV	J2370, J7799	
Phenylephrine hydrochloride (biorphen)	20 mcg	IM	**J2371-J2372**	◀
Phenylephrine 10.16 mg/Ketorolac 2.88	1 ml	VAR	**J1097**	
Phenytoin sodium	per 50 mg	IM, IV	**J1165**	
Photofrin	75 mg	IV	J9600	
Phytonadione (Vitamin K)	per 1 mg	IM, SC, IV	**J3430**	
Piperacillin/Tazobactam Sodium, injection	1.125 g	IV	**J2543**	
Pitocin	up to 10 units	IV, IM	J2590	
Plantinol AQ	10 mg	IV	J9060	
Plasma				
cryoprecipitate reduced	each unit	IV	**P9044**	
pooled multiple donor, frozen	each unit	IV	**P9023, P9070**	
(single donor), pathogen reduced, frozen	each unit	IV	**P9071**	
Plasminogen TVMH	1 mg		**J2998**	
Plas+SD	each unit	IV	P9023	
Platelets, pheresis, pathogen reduced	each unit	IV	**P9073**	
Pathogen(s) test for platelets		OTH	**P9100**	

◀ New   ↩ Revised   ✔ Reinstated   ~~deleted~~ Deleted

DRUG NAME	DOSAGE	METHOD OF ADMINISTRATION	HCPCS CODE
Platinol	10 mg	IV, IM	J9060
Plazomicin	5 mg	IV	J0291
Plerixafor	1 mg	SC	J2562
Plicamycin	2,500 mcg	IV	J9270
Polatuzumab vedotin	1 mg	IV	J9309
Polocaine	per 10 ml	VAR	J0670
Polycillin-N	up to 500 mg	IM, IV	J0290
	per 1.5 gm	IM, IV	J0295
Polygam	500 mg		J1566
Porfimer Sodium	75 mg	IV	J9600
Portrazza	1 mg		J9295
Positron emission tomography radiopharmaceutical, diagnostic			
for non-tumor identification, NOC		IV	A9598
for tumor identification, NOC		IV	A9597
Potassium chloride	per 2 mEq	IV	J3480
Potassium Chloride	up to 1,000 cc		J7120
Pralatrexate	1 mg	IV	J9307
Pralidoxime chloride	up to 1 g	IV, IM, SC	J2730
Predalone-50	up to 1 ml	IM	J2650
Predcor-25	up to 1 ml	IM	J2650
Predcor-50	up to 1 ml	IM	J2650
Predicort-50	up to 1 ml	IM	J2650
Prednisolone acetate	up to 1 ml	IM	J2650
Prednisolone, oral	5 mg	ORAL	J7510
Prednisone, immediate release or delayed release	1 mg	ORAL	J7512
Predoject-50	up to 1 ml	IM	J2650
Pregnyl	per 1,000 USP units	IM	J0725
Premarin Intravenous	per 25 mg	IV, IM	J1410
Prescription, chemotherapeutic, not otherwise specified		ORAL	J8999
Prescription, nonchemotherapeutic, not otherwise specified		ORAL	J8499
Prialt	1 mcg		J2278
Primacor	5 mg	IV	J2260
Primatrix	per square centimeter		Q4110
Primaxin	per 250 mg	IV, IM	J0743
Priscoline HCl	up to 25 mg	IV	J2670
Privigen	500 mg	IV	J1459
Probuphine System Kit			J0570
Procainamide HCl	up to 1 g	IM, IV	J2690
Prochlorperazine	up to 10 mg	IM, IV	J0780
			J8498

◀ **New**   ⟳ **Revised**   ✔ **Reinstated**   ~~deleted~~ **Deleted**

DRUG NAME	DOSAGE	METHOD OF ADMINISTRATION	HCPCS CODE
Prochlorperazine maleate	5 mg	ORAL	Q0164
	5 mg		S0183
Procrit			J0885
			Q4081
Pro-Depo, *see* Hydroxyprogesterone Caproate			
Profasi HP	per 1,000 USP units	IM	J0725
Profilnine Heat-Treated			
non-recombinant	per IU	IV	J7193
recombinant	per IU	IU	J7195, J7200-J7202
complex	per IU	IV	J7194
Profonol	10 mg/ml		J3490
Progestaject	per 50 mg		J2675
Progesterone	per 50 mg	IM	J2675
Prograf			
oral	1 mg	ORAL	J7507
parenteral	5 mg		J7525
Prohance Multipack	per ml		A9576, A9579 ◄
Prokine	50 mcg	IV	J2820
~~Prolastin~~	~~10 mg~~	~~IV~~	~~J0256~~
Proleukin	per single use vial	IM, IV	J9015
Prolia	1 mg		J0897
Prolixin Decanoate	up to 25 mg	IM, SC	J2680
Promazine HCl	up to 25 mg	IM	J2950
Promethazine			J8498
Promethazine HCl			
injection	up to 50 mg	IM, IV	J2550
oral	12.5 mg	ORAL	Q0169
Promethegan			J8498
Pronestyl	up to 1 g	IM, IV	J2690
Proplex SX-T			
non-recombinant	per IU	IV	J7193
recombinant	per IU		J7195, J7200-J7202
complex	per IU	IV	J7194
Proplex T			
non-recombinant	per IU	IV	J7193
recombinant	per IU		J7195, J7200-J7202
complex	per IU	IV	J7194
Propofol	10 mg	IV	J2704

◄ New   ↻ Revised   ✔ Reinstated   ~~deleted~~ Deleted

DRUG NAME	DOSAGE	METHOD OF ADMINISTRATION	HCPCS CODE
Propranolol HCl	up to 1 mg	IV	**J1800**
Prorex-25			
	up to 50 mg	IM, IV	J2550
	12.5 mg	ORAL	Q0169
Prorex-50	up to 50 mg	IM, IV	J2550
	12.5 mg	ORAL	Q0169
Prostaglandin E1	per 1.25 mcg		J0270
Prostaphlin	up to 1 g	IM, IV	J2690
Prostigmin	up to 0.5 mg	IM, IV, SC	J2710
Prostin VR Pediatric	0.5 mg		J0270
Protamine sulfate	per 10 mg	IV	**J2720**
Protein C Concentrate	10 IU	IV	**J2724**
Prothazine	up to 50 mg	IM, IV	J2550
	12.5 mg	ORAL	Q0169
Prothrombin complex concentrate (human), kcentra	per i.u. of factor ix activity	OTH	**J7168**
Protirelin	per 250 mcg	IV	**J2725**
Protonix			J3490
Protopam Chloride	up to 1 g	IV, IM, SC	J2730
Provenge			Q2043
Proventil			
concentrated form	1 mg	INH	J7610, J7611
unit dose form	1 mg	INH	J7609, J7613
Provocholine	per 1 mg		J7674
Prozine-50	up to 25 mg	IM	J2950
Pulmicort Respules			
concentrated form	0.25 mg	INH	J7633, J7634
unit dose	0.5 mg	INH	J7626, J7627
Pulmozyme	per mg		J7639
Pyridoxine HCl	100 mg		**J3415**
Q			
Quelicin	up to 20 mg	IV, IM	J0330
Quinupristin/dalfopristin	500 mg (150/350)	IV	**J2770**
Qutenza	per square cm		J7336
R			
Ramucirumab	5 mg	IV	**J9308**
Ranibizumab	0.1 mg	OTH, IM	**J2778, Q5128**
Ranitidine HCl, injection	25 mg	IV, IM	**J2780**
Rapamune	1 mg	ORAL	J7520
Rasburicase	0.5 mg	IV	**J2783**

◄ New   ↻ Revised   ✔ Reinstated   deleted Deleted

DRUG NAME	DOSAGE	METHOD OF ADMINISTRATION	HCPCS CODE
Ravulizumab-cwvz	10 mg	IV	J1303
Rebif	11 mcg		Q3026
Reclast	1 mg		J3489
Recombinate			
human	per IU	IV	J7190
porcine	per IU	IV	J7191
recombinant	per IU	IV	J7192
Recombivax			J3490
Redisol	up to 1,000 mcg	IM, SC	J3420
Regadenoson	0.1 mg	IV	J2785
Regitine	up to 5 mg	IM, IV	J2760
Reglan	up to 10 mg	IV	J2765
Regular	5 units	SC	J1815
Relefact TRH	per 250 mcg	IV	J2725
Relistor	0.1 mg	SC	J2212
Remicade	10 mg	IM, IV	J1745
Remimazolam	1 mg	IM	J2249 ◀
Remodulin	1 mg		J3285
Renflexis			Q5102
ReoPro	10 mg	IV	J0130
Rep-Pred 40	20 mg	IM	J1020
	40 mg	IM	J1030
	80 mg	IM	J1040
Rep-Pred 80	20 mg	IM	J1020
	40 mg	IM	J1030
	80 mg	IM	J1040
Resectisol			J7799
Reslizumab	1 mg	IV	J2786
Retavase	18.1 mg	IV	J2993
Reteplase	18.8 mg	IV	J2993
Retifanlimab-dlwr	1 mg	IM	J9345 ◀
Retisert			J7311
Retrovir	10 mg	IV	J3485
Revefenacin inhalation solution	—	INH	J7677
Rezafungin	1 mg	IM	J0349 ◀
Rheomacrodex	500 ml	IV	J7100
Rhesonativ	300 mcg	IM	J2790
	50 mg		J2788
Rheumatrex Dose Pack	2.5 mg	ORAL	J8610

◀ **New**   ↻ **Revised**   ✔ **Reinstated**   ~~deleted~~ **Deleted**

DRUG NAME	DOSAGE	METHOD OF ADMINISTRATION	HCPCS CODE
Rho(D)			
immune globulin		IM, IV	J2791
immune globulin, human	1 dose package/ 300 mcg	IM	J2790
	50 mg	IM	J2788
immune globulin, human, solvent detergent	100	IV, IU	J2792
RhoGAM	300 mcg	IM	J2790
	50 mg		J2788
Rhophylac	100 IU	IM, IV	J2791
Riastap	100 mg		J7178
Rifadin			J3490
Rifampin			J3490
Rilonacept	1 mg	SC	J2793
RimabotulinumtoxinB	100 units	IM	J0587
Rimso-50	50 ml		J1212
Ringers lactate infusion	up to 1,000 cc	IV	J7120, J7121
Risankizumab	1 mg	IV	J2327
Risperdal Consta	0.5 mg		J2794
Risperidone	0.5 mg	IM	J2794
Risperidone (perseris)	0.5 mg	IV	J2798
Rituxan	100 mg	IV	J9312
Rituximab	100 mg	IV	J9312
Rituximab-abbs	10 mg	IV	Q5115
Rituximab-arrx, biosimilar, (riabni)	10 mg	IV	Q5123
Rituximab-pvvr, biosimilar, (Ruxience)	10 mg	IV	Q5119
Rixubis			J7200
Robaxin	up to 10 ml	IV, IM	J2800
Rocephin	per 250 mg	IV, IM	J0696
Roferon-A	3 million units	SC, IM	J9213
Rolapitant	0.5 mg	IV	J2797
Rolapitant, oral, 1 mg	1 mg	ORAL	J8670
Romidepsin lyophilized	1 mg	IV	J9319
Romidepsin, non-lyophilized	0.1 mg	IV	J9318
Romiplostim	10 mcg	SC	J2796
Romosozumab-aqqg	1 mg	IV	J3111
Ropivacaine Hydrochloride	1 mg	OTH	J2795
Rubex	10 mg	IV	J9000
Rubramin PC	up to 1,000 mcg	IM, SC	J3420

◀ New   ↻ Revised   ✔ Reinstated   ~~deleted~~ Deleted

DRUG NAME	DOSAGE	METHOD OF ADMINISTRATION	HCPCS CODE
S			
Saizen	1 mg		J2941
Saline solution	10 ml		A4216
5% dextrose	500 ml	IV	**J7042**
infusion	250 cc	IV	**J7050**
	1,000 cc	IV	**J7030**
sterile	500 ml = 1 unit	IV, OTH	**J7040**
Sandimmune	25 mg	ORAL	J7515
	100 mg	ORAL	J7502
	250 mg	OTH	J7516
Sandoglobulin, *see* Immune globulin intravenous (human)			
Sandostatin, Lar Depot	25 mcg		J2354
	1 mg	IM	J2353
Sargramostim (GM-CSF)	50 mcg	IV	**J2820**
Sculptra	0.5 mg	IV	**Q2028**
Sebelelipase alfa	1 mg	IV	**J2840**
Selestoject	per 4 mg	IM, IV	J0702
Sermorelin acetate	1 mcg	SC	**Q0515**
Serostim	1 mg		J2941
Signifor LAR	20 ml		J2502
Siltuximab	10 mg	IV	**J2860**
Simponi Aria	1 mg		J1602
Simulect	20 mg		J0480
Sincalide	5 mcg	IV, IM	**J2805-J2806**
Sinografin	per ml		Q9963
Sinusol-B	per 10 mg	IM, SC, IV	J0945
Sirolimus	1 mg	ORAL	**J7520**
Sirolimus protien-bound	1 mg	IM	**J9331**
Sivextro	1 mg		J3090
Skyla	13.5 mg	OTH	**J7301**
Smz-TMP			J3490
Sodium Chloride	1,000 cc		J7030
	500 ml = 1 unit		J7040
	500 ml		A4217
	250 cc		J7050
Bacteriostatic	10 ml		A4216
Sodium Chloride Concentrate			J7799
Sodium ferricgluconate in sucrose	12.5 mg		**J2916**

◄ **New**   ↻ **Revised**   ✔ **Reinstated**   ~~deleted~~ **Deleted**

DRUG NAME	DOSAGE	METHOD OF ADMINISTRATION	HCPCS CODE
Sodium Hyaluronate			J3490
Euflexxa			**J7323**
Hyalgan			**J7321**
Orthovisc			**J7324**
Sodium Thiosulfate	100 mg	IM	J0208 ◄
Solganal	up to 50 mg	IM	J2910
Soliris	10 mg		J1300
Solu-Cortef	up to 50 mg	IV, IM, SC	J1710
	100 mg		J1720
Solu-Medrol	up to 40 mg	IM, IV	J2920
	up to 125 mg	IM, IV	J2930
Solurex	1 mg	IM, IV, OTH	J1100
Solurex LA	1 mg	IM	J1094
Somatrem	1 mg	SC	**J2940**
Somatropin	1 mg	SC	**J2941**
Somatulin Depot	1 mg		J1930
Sparine	up to 25 mg	IM	J2950
Spasmoject	up to 20 mg	IM	J0500
Spectinomycin HCl	up to 2 g	IM	**J3320**
Spesolimab-sbzo	1 mg	IM	J1747 ◄
Sporanox	50 mg	IV	J1835
Staphcillin, *see* Methicillin sodium			
Stelara	1 mg		J3357
Stilphostrol	250 mg	IV	J9165
Streptase	250,000 IU	IV	J2995
Streptokinase	per 250,000	IU, IV	**J2995**
Streptomycin	up to 1 g	IM	**J3000**
Streptomycin Sulfate	up to 1 g	IM	J3000
Streptozocin	1 gm	IV	**J9320**
Strontium-89 chloride	per millicurie		**A9600**
Sublimaze	0.1 mg	IM, IV	J3010
Succinylcholine chloride	up to 20 mg	IV, IM	**J0330**
Sufentanil Citrate			J3490
Sumarel Dosepro	6 mg		J3030
Sumatriptan succinate	6 mg	SC	**J3030**
Supartz		OTH	**J7321**
Supprelin LA	50 mg		J9226
Surostrin	up to 20 mg	IV, IM	**J0330**
Sus-Phrine	up to 1 ml ampule	SC, IM	J0171

◄ **New**   ↻ **Revised**   ✔ **Reinstated**   ~~deleted~~ **Deleted**

DRUG NAME	DOSAGE	METHOD OF ADMINISTRATION	HCPCS CODE
Sutimlimab-jome	10 mg	IM	J1302
Susvimo	0.1 mg		J2779
Synercid	500 mg (150/350)	IV	J2770
Synkavite	per 1 mg	IM, SC, IV	J3430
Synribo	0.01 mg		J9262
Syntocinon	up to 10 units	IV, IM	J2590
Synvisc and Synvisc-One	1 mg	OTH	J7325
Syrex	10 ml		A4216
Sytobex	1,000 mcg	IM, SC	J3420
T			
Tacrolimus			
(Envarsus XR)	0.25 mg	ORAL	J7503
oral, extended release	0.1 mg	ORAL	J7508
oral, immediate release	1 mg	ORAL	J7507
parenteral	5 mg	IV	J7525
Tafasitamab	2 mg	IV	J9349
Tagraxofusp-erzs	10 mcg	IV	J9269
Taliglucerase Alfa	10 units	IV	J3060
Talimogene laherparepvec	per 1 million plaque forming units	IV	J9325
Talwin	30 mg	IM, SC, IV	J3070
Tamoxifen Citrate			J8999
Taractan, *see* Chlorprothixene			
Taxol	1 mg	IV	J9267
Taxotere	20 mg	IV	J9171
Tazicef	per 500 mg		J0713
Tazidime, *see* Ceftazidime Technetium TC Sestambi	per dose		A9500
			J0713
Tebentafusp-tebn	1 mcg	IM	J9274
Teclistamab-cqyv	0.5 mg	IM	J9380
Tedizolid phosphate	1 mg	IV	J3090
TEEV	1 mg	IM	J3121
Teflaro	1 mg		J0712
Telavancin	10 mg	IV	J3095
Temodar	5 mg	ORAL	J8700, J9328
Temozolomide	1 mg	IV	J9328
	5 mg	ORAL	J8700
Temsirolimus	1 mg	IV	J9330
Tenecteplase	1 mg	IV	J3101

◀ **New**   ↻ **Revised**   ✔ **Reinstated**   ~~deleted~~ **Deleted**

DRUG NAME	DOSAGE	METHOD OF ADMINISTRATION	HCPCS CODE
Teniposide	50 mg		Q2017
Tepadina	15 mg		J9340
Teplizumab-mzwv	5 mcg	IM	J9381 ◀
Teprotumumab-trbw	10 mg	IV	J3241
Tequin	10 mg	IV	J1590
Terbutaline sulfate	up to 1 mg	SC, IV	J3105
concentrated form	per 1 mg	INH	J7680
unit dose form	per 1 mg	INH	J7681
Teriparatide	10 mcg	SC	J3110
Terramycin IM	up to 50 mg	IM	J2460
Testa-C	1 mg		J1071
Testadiate	1 mg	IM	J3121
Testadiate-Depo	1 mg		J1071
Testaject-LA	1 mg		J1071
Testaqua	up to 50 mg	IM	J3140
Test-Estro Cypionates	1 mg		J1071
Test-Estro-C	1 mg		J1071
Testex	up to 100 mg	IM	J3150
Testo AQ	up to 50 mg		J3140
Testoject-50	up to 50 mg	IM	J3140
Testoject-LA	1 mg		J1071
Testone			
LA 100	1 mg	IM	J3121
LA 200	1 mg	IM	J3121
Testopel Pellets			J3490
Testosterone Aqueous	up to 50 mg	IM	J3140
Testosterone cypionate	1 mg	IM	J1071
Testosterone enanthate	1 mg	IM	J3121
Testosterone undecanoate	1 mg	IM	J3145
Testradiol 90/4	1 mg	IM	J3121
Testrin PA	1 mg	IM	J3121
Testro AQ	up to 50 mg		J3140
Tetanus immune globulin, human	up to 250 units	IM	J1670
Tetracycline	up to 250 mg	IM, IV	J0120
Tezepelumab-ekko	1 mg		J2356
Thallous Chloride TI-201	per MCI		A9505
Theelin Aqueous	per 1 mg	IM	J1435
Theophylline	per 40 mg	IV	J2810
Thiamine HCl	100 mg		J3411

◀ **New**   ↻ **Revised**   ✔ **Reinstated**   ~~deleted~~ **Deleted**

DRUG NAME	DOSAGE	METHOD OF ADMINISTRATION	HCPCS CODE
Thiethylperazine maleate			
injection	up to 10 mg	IM	J3280
oral	10 mg	ORAL	Q0174
Thiotepa	15 mg	IV	J9340
Thorazine	up to 50 mg	IM, IV	J3230
Thrombate III	per IU		J7197
Thymoglobulin (*see also* Immune globulin)			
anti-thymocyte globulin, equine	250 mg	IV	J7504
anti-thymocyte globulin, rabbit	25 mg	IV	J7511
Thypinone	per 250 mcg	IV	J2725
Thyrogen	0.9 mg	IM, SC	J3240
Thyrotropin Alfa, injection	0.9 mg	IM, SC	J3240
Ticon			
injection	up to 200 mg	IM	J3250
oral	250 mg	ORAL	Q0173
Tigan			
injection	up to 200 mg	IM	J3250
oral	250 mg	ORAL	Q0173
Tigecycline	1 mg	IV	J3243, J3244
Tiject-20			
injection	up to 200 mg	IM	J3250
oral	250 mg	ORAL	Q0173
Tinzaparin	1,000 IU	SC	J1655
Tirofiban Hydrochloride, injection	0.25 mg	IM, IV	J3246
TNKase	1 mg	IV	J3101
Tobi	300 mg	INH	J7682, J7685
Tobramycin, inhalation solution	300 mg	INH	J7682, J7685
Tobramycin sulfate	up to 80 mg	IM, IV	J3260
Tocilizumab	1 mg	IV	J3262
Tofranil, *see* Imipramine HCl			
Tolazoline HCl	up to 25 mg	IV	J2670
Toposar	10 mg		J9181
Topotecan	0.25 mg	ORAL	J8705
	0.1 mg	IV	J9351
Toradol	per 15 mg	IM, IV	J1885
Torecan			
injection	up to 10 mg	IM	J3280
oral	10 mg	ORAL	Q0174
Torisel	1 mg		J9330

◀ **New**   ⟲ **Revised**   ✔ **Reinstated**   ~~deleted~~ **Deleted**

DRUG NAME	DOSAGE	METHOD OF ADMINISTRATION	HCPCS CODE
Tornalate			
concentrated form	per mg	INH	J7628
unit dose	per mg	INH	J7629
Torsemide	10 mg/ml	IV	J3265
Totacillin-N	up to 500 mg	IM, IV	J0290
	per 1.5 gm	IM, IV	J0295
Trabectedin	0.1 mg	IV	J9352
Trastuzumab	10 mg	IV	J9355
Trastuzumab-anns (kanjinti)	10 mg	IV	Q5117
Trastuzumab-dkst	10 mg	IV	Q5114
Trastuzumab-dttb	10 mg	IV	Q5112
Trastuzumab-pkrb	10 mg	IV	Q5113
Trastuzumab-qyyp (trazimera)	10 mg	IV	Q5116
Trastuzumab and Hyaluronidase	10 mg	IV	J9356
Treanda	1 mg	IV	J3490, J9033
Trelstar	3.75 mg		J3315
Tremelimumab-actl	1 mg	IM	J9347
Treprostinil	1 mg		J3285, J7686
Trexall	2.5 mg	ORAL	J8610
Triam-A	1 mg		J3300
	per 10 mg	IM	J3301
Triamcinolone			
concentrated form	per 1 mg	INH	J7683
unit dose	per 1 mg	INH	J7684
Triamcinolone acetonide	1 mg		J3300
	per 10 mg	IM	J3301
Triamcinolone acetonide XR	1 mg	IM	J3304
Triamcinolone diacetate	per 5 mg	IM	J3302
Triamcinolone hexacetonide	per 5 mg	VAR	J3303
Triesence	1 mg		J3300
	per 10 mg	IM	J3301
Triethylene thio-Phosphoramide/T	15 mg		J9340
Triflupromazine HCl	up to 20 mg	IM, IV	J3400
Tri-Kort	1 mg		J3300
	per 10 mg	IM	J3301
Trilaciclib	1 mg	IV	J1448
Trilafon	4 mg	ORAL	Q0175
	up to 5 mg	IM, IV	J3310
Trilog	1 mg		J3300
	per 10 mg	IM	J3301

◄ New　↻ Revised　✔ Reinstated　deleted **Deleted**

DRUG NAME	DOSAGE	METHOD OF ADMINISTRATION	HCPCS CODE
Trilone	per 5 mg		J3302
Trimethobenzamide HCl			
injection	up to 200 mg	IM	**J3250**
oral	250 mg	ORAL	**Q0173**
Trimetrexate glucuronate	per 25 mg	IV	**J3305**
Triptorelin Pamoate	3.75 mg	SC	**J3315**
Triptorelin XR	3.75 mg	SC	**J3316**
Trisenox	1 mg	IV	J9017
Trobicin	up to 2 g	IM	J3320
Trovan	100 mg	IV	J0200
Tysabri	1 mg		J2323
Tyvaso	1.74 mg		J7686
U			
Ublituximab-xiiy	1 mg	IM	**J2329**
Ultravist 240	per ml		Q9966
Ultravist 300	per ml		Q9967
Ultravist 370	per ml		Q9967
Ultrazine-10	up to 10 mg	IM, IV	J0780
Unasyn	per 1.5 gm	IM, IV	J0295
Unclassified drugs (*see also* Not elsewhere classified)			**J3490**
Unclassified drugs or biological used for ESRD on dialysis		IV	**J3591**
Unspecified oral antiemetic			**Q0181**
Urea	up to 40 g	IV	**J3350**
Ureaphil	up to 40 g	IV	J3350
Urecholine	up to 5 mg	SC	J0520
Urofollitropin	75 IU		**J3355**
Urokinase	5,000 IU vial	IV	**J3364**
	250,000 IU vial	IV	**J3365**
Ustekinumab	1 mg	SC	**J3357**
	1 mg	IV	**J3358**
V			
Valcyte			J3490
Valergen 10	10 mg	IM	J1380
Valergen 20	10 mg	IM	J1380
Valergen 40	up to 10 mg	IM	J1380
Valertest No. 1	1 mg	IM	J3121
Valertest No. 2	1 mg	IM	J3121
Valganciclovir HCL			J8499
Valium	up to 5 mg	IM, IV	J3360
Valrubicin, intravesical	200 mg	OTH	**J9357**
Valstar	200 mg	OTH	J9357

◀ **New**   ⤴ **Revised**   ✔ **Reinstated**   ~~deleted~~ **Deleted**

DRUG NAME	DOSAGE	METHOD OF ADMINISTRATION	HCPCS CODE
Vancocin	500 mg	IV, IM	J3370
Vancoled	500 mg	IV, IM	J3370
Vancomycin HCl	500 mg	IV, IM	J3370, J3371, J3372
Vantas	50 mg		J9226, J9225
Varubi	90 mg		J8670
Vasceze	per 10 mg		J1642
Vasopressin	1 unit	IM	J2598-J2599 ◄
Vasoxyl, *see* Methoxamine HCl			
Vectibix	10 mg		J9303
Vedolizumab	1 mg	IV	J3380
Velaglucerase alfa	100 units	IV	J3385
Velban	1 mg	IV	J9360
Velcade	0.1 mg		J9041
Veletri	0.5 mg		J1325
Velsar	1 mg	IV	J9360
Venofer	1 mg	IV	J1756
Ventavis	20 mcg		Q4074
Ventolin	0.5 mg	INH	J7620
concentrated form	1 mg	INH	J7610, J7611
unit dose form	1 mg	INH	J7609, J7613
VePesid	50 mg	ORAL	J8560
Veritas Collagen Matrix			J3490
Versed	per 1 mg	IM, IV	J2250
Verteporfin	0.1 mg	IV	J3396
Vesprin	up to 20 mg	IM, IV	J3400
Vestronidase alfa-vjbk	1 mg	IV	J3397
VFEND IV	10 mg	IV	J3465
V-Gan 25	up to 50 mg	IM, IV	J2550
	12.5 mg	ORAL	Q0169
V-Gan 50	up to 50 mg	IM, IV	J2550
	12.5 mg	ORAL	Q0169
Viadur	65 mg	OTH	J9219
Vibativ	10 mg		J3095
Viltolarsen	10 mg	IV	J1427
Vinblastine sulfate	1 mg	IV	J9360
Vincasar PFS	1 mg	IV	J9370
Vincristine sulfate	1 mg	IV	J9370
Vincristine sulfate liposome	1 mg	IV	J9371
Vinorelbine tartrate	per 10 mg	IV	J9390
Vispaque	per ml		Q9966, Q9967

◄ New   ⤺ Revised   ✔ Reinstated   ~~deleted~~ **Deleted**

DRUG NAME	DOSAGE	METHOD OF ADMINISTRATION	HCPCS CODE
Vistaject-25	up to 25 mg	IM	J3410
Vistaril	up to 25 mg	IM	J3410
	25 mg	ORAL	Q0177
Vistide	375 mg	IV	J0740
Visudyne	0.1 mg	IV	J3396
Vitamin B-12 cyanocobalamin	up to 1,000 mcg	IM, SC	J3420
Vitamin K, phytonadione, menadione, menadiol sodium diphosphate	per 1 mg	IM, SC, IV	J3430
Vitrase	per 1 USP unit		J3471
Vivaglobin	100 mg		J1562
Vivitrol	1 mg		J2315
Von Willebrand Factor Complex, human	per IU VWF:RCo	IV	J7187
Wilate	per IU VWF	IV	J7183
Vonvendi	per IU VWF	IV	J7179
Voretigene neparvovec-rzyl	1 billion vector genomes	IV	J3398
Voriconazole	10 mg	IV	J3465
Vpriv	100 units		J3385
Vutrisiran	1 mg	IM	J0225
W			
Wehamine	up to 50 mg	IM, IV	J1240
Wehdryl	up to 50 mg	IM, IV	J1200
	50 mg	ORAL	Q0163
Wellcovorin	per 50 mg	IM, IV	J0640
Wilate	per IU	IV	J7183
Win Rho SD	100 IU	IV	J2792
Wyamine Sulfate, see Mephentermine sulfate			
Wycillin	up to 600,000 units	IM, IV	J2510
Wydase	up to 150 units	SC, IV	J3470
X			
Xeloda	150 mg	ORAL	J8520
	500 mg	ORAL	J8521
Xeomin	1 unit		J0588
Xgera	1 mg		J0987
Xgeva	1 mg		J0897
Xiaflex	0.01 mg		J0775
Xipere	1 mg		J3299
Xolair	5 mg		J2357
Xopenex	0.5 mg	INH	J7620
concentrated form	1 mg	INH	J7610, J7611, J7612
unit dose form	1 mg	INH	J7609, J7613, J7614

◄ **New**   ↻ **Revised**   ✔ **Reinstated**   ~~deleted~~ **Deleted**

100

DRUG NAME	DOSAGE	METHOD OF ADMINISTRATION	HCPCS CODE
Xylocaine HCl	10 mg	IV	J2001
Xyntha	per IU	IV	J7185, J7192, J7182, J7188
Y			
Yervoy, *see* Ipilimumab			
Yondelis	0.1 mg		J9352, J9999
Z			
Zaltrap	1 mg		J9400
Zanosar	1 g	IV	J9320
Zantac	25 mg	IV, IM	J2780
Zarxio	1 mcg		Q5101
Zemaira	10 mg	IV	J0256
Zemdri	5 mg	IV	J0291
Zemplar	1 mcg	IM, IV	J2501
Zenapax	25 mg	IV	J7513
Zerbaxa	1 gm		J0695
Zetran	up to 5 mg	IM, IV	J3360
Ziconotide	1 mcg	OTH	**J2278**
Zidovudine	10 mg	IV	**J3485**
Zinacef	per 750 mg	IM, IV	J0697
Zinecard	per 250 mg		J1190
Ziprasidone Mesylate	10 mg	IM	**J3486**
Zithromax	1 gm	ORAL	Q0144
injection	500 mg	IV	J0456
Ziv-Aflibercept	1 mg	IV	**J9400**
Zmax	1 g		Q0144
Zofran	1 mg	IV	J2405
	1 mg	ORAL	Q0162
Zoladex	per 3.6 mg	SC	J9202
Zoledronic Acid	1 mg	IV	**J3489**
Zolicef	500 mg	IV, IM	J0690
Zometra	1 mg		J3489
Zorbtive	1 mg		J2941
Zortress	0.25 mg	ORAL	J7527
Zosyn	1.125 g	IV	J2543
Zovirax	5 mg		J8499
Zyprexa Relprevv	1 mg		J2358
Zyvox	200 mg	IV	J2020

◄ **New**   ⟳ **Revised**   ✓ **Reinstated**   ~~deleted~~ **Deleted**

HCPCS 2024

LEVEL II NATIONAL CODES

2024 HCPCS quarterly updates available on the companion website at: http://www.codingupdates.com

DISCLAIMER

Every effort has been made to make this text complete and accurate, but no guarantee, warranty, or representation is made for its accuracy or completeness. This text is based on the Centers for Medicare and Medicaid Services Healthcare Common Procedure Coding System (HCPCS).

Do not report HCPCS modifiers with MIPS CPT Category II codes, rather, use Performance Measurement Modifiers 1P, 2P, 3P, and 8P, as instructed in the CPT guidelines for Category II codes under 'Modifiers'.

LEVEL II NATIONAL MODIFIERS

* A1   Dressing for one wound
* A2   Dressing for two wounds
* A3   Dressing for three wounds
* A4   Dressing for four wounds
* A5   Dressing for five wounds
* A6   Dressing for six wounds
* A7   Dressing for seven wounds
* A8   Dressing for eight wounds
* A9   Dressing for nine or more wounds
○ AA   Anesthesia services performed personally by anesthesiologist

IOM: 100-04, 12, 90.4

AB   Audiology service furnished personally by an audiologist without a physician/npp order for non-acute hearing assessment unrelated to disequilibrium, or hearing aids, or examinations for the purpose of prescribing, fitting, or changing hearing aids; service may be performed once every 12 months, per beneficiary

○ AD   Medical supervision by a physician: more than four concurrent anesthesia procedures

IOM: 100-04, 12, 90.4

* AE   Registered dietician
* AF   Specialty physician
* AG   Primary physician
○ AH   Clinical psychologist

IOM: 100-04, 12, 170

* AI   Principal physician of record
○ AJ   Clinical social worker

IOM: 100-04, 12, 170; 100-04, 12, 150

* AK   Nonparticipating physician
○ AM   Physician, team member service

Not assigned for Medicare

Cross Reference QM

* AO   Alternate payment method declined by provider of service
* AP   Determination of refractive state was not performed in the course of diagnostic ophthalmological examination

* AQ   Physician providing a service in an unlisted health professional shortage area (HPSA)
* AR   Physician provider services in a physician scarcity area
* AS   Physician assistant, nurse practitioner, or clinical nurse specialist services for assistant at surgery
* AT   Acute treatment (this modifier should be used when reporting service 98940, 98941, 98942)
* AU   Item furnished in conjunction with a urological, ostomy, or tracheostomy supply
* AV   Item furnished in conjunction with a prosthetic device, prosthetic or orthotic
* AW   Item furnished in conjunction with a surgical dressing
* AX   Item furnished in conjunction with dialysis services
* AY   Item or service furnished to an ESRD patient that is not for the treatment of ESRD
⊘ AZ   Physician providing a service in a dental health professional shortage area for the purpose of an electronic health record incentive payment
* BA   Item furnished in conjunction with parenteral enteral nutrition (PEN) services
* BL   Special acquisition of blood and blood products
* BO   Orally administered nutrition, not by feeding tube
* BP   The beneficiary has been informed of the purchase and rental options and has elected to purchase the item
* BR   The beneficiary has been informed of the purchase and rental options and has elected to rent the item
* BU   The beneficiary has been informed of the purchase and rental options and after 30 days has not informed the supplier of his/her decision
* CA   Procedure payable only in the inpatient setting when performed emergently on an outpatient who expires prior to admission
* CB   Service ordered by a renal dialysis facility (RDF) physician as part of the ESRD beneficiary's dialysis benefit, is not part of the composite rate, and is separately reimbursable

---

▶ New   ↻ Revised   ✔ Reinstated   ~~deleted~~ Deleted   ⊘ Not covered or valid by Medicare
○ Special coverage instructions   * Carrier discretion   Ⓑ Bill Part B MAC   Ⓓ Bill DME MAC

* **CC** Procedure code change (Use CC when the procedure code submitted was changed either for administrative reasons or because an incorrect code was filed)

⊙ **CD** AMCC test has been ordered by an ESRD facility or MCP physician that is part of the composite rate and is not separately billable

⊙ **CE** AMCC test has been ordered by an ESRD facility or MCP physician that is a composite rate test but is beyond the normal frequency covered under the rate and is separately reimbursable based on medical necessity

⊙ **CF** AMCC test has been ordered by an ESRD facility or MCP physician that is not part of the composite rate and is separately billable

* **CG** Policy criteria applied

⊙ **CH** 0 percent impaired, limited or restricted

⊙ **CI** At least 1 percent but less than 20 percent impaired, limited or restricted

⊙ **CJ** At least 20 percent but less than 40 percent impaired, limited or restricted

⊙ **CK** At least 40 percent but less than 60 percent impaired, limited or restricted

⊙ **CL** At least 60 percent but less than 80 percent impaired, limited or restricted

⊙ **CM** At least 80 percent but less than 100 percent impaired, limited or restricted

⊙ **CN** 100 percent impaired, limited or restricted

* **CO** Outpatient occupational therapy services furnished in whole or in part by an occupational therapy assistant

* **CR** Catastrophe/Disaster related

* **CS** Cost-sharing waived for specified covid-19 testing-related services that result in and order for or administration of a covid-19 test and/or used for cost-sharing waived preventive services furnished via telehealth in rural health clinics and federally qualified health centers during the covid-19 public health emergency

* **CT** Computed tomography services furnished using equipment that does not meet each of the attributes of the national electrical manufacturers association (NEMA) XR-29-2013 standard

Coding Clinic: 2017, Q1, P6

* **CQ** Outpatient physical therapy services furnished in whole or in part by a physical therapist assistant

* **DA** Oral health assessment by a licensed health professional other than a dentist

* **E1** Upper left, eyelid
Coding Clinic: 2016, Q3, P3

* **E2** Lower left, eyelid
Coding Clinic: 2016, Q3, P3

* **E3** Upper right, eyelid
Coding Clinic: 2011, Q3, P6

* **E4** Lower right, eyelid

⊙ **EA** Erythropoetic stimulating agent (ESA) administered to treat anemia due to anti-cancer chemotherapy
CMS requires claims for non-ESRD ESAs (J0881 and J0885) to include one of three modifiers: EA, EB, EC.

⊙ **EB** Erythropoetic stimulating agent (ESA) administered to treat anemia due to anti-cancer radiotherapy
CMS requires claims for non-ESRD ESAs (J0881 and J0885) to include one of three modifiers: EA, EB, EC.

⊙ **EC** Erythropoetic stimulating agent (ESA) administered to treat anemia not due to anti-cancer radiotherapy or anti-cancer chemotherapy
CMS requires claims for non-ESRD ESAs (J0881 and J0885) to include one of three modifiers: EA, EB, EC.

⊙ **ED** Hematocrit level has exceeded 39% (or hemoglobin level has exceeded 13.0 g/dl) for 3 or more consecutive billing cycles immediately prior to and including the current cycle

⊙ **EE** Hematocrit level has not exceeded 39% (or hemoglobin level has not exceeded 13.0 g/dl) for 3 or more consecutive billing cycles immediately prior to and including the current cycle

⊙ **EJ** Subsequent claims for a defined course of therapy, e.g., EPO, sodium hyaluronate, infliximab

⊙ **EM** Emergency reserve supply (for ESRD benefit only)

* **EP** Service provided as part of Medicaid early periodic screening diagnosis and treatment (EPSDT) program

* **ER** Items and services furnished by a provider-based, off-campus emergency department

* **ET** Emergency services

* **EX** Expatriate beneficiary

LEVEL II NATIONAL MODIFIERS CC – EX

🐾 MIPS　[Op] Quantity Physician　[Qh] Quantity Hospital　♀ Female only　♂ Male only　[A] Age　♿ DMEPOS　A2-Z3 ASC Payment Indicator　A-Y ASC Status Indicator　Coding Clinic

105

* **EY**   No physician or other licensed health care provider order for this item or service

    Items billed before a signed and dated order has been received by the supplier must be submitted with an EY modifier added to each related HCPCS code.

* **F1**   Left hand, second digit
* **F2**   Left hand, third digit
* **F3**   Left hand, fourth digit
* **F4**   Left hand, fifth digit
* **F5**   Right hand, thumb
* **F6**   Right hand, second digit
* **F7**   Right hand, third digit
* **F8**   Right hand, fourth digit
* **F9**   Right hand, fifth digit
* **FA**   Left hand, thumb
⊘ **FB**   Item provided without cost to provider, supplier or practitioner, or full credit received for replaced device (examples, but not limited to, covered under warranty, replaced due to defect, free samples)
⊚ **FC**   Partial credit received for replaced device
* **FP**   Service provided as part of family planning program
* **FQ**   The service was furnished using audio-only communication technology
* **FR**   The supervising practitioner was present through two-way, audio/video communication technology
* **FS**   Split (or shared) evaluation and management visit
* **FT**   Unrelated evaluation and management (e/m) visit during a postoperative period, or on the same day as a procedure or another E/M visit. (report when an e/m visit is furnished within the global period but is unrelated, or when one or more additional E/M visits furnished on the same day are unrelated)
* **FX**   X-ray taken using film

    Coding Clinic: 2017, Q1, P6

* **FY**   X-ray taken using computed radiography technology/cassette-based imaging
* **G0**   Telehealth services for diagnosis, evaluation, or treatment, of symptoms of an acute stroke
* **G1**   Most recent URR reading of less than 60

    IOM: 100-04, 8, 50.9

* **G2**   Most recent URR reading of 60 to 64.9

    IOM: 100-04, 8, 50.9

* **G3**   Most recent URR reading of 65 to 69.9

    IOM: 100-04, 8, 50.9

* **G4**   Most recent URR reading of 70 to 74.9

    IOM: 100-04, 8, 50.9

* **G5**   Most recent URR reading of 75 or greater

    IOM: 100-04, 8, 50.9

* **G6**   ESRD patient for whom less than six dialysis sessions have been provided in a month

    IOM: 100-04, 8, 50.9

⊚ **G7**   Pregnancy resulted from rape or incest or pregnancy certified by physician as life threatening

    IOM: 100-02, 15, 20.1; 100-03, 3, 170.3

* **G8**   Monitored anesthesia care (MAC) for deep complex, complicated, or markedly invasive surgical procedure
* **G9**   Monitored anesthesia care for patient who has history of severe cardiopulmonary condition
* **GA**   Waiver of liability statement issued as required by payer policy, individual case

    An item/service is expected to be denied as not reasonable and necessary and an ABN is on file. Modifier GA can be used on either a specific or a miscellaneous HCPCS code. Modifiers GA and GY should never be reported together on the same line for the same HCPCS code.

* **GB**   Claim being resubmitted for payment because it is no longer covered under a global payment demonstration
⊚ **GC**   This service has been performed in part by a resident under the direction of a teaching physician

    IOM: 100-04, 12, 90.4, 100

⊚ **GE**   This service has been performed by a resident without the presence of a teaching physician under the primary care exception
* **GF**   Non-physician (e.g., nurse practitioner (NP), certified registered nurse anesthetist (CRNA), certified registered nurse (CRN), clinical nurse specialist (CNS), physician assistant (PA)) services in a critical access hospital
* **GG**   Performance and payment of a screening mammogram and diagnostic mammogram on the same patient, same day

---

▶ New   ↩ Revised   ✔ Reinstated   ~~deleted~~ Deleted   ⊘ Not covered or valid by Medicare
⊚ Special coverage instructions   * Carrier discretion   Ⓑ Bill Part B MAC   Ⓓ Bill DME MAC

* **GH** Diagnostic mammogram converted from screening mammogram on same day

* **GJ** "Opt out" physician or practitioner emergency or urgent service

* **GK** Reasonable and necessary item/service associated with a GA or GZ modifier

An upgrade is defined as an item that goes beyond what is medically necessary under Medicare's coverage requirements. An item can be considered an upgrade even if the physician has signed an order for it. When suppliers know that an item will not be paid in full because it does not meet the coverage criteria stated in the LCD, the supplier can still obtain partial payment at the time of initial determination if the claim is billed using one of the upgrade modifiers (GK or GL). (https://www.cms.gov/manuals/downloads/clm104c01.pdf)

* **GL** Medically unnecessary upgrade provided instead of non-upgraded item, no charge, no Advance Beneficiary Notice (ABN)

* **GM** Multiple patients on one ambulance trip

* **GN** Services delivered under an outpatient speech language pathology plan of care

* **GO** Services delivered under an outpatient occupational therapy plan of care

* **GP** Services delivered under an outpatient physical therapy plan of care

* **GQ** Via asynchronous telecommunications system

* **GR** This service was performed in whole or in part by a resident in a Department of Veterans Affairs medical center or clinic, supervised in accordance with VA policy

⊚ **GS** Dosage of erythropoietin-stimulating agent has been reduced and maintained in response to hematocrit or hemoglobin level

⊚ **GT** Via interactive audio and video telecommunication systems

* **GU** Waiver of liability statement issued as required by payer policy, routine notice

⊚ **GV** Attending physician not employed or paid under arrangement by the patient's hospice provider

⊚ **GW** Service not related to the hospice patient's terminal condition

* **GX** Notice of liability issued, voluntary under payer policy

GX modifier must be submitted with non-covered charges only. This modifier differentiates from the required uses in conjunction with ABN. (https://www.cms.gov/manuals/downloads/clm104c01.pdf)

⊘ **GY** Item or service statutorily excluded, does not meet the definition of any Medicare benefit or, for non-Medicare insurers, is not a contract benefit

Examples of "statutorily excluded" include: Infusion drug not administered using a durable infusion pump, a wheelchair that is for use for mobility outside the home or hearing aids. GA and GY should never be coded together on the same line for the same HCPCS code. (https://www.cms.gov/manuals/downloads/clm104c01.pdf)

⊘ **GZ** Item or service expected to be denied as not reasonable or necessary

Used when an ABN is not on file and can be used on either a specific or a miscellaneous HCPCS code. It would never be correct to place any combination of GY, GZ or GA modifiers on the same claim line and will result in rejected or denied claim for invalid coding. (https://www.cms.gov/manuals/downloads/clm104c01.pdf)

⊘ **H9** Court-ordered

⊘ **HA** Child/adolescent program

⊘ **HB** Adult program, nongeriatric

⊘ **HC** Adult program, geriatric

⊘ **HD** Pregnant/parenting women's program

⊘ **HE** Mental health program

⊘ **HF** Substance abuse program

⊘ **HG** Opioid addiction treatment program

⊘ **HH** Integrated mental health/substance abuse program

⊘ **HI** Integrated mental health and intellectual disability/developmental disabilities program

⊘ **HJ** Employee assistance program

⊘ **HK** Specialized mental health programs for high-risk populations

⊘ **HL** Intern

⊘ **HM** Less than bachelors degree level

⊘ **HN** Bachelors degree level

⊘ **HO** Masters degree level

⊘ **HP** Doctoral level

⊘ **HQ** Group setting

⊘ **HR** Family/couple with client present

🏷 MIPS   **Qp** Quantity Physician   **Qh** Quantity Hospital   ♀ Female only

♂ Male only   **A** Age   ♿ DMEPOS   A2-Z3 ASC Payment Indicator   A-Y ASC Status Indicator   Coding Clinic

⊘ **HS** Family/couple without client present

⊘ **HT** Multi-disciplinary team

⊘ **HU** Funded by child welfare agency

⊘ **HV** Funded by state addictions agency

⊘ **HW** Funded by state mental health agency

⊘ **HX** Funded by county/local agency

⊘ **HY** Funded by juvenile justice agency

⊘ **HZ** Funded by criminal justice agency

∗ **J1** Competitive acquisition program no-pay submission for a prescription number

∗ **J2** Competitive acquisition program, restocking of emergency drugs after emergency administration

∗ **J3** Competitive acquisition program (CAP), drug not available through CAP as written, reimbursed under average sales price methodology

∗ **J4** DMEPOS item subject to DMEPOS competitive bidding program that is furnished by a hospital upon discharge

∗ **J5** Off-the-shelf orthotic subject to dmepos competitive bidding program that is furnished as part of a physical therapist or occupational therapist professional service

∗ **JA** Administered intravenously

This modifier is informational only (not a payment modifier) and may be submitted with all injection codes. According to Medicare, reporting this modifier is voluntary. (CMS Pub. 100-04, chapter 8, section 60.2.3.1 and Pub. 100-04, chapter 17, section 80.11)

∗ **JB** Administered subcutaneously

∗ **JC** Skin substitute used as a graft

∗ **JD** Skin substitute not used as a graft

∗ **JE** Administered via dialysate

∗ **JG** Drug or biological acquired with 340B drug pricing program discount, reported for informational purposes

▶ **JK** One month supply or less of drug or biological

▶ **JL** Three month supply of drug or biological

∗ **JW** Drug amount discarded/not administered to any patient

Use JW to identify unused drugs or biologicals from single use vial/package that are appropriately discarded. Bill on separate line for payment of discarded drug/biological.

IOM: 100-4, 17, 40

Coding Clinic: 2023, Q3, P14-19; 2016, Q4, P4-7; 2010, Q3, P10

JZ Zero drug amount discarded/not administered to any patient

Coding Clinic: 2023, Q3, P14-19

∗ **K0** Lower extremity prosthesis functional Level 0 - does not have the ability or potential to ambulate or transfer safely with or without assistance and a prosthesis does not enhance their quality of life or mobility.

∗ **K1** Lower extremity prosthesis functional Level 1 - has the ability or potential to use a prosthesis for transfers or ambulation on level surfaces at fixed cadence. Typical of the limited and unlimited household ambulator.

∗ **K2** Lower extremity prosthesis functional Level 2 - has the ability or potential for ambulation with the ability to traverse low level environmental barriers such as curbs, stairs or uneven surfaces. Typical of the limited community ambulator.

∗ **K3** Lower extremity prosthesis functional Level 3 - has the ability or potential for ambulation with variable cadence. Typical of the community ambulator who has the ability to traverse most environmental barriers and may have vocational, therapeutic, or exercise activity that demands prosthetic utilization beyond simple locomotion.

∗ **K4** Lower extremity prosthesis functional Level 4 - has the ability or potential for prosthetic ambulation that exceeds the basic ambulation skills, exhibiting high impact, stress, or energy levels, typical of the prosthetic demands of the child, active adult, or athlete.

∗ **KA** Add on option/accessory for wheelchair

∗ **KB** Beneficiary requested upgrade for ABN, more than 4 modifiers identified on claim

∗ **KC** Replacement of special power wheelchair interface

∗ **KD** Drug or biological infused through DME

∗ **KE** Bid under round one of the DMEPOS competitive bidding program for use with non-competitive bid base equipment

---

▶ **New**   ↻ **Revised**   ✓ **Reinstated**   ~~deleted~~ **Deleted**   ⊘ **Not covered or valid by Medicare**

⊛ **Special coverage instructions**   ∗ **Carrier discretion**   Ⓑ **Bill Part B MAC**   Ⓑ **Bill DME MAC**

✷ **KF** Item designated by FDA as Class III device

✷ **KG** DMEPOS item subject to DMEPOS competitive bidding program number 1

✷ **KH** DMEPOS item, initial claim, purchase or first month rental

✷ **KI** DMEPOS item, second or third month rental

✷ **KJ** DMEPOS item, parenteral enteral nutrition (PEN) pump or capped rental, months four to fifteen

✷ **KK** DMEPOS item subject to DMEPOS competitive bidding program number 2

✷ **KL** DMEPOS item delivered via mail

✷ **KM** Replacement of facial prosthesis including new impression/moulage

✷ **KN** Replacement of facial prosthesis using previous master model

✷ **KO** Single drug unit dose formulation

✷ **KP** First drug of a multiple drug unit dose formulation

✷ **KQ** Second or subsequent drug of a multiple drug unit dose formulation

✷ **KR** Rental item, billing for partial month

⚙ **KS** Glucose monitor supply for diabetic beneficiary not treated with insulin

✷ **KT** Beneficiary resides in a competitive bidding area and travels outside that competitive bidding area and receives a competitive bid item

✷ **KU** DMEPOS item subject to DMEPOS competitive bidding program number 3

✷ **KV** DMEPOS item subject to DMEPOS competitive bidding program that is furnished as part of a professional service

✷ **KW** DMEPOS item subject to DMEPOS competitive bidding program number 4

✷ **KX** Requirements specified in the medical policy have been met

Used for physical, occupational, or speech-language therapy to request an exception to therapy payment caps and indicate the services are reasonable and necessary and that there is documentation of medical necessity in the patient's medical record. (Pub 100-04 Attachment - Business Requirements Centers for Medicare and Medicaid Services, Transmittal 2457, April 27, 2012)

Medicare requires modifier KX for implanted permanent cardiac pacemakers, single chamber or duel chamber, for one of the following CPT codes: 33206, 33207, 33208.

✷ **KY** DMEPOS item subject to DMEPOS competitive bidding program number 5

✷ **KZ** New coverage not implemented by managed care

✷ **LC** Left circumflex coronary artery

✷ **LD** Left anterior descending coronary artery

✷ **LL** Lease/rental (use the LL modifier when DME equipment rental is to be applied against the purchase price)

✷ **LM** Left main coronary artery

✷ **LR** Laboratory round trip

⚙ **LS** FDA-monitored intraocular lens implant

✷ **LT** Left side (used to identify procedures performed on the left side of the body)

Modifiers LT and RT identify procedures which can be performed on paired organs. Used for procedures performed on one side only. Should also be used when the procedures are similar but not identical and are performed on paired body parts.
Coding Clinic: 2016, Q3, P5

↩ **LU** Fractionated payment of CAR-T therapy

✷ **M2** Medicare secondary payer (MSP)

✷ **MA** Ordering professional is not required to consult a clinical decision support mechanism due to service being rendered to a patient with a suspected or confirmed emergency medical condition

✷ **MB** Ordering professional is not required to consult a clinical decision support mechanism due to the significant hardship exception of insufficient internet access

✷ **MC** Ordering professional is not required to consult a clinical decision support mechanism due to the significant hardship exception of electronic health record or clinical decision support mechanism vendor issues

✷ **MD** Ordering professional is not required to consult a clinical decision support mechanism due to the significant hardship exception of extreme and uncontrollable circumstances

✷ **ME** The order for this service adheres to appropriate use criteria in the clinical decision support mechanism consulted by the ordering professional

LEVEL II NATIONAL MODIFIERS KF — ME

🔊 MIPS Qp Quantity Physician Qh Quantity Hospital ♀ Female only ♂ Male only A Age ♿ DMEPOS A2-Z3 ASC Payment Indicator A-Y ASC Status Indicator Coding Clinic

109

* **MF**   The order for this service does not adhere to the appropriate use criteria in the clinical decision support mechanism consulted by the ordering professional

* **MG**   The order for this service does not have applicable appropriate use criteria in the qualified clinical decision support mechanism consulted by the ordering professional

* **MH**   Unknown if ordering professional consulted a clinical decision support mechanism for this service, related information was not provided to the furnishing professional or provider

* **MS**   Six month maintenance and servicing fee for reasonable and necessary parts and labor which are not covered under any manufacturer or supplier warranty

▶ **N1**   Group 1 oxygen coverage criteria met

▶ **N2**   Group 2 oxygen coverage criteria met

▶ **N3**   Group 3 oxygen coverage criteria met

* **NB**   Nebulizer system, any type, FDA-cleared for use with specific drug

* **NR**   New when rented (use the NR modifier when DME which was new at the time of rental is subsequently purchased)

* **NU**   New equipment

* **P1**   A normal healthy patient

* **P2**   A patient with mild systemic disease

* **P3**   A patient with severe systemic disease

* **P4**   A patient with severe systemic disease that is a constant threat to life

* **P5**   A moribund patient who is not expected to survive without the operation

* **P6**   A declared brain-dead patient whose organs are being removed for donor purposes

⊘ **PA**   Surgical or other invasive procedure on wrong body part

⊘ **PB**   Surgical or other invasive procedure on wrong patient

⊘ **PC**   Wrong surgery or other invasive procedure on patient

* **PD**   Diagnostic or related non diagnostic item or service provided in a wholly owned or operated entity to a patient who is admitted as an inpatient within 3 days

* **PI**   Positron emission tomography (PET) or PET/computed tomography (CT) to inform the initial treatment strategy of tumors that are biopsy proven or strongly suspected of being cancerous based on other diagnostic testing

* **PL**   Progressive addition lenses

* **PM**   Post mortem

* **PN**   Non-excepted service provided at an off-campus, outpatient, provider-based department of a hospital

* **PO**   Expected services provided at off-campus, outpatient, provider-based department of a hospital

* **PS**   Positron emission tomography (PET) or PET/computed tomography (CT) to inform the subsequent treatment strategy of cancerous tumors when the beneficiary's treating physician determines that the PET study is needed to inform subsequent anti-tumor strategy

* **PT**   Colorectal cancer screening test; converted to diagnostic text or other procedure

Assign this modifier with the appropriate CPT procedure code for colonoscopy, flexible sigmoidoscopy, or barium enema when the service is initiated as a colorectal cancer screening service but then becomes a diagnostic service. MLN Matters article MM7012 (PDF, 75 KB) Reference Medicare Transmittal 3232 April 3, 2015.

Coding Clinic: 2011, Q1, P10

⊙ **Q0**   Investigational clinical service provided in a clinical research study that is in an approved clinical research study

⊙ **Q1**   Routine clinical service provided in a clinical research study that is in an approved clinical research study

* **Q2**   Demonstration procedure/service

* **Q3**   Live kidney donor surgery and related services

* **Q4**   Service for ordering/referring physician qualifies as a service exemption

⊙ **Q5**   Service furnished under a reciprocal billing arrangement by a substitute physician or by a substitute physical therapist furnishing outpatient physical therapy services in a health professional shortage area, a medically underserved area, or a rural area

IOM: 100-04, 1, 30.2.10

▶ **New**   ↻ **Revised**   ✔ **Reinstated**   deleted **Deleted**   ⊘ **Not covered or valid by Medicare**
⊙ **Special coverage instructions**   * **Carrier discretion**   Ⓑ **Bill Part B MAC**   Ⓑ **Bill DME MAC**

MF – Q5   LEVEL II NATIONAL MODIFIERS

⊘ **Q6** Service furnished under a fee-for-time compensation arrangement by a substitute physician or by a substitute physical therapist furnishing outpatient physical therapy services in a health professional shortage area, a medically underserved area, or a rural area

IOM: 100-04, 1, 30.2.11

∗ **Q7** One Class A finding

∗ **Q8** Two Class B findings

∗ **Q9** One Class B and two Class C findings

∗ **QA** Prescribed amounts of stationary oxygen for daytime use while at rest and nighttime use differ and the average of the two amounts is less than 1 liter per minute (lpm)

∗ **QB** Prescribed amounts of stationary oxygen for daytime use while at rest and nighttime use differ and the average of the two amounts exceeds 4 liters per minute (lpm) and portable oxygen is prescribed

∗ **QC** Single channel monitoring

∗ **QD** Recording and storage in solid state memory by a digital recorder

∗ **QE** Prescribed amount of stationary oxygen while at rest is less than 1 liter per minute (LPM)

∗ **QF** Prescribed amount of stationary oxygen while at rest exceeds 4 liters per minute (LPM) and portable oxygen is prescribed

∗ **QG** Prescribed amount of stationary oxygen while at rest is greater than 4 liters per minute (LPM)

∗ **QH** Oxygen conserving device is being used with an oxygen delivery system

⊘ **QJ** Services/items provided to a prisoner or patient in state or local custody, however, the state or local government, as applicable, meets the requirements in 42 CFR 411.4 (B)

⊘ **QK** Medical direction of two, three, or four concurrent anesthesia procedures involving qualified individuals

IOM: 100-04, 12, 50K, 90

∗ **QL** Patient pronounced dead after ambulance called

∗ **QM** Ambulance service provided under arrangement by a provider of services

∗ **QN** Ambulance service furnished directly by a provider of services

⊘ **QP** Documentation is on file showing that the laboratory test(s) was ordered individually or ordered as a CPT-recognized panel other than automated profile codes 80002-80019, G0058, G0059, and G0060

∗ **QQ** Ordering professional consulted a qualified clinical decision support mechanism for this service and the related data was provided to the furnishing professional

∗ **QR** Prescribed amounts of stationary oxygen for daytime use while at rest and nighttime use differ and the average of the two amounts is greater than 4 liters per minute (lpm)

⊘ **QS** Monitored anesthesia care service

IOM: 100-04, 12, 30.6, 501

∗ **QT** Recording and storage on tape by an analog tape recorder

∗ **QW** CLIA-waived test

∗ **QX** CRNA service: with medical direction by a physician

⊘ **QY** Medical direction of one certified registered nurse anesthetist (CRNA) by an anesthesiologist

IOM: 100-04, 12, 50K, 90

∗ **QZ** CRNA service: without medical direction by a physician

∗ **RA** Replacement of a DME, orthotic or prosthetic item

Contractors will deny claims for replacement parts when furnished in conjunction with the repair of a capped rental item and billed with modifier RB, including claims for parts submitted using code E1399, that are billed during the capped rental period (i.e., the last day of the 13th month of continuous use or before). Repair includes all maintenance, servicing, and repair of capped rental DME because it is included in the allowed rental payment amounts. (Pub 100-20 One-Time Notification Centers for Medicare & Medicaid Services, Transmittal: 901, May 13, 2011)

∗ **RB** Replacement of a part of a DME, orthotic or prosthetic item furnished as part of a repair

∗ **RC** Right coronary artery

∗ **RD** Drug provided to beneficiary, but not administered "incident-to"

🐾 MIPS	Qp Quantity Physician	Qh Quantity Hospital	♀ Female only
♂ Male only	A Age	⅙ DMEPOS	A2-Z3 ASC Payment Indicator	A-Y ASC Status Indicator	Coding Clinic

✳ **RE** Furnished in full compliance with FDA-mandated risk evaluation and mitigation strategy (REMS)

✳ **RI** Ramus intermedius coronary artery

✳ **RR** Rental (use the 'RR' modifier when DME is to be rented)

✳ **RT** Right side (used to identify procedures performed on the right side of the body)

Modifiers LT and RT identify procedures which can be performed on paired organs. Used for procedures performed on one side only. Should also be used when the procedures are similar but not identical and are performed on paired body parts.

Coding Clinic: 2016, Q3, P5

⊘ **SA** Nurse practitioner rendering service in collaboration with a physician

⊘ **SB** Nurse midwife

✳ **SC** Medically necessary service or supply

⊘ **SD** Services provided by registered nurse with specialized, highly technical home infusion training

⊘ **SE** State and/or federally funded programs/services

✳ **SF** Second opinion ordered by a professional review organization (PRO) per Section 9401, P.L. 99-272 (100% reimbursement – no Medicare deductible or coinsurance)

✳ **SG** Ambulatory surgical center (ASC) facility service

Only valid for surgical codes. After 1/1/08 not required for ASC facility charges.

⊘ **SH** Second concurrently administered infusion therapy

⊘ **SJ** Third or more concurrently administered infusion therapy

⊘ **SK** Member of high risk population (use only with codes for immunization)

⊘ **SL** State supplied vaccine

⊘ **SM** Second surgical opinion

⊘ **SN** Third surgical opinion

⊘ **SQ** Item ordered by home health

⊘ **SS** Home infusion services provided in the infusion suite of the IV therapy provider

⊘ **ST** Related to trauma or injury

⊘ **SU** Procedure performed in physician's office (to denote use of facility and equipment)

⊘ **SV** Pharmaceuticals delivered to patient's home but not utilized

✳ **SW** Services provided by a certified diabetic educator

⊘ **SY** Persons who are in close contact with member of high-risk population (use only with codes for immunization)

✳ **T1** Left foot, second digit

✳ **T2** Left foot, third digit

✳ **T3** Left foot, fourth digit

✳ **T4** Left foot, fifth digit

✳ **T5** Right foot, great toe

✳ **T6** Right foot, second digit

✳ **T7** Right foot, third digit

✳ **T8** Right foot, fourth digit

✳ **T9** Right foot, fifth digit

✳ **TA** Left foot, great toe

✳ **TB** Drug or biological acquired with 340B drug pricing program discount, reported for informational purposes for select entities

✳ **TC** Technical component; under certain circumstances, a charge may be made for the technical component alone; under those circumstances the technical component charge is identified by adding modifier TC to the usual procedure number; technical component charges are institutional charges and not billed separately by physicians; however, portable x-ray suppliers only bill for technical component and should utilize modifier TC; the charge data from portable x-ray suppliers will then be used to build customary and prevailing profiles.

⊘ **TD** RN

⊘ **TE** LPN/LVN

⊘ **TF** Intermediate level of care

⊘ **TG** Complex/high tech level of care

⊘ **TH** Obstetrical treatment/services, prenatal or postpartum

⊘ **TJ** Program group, child and/or adolescent

⊘ **TK** Extra patient or passenger, non-ambulance

⊘ **TL** Early intervention/individualized family service plan (IFSP)

⊘ **TM** Individualized education program (IEP)

⊘ **TN** Rural/outside providers' customary service area

⊘ **TP** Medical transport, unloaded vehicle

▶ New ↻ Revised ✔ Reinstated deleted Deleted ⊘ Not covered or valid by Medicare ⊙ Special coverage instructions ✳ Carrier discretion Ⓑ Bill Part B MAC Ⓑ Bill DME MAC

⊘ **TQ** Basic life support transport by a volunteer ambulance provider

⊘ **TR** School-based individual education program (IEP) services provided outside the public school district responsible for the student

✳ **TS** Follow-up service

⊘ **TT** Individualized service provided to more than one patient in same setting

⊘ **TU** Special payment rate, overtime

⊘ **TV** Special payment rates, holidays/ weekends

⊘ **TW** Back-up equipment

⊘ **U1** Medicaid Level of Care 1, as defined by each State

⊘ **U2** Medicaid Level of Care 2, as defined by each State

⊘ **U3** Medicaid Level of Care 3, as defined by each State

⊘ **U4** Medicaid Level of Care 4, as defined by each State

⊘ **U5** Medicaid Level of Care 5, as defined by each State

⊘ **U6** Medicaid Level of Care 6, as defined by each State

⊘ **U7** Medicaid Level of Care 7, as defined by each State

⊘ **U8** Medicaid Level of Care 8, as defined by each State

⊘ **U9** Medicaid Level of Care 9, as defined by each State

⊘ **UA** Medicaid Level of Care 10, as defined by each State

⊘ **UB** Medicaid Level of Care 11, as defined by each State

⊘ **UC** Medicaid Level of Care 12, as defined by each State

⊘ **UD** Medicaid Level of Care 13, as defined by each State

✳ **UE** Used durable medical equipment

⊘ **UF** Services provided in the morning

⊘ **UG** Services provided in the afternoon

⊘ **UH** Services provided in the evening

✳ **UJ** Services provided at night

⊘ **UK** Services provided on behalf of the client to someone other than the client (collateral relationship)

✳ **UN** Two patients served

✳ **UP** Three patients served

✳ **UQ** Four patients served

✳ **UR** Five patients served

✳ **US** Six or more patients served

✳ **V1** Demonstration Modifier 1

✳ **V2** Demonstration Modifier 2

✳ **V3** Demonstration Modifier 3

✳ **V4** Demonstration modifier 4

✳ **V5** Vascular catheter (alone or with any other vascular access)

✳ **V6** Arteriovenous graft (or other vascular access not including a vascular catheter)

✳ **V7** Arteriovenous fistula only (in use with two needles)

✳ **VM** Medicare diabetes prevention program (MDPP) virtual make-up session

✳ **VP** Aphakic patient

✳ **X1** Continuous/broad services: for reporting services by clinicians, who provide the principal care for a patient, with no planned endpoint of the relationship; services in this category represent comprehensive care, dealing with the entire scope of patient problems, either directly or in a care coordination role; reporting clinician service examples include, but are not limited to: primary care, and clinicians providing comprehensive care to patients in addition to specialty care

✳ **X2** Continuous/focused services: for reporting services by clinicians whose expertise is needed for the ongoing management of a chronic disease or a condition that needs to be managed and followed with no planned endpoint to the relationship; reporting clinician service examples include but are not limited to: a rheumatologist taking care of the patient's rheumatoid arthritis longitudinally but not providing general primary care services

✳ **X3** Episodic/broad services: for reporting services by clinicians who have broad responsibility for the comprehensive needs of the patient that is limited to a defined period and circumstance such as a hospitalization; reporting clinician service examples include but are not limited to the hospitalist's services rendered providing comprehensive and general care to a patient while admitted to the hospital

---

🐾 MIPS   🆀🅿 Quantity Physician   🆀🅷 Quantity Hospital   ♀ Female only

♂ Male only   🅐 Age   ♿ DMEPOS   A2-Z3 ASC Payment Indicator   A-Y ASC Status Indicator   Coding Clinic

* **X4**   Episodic/focused services: for reporting services by clinicians who provide focused care on particular types of treatment limited to a defined period and circumstance; the patient has a problem, acute or chronic, that will be treated with surgery, radiation, or some other type of generally time-limited intervention; reporting clinician service examples include but are not limited to, the orthopedic surgeon performing a knee replacement and seeing the patient through the postoperative period

* **X5**   Diagnostic services requested by another clinician: for reporting services by a clinician who furnishes care to the patient only as requested by another clinician or subsequent and related services requested by another clinician; this modifier is reported for patient relationships that may not be adequately captured by the above alternative categories; reporting clinician service examples include but are not limited to, the radiologist's interpretation of an imaging study requested by another clinician

* **XE**   Separate encounter, a service that is distinct because it occurred during a separate encounter

* **XP**   Separate practitioner, a service that is distinct because it was performed by a different practitioner

* **XS**   Separate structure, a service that is distinct because it was performed on a separate organ/structure

* **XU**   Unusual non-overlapping service, the use of a service that is distinct because it does not overlap usual components of the main service

Ambulance Modifiers

Modifiers that are used on claims for ambulance services are created by combining two alpha characters. Each alpha character, with the exception of X, represents an origin (source) code or a destination code. The pair of alpha codes creates one modifier. The first position alpha-code = origin; the second position alpha-code = destination. On form CMS-1491, used to report ambulance services, Item 12 should contain the origin code and Item 13 should contain the destination code. Origin and destination codes and their descriptions are as follows:

D	Diagnostic or therapeutic site other than P or H when these are used as origin codes
E	Residential, domiciliary, custodial facility (other than an 1819 facility)
G	Hospital-based ESRD facility
H	Hospital
I	Site of transfer (e.g., airport or helicopter pad) between modes of ambulance transport
J	Freestanding ESRD facility
N	Skilled nursing facility
P	Physician's office
R	Residence
S	Scene of accident or acute event
X	Intermediate stop at physician's office on way to hospital (destination code only)

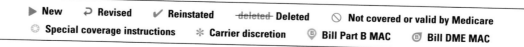

TRANSPORT SERVICES INCLUDING AMBULANCE (A0000–A0999)

⊘ **A0021** Ambulance service, outside state per mile, transport (Medicaid only) Ⓑ Qp Qh E1

Cross Reference A0030

⊘ **A0080** Non-emergency transportation, per mile - vehicle provided by volunteer (individual or organization), with no vested interest Ⓑ Qp Qh E1

⊘ **A0090** Non-emergency transportation, per mile - vehicle provided by individual (family member, self, neighbor) with vested interest Ⓑ Qp Qh E1

⊘ **A0100** Non-emergency transportation; taxi Ⓑ Qp Qh E1

⊘ **A0110** Non-emergency transportation and bus, intra- or interstate carrier Ⓑ Qp Qh E1

⊘ **A0120** Non-emergency transportation: mini-bus, mountain area transports, or other transportation systems Ⓑ Qp Qh E1

⊘ **A0130** Non-emergency transportation: wheelchair van Ⓑ Qp Qh E1

⊘ **A0140** Non-emergency transportation and air travel (private or commercial), intra- or interstate Ⓑ Qp Qh E1

⊘ **A0160** Non-emergency transportation: per mile - caseworker or social worker Ⓑ Qp Qh E1

⊘ **A0170** Transportation: ancillary: parking fees, tolls, other Ⓑ Qp Qh E1

⊘ **A0180** Non-emergency transportation: ancillary: lodging - recipient Ⓑ Qp Qh E1

⊘ **A0190** Non-emergency transportation: ancillary: meals - recipient Ⓑ Qp Qh E1

⊘ **A0200** Non-emergency transportation: ancillary: lodging - escort Ⓑ Qp Qh E1

⊘ **A0210** Non-emergency transportation: ancillary: meals - escort Ⓑ Qp Qh E1

⊘ **A0225** Ambulance service, neonatal transport, base rate, emergency transport, one way Ⓑ Qp Qh E1

⊘ **A0380** BLS mileage (per mile) Ⓑ Qp Qh E1

Cross Reference A0425

⊘ **A0382** BLS routine disposable supplies Ⓑ Qp Qh E1

⊘ **A0384** BLS specialized service disposable supplies; defibrillation (used by ALS ambulances and BLS ambulances in jurisdictions where defibrillation is permitted in BLS ambulances) Ⓑ Qp Qh E1

⊘ **A0390** ALS mileage (per mile) Ⓑ Qp Qh E1

Cross Reference A0425

⊘ **A0392** ALS specialized service disposable supplies; defibrillation (to be used only in jurisdictions where defibrillation cannot be performed in BLS ambulances) Ⓑ Qp Qh E1

⊘ **A0394** ALS specialized service disposable supplies; IV drug therapy Ⓑ Qp Qh E1

⊘ **A0396** ALS specialized service disposable supplies; esophageal intubation Ⓑ Qp Qh E1

⊘ **A0398** ALS routine disposable supplies Ⓑ Qp Qh E1

⊘ **A0420** Ambulance waiting time (ALS or BLS), one half (½) hour increments Ⓑ Qp Qh E1

Waiting Time Table

UNITS	TIME	UNITS	TIME
1	½ to 1 hr.	6	3 to 3½ hrs.
2	1 to 1½ hrs.	7	3½ to 4 hrs.
3	1½ to 2 hrs.	8	4 to 4½ hrs.
4	2 to 2½ hrs.	9	4½ to 5 hrs.
5	2½ to 3 hrs.	10	5 to 5½ hrs.

⊘ **A0422** Ambulance (ALS or BLS) oxygen and oxygen supplies, life sustaining situation Ⓑ Qp Qh E1

⊘ **A0424** Extra ambulance attendant, ground (ALS or BLS) or air (fixed or rotary winged); (requires medical review) Ⓑ Qp Qh E1

✳ **A0425** Ground mileage, per statute mile Ⓑ Qp Qh A

✳ **A0426** Ambulance service, advanced life support, non-emergency transport, Level 1 (ALS 1) Ⓑ Qp Qh A

✳ **A0427** Ambulance service, advanced life support, emergency transport, Level 1 (ALS 1-Emergency) Ⓑ Qp Qh A

✳ **A0428** Ambulance service, basic life support, non-emergency transport (BLS) Ⓑ Qp Qh A

✳ **A0429** Ambulance service, basic life support, emergency transport (BLS-Emergency) Ⓑ Qp Qh A

✳ **A0430** Ambulance service, conventional air services, transport, one way (fixed wing) Ⓑ Qp Qh A

✳ **A0431** Ambulance service, conventional air services, transport, one way (rotary wing) Ⓑ Qp Qh A

* **A0432** Paramedic intercept (PI), rural area, transport furnished by a volunteer ambulance company, which is prohibited by state law from billing third party payers Ⓑ Qp Qh   A

* **A0433** Advanced life support, Level 2 (ALS2) Ⓑ Qp Qh   A

* **A0434** Specialty care transport (SCT) Ⓑ Qp Qh   A

* **A0435** Fixed wing air mileage, per statute mile Ⓑ Qp Qh   A

* **A0436** Rotary wing air mileage, per statute mile Ⓑ Qp Qh   A

⊘ **A0888** Noncovered ambulance mileage, per mile (e.g., for miles traveled beyond closest appropriate facility) Ⓑ Qp Qh   E1

MCM: 2125

⊘ **A0998** Ambulance response and treatment, no transport Ⓑ Qp Qh   E1

IOM: 100-02, 10, 20

⊛ **A0999** Unlisted ambulance service Ⓑ   A

IOM: 100-02, 10, 20

MEDICAL AND SURGICAL SUPPLIES
(A2001-A8004)

Wound Supplies

A2001 Innovamatrix ac, per square centimeter   N1

A2002 Mirragen advanced wound matrix, per square centimeter   N1

~~A2003~~ ~~Bio connekt wound matrix, per square centimeter~~   ~~N1~~

A2004 Xcellistem, 1 mg   N1

A2005 Microlyte matrix, per square centimeter   N1

A2006 Novosorb synpath dermal matrix, per square centimeter   N1

A2007 Restrata, per square centimeter   N1

A2008 Theragenesis, per square centimeter   N1

A2009 Symphony, per square centimeter   N1

A2010 Apis, per square centimeter   N1

A2011 Supra sdrm, per square centimeter   N1

A2012 Suprathel, per square centimeter   N1

A2013 Innovamatrix fs, per square centimeter   N1

A2014 Omeza collagen matrix, per 100 mg   N1

A2015 Phoenix wound matrix, per square centimeter   N1

A2016 Permeaderm B, per square centimeter   N1

A2017 Permeaderm glove, each   N1

A2018 Permeaderm C, per square centimeter   N1

▶ **A2019** Kerecis omega3 marigen shield, per square centimeter   N1

▶ **A2020** Ac5 advanced wound system (ac5)   N1

▶ **A2021** Neomatrix, per square centimeter   N1

▶ **A2022** Innovaburn or innovamatrix xl, per square centimeter   N1

▶ **A2023** Innovamatrix pd, 1 mg   N1

▶ **A2024** Resolve matrix, per square centimeter   N1

▶ **A2025** Miro3d, per cubic centimeter   N1

▶ **A4100** Skin substitute, FDA cleared as a device, not otherwise specified   N1

Injection and Infusion

* **A4206** Syringe with needle, sterile 1 cc or less, each Ⓑ Ⓓ   N

* **A4207** Syringe with needle, sterile 2 cc, each Ⓑ Ⓓ   N

* **A4208** Syringe with needle, sterile 3 cc, each Ⓑ Ⓓ   N

* **A4209** Syringe with needle, sterile 5 cc or greater, each Ⓑ Ⓓ   N

⊘ **A4210** Needle-free injection device, each Ⓑ Qp Qh   E1

IOM: 100-03, 4, 280.1

⊛ **A4211** Supplies for self-administered injections Ⓓ Ⓑ Qp Qh   N

IOM: 100-02, 15, 50

* **A4212** Non-coring needle or stylet with or without catheter Ⓑ Qp Qh   N

* **A4213** Syringe, sterile, 20 cc or greater, each Ⓑ Ⓓ   N

* **A4215** Needle, sterile, any size, each Ⓑ Ⓓ   N

⊛ **A4216** Sterile water, saline and/or dextrose diluent/flush, 10 ml Ⓑ Ⓓ ♿   N

Other: Sodium Chloride, Bacteriostatic, Syrex

IOM: 100-02, 15, 50

⊛ **A4217** Sterile water/saline, 500 ml Ⓑ Ⓓ ♿   N

Other: Sodium Chloride

IOM: 100-02, 15, 50

⊛ **A4218** Sterile saline or water, metered dose dispenser, 10 ml Ⓑ Ⓓ   N

Other: Sodium Chloride

▶ **New**   ↻ **Revised**   ✔ **Reinstated**   ~~deleted~~ **Deleted**   ⊘ **Not covered or valid by Medicare**
⊛ **Special coverage instructions**   * **Carrier discretion**   Ⓑ **Bill Part B MAC**   Ⓓ **Bill DME MAC**

Figure 1 Insulin pump.

⚙ **A4220** Refill kit for implantable infusion pump Ⓑ Qp Qh   N

Do not report with 95990 or 95991 since Medicare payment for these codes includes the refill kit.

IOM: 100-03, 4, 280.1

✳ **A4221** Supplies for maintenance of non-insulin drug infusion catheter, per week (list drugs separately) Ⓑ Qp Qh ♿   N

Includes dressings for catheter site and flush solutions not directly related to drug infusion.

✳ **A4222** Infusion supplies for external drug infusion pump, per cassette or bag (list drug separately) Ⓑ Qp Qh ♿   N

Includes cassette or bag, diluting solutions, tubing and/or administration supplies, port cap changes, compounding charges, and preparation charges.

✳ **A4223** Infusion supplies not used with external infusion pump, per cassette or bag (list drugs separately) Ⓑ   N

IOM: 100-03, 4, 280.1

✳ **A4224** Supplies for maintenance of insulin infusion catheter, per week Ⓑ Qp Qh ♿   N

⚙ **A4225** Supplies for external insulin infusion pump, syringe type cartridge, sterile, each Ⓑ Qp Qh ♿   N

IOM: 100-03, 1, 50.3

✳ **A4226** Supplies for maintenance of insulin infusion pump with dosage rate adjustment using therapeutic continuous glucose sensing, per week   N

⚙ **A4230** Infusion set for external insulin pump, non-needle cannula type Ⓑ   N

Requires prior authorization and copy of invoice.

IOM: 100-03, 4, 280.1

⚙ **A4231** Infusion set for external insulin pump, needle type Ⓑ   N

Requires prior authorization and copy of invoice.

IOM: 100-03, 4, 280.1

⊘ **A4232** Syringe with needle for external insulin pump, sterile, 3 cc Ⓑ Qp Qh   E1

Reports insulin reservoir for use with external insulin infusion pump (E0784); may be glass or plastic; includes needle for drawing up insulin. Does not include insulin for use in reservoir.

IOM: 100-03, 4, 280.1

Replacement Batteries

✳ **A4233** Replacement battery, alkaline (other than J cell), for use with medically necessary home blood glucose monitor owned by patient, each Ⓑ Qh ♿   E1

✳ **A4234** Replacement battery, alkaline, J cell, for use with medically necessary home blood glucose monitor owned by patient, each Ⓑ Qh ♿   E1

✳ **A4235** Replacement battery, lithium, for use with medically necessary home blood glucose monitor owned by patient, each Ⓑ Qp Qh ♿   E1

✳ **A4236** Replacement battery, silver oxide, for use with medically necessary home blood glucose monitor owned by patient, each Ⓑ Qh ♿   E1

Miscellaneous Supplies

✳ **A4238** Supply allowance for adjunctive, non-implanted continuous glucose monitor (cgm), includes all supplies and accessories, 1 month supply = 1 unit of service ♿   Y

✳ **A4239** Supply allowance for non-adjunctive, non-implanted continuous glucose monitor (cgm), includes all supplies and accessories, 1 month supply = 1 unit of service ♿   Y

✳ **A4244** Alcohol or peroxide, per pint Ⓑ Ⓑ   N

✳ **A4245** Alcohol wipes, per box Ⓑ Ⓑ   N

✳ **A4246** Betadine or Phisohex solution, per pint Ⓑ Ⓑ   N

✳ **A4247** Betadine or iodine swabs/wipes, per box Ⓑ Ⓑ   N

✳ **A4248** Chlorhexidine containing antiseptic, 1 ml Ⓑ Ⓑ   N

⊘ **A4250** Urine test or reagent strips or tablets (100 tablets or strips) Ⓑ Ⓑ Qp Qh   E1

IOM: 100-02, 15, 110

⊘ **A4252** Blood ketone test or reagent strip, each ⑬ Qp Qh E1

Medicare Statute 1861(n)

⊛ **A4253** Blood glucose test or reagent strips for home blood glucose monitor, per 50 strips ⑬ Qp Qh ₺ N

Test strips (1 unit = 50 strips); non-insulin treated (every 3 months) 100 test strips (1×/day testing), 100 lancets (1×/day testing); modifier KS

IOM: 100-03, 1, 40.2

⊛ **A4255** Platforms for home blood glucose monitor, 50 per box ⑬ Qp Qh ₺ N

IOM: 100-03, 1, 40.2

⊛ **A4256** Normal, low and high calibrator solution/chips ⑬ Qp Qh ₺ N

IOM: 100-03, 1, 40.2

⊛ **A4257** Replacement lens shield cartridge for use with laser skin piercing device, each ⑬ Qp Qh ₺ E1

⊛ **A4258** Spring-powered device for lancet, each ⑬ Qp Qh ₺ N

IOM: 100-03, 1, 40.2

⊛ **A4259** Lancets, per box of 100 ⑬ Qp Qh ₺ N

IOM: 100-03, 1, 40.2

⊘ **A4261** Cervical cap for contraceptive use ⑬ Qp Qh ♀ E1

Medicare Statute 1862A1

⊛ **A4262** Temporary, absorbable lacrimal duct implant, each ⑬ Qp Qh N

IOM: 100-04, 12, 20.3, 30.4

⊛ **A4263** Permanent, long term, non-dissolvable lacrimal duct implant, each ⑬ Qp Qh N

Bundled with insertion if performed in physician office.

IOM: 100-04, 12, 30.4

⊘ **A4264** Permanent implantable contraceptive intratubal occlusion device(s) and delivery system ⑤ Qp Qh ♀ E1

Reports the Essure device.

⊛ **A4265** Paraffin, per pound ⑬ ⑬ Qp Qh ₺ N

IOM: 100-03, 4, 280.1

⊘ **A4266** Diaphragm for contraceptive use ⑬ Qp Qh ♀ E1

⊘ **A4267** Contraceptive supply, condom, male, each ⑬ Qp Qh ♂ E1

⊘ **A4268** Contraceptive supply, condom, female, each ⑬ Qp Qh ♀ E1

⊘ **A4269** Contraceptive supply, spermicide (e.g., foam, gel), each ⑬ Qp Qh E1

⊛ **A4270** Disposable endoscope sheath, each ⑬ Qp Qh N

⊛ **A4280** Adhesive skin support attachment for use with external breast prosthesis, each ⑬ Qh ♀ ₺ N

⊛ **A4281** Tubing for breast pump, replacement ⑬ ♀ E1

⊛ **A4282** Adapter for breast pump, replacement ⑬ ♀ E1

⊛ **A4283** Cap for breast pump bottle, replacement ⑬ ♀ E1

⊛ **A4284** Breast shield and splash protector for use with breast pump, replacement ⑬ ♀ E1

⊛ **A4285** Polycarbonate bottle for use with breast pump, replacement ⑬ ♀ E1

⊛ **A4286** Locking ring for breast pump, replacement ⑬ ♀ E1

⊛ **A4290** Sacral nerve stimulation test lead, each ⑬ N

Service not separately priced by Part B (e.g., services not covered, bundled, used by Part A only)

Implantable Catheters

⊛ **A4300** Implantable access catheter, (e.g., venous, arterial, epidural subarachnoid, or peritoneal, etc.) external access ⑬ Qp Qh N

IOM: 100-02, 15, 120

⊛ **A4301** Implantable access total; catheter, port/reservoir (e.g., venous, arterial, epidural, subarachnoid, peritoneal, etc.) ⑤ Qp Qh N

Disposable Drug Delivery System

⊛ **A4305** Disposable drug delivery system, flow rate of 50 ml or greater per hour ⑬ ⑬ Qp Qh N

⊛ **A4306** Disposable drug delivery system, flow rate of less than 50 ml per hour ⑬ ⑬ Qp Qh N

Incontinence Appliances and Care Supplies

⊛ **A4310** Insertion tray without drainage bag and without catheter (accessories only) ⑬ ⑬ Qp Qh ₺ N

IOM: 100-02, 15, 120

⊛ **A4311** Insertion tray without drainage bag with indwelling catheter, Foley type, two-way latex with coating (Teflon, silicone, silicone elastomer, or hydrophilic, etc.) ⑬ ⑬ Qp Qh ₺ N

IOM: 100-02, 15, 120

▶ **New**   ↻ **Revised**   ✔ **Reinstated**   ~~deleted~~ **Deleted**   ⊘ **Not covered or valid by Medicare**
⊛ **Special coverage instructions**   ✳ **Carrier discretion**   ⑬ **Bill Part B MAC**   ⑬ **Bill DME MAC**

Holes at end of catheter

Channel for water to expand balloon

Channel for urine

Figure 2 Foley catheter.

A4312 Insertion tray without drainage bag with indwelling catheter, Foley type, two-way, all silicone N

Must meet criteria for indwelling catheter and medical record must justify need for:

• Recurrent encrustation

• Inability to pass a straight catheter

• Sensitivity to latex

Must be medically necessary.

IOM: 100-02, 15, 120

A4313 Insertion tray without drainage bag with indwelling catheter, Foley type, three-way, for continuous irrigation N

Must meet criteria for indwelling catheter and medical record must justify need for:

• Recurrent encrustation

• Inability to pass a straight catheter

• Sensitivity to latex

Must be medically necessary.

IOM: 100-02, 15, 120

A4314 Insertion tray with drainage bag with indwelling catheter, Foley type, two-way latex with coating (Teflon, silicone, silicone elastomer or hydrophilic, etc.) N

IOM: 100-02, 15, 120

A4315 Insertion tray with drainage bag with indwelling catheter, Foley type, two-way, all silicone N

IOM: 100-02, 15, 120

A4316 Insertion tray with drainage bag with indwelling catheter, Foley type, three-way, for continuous irrigation N

IOM: 100-02, 15, 120

A4320 Irrigation tray with bulb or piston syringe, any purpose N

IOM: 100-02, 15, 120

A4321 Therapeutic agent for urinary catheter irrigation N

IOM: 100-02, 15, 120

A4322 Irrigation syringe, bulb, or piston, each N

IOM: 100-02, 15, 120

A4326 Male external catheter with integral collection chamber, any type, each N

IOM: 100-02, 15, 120

A4327 Female external urinary collection device; meatal cup, each N

IOM: 100-02, 15, 120

A4328 Female external urinary collection device; pouch, each N

IOM: 100-02, 15, 120

A4330 Perianal fecal collection pouch with adhesive, each N

IOM: 100-02, 15, 120

A4331 Extension drainage tubing, any type, any length, with connector/adaptor, for use with urinary leg bag or urostomy pouch, each N

IOM: 100-02, 15, 120

A4332 Lubricant, individual sterile packet, each N

IOM: 100-02, 15, 120

A4333 Urinary catheter anchoring device, adhesive skin attachment, each N

IOM: 100-02, 15, 120

A4334 Urinary catheter anchoring device, leg strap, each N

IOM: 100-02, 15, 120

A4335 Incontinence supply; miscellaneous N

IOM: 100-02, 15, 120

🔊 MIPS	**Qp** Quantity Physician	**Qh** Quantity Hospital	♀ Female only
♂ Male only	**A** Age	🦽 DMEPOS	A2-Z3 ASC Payment Indicator	A-Y ASC Status Indicator	Coding Clinic

⊚ **A4336** Incontinence supply, urethral insert, any type, each Ⓑ Ⓑ ও   N
IOM: 100-02, 15, 120

⊚ **A4337** Incontinence supply, rectal insert, any type, each Ⓥ Ⓑ Qp Qh   N
IOM: 100-02, 15, 120

⊚ **A4338** Indwelling catheter; Foley type, two-way latex with coating (Teflon, silicone, silicone elastomer, or hydrophilic, etc.), each Ⓑ Ⓖ Qp Qh   N
IOM: 100-02, 15, 120

⊚ **A4340** Indwelling catheter; specialty type (e.g., coude, mushroom, wing, etc.), each Ⓥ Ⓖ Qp Qh   N

Must meet criteria for indwelling catheter and medical record must justify need for:

- Recurrent encrustation
- Inability to pass a straight catheter
- Sensitivity to latex

Must be medically necessary.
IOM: 100-02, 15, 120

▶ **A4341** Indwelling intraurethral drainage device with valve, patient inserted, replacement only, each   N

▶ **A4342** Accessories for patient inserted indwelling intraurethral drainage device with valve, replacement only, each   N

↻⊚ **A4344** Indwelling catheter, Foley type, two-way, all silicone, or polyurethane each Ⓥ Ⓖ Qp Qh &   N1 N

Must meet criteria for indwelling catheter and medical record must justify need for:

- Recurrent encrustation
- Inability to pass a straight catheter
- Sensitivity to latex

Must be medically necessary.
IOM: 100-02, 15, 120

⊚ **A4346** Indwelling catheter; Foley type, three way for continuous irrigation, each Ⓥ Ⓖ Qp Qh &   N
IOM: 100-02, 15, 120

⊚ **A4349** Male external catheter, with or without adhesive, disposable, each Ⓥ Ⓖ ♂ & N
IOM: 100-02, 15, 120

⊚ **A4351** Intermittent urinary catheter; straight tip, with or without coating (Teflon, silicone, silicone elastomer, or hydrophilic, etc.), each Ⓥ Ⓖ Qp Qh &   N
IOM: 100-02, 15, 120

⊚ **A4352** Intermittent urinary catheter; coude (curved) tip, with or without coating (Teflon, silicone, silicone elastomeric, or hydrophilic, etc.), each Ⓥ Ⓖ Qp Qh &   N
IOM: 100-02, 15, 120

⊚ **A4353** Intermittent urinary catheter, with insertion supplies Ⓥ Ⓖ Qh &   N
IOM: 100-02, 15, 120

⊚ **A4354** Insertion tray with drainage bag but without catheter Ⓑ Ⓖ Qp Qh &   N
IOM: 100-02, 15, 120

⊚ **A4355** Irrigation tubing set for continuous bladder irrigation through a three-way indwelling Foley catheter, each Ⓑ Ⓖ Qp Qh &   N
IOM: 100-02, 15, 120

External Urinary Supplies

⊚ **A4356** External urethral clamp or compression device (not to be used for catheter clamp), each Ⓑ Ⓖ Qp Qh &   N
IOM: 100-02, 15, 120

⊚ **A4357** Bedside drainage bag, day or night, with or without anti-reflux device, with or without tube, each Ⓑ Ⓖ Qp Qh &   N
IOM: 100-02, 15, 120

⊚ **A4358** Urinary drainage bag, leg or abdomen, vinyl, with or without tube, with straps, each Ⓥ Ⓖ Qp &   N
IOM: 100-02, 15, 120

⊚ **A4360** Disposable external urethral clamp or compression device, with pad and/or pouch, each Ⓑ Ⓖ &   N

Ostomy Supplies

⊚ **A4361** Ostomy faceplate, each Ⓑ Ⓖ Qp Qh &   N
IOM: 100-02, 15, 120

⊚ **A4362** Skin barrier; solid, 4 × 4 or equivalent; each Ⓑ Ⓖ Qp Qh &   N
IOM: 100-02, 15, 120

⊚ **A4363** Ostomy clamp, any type, replacement only, each Ⓥ Ⓖ Qp Qh &   E1

⊚ **A4364** Adhesive, liquid or equal, any type, per oz Ⓥ Ⓑ Qp Qh &   N

Fee schedule category: Ostomy, tracheostomy, and urologicals items.
IOM: 100-02, 15, 120

▶ New   ↻ Revised   ✔ Reinstated   ~~deleted~~ Deleted   ⊘ Not covered or valid by Medicare
⊚ Special coverage instructions   ✳ Carrier discretion   Ⓑ Bill Part B MAC   Ⓖ Bill DME MAC

Figure 3 Ostomy pouch.

* **A4366** Ostomy vent, any type, each Ⓑ Ⓑ Qh ♿   N

☼ **A4367** Ostomy belt, each Ⓑ Ⓑ Qp Qh ♿   N

IOM: 100-02, 15, 120

* **A4368** Ostomy filter, any type, each Ⓑ Ⓑ Qp Qh ♿   N

☼ **A4369** Ostomy skin barrier, liquid (spray, brush, etc.), per oz Ⓟ Ⓑ Ⓑ ♿   N

IOM: 100-02, 15, 120

☼ **A4371** Ostomy skin barrier, powder, per oz Ⓑ Ⓑ ♿   N

IOM: 100-02, 15, 120

☼ **A4372** Ostomy skin barrier, solid 4 × 4 or equivalent, standard wear, with built-in convexity, each Ⓑ Ⓑ Qh ♿   N

IOM: 100-02, 15, 120

☼ **A4373** Ostomy skin barrier, with flange (solid, flexible, or accordion), with built-in convexity, any size, each Ⓑ Ⓑ Qh ♿ N

IOM: 100-02, 15, 120

☼ **A4375** Ostomy pouch, drainable, with faceplate attached, plastic, each Ⓑ Ⓑ Qp Qh ♿ N

IOM: 100-02, 15, 120

☼ **A4376** Ostomy pouch, drainable, with faceplate attached, rubber, each Ⓑ Ⓑ Qp Qh ♿   N

IOM: 100-02, 15, 120

☼ **A4377** Ostomy pouch, drainable, for use on faceplate, plastic, each Ⓟ Ⓑ Qp Qh ♿   N

IOM: 100-02, 15, 120

☼ **A4378** Ostomy pouch, drainable, for use on faceplate, rubber, each Ⓑ Ⓑ Qp Qh ♿   N

IOM: 100-02, 15, 120

☼ **A4379** Ostomy pouch, urinary, with faceplate attached, plastic, each Ⓟ Ⓑ Qp Qh ♿   N

☼ **A4380** Ostomy pouch, urinary, with faceplate attached, rubber, each Ⓑ Ⓑ Qp Qh ♿   N

IOM: 100-02, 15, 120

☼ **A4381** Ostomy pouch, urinary, for use on faceplate, plastic, each Ⓟ Ⓑ Qp Qh ♿   N

IOM: 100-02, 15, 120

☼ **A4382** Ostomy pouch, urinary, for use on faceplate, heavy plastic, each Ⓟ Ⓑ Qp Qh ♿   N

IOM: 100-02, 15, 120

☼ **A4383** Ostomy pouch, urinary, for use on faceplate, rubber, each Ⓟ Ⓑ Qp Qh ♿   N

IOM: 100-02, 15, 120

☼ **A4384** Ostomy faceplate equivalent, silicone ring, each Ⓟ Ⓑ Qp Qh ♿   N

IOM: 100-02, 15, 120

☼ **A4385** Ostomy skin barrier, solid 4 × 4 or equivalent, extended wear, without built-in convexity, each Ⓑ Ⓑ Qp Qh ♿   N

IOM: 100-02, 15, 120

☼ **A4387** Ostomy pouch closed, with barrier attached, with built-in convexity (1 piece), each Ⓟ Ⓑ Qh ♿   N

IOM: 100-02, 15, 120

☼ **A4388** Ostomy pouch, drainable, with extended wear barrier attached (1 piece), each Ⓑ Ⓑ Qh ♿   N

IOM: 100-02, 15, 120

☼ **A4389** Ostomy pouch, drainable, with barrier attached, with built-in convexity (1 piece), each Ⓟ Ⓑ Qp Qh ♿   N

IOM: 100-02, 15, 120

☼ **A4390** Ostomy pouch, drainable, with extended wear barrier attached, with built-in convexity (1 piece), each Ⓟ Ⓑ Qh ♿   N

IOM: 100-02, 15, 120

☼ **A4391** Ostomy pouch, urinary, with extended wear barrier attached (1 piece), each Ⓟ Ⓑ Qh ♿   N

IOM: 100-02, 15, 120

☼ **A4392** Ostomy pouch, urinary, with standard wear barrier attached, with built-in convexity (1 piece), each Ⓟ Ⓑ Qp Qh ♿   N

IOM: 100-02, 15, 120

☼ **A4393** Ostomy pouch, urinary, with extended wear barrier attached, with built-in convexity (1 piece), each Ⓟ Ⓑ Qh ♿ N

IOM: 100-02, 15, 120

☼ MIPS   Qp Quantity Physician   Qh Quantity Hospital   ♀ Female only

♂ Male only   Ⓐ Age   ♿ DMEPOS   A2-Z3 ASC Payment Indicator   A-Y ASC Status Indicator   Coding Clinic

⊛ **A4394** Ostomy deodorant, with or without lubricant, for use in ostomy pouch, per fluid ounce Ⓑ Ⓓ ♿ N

IOM: 100-02, 15, 20

⊛ **A4395** Ostomy deodorant for use in ostomy pouch, solid, per tablet Ⓑ Ⓓ ♿ N

IOM: 100-02, 15, 20

⊛ **A4396** Ostomy belt with peristomal hernia support Ⓑ Ⓓ Qh ♿ N

IOM: 100-02, 15, 120

⊛ **A4398** Ostomy irrigation supply; bag, each Ⓑ Ⓓ Qp Qh ♿ N

IOM: 100-02, 15, 120

⊛ **A4399** Ostomy irrigation supply; cone/catheter, with or without brush Ⓑ Ⓓ Qp Qh ♿ N

IOM: 100-02, 15, 120

⊛ **A4400** Ostomy irrigation set Ⓑ Ⓓ Qp Qh ♿ N

IOM: 100-02, 15, 120

⊛ **A4402** Lubricant, per ounce Ⓑ Ⓓ Qp Qh ♿ N

IOM: 100-02, 15, 120

⊛ **A4404** Ostomy ring, each Ⓑ Ⓓ Qp Qh ♿ N

IOM: 100-02, 15, 120

⊛ **A4405** Ostomy skin barrier, non-pectin based, paste, per ounce Ⓑ Ⓓ ♿ N

IOM: 100-02, 15, 120

⊛ **A4406** Ostomy skin barrier, pectin-based, paste, per ounce Ⓑ Ⓓ ♿ N

IOM: 100-02, 15, 120

⊛ **A4407** Ostomy skin barrier, with flange (solid, flexible, or accordion), extended wear, with built-in convexity, 4 × 4 inches or smaller, each Ⓑ Ⓓ Qp Qh ♿ N

IOM: 100-02, 15, 120

⊛ **A4408** Ostomy skin barrier, with flange (solid, flexible, or accordion), extended wear, with built-in convexity, larger than 4 × 4 inches, each Ⓑ Ⓓ Qh ♿ N

IOM: 100-02, 15, 120

⊛ **A4409** Ostomy skin barrier, with flange (solid, flexible, or accordion), extended wear, without built-in convexity, 4 × 4 inches or smaller, each Ⓑ Ⓓ Qh ♿ N

IOM: 100-02, 15, 120

⊛ **A4410** Ostomy skin barrier, with flange (solid, flexible, or accordion), extended wear, without built-in convexity, larger than 4 × 4 inches, each Ⓑ Ⓓ Qp Qh ♿ N

IOM: 100-02, 15, 120

⊛ **A4411** Ostomy skin barrier, solid 4 × 4 or equivalent, extended wear, with built-in convexity, each Ⓑ Ⓓ Qh ♿ N

⊛ **A4412** Ostomy pouch, drainable, high output, for use on a barrier with flange (2 piece system), without filter, each Ⓑ Ⓓ Qh ♿ N

IOM: 100-02, 15, 120

⊛ **A4413** Ostomy pouch, drainable, high output, for use on a barrier with flange (2 piece system), with filter, each Ⓑ Ⓓ Qp Qh ♿ N

IOM: 100-02, 15, 120

⊛ **A4414** Ostomy skin barrier, with flange (solid, flexible, or accordion), without built-in convexity, 4 × 4 inches or smaller, each Ⓑ Ⓓ Qh ♿ N

IOM: 100-02, 15, 120

⊛ **A4415** Ostomy skin barrier, with flange (solid, flexible, or accordion), without built-in convexity, larger than 4 × 4 inches, each Ⓑ Ⓓ Qh ♿ N

IOM: 100-02, 15, 120

✳ **A4416** Ostomy pouch, closed, with barrier attached, with filter (1 piece), each Ⓑ Ⓓ Qp Qh ♿ N

✳ **A4417** Ostomy pouch, closed, with barrier attached, with built-in convexity, with filter (1 piece), each Ⓑ Ⓓ Qh ♿ N

✳ **A4418** Ostomy pouch, closed; without barrier attached, with filter (1 piece), each Ⓑ Ⓓ Qh ♿ N

✳ **A4419** Ostomy pouch, closed; for use on barrier with non-locking flange, with filter (2 piece), each Ⓑ Ⓓ Qp Qh ♿ N

✳ **A4420** Ostomy pouch, closed; for use on barrier with locking flange (2 piece), each Ⓑ Ⓓ Qh ♿ N

✳ **A4421** Ostomy supply; miscellaneous Ⓑ Ⓓ N

⊛ **A4422** Ostomy absorbent material (sheet/pad/crystal packet) for use in ostomy pouch to thicken liquid stomal output, each Ⓑ Ⓓ ♿ N

IOM: 100-02, 15, 120

✳ **A4423** Ostomy pouch, closed; for use on barrier with locking flange, with filter (2 piece), each Ⓑ Ⓓ Qp Qh ♿ N

✳ **A4424** Ostomy pouch, drainable, with barrier attached, with filter (1 piece), each Ⓑ Ⓓ Qh ♿ N

✳ **A4425** Ostomy pouch, drainable; for use on barrier with non-locking flange, with filter (2 piece system), each Ⓑ Ⓓ Qh ♿ N

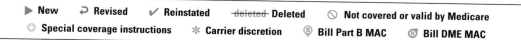

▶ New　↻ Revised　✔ Reinstated　~~deleted~~ Deleted　⃠ Not covered or valid by Medicare
⊛ Special coverage instructions　✳ Carrier discretion　Ⓑ Bill Part B MAC　Ⓓ Bill DME MAC

A4394 – A4425　MEDICAL AND SURGICAL SUPPLIES

* **A4426** Ostomy pouch, drainable; for use on barrier with locking flange (2 piece system), each Ⓑ Ⓖ Qp Qh ♿   N

* **A4427** Ostomy pouch, drainable; for use on barrier with locking flange, with filter (2 piece system), each Ⓑ Ⓖ Qh ♿   N

* **A4428** Ostomy pouch, urinary, with extended wear barrier attached, with faucet-type tap with valve (1 piece), each Ⓑ Ⓖ Qh ♿   N

* **A4429** Ostomy pouch, urinary, with barrier attached, with built-in convexity, with faucet-type tap with valve (1 piece), each Ⓑ Ⓖ Qp Qh ♿   N

* **A4430** Ostomy pouch, urinary, with extended wear barrier attached, with built-in convexity, with faucet-type tap with valve (1 piece), each Ⓑ Ⓖ Qh ♿   N

* **A4431** Ostomy pouch, urinary; with barrier attached, with faucet-type tap with valve (1 piece), each Ⓑ Ⓖ Qh ♿   N

* **A4432** Ostomy pouch, urinary; for use on barrier with non-locking flange, with faucet-type tap with valve (2 piece), each Ⓑ Ⓖ Qp Qh ♿   N

* **A4433** Ostomy pouch, urinary; for use on barrier with locking flange (2 piece), each Ⓑ Ⓖ Qh ♿   N

* **A4434** Ostomy pouch, urinary; for use on barrier with locking flange, with faucet-type tap with valve (2 piece), each Ⓑ Ⓖ Qh ♿   N

* **A4435** Ostomy pouch, drainable, high output, with extended wear barrier (one-piece system), with or without filter, each Ⓑ Ⓖ Qp Qh ♿   N

* **A4436** Irrigation supply; sleeve, reusable, per month ♿   N

* **A4437** Irrigation supply; sleeve, disposable, per month ♿   N

Miscellaneous Supplies

⊘ **A4450** Tape, non-waterproof, per 18 square inches Ⓑ Ⓖ ♿   N

If used with surgical dressings, billed with AW modifier (in addition to appropriate A1-A9 modifier).

IOM: 100-02, 15, 120

⊘ **A4452** Tape, waterproof, per 18 square inches Ⓑ Ⓖ ♿   N

If used with surgical dressings, billed with AW modifier (in addition to appropriate A1-A9 modifier).

IOM: 100-02, 15, 120

⊘ **A4453** Rectal catheter for use with the manual pump-operated enema system, replacement only   N

If used with surgical dressings, billed with AW modifier (in addition to appropriate A1-A9 modifier).

⊘ **A4455** Adhesive remover or solvent (for tape, cement or other adhesive), per ounce Ⓑ Ⓖ Qp Qh ♿   N

IOM: 100-02, 15, 120

⊘ **A4456** Adhesive remover, wipes, any type, each Ⓑ Ⓖ ♿   N

May be reimbursed for male or female clients to home health DME providers and DME medical suppliers in the home setting.

IOM: 100-02, 15, 120

* **A4458** Enema bag with tubing, reusable Ⓖ   N

* **A4459** Manual pump-operated enema system, includes balloon, catheter and all accessories, reusable, any type Ⓖ Qp Qh   N

* **A4461** Surgical dressing holder, non-reusable, each Ⓑ Ⓖ Qp Qh ♿   N

* **A4463** Surgical dressing holder, reusable, each Ⓑ Ⓖ Qh ♿   N

* **A4465** Non-elastic binder for extremity Ⓑ Qp Qh   N

⊘ **A4467** Belt, strap, sleeve, garment, or covering, any type Ⓑ Qp Qh   E1

⊘ **A4470** Gravlee jet washer Ⓑ Qp Qh   N

Symptoms suggestive of endometrial disease must be present for this disposable diagnostic tool to be covered.

IOM: 100-02, 16, 90; 100-03, 4, 230.5

⊘ **A4480** VABRA aspirator Ⓑ Qp Qh   N

Symptoms suggestive of endometrial disease must be present for this disposable diagnostic tool to be covered.

IOM: 100-02, 16, 90; 100-03, 4, 230.6

⊘ **A4481** Tracheostoma filter, any type, any size, each Ⓑ Ⓖ Qh ♿   N

IOM: 100-02, 15, 120

⊘ **A4483** Moisture exchanger, disposable, for use with invasive mechanical ventilation Ⓖ ♿   N

IOM: 100-02, 15, 120

⊘ **A4490** Surgical stockings above knee length, each Ⓑ Qp Qh   E1

IOM: 100-02, 15, 100; 100-02, 15, 110; 100-03, 4, 280.1

⊘ **A4495** Surgical stockings thigh length, each Ⓑ Qp Qh   E1

IOM: 100-02, 15, 100; 100-02, 15, 110; 100-03, 4, 280.1

🐍 **MIPS**   Qp **Quantity Physician**   Qh **Quantity Hospital**   ♀ **Female only**

♂ **Male only**   Ⓐ **Age**   ♿ **DMEPOS**   A2-Z3 **ASC Payment Indicator**   A-Y **ASC Status Indicator**   Coding Clinic

⊘ **A4500** Surgical stockings below knee length, each Ⓑ ⓠp ⓠh   E1

IOM: 100-02, 15, 100; 100-02, 15, 110; 100-03, 4, 280.1

⊘ **A4510** Surgical stockings full length, each Ⓑ ⓠp ⓠh   E1

IOM: 100-02, 15, 100; 100-02, 15, 110; 100-03, 4, 280.1

⊘ **A4520** Incontinence garment, any type (e.g., brief, diaper), each Ⓑ ⓠp ⓠh   E1

IOM: 100-03, 4, 280.1

⊛ **A4550** Surgical trays Ⓑ ⓠp ⓠh   B

No longer payable by Medicare; included in practice expense for procedures. Some private payers may pay, most private payers follow Medicare guidelines.

IOM: 100-04, 12, 20.3, 30.4

⊘ **A4553** Non-disposable underpads, all sizes Ⓑ ⓠp ⓠh   E1

IOM: 100-03, 4, 280.1

⊘ **A4554** Disposable underpads, all sizes Ⓑ ⓠp ⓠh   E1

IOM: 100-03, 4, 280.1

⊘ **A4555** Electrode/transducer for use with electrical stimulation device used for cancer treatment, replacement only Ⓓ Ⓑ ⓠp ⓠh   E1

∗ **A4556** Electrodes (e.g., apnea monitor), per pair Ⓓ Ⓑ ⓠp ⓠh ♿   N

∗ **A4557** Lead wires (e.g., apnea monitor), per pair Ⓓ Ⓑ ⓠp ⓠh ♿   N

∗ **A4558** Conductive gel or paste, for use with electrical device (e.g., TENS, NMES), per oz Ⓑ Ⓓ ⓠp ⓠh ♿   N

∗ **A4559** Coupling gel or paste, for use with ultrasound device, per oz Ⓑ Ⓓ ♿   N

▶ **A4560** Neuromuscular electrical stimulator (NMES), disposable, replacement only   N

∗ **A4561** Pessary, rubber, any type Ⓑ ⓠp ⓠh ♀ ♿   N

∗ **A4562** Pessary, non-rubber, any type Ⓑ ⓠp ⓠh ♀ ♿   N

∗ **A4563** Rectal control system for vaginal insertion, for long term use, includes pump and all supplies and accessories, any type each Ⓑ ♿   N

∗ **A4565** Slings Ⓑ ⓠp ⓠh ♿   N

⊘ **A4566** Shoulder sling or vest design, abduction restrainer, with or without swathe control, prefabricated, includes fitting and adjustment Ⓑ ⓠp ⓠh   E1

⊘ **A4570** Splint Ⓑ ⓠp ⓠh   E1

IOM: 100-02, 6, 10; 100-02, 15, 100; 100-04, 4, 240

Figure 4 Arm sling.

∗ **A4575** Topical hyperbaric oxygen chamber, disposable Ⓑ ⓠp ⓠh   A

⊘ **A4580** Cast supplies (e.g., plaster) Ⓑ ⓠp ⓠh   E1

IOM: 100-02, 6, 10; 100-02, 15, 100; 100-04, 4, 240

⊘ **A4590** Special casting material (e.g., fiberglass) Ⓑ ⓠp ⓠh   E1

IOM: 100-02, 6, 10; 100-02, 15, 100; 100-04, 4, 240

⊛ **A4595** Electrical stimulator supplies, 2 lead, per month (e.g., TENS, NMES) Ⓓ Ⓑ ⓠp ⓠh ♿   N

IOM: 100-03, 2, 160.13

A4596 Cranial electrotherapy stimulation (CES) system supplies and accessories, per month ♿

∗ **A4600** Sleeve for intermittent limb compression device, replacement only, each Ⓓ   E1

∗ **A4601** Lithium ion battery, rechargeable, for non-prosthetic use, replacement Ⓓ   E1

∗ **A4602** Replacement battery for external infusion pump owned by patient, lithium, 1.5 volt, each Ⓓ ⓠp ⓠh ♿   N

∗ **A4604** Tubing with integrated heating element for use with positive airway pressure device Ⓑ ⓠh ♿   N

∗ **A4605** Tracheal suction catheter, closed system, each Ⓓ ⓠh ♿   N

∗ **A4606** Oxygen probe for use with oximeter device, replacement Ⓓ ⓠp ⓠh   N

∗ **A4608** Transtracheal oxygen catheter, each Ⓑ ♿   N

Figure 5   Nasal cannula.

Figure 6   Tracheostomy cannula.

Supplies for Respiratory and Oxygen Equipment

⊘ **A4611**   Battery, heavy duty; replacement for patient owned ventilator Ⓑ Qp Qh   E1

Medicare Statute 1834(a)(3)(a)

⊘ **A4612**   Battery cables; replacement for patient-owned ventilator Ⓑ Qh   E1

Medicare Statute 1834(a)(3)(a)

⊘ **A4613**   Battery charger; replacement for patient-owned ventilator Ⓑ Qh   E1

Medicare Statute 1834(a)(3)(a)

✳ **A4614**   Peak expiratory flow rate meter, hand held Ⓑ Ⓑ Qp Qh ⅙   N

⊛ **A4615**   Cannula, nasal Ⓑ Ⓑ ⅙   N

IOM: 100-03, 2, 160.6; 100-04, 20, 100.2

⊛ **A4616**   Tubing (oxygen), per foot Ⓑ Ⓑ ⅙   N

IOM: 100-03, 2, 160.6; 100-04, 20, 100.2

⊛ **A4617**   Mouth piece Ⓑ Ⓑ ⅙   N

IOM: 100-03, 2, 160.6; 100-04, 20, 100.2

⊛ **A4618**   Breathing circuits Ⓑ Ⓑ Qp Qh ⅙   N

IOM: 100-03, 2, 160.6; 100-04, 20, 100.2

⊛ **A4619**   Face tent Ⓑ Ⓑ ⅙   N

IOM: 100-03, 2, 160.6; 100-04, 20, 100.2

⊛ **A4620**   Variable concentration mask Ⓑ Ⓑ ⅙   N

IOM: 100-03, 2, 160.6; 100-04, 20, 100.2

⊛ **A4623**   Tracheostomy, inner cannula Ⓑ Ⓑ Qh ⅙   N

IOM: 100-02, 15, 120; 100-03, 1, 20.9

✳ **A4624**   Tracheal suction catheter, any type, other than closed system, each Ⓑ Ⓑ Qh ⅙   N

Sterile suction catheters are medically necessary only for tracheostomy suctioning. Limitations include three suction catheters per day when covered for medically necessary tracheostomy suctioning. Assign DX V44.0 or V55.0 on the claim form. (CMS Manual System, Pub. 100-3, NCD manual, Chapter 1, Section 280-1)

⊛ **A4625**   Tracheostomy care kit for new tracheostomy Ⓑ Ⓑ Qp Qh ⅙   N

Dressings used with tracheostomies are included in the allowance for the code. This starter kit is covered after a surgical tracheostomy. (https://www.noridianmedicare.com/dme/coverage/docs/lcds/current_lcds/tracheostomy_care_supplies.htm)

IOM: 100-02, 15, 120

⊛ **A4626**   Tracheostomy cleaning brush, each Ⓑ Ⓑ ⅙   N

IOM: 100-02, 15, 120

⊘ **A4627**   Spacer, bag, or reservoir, with or without mask, for use with metered dose inhaler Ⓑ Ⓑ Qp Qh   E1

IOM: 100-02, 15, 110

↻ ✳ **A4628**   Oral and/or oropharyngeal suction catheter, each Ⓑ Ⓑ Qh ⅙   N

No more than three catheters per week are covered for medically necessary oropharyngeal suctioning because the catheters can be reused if cleansed and disinfected. (MS Manual System, Pub. 100-3, NCD manual, Chapter 1, Section 280-1)

⊛ **A4629**   Tracheostomy care kit for established tracheostomy Ⓑ Ⓑ Qh ⅙   N

IOM: 100-02, 15, 120

Replacement Parts

⚙ **A4630** Replacement batteries, medically necessary, transcutaneous electrical stimulator, owned by patient ⑧ ♿   E1

IOM: 100-03, 3, 160.7

* **A4633** Replacement bulb/lamp for ultraviolet light therapy system, each ⑧ Qp Qh ♿   E1

* **A4634** Replacement bulb for therapeutic light box, tabletop model ⑧   N

⚙ **A4635** Underarm pad, crutch, replacement, each ⑧ Qp Qh ♿   E1

IOM: 100-03, 4, 280.1

⚙ **A4636** Replacement, handgrip, cane, crutch, or walker, each ⑧ Qh ♿   E1

IOM: 100-03, 4, 280.1

⚙ **A4637** Replacement, tip, cane, crutch, walker, each ⑧ Qh ♿   E1

IOM: 100-03, 4, 280.1

* **A4638** Replacement battery for patient-owned ear pulse generator, each ⑧ Qp Qh ♿   E1

* **A4639** Replacement pad for infrared heating pad system, each ⑧ ♿   E1

⚙ **A4640** Replacement pad for use with medically necessary alternating pressure pad owned by patient ⑧ Qp Qh ♿   E1

IOM: 100-03, 4, 280.1; 100-08, 5, 5.2.3

Supplies for Radiological Procedures

* **A4641** Radiopharmaceutical, diagnostic, not otherwise classified ⑧   N

Is not an applicable tracer for PET scans

* **A4642** Indium In-111 satumomab pendetide, diagnostic, per study dose, up to 6 millicuries ⑧ Qp Qh   N

Miscellaneous Supplies

* **A4648** Tissue marker, implantable, any type, each ⑧ Qp Qh   N

Coding Clinic: 2018, Q2, P4,5; 2013, Q3, P9

* **A4649** Surgical supply miscellaneous ⚙ ⑧ Qp   N

* **A4650** Implantable radiation dosimeter, each ⑧ Qp Qh   N

⚙ **A4651** Calibrated microcapillary tube, each ⑧   N

IOM: 100-04, 3, 40.3

⚙ **A4652** Microcapillary tube sealant ⑧   N

IOM: 100-04, 3, 40.3

Supplies for Dialysis

* **A4653** Peritoneal dialysis catheter anchoring device, belt, each ⑧ Qp Qh   N

⚙ **A4657** Syringe, with or without needle, each ⑧ Qp Qh   N

IOM: 100-04, 8, 90.3.2

⚙ **A4660** Sphygmomanometer/blood pressure apparatus with cuff and stethoscope ⑧ Qp Qh   N

IOM: 100-04, 8, 90.3.2

⚙ **A4663** Blood pressure cuff only ⑧ Qp Qh   N

IOM: 100-04, 8, 90.3.2

⊘ **A4670** Automatic blood pressure monitor ⑧ Qp Qh   E1

IOM: 100-04, 8, 90.3.2

⚙ **A4671** Disposable cycler set used with cycler dialysis machine, each ⑧ Qp Qh   B

IOM: 100-04, 8, 90.3.2

⚙ **A4672** Drainage extension line, sterile, for dialysis, each ⑧ Qp Qh   B

IOM: 100-04, 8, 90.3.2

⚙ **A4673** Extension line with easy lock connectors, used with dialysis ⑧ Qp Qh   B

IOM: 100-04, 8, 90.3.2

⚙ **A4674** Chemicals/antiseptics solution used to clean/sterilize dialysis equipment, per 8 oz ⑧ Qp Qh   B

IOM: 100-04, 8, 90.3.2

⚙ **A4680** Activated carbon filters for hemodialysis, each ⑧ Qp Qh   N

IOM: 100-04, 8, 90.3.2

⚙ **A4690** Dialyzers (artificial kidneys), all types, all sizes, for hemodialysis, each ⑧ Qp Qh   N

IOM: 100-04, 8, 90.3.2

⚙ **A4706** Bicarbonate concentrate, solution, for hemodialysis, per gallon ⑧ Qp Qh   N

IOM: 100-04, 8, 90.3.2

⚙ **A4707** Bicarbonate concentrate, powder, for hemodialysis, per packet ⑧ Qp Qh   N

IOM: 100-04, 8, 90.3.2

▶ New   ↻ Revised   ✔ Reinstated   deleted Deleted   ⊘ Not covered or valid by Medicare
⚙ Special coverage instructions   * Carrier discretion   ⑧ Bill Part B MAC   ⑧ Bill DME MAC

⊘ **A4708**   Acetate concentrate solution, for hemodialysis, per gallon ⑧ Qp Qh   N

IOM: 100-04, 8, 90.3.2

⊘ **A4709**   Acid concentrate, solution, for hemodialysis, per gallon ⑧ Qp Qh   N

IOM: 100-04, 8, 90.3.2

⊘ **A4714**   Treated water (deionized, distilled, or reverse osmosis) for peritoneal dialysis, per gallon ⑧ Qp Qh   N

IOM: 100-03, 4, 230.7; 100-04, 3, 40.3

⊘ **A4719**   "Y set" tubing for peritoneal dialysis ⑧ Qp Qh   N

IOM: 100-04, 8, 90.3.2

⊘ **A4720**   Dialysate solution, any concentration of dextrose, fluid volume greater than 249 cc, but less than or equal to 999 cc, for peritoneal dialysis ⑧ Qp Qh   N

Do not use AX modifier.

IOM: 100-04, 8, 90.3.2

⊘ **A4721**   Dialysate solution, any concentration of dextrose, fluid volume greater than 999 cc but less than or equal to 1999 cc, for peritoneal dialysis ⑧ Qp Qh   N

IOM: 100-04, 8, 90.3.2

⊘ **A4722**   Dialysate solution, any concentration of dextrose, fluid volume greater than 1999 cc but less than or equal to 2999 cc, for peritoneal dialysis ⑧ Qp Qh   N

IOM: 100-04, 8, 90.3.2

⊘ **A4723**   Dialysate solution, any concentration of dextrose, fluid volume greater than 2999 cc but less than or equal to 3999 cc, for peritoneal dialysis ⑧ Qp Qh   N

IOM: 100-04, 8, 90.3.2

⊘ **A4724**   Dialysate solution, any concentration of dextrose, fluid volume greater than 3999 cc but less than or equal to 4999 cc for peritoneal dialysis ⑧ Qp Qh   N

IOM: 100-04, 8, 90.3.2

⊘ **A4725**   Dialysate solution, any concentration of dextrose, fluid volume greater than 4999 cc but less than or equal to 5999 cc, for peritoneal dialysis ⑧ Qp Qh   N

IOM: 100-04, 8, 90.3.2

⊘ **A4726**   Dialysate solution, any concentration of dextrose, fluid volume greater than 5999 cc, for peritoneal dialysis ⑧ Qp Qh   N

IOM: 100-04, 8, 90.3.2

✳ **A4728**   Dialysate solution, non-dextrose containing, 500 ml ⑧ Qp Qh   B

⊘ **A4730**   Fistula cannulation set for hemodialysis, each ⑧ Qp Qh   N

IOM: 100-04, 8, 90.3.2

⊘ **A4736**   Topical anesthetic, for dialysis, per gram ⑧ Qp Qh   N

IOM: 100-04, 8, 90.3.2

⊘ **A4737**   Injectable anesthetic, for dialysis, per 10 ml ⑧ Qp Qh   N

IOM: 100-04, 8, 90.3.2

⊘ **A4740**   Shunt accessory, for hemodialysis, any type, each ⑧ Qp Qh   N

IOM: 100-04, 8, 90.3.2

⊘ **A4750**   Blood tubing, arterial or venous, for hemodialysis, each ⑧ Qp Qh   N

IOM: 100-04, 8, 90.3.2

⊘ **A4755**   Blood tubing, arterial and venous combined, for hemodialysis, each ⑧ Qp Qh   N

IOM: 100-04, 8, 90.3.2

⊘ **A4760**   Dialysate solution test kit, for peritoneal dialysis, any type, each ⑧ Qp Qh   N

IOM: 100-04, 8, 90.3.2

⊘ **A4765**   Dialysate concentrate, powder, additive for peritoneal dialysis, per packet ⑧ Qp Qh   N

IOM: 100-04, 8, 90.3.2

⊘ **A4766**   Dialysate concentrate, solution, additive for peritoneal dialysis, per 10 ml ⑧ Qp Qh   N

IOM: 100-04, 8, 90.3.2

⊘ **A4770**   Blood collection tube, vacuum, for dialysis, per 50 ⑧ Qp Qh   N

IOM: 100-04, 8, 90.3.2

⊘ **A4771**   Serum clotting time tube, for dialysis, per 50 ⑧ Qp Qh   N

IOM: 100-04, 8, 90.3.2

⊘ **A4772**   Blood glucose test strips, for dialysis, per 50 ⑧ Qp Qh   N

IOM: 100-04, 8, 90.3.2

⊘ **A4773**   Occult blood test strips, for dialysis, per 50 ⑧ Qp Qh   N

IOM: 100-04, 8, 90.3.2

⊘ **A4774**   Ammonia test strips, for dialysis, per 50 ⑧ Qp Qh   N

IOM: 100-04, 8, 90.3.2

⊘ **A4802**   Protamine sulfate, for hemodialysis, per 50 mg ⑧ Qp Qh   N

IOM: 100-04, 8, 90.3.2

⊛ **A4860** Disposable catheter tips for peritoneal dialysis, per 10 ⑧ **Qp** **Qh**   N

IOM: 100-04, 8, 90.3.2

⊛ **A4870** Plumbing and/or electrical work for home hemodialysis equipment ⑨ **Qp** **Qh**   N

IOM: 100-04, 8, 90.3.2

⊛ **A4890** Contracts, repair and maintenance, for hemodialysis equipment ⑨ **Qp** **Qh**   N

IOM: 100-02, 15, 110.2

⊛ **A4911** Drain bag/bottle, for dialysis, each ⑨ **Qp** **Qh**   N

⊛ **A4913** Miscellaneous dialysis supplies, not otherwise specified ⑧ **Qp** **Qh**   N

Items not related to dialysis must not be billed with the miscellaneous codes A4913 or E1699.

⊛ **A4918** Venous pressure clamp, for hemodialysis, each ⑨ **Qp** **Qh**   N

⊛ **A4927** Gloves, non-sterile, per 100 ⑨ **Qp** **Qh**   N

⊛ **A4928** Surgical mask, per 20 ⑧ **Qp** **Qh**   N

⊛ **A4929** Tourniquet for dialysis, each ⑧ **Qp** **Qh**   N

⊛ **A4930** Gloves, sterile, per pair ⑧ **Qp** **Qh**   N

✳ **A4931** Oral thermometer, reusable, any type, each ⑨ **Qp** **Qh**   N

✳ **A4932** Rectal thermometer, reusable, any type, each ⑨ **Qp** **Qh**   N

Additional Ostomy Supplies

⊛ **A5051** Ostomy pouch, closed; with barrier attached (1 piece), each ⑧ ⑧ **Qp** **Qh** ♿   N

IOM: 100-02, 15, 120

⊛ **A5052** Ostomy pouch, closed; without barrier attached (1 piece), each ⑧ ⑧ **Qp** **Qh** ♿   N

IOM: 100-02, 15, 120

⊛ **A5053** Ostomy pouch, closed; for use on faceplate, each ⑧ ⑧ **Qp** **Qh** ♿   N

IOM: 100-02, 15, 120

⊛ **A5054** Ostomy pouch, closed; for use on barrier with flange (2 piece), each ⑧ ⑧ **Qp** ♿   N

IOM: 100-02, 15, 120

⊛ **A5055** Stoma cap ⑧ ⑧ **Qp** **Qh** ♿   N

IOM: 100-02, 15, 120

⊛ **A5056** Ostomy pouch, drainable, with extended wear barrier attached, with filter (1 piece), each ⑧ ⑧ **Qp** **Qh** ♿   N

IOM: 100-02, 15, 120

⊛ **A5057** Ostomy pouch, drainable, with extended wear barrier attached, with built in convexity, with filter (1 piece), each ⑧ ⑧ **Qp** **Qh** ♿   N

IOM: 100-02, 15, 120

✳ **A5061** Ostomy pouch, drainable; with barrier attached (1 piece), each ⑧ ⑧ **Qp** **Qh** ♿   N

IOM: 100-02, 15, 120

⊛ **A5062** Ostomy pouch, drainable; without barrier attached (1 piece), each ⑨ ⑧ **Qp** **Qh** ♿   N

IOM: 100-02, 15, 120

⊛ **A5063** Ostomy pouch, drainable; for use on barrier with flange (2 piece system), each ⑨ ⑧ **Qp** **Qh** ♿   N

IOM: 100-02, 15, 120

⊛ **A5071** Ostomy pouch, urinary; with barrier attached (1 piece), each ⑨ ⑨ **Qp** **Qh** ♿   N

IOM: 100-02, 15, 120

⊛ **A5072** Ostomy pouch, urinary; without barrier attached (1 piece), each ⑨ ⑧ **Qp** **Qh** ♿   N

IOM: 100-02, 15, 120

⊛ **A5073** Ostomy pouch, urinary; for use on barrier with flange (2 piece), each ⑨ ⑧ **Qp** **Qh** ♿   N

IOM: 100-02, 15, 120

⊛ **A5081** Stoma plug or seal, any type ⑨ ⑧ ⑧ **Qp** **Qh** ♿   N

IOM: 100-02, 15, 120

⊛ **A5082** Continent device; catheter for continent stoma ⑧ ⑨ **Qp** **Qh** ♿   N

IOM: 100-02, 15, 120

✳ **A5083** Continent device, stoma absorptive cover for continent stoma ⑨ ⑧ **Qh** ♿   N

⊛ **A5093** Ostomy accessory; convex insert ⑧ ⑨ **Qp** **Qh** ♿   N

IOM: 100-02, 15, 120

▶ New   ↻ Revised   ✔ Reinstated   ~~deleted~~ Deleted   ⊘ Not covered or valid by Medicare
⊛ Special coverage instructions   ✳ Carrier discretion   ⑧ Bill Part B MAC   ⑨ Bill DME MAC

Additional Incontinence and Ostomy Supplies

◎ **A5102** Bedside drainage bottle with or without tubing, rigid or expandable, each ⑧ ⑧ **Qp** **Qh**   N

IOM: 100-02, 15, 120

◎ **A5105** Urinary suspensory, with leg bag, with or without tube, each ⑧ ⑧ **Qp** **Qh**   N

IOM: 100-02, 15, 120

◎ **A5112** Urinary drainage bag, leg bag, leg or abdomen, latex, with or without tube, with straps, each ⑧ ⑧ **Qp** **Qh**   N

IOM: 100-02, 15, 120

◎ **A5113** Leg strap; latex, replacement only, per set ⑧ ⑧ **Qp** **Qh**   E1

IOM: 100-02, 15, 120

◎ **A5114** Leg strap; foam or fabric, replacement only, per set ⑧ ⑧ **Qp** **Qh**   E1

IOM: 100-02, 15, 120

◎ **A5120** Skin barrier, wipes or swabs, each ⑧ ⑧ **Qp** **Qh**   N

IOM: 100-02, 15, 120

◎ **A5121** Skin barrier; solid, 6 × 6 or equivalent, each ⑧ ⑧ **Qp** **Qh**   N

IOM: 100-02, 15, 120

◎ **A5122** Skin barrier; solid, 8 × 8 or equivalent, each ⑧ ⑧ **Qp** **Qh**   N

IOM: 100-02, 15, 120

◎ **A5126** Adhesive or non-adhesive; disk or foam pad ⑧ ⑧ **Qp** **Qh**   N

IOM: 100-02, 15, 120

◎ **A5131** Appliance cleaner, incontinence and ostomy appliances, per 16 oz ⑧ ⑧ **Qp** **Qh**   N

IOM: 100-02, 15, 120

◎ **A5200** Percutaneous catheter/tube anchoring device, adhesive skin attachment ⑧ ⑧ **Qh**   N

IOM: 100-02, 15, 120

Diabetic Shoes, Fitting, and Modifications

◎ **A5500** For diabetics only, fitting (including follow-up), custom preparation and supply of off-the-shelf depth-inlay shoe manufactured to accommodate multi-density insert(s), per shoe ⑧ **Qp** **Qh**   Y

IOM: 100-02, 15, 140

◎ **A5501** For diabetics only, fitting (including follow-up), custom preparation and supply of shoe molded from cast(s) of patient's foot (custom-molded shoe), per shoe ⑧ **Qp** **Qh**   Y

The diabetic patient must have at least one of the following conditions: peripheral neuropathy with evidence of callus formation, pre-ulcerative calluses, previous ulceration, foot deformity, previous amputation or poor circulation.

IOM: 100-02, 15, 140

◎ **A5503** For diabetics only, modification (including fitting) of off-the-shelf depth-inlay shoe or custom-molded shoe with roller or rigid rocker bottom, per shoe ⑧ **Qp** **Qh**   Y

IOM: 100-02, 15, 140

◎ **A5504** For diabetics only, modification (including fitting) of off-the-shelf depth-inlay shoe or custom-molded shoe with wedge(s), per shoe ⑧ **Qp** **Qh**   Y

IOM: 100-02, 15, 140

◎ **A5505** For diabetics only, modification (including fitting) of off-the-shelf depth-inlay shoe or custom-molded shoe with metatarsal bar, per shoe ⑧ **Qp** **Qh** Y

IOM: 100-02, 15, 140

◎ **A5506** For diabetics only, modification (including fitting) of off-the-shelf depth-inlay shoe or custom-molded shoe with off-set heel(s), per shoe ⑧ **Qp** **Qh**   Y

IOM: 100-02, 15, 140

◎ **A5507** For diabetics only, not otherwise specified modification (including fitting) of off-the-shelf depth-inlay shoe or custom-molded shoe, per shoe ⑧ **Qp** **Qh**   Y

Only used for not otherwise specified therapeutic modifications to shoe or for repairs to a diabetic shoe(s)

IOM: 100-02, 15, 140

◎ **A5508** For diabetics only, deluxe feature of off-the-shelf depth-inlay shoe or custom-molded shoe, per shoe ⑧ **Qp** **Qh**   Y

IOM: 100-02, 15, 40

◎ **A5510** For diabetics only, direct formed, compression molded to patient's foot without external heat source, multiple-density insert(s) prefabricated, per shoe ⑧ **Qp** **Qh**   N

IOM: 100-02, 15, 140

✳ **A5512** For diabetics only, multiple density insert, direct formed, molded to foot after external heat source of 230 degrees Fahrenheit or higher, total contact with patient's foot, including arch, base layer minimum of 1/4 inch material of shore a 35 durometer or 3/16 inch material of shore a 40 durometer (or higher), prefabricated, each ⑨ Qp Qh ♿   Y

✳ **A5513** For diabetics only, multiple density insert, custom molded from model of patient's foot, total contact with patient's foot, including arch, base layer minimum of 3/16 inch material of shore a 35 durometer (or higher), includes arch filler and other shaping material, custom fabricated, each ⑨ Qp Qh ♿   Y

✿ **A5514** For diabetics only, multiple density insert, made by direct carving with cam technology from a rectified CAD model created from a digitized scan of the patient, total contact with patient's foot, including arch, base layer minimum of 3/16 inch material of shore a 35 durometer (or higher), includes arch filler and other shaping material, custom fabricated, each ⑨ ♿   Y

Dressings

⊘ **A6000** Non-contact wound warming wound cover for use with the non-contact wound warming device and warming card ⑧ Qp Qh   E1

IOM: 100-02, 16, 20

✿ **A6010** Collagen based wound filler, dry form, sterile, per gram of collagen ⑨ ⑧ ♿   N

IOM: 100-02, 15, 100

✿ **A6011** Collagen based wound filler, gel/paste, per gram of collagen ⑧ ⑨ ♿   N

IOM: 100-02, 15, 100

✿ **A6021** Collagen dressing, sterile, size 16 sq. in. or less, each ⑧ ⑨ ♿   N

IOM: 100-02, 15, 100

✿ **A6022** Collagen dressing, sterile, size more than 16 sq. in. but less than or equal to 48 sq. in., each ⑧ ⑨ Qp ♿   N

IOM: 100-02, 15, 100

✿ **A6023** Collagen dressing, sterile, size more than 48 sq. in., each ⑧ ⑨ ♿   N

IOM: 100-02, 15, 100

✿ **A6024** Collagen dressing wound filler, sterile, per 6 inches ⑧ ⑨ ♿   N

IOM: 100-02, 15, 100

✳ **A6025** Gel sheet for dermal or epidermal application (e.g., silicone, hydrogel, other), each ⑧ ⑨   N

If used for the treatment of keloids or other scars, a silicone gel sheet will not meet the definition of the surgical dressing benefit and will be denied as noncovered.

✿ **A6154** Wound pouch, each ⑧ ⑨ Qp Qh ♿ N

Waterproof collection device with drainable port that adheres to skin around wound. Usual dressing change is up to 3 times per week.

IOM: 100-02, 15, 100

✿ **A6196** Alginate or other fiber gelling dressing, wound cover, sterile, pad size 16 sq. in. or less, each dressing ⑧ ⑨ Qp ♿   N

IOM: 100-02, 15, 100

✿ **A6197** Alginate or other fiber gelling dressing, wound cover, sterile, pad size more than 16 sq. in., but less than or equal to 48 sq. in., each dressing ⑧ ⑨ Qp ♿ N

IOM: 100-02, 15, 100

✿ **A6198** Alginate or other fiber gelling dressing, wound cover, sterile, pad size more than 48 sq. in., each dressing ⑧ ⑨ Qp   N

IOM: 100-02, 15, 100

✿ **A6199** Alginate or other fiber gelling dressing, wound filler, sterile, per 6 inches ⑧ ⑨ Qp ♿   N

IOM: 100-02, 15, 100

✿ **A6203** Composite dressing, sterile, pad size 16 sq. in. or less, with any size adhesive border, each dressing ⑧ ⑨ Qp ♿   N

Usual composite dressing change is up to 3 times per week, one wound cover per dressing change.

IOM: 100-02, 15, 100

✿ **A6204** Composite dressing, sterile, pad size more than 16 sq. in. but less than or equal to 48 sq. in., with any size adhesive border, each dressing ⑧ ⑨ Qp ♿   N

Usual composite dressing change is up to 3 times per week, one wound cover per dressing change.

IOM: 100-02, 15, 100

▶ New   ↺ Revised   ✔ Reinstated   ~~deleted~~ Deleted   ⊘ Not covered or valid by Medicare
✿ Special coverage instructions   ✳ Carrier discretion   ⑧ Bill Part B MAC   ⑨ Bill DME MAC

☼ **A6205** Composite dressing, sterile, pad size more than 48 sq. in., with any size adhesive border, each dressing ⑨ ⑧ **Qp** **Qh**   N

Usual composite dressing change is up to 3 times per week, one wound cover per dressing change.

IOM: 100-02, 15, 100

☼ **A6206** Contact layer, sterile, 16 sq. in. or less, each dressing ⑨ ⑧ **Qp**   N

Contact layers are porous to allow wound fluid to pass through for absorption by separate overlying dressing and are not intended to be changed with each dressing change. Usual dressing change is up to once per week.

IOM: 100-02, 15, 100

☼ **A6207** Contact layer, sterile, more than 16 sq. in. but less than or equal to 48 sq. in., each dressing ⑨ ⑧ **Qp** &   N

Contact layer dressings are used to line the entire wound; they are not intended to be changed with each dressing change. Usual dressing change is up to once per week.

IOM: 100-02, 15, 100

☼ **A6208** Contact layer, sterile, more than 48 sq. in., each dressing ⑨ ⑧ **Qp**   N

Contact layer dressings are used to line the entire wound; they are not intended to be changed with each dressing change. Usual dressing change is up to once per week.

IOM: 100-02, 15, 100

☼ **A6209** Foam dressing, wound cover, sterile, pad size 16 sq. in. or less, without adhesive border, each dressing ⑨ ⑧ **Qp** &   N

Made of open cell, medical grade expanded polymer; with nonadherent property over wound site.

IOM: 100-02, 15, 100

☼ **A6210** Foam dressing, wound cover, sterile, pad size more than 16 sq. in. but less than or equal to 48 sq. in., without adhesive border, each dressing ⑧ ⑨ **Qp** &   N

Foam dressings are covered items when used on full thickness wounds (e.g., stage III or IV ulcers) with moderate to heavy exudates. Usual dressing change for a foam wound cover when used as primary dressing is up to 3 times per week. When foam wound cover is used as a secondary dressing for wounds with very heavy exudates, dressing change may be up to 3 times per week. Usual dressing change for foam wound fillers is up to once per day (A6209-A6215).

IOM: 100-02, 15, 100

☼ **A6211** Foam dressing, wound cover, sterile, pad size more than 48 sq. in., without adhesive border, each dressing ⑧ ⑨ **Qp** &   N

IOM: 100-02, 15, 100

☼ **A6212** Foam dressing, wound cover, sterile, pad size 16 sq. in. or less, with any size adhesive border, each dressing ⑧ ⑨ **Qp** &   N

IOM: 100-02, 15, 100

☼ **A6213** Foam dressing, wound cover, sterile, pad size more than 16 sq. in. but less than or equal to 48 sq. in., with any size adhesive border, each dressing ⑧ ⑨ **Qp**   N

IOM: 100-02, 15, 100

☼ **A6214** Foam dressing, wound cover, sterile, pad size more than 48 sq. in., with any size adhesive border, each dressing ⑧ ⑨ **Qp** &   N

IOM: 100-02, 15, 100

☼ **A6215** Foam dressing, wound filler, sterile, per gram ⑧ ⑨ **Qp**   N

IOM: 100-02, 15, 100

☼ **A6216** Gauze, non-impregnated, non-sterile, pad size 16 sq. in. or less, without adhesive border, each dressing ⑨ ⑧ **Qp** &   N

IOM: 100-02, 15, 100

☼ **A6217** Gauze, non-impregnated, non-sterile, pad size more than 16 sq. in. but less than or equal to 48 sq. in., without adhesive border, each dressing ⑧ ⑨ **Qp** &   N

IOM: 100-02, 15, 100

⊛ **A6218** Gauze, non-impregnated, non-sterile, pad size more than 48 sq. in., without adhesive border, each dressing Ⓑ Ⓓ **Qp** N

IOM: 100-02, 15, 100

⊛ **A6219** Gauze, non-impregnated, sterile, pad size 16 sq. in. or less, with any size adhesive border, each dressing Ⓑ Ⓓ **Qp** ♿ N

IOM: 100-02, 15, 100

⊛ **A6220** Gauze, non-impregnated, sterile, pad size more than 16 sq. in. but less than or equal to 48 sq. in., with any size adhesive border, each dressing Ⓑ Ⓓ **Qp** ♿ N

IOM: 100-02, 15, 100

⊛ **A6221** Gauze, non-impregnated, sterile, pad size more than 48 sq. in., with any size adhesive border, each dressing Ⓑ Ⓓ N

IOM: 100-02, 15, 100

⊛ **A6222** Gauze, impregnated with other than water, normal saline, or hydrogel, sterile, pad size 16 sq. in. or less, without adhesive border, each dressing Ⓑ Ⓓ **Qp** ♿ N

Substances may have been incorporated into dressing material (i.e., iodinated agents, petrolatum, zinc paste, crystalline sodium chloride, chlorhexadine gluconate [CHG], bismuth tribromophenate [BTP], water, aqueous saline, hydrogel, or agents).

IOM: 100-02, 15, 100

⊛ **A6223** Gauze, impregnated with other than water, normal saline, or hydrogel, sterile, pad size more than 16 sq. in. but less than or equal to 48 sq. in., without adhesive border, each dressing Ⓥ Ⓑ **Qp** ♿ N

IOM: 100-02, 15, 100

⊛ **A6224** Gauze, impregnated with other than water, normal saline, or hydrogel, sterile, pad size more than 48 sq. in., without adhesive border, each dressing Ⓥ Ⓑ **Qp** ♿ N

IOM: 100-02, 15, 100

⊛ **A6228** Gauze, impregnated, water or normal saline, sterile, pad size 16 sq. in. or less, without adhesive border, each dressing Ⓥ Ⓑ **Qp** **Qh** N

IOM: 100-02, 15, 100

⊛ **A6229** Gauze, impregnated, water or normal saline, sterile, pad size more than 16 sq. in. but less than or equal to 48 sq. in., without adhesive border, each dressing Ⓥ Ⓑ Ⓓ **Qp** ♿ N

IOM: 100-02, 15, 100

⊛ **A6230** Gauze, impregnated, water or normal saline, sterile, pad size more than 48 sq. in., without adhesive border, each dressing Ⓥ Ⓑ Ⓓ **Qp** **Qh** N

IOM: 100-02, 15, 100

⊛ **A6231** Gauze, impregnated, hydrogel, for direct wound contact, sterile, pad size 16 sq. in. or less, each dressing Ⓥ Ⓓ **Qp** ♿ N

IOM: 100-02, 15, 100

⊛ **A6232** Gauze, impregnated, hydrogel, for direct wound contact, sterile, pad size greater than 16 sq. in., but less than or equal to 48 sq. in., each dressing Ⓥ Ⓑ ♿ N

IOM: 100-02, 15, 100

⊛ **A6233** Gauze, impregnated, hydrogel, for direct wound contact, sterile, pad size more than 48 sq. in., each dressing Ⓥ Ⓑ ♿ N

IOM: 100-02, 15, 100

⊛ **A6234** Hydrocolloid dressing, wound cover, sterile, pad size 16 sq. in. or less, without adhesive border, each dressing Ⓑ Ⓓ **Qp** ♿ N

This type of dressing is usually used on wounds with light to moderate exudate with an average of three dressing changes per week.

IOM: 100-02, 15, 100

⊛ **A6235** Hydrocolloid dressing, wound cover, sterile, pad size more than 16 sq. in. but less than or equal to 48 sq. in., without adhesive border, each dressing Ⓥ Ⓑ **Qp** ♿ N

IOM: 100-02, 15, 100

⊛ **A6236** Hydrocolloid dressing, wound cover, sterile, pad size more than 48 sq. in., without adhesive border, each dressing Ⓥ Ⓑ Ⓓ **Qp** **Qh** ♿ N

IOM: 100-02, 15, 100

⊛ **A6237** Hydrocolloid dressing, wound cover, sterile, pad size 16 sq. in. or less, with any size adhesive border, each dressing Ⓥ Ⓑ Ⓓ **Qp** ♿ N

IOM: 100-02, 15, 100

▶ **New** ↻ **Revised** ✓ **Reinstated** ~~deleted~~ **Deleted** ⊘ **Not covered or valid by Medicare**
⊛ **Special coverage instructions** ✶ **Carrier discretion** Ⓑ **Bill Part B MAC** Ⓓ **Bill DME MAC**

⊘ **A6238** Hydrocolloid dressing, wound cover, sterile, pad size more than 16 sq. in. but less than or equal to 48 sq. in., with any size adhesive border, each dressing ⑧ ⑧ [Qp] [Qh] ♿   N

IOM: 100-02, 15, 100

⊘ **A6239** Hydrocolloid dressing, wound cover, sterile, pad size more than 48 sq. in., with any size adhesive border, each dressing ⑧ ⑧ [Qp] [Qh]   N

IOM: 100-02, 15, 100

⊘ **A6240** Hydrocolloid dressing, wound filler, paste, sterile, per ounce ⑧ ⑧ [Qp] [Qh] ♿   N

IOM: 100-02, 15, 100

⊘ **A6241** Hydrocolloid dressing, wound filler, dry form, sterile, per gram ⑧ ⑧ [Qp] [Qh] ♿   N

IOM: 100-02, 15, 100

⊘ **A6242** Hydrogel dressing, wound cover, sterile, pad size 16 sq. in. or less, without adhesive border, each dressing ⑧ ⑧ [Qp] ♿   N

Considered medically necessary when used on full thickness wounds with minimal or no exudate (e.g., stage III or IV ulcers).

Usually up to one dressing change per day is considered medically necessary, but if well documented and medically necessary, the payer may allow more frequent dressing changes.

IOM: 100-02, 15, 100

⊘ **A6243** Hydrogel dressing, wound cover, sterile, pad size more than 16 sq. in. but less than or equal to 48 sq. in., without adhesive border, each dressing ⑧ ⑧ [Qp] ♿   N

IOM: 100-02, 15, 100

⊘ **A6244** Hydrogel dressing, wound cover, sterile, pad size more than 48 sq. in., without adhesive border, each dressing ⑧ ⑧ [Qp] [Qh] ♿   N

IOM: 100-02, 15, 100

⊘ **A6245** Hydrogel dressing, wound cover, sterile, pad size 16 sq. in. or less, with any size adhesive border, each dressing ⑧ ⑧ [Qp] ♿   N

Coverage of a non-elastic gradient compression wrap is limited to one per 6 months per leg.

IOM: 100-02, 15, 100

⊘ **A6246** Hydrogel dressing, wound cover, sterile, pad size more than 16 sq. in. but less than or equal to 48 sq. in., with any size adhesive border, each dressing ⑧ ⑧ [Qp] [Qh] ♿   N

IOM: 100-02, 15, 100

⊘ **A6247** Hydrogel dressing, wound cover, sterile, pad size more than 48 sq. in., with any size adhesive border, each dressing ⑧ ⑧ [Qp] [Qh] ♿   N

IOM: 100-02, 15, 100

⊘ **A6248** Hydrogel dressing, wound filler, gel, per fluid ounce ⑧ ⑧ [Qp] ♿   N

IOM: 100-02, 15, 100

⊘ **A6250** Skin sealants, protectants, moisturizers, ointments, any type, any size ⑧ ⑧ [Qp] [Qh]   N

IOM: 100-02, 15, 100

⊘ **A6251** Specialty absorptive dressing, wound cover, sterile, pad size 16 sq. in. or less, without adhesive border, each dressing ⑧ ⑧ [Qp] ♿   N

IOM: 100-02, 15, 100

⊘ **A6252** Specialty absorptive dressing, wound cover, sterile, pad size more than 16 sq. in. but less than or equal to 48 sq. in., without adhesive border, each dressing ⑧ ⑧ [Qp] ♿   N

IOM: 100-02, 15, 100

⊘ **A6253** Specialty absorptive dressing, wound cover, sterile, pad size more than 48 sq. in., without adhesive border, each dressing ⑧ ⑧ [Qp] ♿   N

IOM: 100-02, 15, 100

⊘ **A6254** Specialty absorptive dressing, wound cover, sterile, pad size 16 sq. in. or less, with any size adhesive border, each dressing ⑧ ⑧ [Qp] ♿   N

IOM: 100-02, 15, 100

⊘ **A6255** Specialty absorptive dressing, wound cover, sterile, pad size more than 16 sq. in. but less than or equal to 48 sq. in., with any size adhesive border, each dressing ⑧ ⑧ [Qp] ♿   N

IOM: 100-02, 15, 100

⊘ **A6256** Specialty absorptive dressing, wound cover, sterile, pad size more than 48 sq. in., with any size adhesive border, each dressing ⑧ ⑧ [Qp] [Qh]   N

Considered medically necessary when used for moderately or highly exudative wounds (e.g., stage III or IV ulcers).

IOM: 100-02, 15, 100

🔖 MIPS	[Qp] Quantity Physician	[Qh] Quantity Hospital	♀ Female only
♂ Male only [A] Age ♿ DMEPOS A2-Z3 ASC Payment Indicator A-Y ASC Status Indicator			Coding Clinic

⊕ **A6257** Transparent film, sterile, 16 sq. in. or less, each dressing ⑧ ⑧ Qp ⬚ N

Considered medically necessary when used on open partial thickness wounds with minimal exudate or closed wounds.

IOM: 100-02, 15, 100

⊕ **A6258** Transparent film, sterile, more than 16 sq. in. but less than or equal to 48 sq. in., each dressing ⑧ ⑧ Qp ⬚ N

IOM: 100-02, 15, 100

⊕ **A6259** Transparent film, sterile, more than 48 sq. in., each dressing ⑧ ⑧ Qp Qh ⬚ N

IOM: 100-02, 15, 100

⊕ **A6260** Wound cleansers, any type, any size ⑧ ⑧ Qp N

IOM: 100-02, 15, 100

⊕ **A6261** Wound filler, gel/paste, per fluid ounce, not otherwise specified ⑧ ⑧ Qp Qh N

Units of service for wound fillers are 1 gram, 1 fluid ounce, 6 inch length, or 1 yard depending on product.

IOM: 100-02, 15, 100

⊕ **A6262** Wound filler, dry form, per gram, not otherwise specified ⑧ ⑧ Qp Qh N

Dry forms (e.g., powder, granules, beads) are used to eliminate dead space in an open wound.

IOM: 100-02, 15, 100

⊕ **A6266** Gauze, impregnated, other than water, normal saline, or zinc paste, sterile, any width, per linear yard ⑧ ⑧ Qp ⬚ N

IOM: 100-02, 15, 100

⊕ **A6402** Gauze, non-impregnated, sterile, pad size 16 sq. in. or less, without adhesive border, each dressing ⑧ ⑧ Qp ⬚ N

IOM: 100-02, 15, 100

⊕ **A6403** Gauze, non-impregnated, sterile, pad size more than 16 sq. in., less than or equal to 48 sq. in., without adhesive border, each dressing ⑧ ⑧ Qp N

IOM: 100-02, 15, 100

⊕ **A6404** Gauze, non-impregnated, sterile, pad size more than 48 sq. in., without adhesive border, each dressing ⑧ ⑧ Qp Qh N

IOM: 100-02, 15, 100

∗ **A6407** Packing strips, non-impregnated, sterile, up to 2 inches in width, per linear yard ⑧ ⑧ ⬚ N

IOM: 100-02, 15, 100

⊕ **A6410** Eye pad, sterile, each ⑧ ⑧ Qp Qh ⬚ N

IOM: 100-02, 15, 100

⊕ **A6411** Eye pad, non-sterile, each ⑧ ⑧ Qh ⬚ N

IOM: 100-02, 15, 100

∗ **A6412** Eye patch, occlusive, each ⑧ ⑧ N

Bandages

⊘ **A6413** Adhesive bandage, first-aid type, any size, each ⑧ ⑧ Qp Qh E1

First aid type bandage is a wound cover with a pad size of less than 4 sq. in. Does not meet the definition of the surgical dressing benefit and will be denied as non-covered.

Medicare Statute 1861(s)(5)

∗ **A6441** Padding bandage, non-elastic, non-woven/non-knitted, width greater than or equal to three inches and less than five inches, per yard ⑧ ⑧ ⬚ N

∗ **A6442** Conforming bandage, non-elastic, knitted/woven, non-sterile, width less than three inches, per yard ⑧ ⑧ ⬚ N

Non-elastic, moderate or high compression that is typically sustained for one week

∗ **A6443** Conforming bandage, non-elastic, knitted/woven, non-sterile, width greater than or equal to three inches and less than five inches, per yard ⑧ ⑧ ⬚ N

∗ **A6444** Conforming bandage, non-elastic, knitted/woven, non-sterile, width greater than or equal to five inches, per yard ⑧ ⑧ ⬚ N

∗ **A6445** Conforming bandage, non-elastic, knitted/woven, sterile, width less than three inches, per yard ⑧ ⑧ ⬚ N

∗ **A6446** Conforming bandage, non-elastic, knitted/woven, sterile, width greater than or equal to three inches and less than five inches, per yard ⑧ ⑧ ⬚ N

∗ **A6447** Conforming bandage, non-elastic, knitted/woven, sterile, width greater than or equal to five inches, per yard ⑧ ⑧ ⬚ N

∗ **A6448** Light compression bandage, elastic, knitted/woven, width less than three inches, per yard ⑧ ⑧ ⬚ N

Used to hold wound cover dressings in place over a wound. Example is an ACE type elastic bandage.

∗ **A6449** Light compression bandage, elastic, knitted/woven, width greater than or equal to three inches and less than five inches, per yard ⑧ ⑧ ⬚ N

▶ New   ↻ Revised   ✔ Reinstated   ~~deleted~~ Deleted   ⊘ Not covered or valid by Medicare
⊕ Special coverage instructions   ∗ Carrier discretion   ⑧ Bill Part B MAC   ⑧ Bill DME MAC

✱ **A6450** Light compression bandage, elastic, knitted/woven, width greater than or equal to five inches, per yard ⑧ ⑥ 🦽 N

✱ **A6451** Moderate compression bandage, elastic, knitted/woven, load resistance of 1.25 to 1.34 foot pounds at 50% maximum stretch, width greater than or equal to three inches and less than five inches, per yard ⑧ ⑥ 🦽 N

Elastic bandages that produce moderate compression that is typically sustained for one week

Medicare considers coverage if part of a multi-layer compression bandage system for the treatment of a venous stasis ulcer. Do not assign for strains or sprains.

✱ **A6452** High compression bandage, elastic, knitted/woven, load resistance greater than or equal to 1.35 foot pounds at 50% maximum stretch, width greater than or equal to three inches and less than five inches, per yard ⑧ ⑥ 🦽 N

Elastic bandages that produce high compression that is typically sustained for one week

✱ **A6453** Self-adherent bandage, elastic, non-knitted/non-woven, width less than three inches, per yard ⑧ ⑥ 🦽 N

✱ **A6454** Self-adherent bandage, elastic, non-knitted/non-woven, width greater than or equal to three inches and less than five inches, per yard ⑧ ⑥ 🦽 N

✱ **A6455** Self-adherent bandage, elastic, non-knitted/non-woven, width greater than or equal to five inches, per yard ⑧ ⑥ 🦽 N

✱ **A6456** Zinc paste impregnated bandage, non-elastic, knitted/woven, width greater than or equal to three inches and less than five inches, per yard ⑧ ⑥ 🦽 N

✱ **A6457** Tubular dressing with or without elastic, any width, per linear yard ⑧ ⑥ 🦽 N

✱ **A6460** Synthetic resorbable wound dressing, sterile, pad size 16 sq. in. or less, without adhesive border, each dressing ⑧ N

✱ **A6461** Synthetic resorbable wound dressing, sterile, pad size more than 16 sq. in. but less than or equal to 48 sq. in., without adhesive border, each dressing ⑧ N

Compression Garments

⊘ **A6501** Compression burn garment, bodysuit (head to foot), custom fabricated ⑧ ⑥ Qp Qh 🦽 N

Garments used to reduce hypertrophic scarring and joint contractures following burn injury

IOM: 100-02, 15, 100

⊘ **A6502** Compression burn garment, chin strap, custom fabricated ⑧ ⑥ Qp Qh 🦽 N

IOM: 100-02, 15, 100

⊘ **A6503** Compression burn garment, facial hood, custom fabricated ⑧ ⑥ Qp Qh 🦽 N

IOM: 100-02, 15, 100

⊘ **A6504** Compression burn garment, glove to wrist, custom fabricated ⑧ ⑥ Qp Qh 🦽 N

IOM: 100-02, 15, 100

⊘ **A6505** Compression burn garment, glove to elbow, custom fabricated ⑧ ⑥ Qp Qh 🦽 N

IOM: 100-02, 15, 100

⊘ **A6506** Compression burn garment, glove to axilla, custom fabricated ⑧ ⑥ Qp Qh 🦽 N

IOM: 100-02, 15, 100

⊘ **A6507** Compression burn garment, foot to knee length, custom fabricated ⑧ ⑥ Qp Qh 🦽 N

IOM: 100-02, 15, 100

⊘ **A6508** Compression burn garment, foot to thigh length, custom fabricated ⑧ ⑥ Qp Qh 🦽 N

IOM: 100-02, 15, 100

⊘ **A6509** Compression burn garment, upper trunk to waist including arm openings (vest), custom fabricated ⑧ ⑥ Qp Qh 🦽 N

IOM: 100-02, 15, 100

⊘ **A6510** Compression burn garment, trunk, including arms down to leg openings (leotard), custom fabricated ⑧ ⑥ Qp Qh 🦽 N

IOM: 100-02, 15, 100

⊘ **A6511** Compression burn garment, lower trunk including leg openings (panty), custom fabricated ⑧ ⑥ Qp Qh 🦽 N

IOM: 100-02, 15, 100

⊘ **A6512** Compression burn garment, not otherwise classified ⑧ ⑥ N

IOM: 100-02, 15, 100

🝔 MIPS	Qp **Quantity Physician**	Qh **Quantity Hospital**	♀ **Female only**
♂ **Male only**	A **Age**	🦽 **DMEPOS**	A2-Z3 **ASC Payment Indicator**	A-Y **ASC Status Indicator**	Coding Clinic

✳ **A6513** Compression burn mask, face and/or neck, plastic or equal, custom fabricated ⑧ Qp Qh ♿   **B**

⊘ **A6530** Gradient compression stocking, below knee, 18-30 mmHg, each ⑧ Qp Qh   **E1**

IOM: 100-03, 4, 280.1

⊛ **A6531** Gradient compression stocking, below knee, 30-40 mmHg, each ⑧ Qp Qh ♿   **N**

Covered when used in treatment of open venous stasis ulcer. Modifiers A1-A9 are not assigned. Must be billed with AW, RT, or LT.

IOM: 100-02, 15, 100

⊛ **A6532** Gradient compression stocking, below knee, 40-50 mmHg, each ⑧ Qp Qh ♿   **N**

Covered when used in treatment of open venous stasis ulcer. Modifiers A1-A9 are not assigned. Must be billed with AW, RT, or LT.

IOM: 100-02, 15, 100

⊘ **A6533** Gradient compression stocking, thigh length, 18-30 mmHg, each ⑧ Qp Qh   **E1**

IOM: 100-02, 15, 130; 100-03, 4, 280.1

⊘ **A6534** Gradient compression stocking, thigh length, 30-40 mmHg, each ⑧ Qp Qh   **E1**

IOM: 100-02, 15, 130; 100-03, 4, 280.1

⊘ **A6535** Gradient compression stocking, thigh length, 40-50 mmHg, each ⑧ Qp Qh   **E1**

IOM: 100-02, 15, 130; 100-03, 4, 280.1

⊘ **A6536** Gradient compression stocking, full length/chap style, 18-30 mmHg, each ⑧ Qp Qh   **E1**

IOM: 100-02, 15, 130; 100-03, 4, 280.1

⊘ **A6537** Gradient compression stocking, full length/chap style, 30-40 mmHg, each ⑧ Qp Qh   **E1**

IOM: 100-02, 15, 130; 100-03, 4, 280.1

⊘ **A6538** Gradient compression stocking, full length/chap style, 40-50 mmHg, each ⑧ Qp Qh   **E1**

IOM: 100-02, 15, 130; 100-03, 4, 280.1

⊘ **A6539** Gradient compression stocking, waist length, 18-30 mmHg, each ⑧ Qp Qh   **E1**

IOM: 100-02, 15, 130; 100-03, 4, 280.1

⊘ **A6540** Gradient compression stocking, waist length, 30-40 mmHg, each ⑧ Qp Qh   **E1**

IOM: 100-02, 15, 130; 100-03, 4, 280.1

⊘ **A6541** Gradient compression stocking, waist length, 40-50 mmHg, each ⑧ Qp Qh   **E1**

IOM: 100-02, 15, 130; 100-03, 4, 280.1

⊘ **A6544** Gradient compression stocking, garter belt ⑧ Qp Qh   **E1**

IOM: 100-02, 15, 130; 100-03, 4, 280.1

⊛ **A6545** Gradient compression wrap, non-elastic, below knee, 30-50 mm hg, each ⑧ Qp Qh ♿   **N**

Modifiers RT and/or LT must be appended. When assigned for bilateral items (left/right) on the same date of service, bill both items on the same claim line using RT/LT modifiers and 2 units of service.

IOM: 10-02, 15, 100

⊘ **A6549** Gradient compression stocking/sleeve, not otherwise specified ⑧ Qp Qh   **E1**

IOM: 100-02, 15, 130; 100-03, 4, 280.1

Wound Care

✳ **A6550** Wound care set, for negative pressure wound therapy electrical pump, includes all supplies and accessories ⑧ Qh ♿   **N**

Urinary Catheters

▶ **A6590** External urinary catheters; disposable, with wicking material, for use with suction pump, per month

▶ **A6591** External urinary catheter; non-disposable, for use with suction pump, per month

Respiratory Supplies

✳ **A7000** Canister, disposable, used with suction pump, each ⑧ Qp Qh &   **Y**

✳ **A7001** Canister, non-disposable, used with suction pump, each ⑧ Qh &   **Y**

✳ **A7002** Tubing, used with suction pump, each ⑧ Qh &   **Y**

✳ **A7003** Administration set, with small volume nonfiltered pneumatic nebulizer, disposable ⑧ Qp Qh &   **Y**

✳ **A7004** Small volume nonfiltered pneumatic nebulizer, disposable ⑧ Qh &   **Y**

✳ **A7005** Administration set, with small volume nonfiltered pneumatic nebulizer, non-disposable ⑧ Qp Qh &   **Y**

▶ **New**   ⏎ **Revised**   ✓ **Reinstated**   ~~deleted~~ **Deleted**   ⊘ **Not covered or valid by Medicare**

⊛ **Special coverage instructions**   ✳ **Carrier discretion**   ⑧ **Bill Part B MAC**   ⑧ **Bill DME MAC**

* **A7006** Administration set, with small volume filtered pneumatic nebulizer ⑬ Qp Qh ⅋   Y

* **A7007** Large volume nebulizer, disposable, unfilled, used with aerosol compressor ⑬ Qh ⅋   Y

* **A7008** Large volume nebulizer, disposable, prefilled, used with aerosol compressor ⑬ ⅋   Y

* **A7009** Reservoir bottle, nondisposable, used with large volume ultrasonic nebulizer ⑬ ⅋   Y

* **A7010** Corrugated tubing, disposable, used with large volume nebulizer, 100 feet ⑬ Qh ⅋   Y

* **A7012** Water collection device, used with large volume nebulizer ⑬ Qh ⅋   Y

* **A7013** Filter, disposable, used with aerosol compressor or ultrasonic generator ⑬ Qp Qh ⅋   Y

* **A7014** Filter, non-disposable, used with aerosol compressor or ultrasonic generator ⑬ Qp Qh ⅋   Y

* **A7015** Aerosol mask, used with DME nebulizer ⑬ Qh ⅋   Y

* **A7016** Dome and mouthpiece, used with small volume ultrasonic nebulizer ⑬ Qp Qh ⅋   Y

* **A7017** Nebulizer, durable, glass or autoclavable plastic, bottle type, not used with oxygen ⑬ Qp Qh ⅋   Y

  IOM: 100-03, 4, 280.1

* **A7018** Water, distilled, used with large volume nebulizer, 1000 ml ⑬ Qh ⅋   Y

* **A7020** Interface for cough stimulating device, includes all components, replacement only ⑬ Qp Qh ⅋   Y

* **A7025** High frequency chest wall oscillation system vest, replacement for use with patient owned equipment, each ⑬ Qp Qh ⅋   N

* **A7026** High frequency chest wall oscillation system hose, replacement for use with patient owned equipment, each ⑬ Qp Qh ⅋   Y

* **A7027** Combination oral/nasal mask, used with continuous positive airway pressure device, each ⑬ Qp Qh ⅋   Y

* **A7028** Oral cushion for combination oral/ nasal mask, replacement only, each ⑬ Qp Qh ⅋   Y

* **A7029** Nasal pillows for combination oral/ nasal mask, replacement only, pair ⑬ Qp Qh ⅋   Y

* **A7030** Full face mask used with positive airway pressure device, each ⑬ Qh ⅋   Y

* **A7031** Face mask interface, replacement for full face mask, each ⑬ Qh ⅋   Y

* **A7032** Cushion for use on nasal mask interface, replacement only, each ⑬ Qp Qh ⅋   Y

* **A7033** Pillow for use on nasal cannula type interface, replacement only, pair ⑬ Qh ⅋   Y

* **A7034** Nasal interface (mask or cannula type) used with positive airway pressure device, with or without head strap ⑬ Qh ⅋   Y

* **A7035** Headgear used with positive airway pressure device ⑬ Qp Qh ⅋   Y

* **A7036** Chinstrap used with positive airway pressure device ⑬ Qp Qh ⅋   Y

* **A7037** Tubing used with positive airway pressure device ⑬ Qp Qh ⅋   Y

* **A7038** Filter, disposable, used with positive airway pressure device ⑬ Qh ⅋   Y

* **A7039** Filter, non disposable, used with positive airway pressure device ⑬ Qp Qh ⅋   Y

* **A7040** One way chest drain valve ⑬ Qp Qh ⅋   N

* **A7041** Water seal drainage container and tubing for use with implanted chest tube ⑬ Qp Qh ⅋   N

* **A7044** Oral interface used with positive airway pressure device, each ⑬ Qp Qh ⅋   Y

* **A7045** Exhalation port with or without swivel used with accessories for positive airway devices, replacement only ⑬ Qh ⅋   Y

  IOM: 100-03, 4, 230.17

* **A7046** Water chamber for humidifier, used with positive airway pressure device, replacement, each ⑬ Qh ⅋   Y

  IOM: 100-03, 4, 230.17

* **A7047** Oral interface used with respiratory suction pump, each ⑬ Qp Qh ⅋   N

* **A7048** Vacuum drainage collection unit and tubing kit, including all supplies needed for collection unit change, for use with implanted catheter, each ⑬ Qp Qh ⅋   N

▶ **A7049** Expiratory positive airway pressure intranasal resistance valve

---

🏷 MIPS   Qp **Quantity Physician**   Qh **Quantity Hospital**   ♀ **Female only**
♂ **Male only**   Ⓐ **Age**   ⅋ **DMEPOS**   A2-Z3 **ASC Payment Indicator**   A-Y **ASC Status Indicator**   Coding Clinic

Tracheostomy Supplies

⊙ **A7501** Tracheostoma valve, including diaphragm, each ⑥ Qp Qh &
N

IOM: 100-02, 15, 120

⊙ **A7502** Replacement diaphragm/faceplate for tracheostoma valve, each ⑧ Qh &
N

IOM: 100-02, 15, 120

⊙ **A7503** Filter holder or filter cap, reusable, for use in a tracheostoma heat and moisture exchange system, each ⑧ Qh &
N

IOM: 100-02, 15, 120

⊙ **A7504** Filter for use in a tracheostoma heat and moisture exchange system, each ⑧ Qp Qh &
N

IOM: 100-02, 15, 120

⊙ **A7505** Housing, reusable without adhesive, for use in a heat and moisture exchange system and/or with a tracheostoma valve, each ⑧ Qh &
N

IOM: 100-02, 15, 120

⊙ **A7506** Adhesive disc for use in a heat and moisture exchange system and/or with tracheostoma valve, any type, each ⑧ Qh &
N

IOM: 100-02, 15, 120

⊙ **A7507** Filter holder and integrated filter without adhesive, for use in a tracheostoma heat and moisture exchange system, each ⑧ Qp Qh &
N

IOM: 100-02, 15, 120

⊙ **A7508** Housing and integrated adhesive, for use in a tracheostoma heat and moisture exchange system and/or with a tracheostoma valve, each ⑧ Qh &
N

IOM: 100-02, 15, 120

⊙ **A7509** Filter holder and integrated filter housing, and adhesive, for use as a tracheostoma heat and moisture exchange system, each ⑧ Qh &
N

IOM: 100-02, 15, 120

✳ **A7520** Tracheostomy/laryngectomy tube, non-cuffed, polyvinylchloride (PVC), silicone or equal, each ⑧ Qp Qh &
N

✳ **A7521** Tracheostomy/laryngectomy tube, cuffed, polyvinylchloride (PVC), silicone or equal, each ⑧ Qh &
N

✳ **A7522** Tracheostomy/laryngectomy tube, stainless steel or equal (sterilizable and reusable), each ⑧ Qh &
N

Figure 7 Helmet.

✳ **A7523** Tracheostomy shower protector, each ⑧
N

✳ **A7524** Tracheostoma stent/stud/button, each ⑧ Qp Qh &
N

✳ **A7525** Tracheostomy mask, each ⑧ Qh &
N

✳ **A7526** Tracheostomy tube collar/holder, each ⑧ Qh &
N

✳ **A7527** Tracheostomy/laryngectomy tube plug/stop, each ⑧ Qp Qh &
N

Helmets

✳ **A8000** Helmet, protective, soft, prefabricated, includes all components and accessories ⑧ &
Y

✳ **A8001** Helmet, protective, hard, prefabricated, includes all components and accessories ⑧ &
Y

✳ **A8002** Helmet, protective, soft, custom fabricated, includes all components and accessories ⑧ &
Y

✳ **A8003** Helmet, protective, hard, custom fabricated, includes all components and accessories ⑧ &
Y

✳ **A8004** Soft interface for helmet, replacement only ⑧ &
Y

ADMINISTRATIVE, MISCELLANEOUS, AND INVESTIGATIONAL (A9000-A9999)

NOTE: The following codes do not imply that codes in other sections are necessarily covered.

Miscellaneous Supplies

⊙ **A9150** Non-prescription drugs ⑧
B

IOM: 100-02, 15, 50

⊘ **A9152** Single vitamin/mineral/trace element, oral, per dose, not otherwise specified ⑧ Qp Qh
E1

▶ **New** ↻ **Revised** ✔ **Reinstated** ~~deleted~~ **Deleted** ⊘ **Not covered or valid by Medicare**
⊙ **Special coverage instructions** ✳ **Carrier discretion** ⑧ **Bill Part B MAC** ⑥ **Bill DME MAC**

⊘ **A9153** Multiple vitamins, with or without minerals and trace elements, oral, per dose, not otherwise specified Ⓑ Qp Qh E1

✳ **A9155** Artificial saliva, 30 ml Ⓑ Qp Qh B

▶ **A9156** Oral mucoadhesive, any type (liquid, gel, paste, etc.), per 1 ml N1

⊘ **A9180** Pediculosis (lice infestation) treatment, topical, for administration by patient/caretaker Ⓑ Qp Qh E1

▶ **A9268** Programmer for transient, orally ingested capsule

▶ **A9269** Programable, transient, orally ingested capsule, for use with external programmer, per month

⊘ **A9270** Non-covered item or service Ⓑ Qp Qh E1

IOM: 100-02, 16, 20

⊘ **A9272** Wound suction, disposable, includes dressing, all accessories and components, any type, each Ⓑ Qp Qh E1

Medicare Statute 1861(n)

⊘ **A9273** Cold or hot water bottle, ice cap or collar, heat and/or cold wrap, any type Ⓑ Qp Qh E1

⊘ **A9274** External ambulatory insulin delivery system, disposable, each, includes all supplies and accessories Ⓑ Qp Qh E1

Medicare Statute 1861(n)

⊘ **A9275** Home glucose disposable monitor, includes test strips Ⓑ Qp Qh E1

⊘ **A9276** Sensor; invasive (e.g., subcutaneous), disposable, for use with non-durable medical equipment interstitial continuous glucose monitoring system, one unit = 1 day supply Ⓑ Qp Qh E1

Medicare Statute 1861(n)

⊘ **A9277** Transmitter; external, for use with non-durable medical equipment interstitial continuous glucose monitoring system Ⓑ Qp Qh E1

Medicare Statute 1861(n)

⊘ **A9278** Receiver (monitor); external, for use with non-durable medical equipment interstitial continuous glucose monitoring system Ⓑ Qp Qh E1

Medicare Statute 1861(n)

⊘ **A9279** Monitoring feature/device, stand-alone or integrated, any type, includes all accessories, components and electronics, not otherwise classified Ⓑ Qp Qh E1

Medicare Statute 1861(n)

⊘ **A9280** Alert or alarm device, not otherwise classified Ⓑ Qp Qh E1

Medicare Statute 1861

⊘ **A9281** Reaching/grabbing device, any type, any length, each Ⓑ Qp Qh E1

Medicare Statute 1862 SSA

⊘ **A9282** Wig, any type, each Ⓑ Qp Qh E1

Medicare Statute 1862 SSA

⊘ **A9283** Foot pressure off loading/supportive device, any type, each Ⓑ Qp Qh E1

Medicare Statute 1862A(i)13

⊛ **A9284** Spirometer, non-electronic, includes all accessories Ⓑ Qp Qh N

✳ **A9285** Inversion/eversion correction device Ⓑ Qp Qh A

⊘ **A9286** Hygienic item or device, disposable or non-disposable, any type, each Ⓑ Qp Qh E1

Medicare Statute 1834

A9291 Prescription digital cognitive and/or behavioral therapy, FDA cleared, per course of treatment E1

▶ **A9292** Prescription digital visual therapy, software-only, FDA cleared, per course of treatment

⊘ **A9300** Exercise equipment Ⓑ Qp Qh E1

IOM: 100-02, 15, 110.1; 100-03, 4, 280.1

Supplies for Radiology Procedures (Radiopharmaceuticals)

✳ **A9500** Technetium Tc-99m sestamibi, diagnostic, per study dose Ⓑ Qp Qh N1 N

Should be filed on same claim as procedure code reporting radiopharmaceutical. Verify with payer definition of a "study."

Coding Clinic: 2006, Q2, P5

✳ **A9501** Technetium Tc-99m teboroxime, diagnostic, per study dose Ⓑ Qp Qh N1 N

✳ **A9502** Technetium Tc-99m tetrofosmin, diagnostic, per study dose Ⓑ Qp Qh N1 N

Coding Clinic: 2006, Q2, P5

✳ **A9503** Technetium Tc-99m medronate, diagnostic, per study dose, up to 30 millicuries Ⓑ Qp Qh N1 N

✳ **A9504** Technetium Tc-99m apcitide, diagnostic, per study dose, up to 20 millicuries Ⓑ Qp Qh N1 N

🖑 MIPS   Qp **Quantity Physician**   Qh **Quantity Hospital**   ♀ **Female only**

♂ **Male only**   Ⓐ **Age**   ♿ **DMEPOS**   A2-Z3 **ASC Payment Indicator**   A-Y **ASC Status Indicator**   Coding Clinic

* **A9505** Thallium Tl-201 thallous chloride, diagnostic, per millicurie Ⓑ Qp Qh   N1 N

* **A9507** Indium In-111 capromab pendetide, diagnostic, per study dose, up to 10 millicuries Ⓟ Qp Qh   N1 N

* **A9508** Iodine I-131 iobenguane sulfate, diagnostic, per 0.5 millicurie Ⓑ Qp Qh   N1 N

* **A9509** Iodine I-123 sodium iodide, diagnostic, per millicurie Ⓑ Qp Qh   N1 N

* **A9510** Technetium Tc-99m disofenin, diagnostic, per study dose, up to 15 millicuries Ⓑ Qp Qh   N1 N

* **A9512** Technetium Tc-99m pertechnetate, diagnostic, per millicurie Ⓑ Qp Qh   N1 N

◎ **A9513** Lutetium lu 177, dotatate, therapeutic, 1 millicurie   G

* **A9515** Choline C-11, diagnostic, per study dose up to 20 millicuries Qp Qh   K2 G

* **A9516** Iodine I-123 sodium iodide, diagnostic, per 100 microcuries, up to 999 microcuries Ⓟ Qp Qh   N1 N

* **A9517** Iodine I-131 sodium iodide capsule(s), therapeutic, per millicurie Ⓑ Qp Qh   K

* **A9520** Technetium Tc-99m tilmanocept, diagnostic, up to 0.5 millicuries Ⓟ Qp Qh   N1 N

* **A9521** Technetium Tc-99m exametazime, diagnostic, per study dose, up to 25 millicuries Ⓑ Qp Qh   N1 N

* **A9524** Iodine I-131 iodinated serum albumin, diagnostic, per 5 microcuries Ⓑ Qp Qh   N1 N

* **A9526** Nitrogen N-13 ammonia, diagnostic, per study dose, up to 40 millicuries Ⓑ Qp Qh   N1 N

* **A9527** Iodine I-125, sodium iodide solution, therapeutic, per millicurie Ⓑ Qp Qh   H2 U

* **A9528** Iodine I-131 sodium iodide capsule(s), diagnostic, per millicurie Ⓟ Qp Qh   N1 N

* **A9529** Iodine I-131 sodium iodide solution, diagnostic, per millicurie Ⓟ Qp Qh   N1 N

* **A9530** Iodine I-131 sodium iodide solution, therapeutic, per millicurie Ⓑ Qp Qh   K

* **A9531** Iodine I-131 sodium iodide, diagnostic, per microcurie (up to 100 microcuries) Ⓑ Qp Qh   N1 N

* **A9532** Iodine I-125 serum albumin, diagnostic, per 5 microcuries Ⓑ Qp Qh   N1 N

* **A9536** Technetium Tc-99m depreotide, diagnostic, per study dose, up to 35 millicuries Ⓑ Qp Qh   N1 N

* **A9537** Technetium Tc-99m mebrofenin, diagnostic, per study dose, up to 15 millicuries Ⓑ Qp Qh   N1 N

* **A9538** Technetium Tc-99m pyrophosphate, diagnostic, per study dose, up to 25 millicuries Ⓑ Qp Qh   N1 N

* **A9539** Technetium Tc-99m pentetate, diagnostic, per study dose, up to 25 millicuries Ⓑ Qp Qh   N1 N

* **A9540** Technetium Tc-99m macroaggregated albumin, diagnostic, per study dose, up to 10 millicuries Ⓑ Qp Qh   N1 N

* **A9541** Technetium Tc-99m sulfur colloid, diagnostic, per study dose, up to 20 millicuries Ⓑ Qp Qh   N1 N

* **A9542** Indium In-111 ibritumomab tiuxetan, diagnostic, per study dose, up to 5 millicuries Ⓑ Qp Qh   N1 N

   Specifically for diagnostic use.

* **A9543** Yttrium Y-90 ibritumomab tiuxetan, therapeutic, per treatment dose, up to 40 millicuries Ⓑ Qp Qh   K

   Specifically for therapeutic use.

* **A9546** Cobalt Co-57/58, cyanocobalamin, diagnostic, per study dose, up to 1 microcurie Ⓑ Qp Qh   N1 N

* **A9547** Indium In-111 oxyquinoline, diagnostic, per 0.5 millicurie Ⓑ Qp Qh   N1 N

* **A9548** Indium In-111 pentetate, diagnostic, per 0.5 millicurie Ⓑ Qp Qh   N1 N

* **A9550** Technetium Tc-99m sodium gluceptate, diagnostic, per study dose, up to 25 millicuries Ⓟ Qp Qh   N1 N

* **A9551** Technetium Tc-99m succimer, diagnostic, per study dose, up to 10 millicuries Ⓑ Qp Qh   N1 N

* **A9552** Fluorodeoxyglucose F-18 FDG, diagnostic, per study dose, up to 45 millicuries Ⓑ Qp Qh   N1 N

   Coding Clinic: 2008, Q3, P7

* **A9553** Chromium Cr-51 sodium chromate, diagnostic, per study dose, up to 250 microcuries Ⓑ Qp Qh   N1 N

* **A9554** Iodine I-125 sodium Iothalamate, diagnostic, per study dose, up to 10 microcuries Ⓟ Qp Qh   N1 N

* **A9555** Rubidium Rb-82, diagnostic, per study dose, up to 60 millicuries Ⓑ Qp Qh   N1 N

▶ **New**   ↻ **Revised**   ✔ **Reinstated**   ~~deleted~~ **Deleted**   ⊘ **Not covered or valid by Medicare**
◎ **Special coverage instructions**   ✳ **Carrier discretion**   Ⓑ **Bill Part B MAC**   Ⓓ **Bill DME MAC**

* **A9556** Gallium Ga-67 citrate, diagnostic, per millicurie Ⓑ Qp Qh   N1 N

* **A9557** Technetium Tc-99m bicisate, diagnostic, per study dose, up to 25 millicuries Ⓑ Qp Qh   N1 N

* **A9558** Xenon Xe-133 gas, diagnostic, per 10 millicuries Ⓑ Qp Qh   N1 N

* **A9559** Cobalt Co-57 cyanocobalamin, oral, diagnostic, per study dose, up to 1 microcurie Ⓑ Qp Qh   N1 N

* **A9560** Technetium Tc-99m labeled red blood cells, diagnostic, per study dose, up to 30 millicuries Ⓑ Qp Qh   N1 N

    Coding Clinic: 2008, Q3, P7

* **A9561** Technetium Tc-99m oxidronate, diagnostic, per study dose, up to 30 millicuries Ⓑ Qp Qh   N1 N

* **A9562** Technetium Tc-99m mertiatide, diagnostic, per study dose, up to 15 millicuries Ⓑ Qp Qh   N1 N

* **A9563** Sodium phosphate P-32, therapeutic, per millicurie Ⓑ Qp Qh   K

* **A9564** Chromic phosphate P-32 suspension, therapeutic, per millicurie Ⓑ Qp Qh   E1

* **A9566** Technetium Tc-99m fanolesomab, diagnostic, per study dose, up to 25 millicuries Ⓑ Qp Qh   N1 N

* **A9567** Technetium Tc-99m pentetate, diagnostic, aerosol, per study dose, up to 75 millicuries Ⓑ Qp Qh   N1 N

* **A9568** Technetium TC-99m arcitumomab, diagnostic, per study dose, up to 45 millicuries Ⓑ Qp Qh   N1 N

* **A9569** Technetium Tc-99m exametazime labeled autologous white blood cells, diagnostic, per study dose Ⓑ Qp Qh   N1 N

* **A9570** Indium In-111 labeled autologous white blood cells, diagnostic, per study dose Ⓑ Qp Qh   N1 N

* **A9571** Indium In-111 labeled autologous platelets, diagnostic, per study dose Ⓑ Qp Qh   N1 N

* **A9572** Indium In-111 pentetreotide, diagnostic, per study dose, up to 6 millicuries Ⓑ Qp Qh   N1 N

▶ ⊙ **A9573** Injection, gadopiclenol, 1 ml   N1 N

* **A9575** Injection, gadoterate meglumine, 0.1 ml Ⓑ Qp Qh   N1 N

    Other: Clariscan, Gadoterate Meglumine

* **A9576** Injection, gadoteridol, (ProHance Multipack), per ml Ⓑ Qp Qh   N1 N

* **A9577** Injection, gadobenate dimeglumine (MultiHance), per ml Ⓑ Qp Qh   N1 N

* **A9578** Injection, gadobenate dimeglumine (MultiHance Multipack), per ml Ⓑ Qp Qh   N1 N

* **A9579** Injection, gadolinium-based magnetic resonance contrast agent, not otherwise specified (NOS), per ml Ⓑ Qp Qh   N1 N

    Other: Magnevist, Prohance

* **A9580** Sodium fluoride F-18, diagnostic, per study dose, up to 30 millicuries Ⓑ Qp Qh   N1 N

* **A9581** Injection, gadoxetate disodium, 1 ml Ⓑ Qp Qh   N1 N

    Local Medicare contractors may require the use of modifier JW to identify unused product from single-dose vials that are appropriately discarded.

    Other: Eovist

* **A9582** Iodine I-123 iobenguane, diagnostic, per study dose, up to 15 millicuries Ⓑ Qp Qh   N1 N

    Molecular imaging agent that assists in the identification of rare neuroendocrine tumors.

* **A9583** Injection, gadofosveset trisodium, 1 ml Ⓑ Qp Qh   N1 N

* **A9584** Iodine 1-123 ioflupane, diagnostic, per study dose, up to 5 millicuries Ⓑ Qp Qh   N1 N

    Coding Clinic: 2012, Q1, P9

* **A9585** Injection, gadobutrol, 0.1 ml Ⓑ Qp Qh   N1 N

    Other: Gadavist

    Coding Clinic: 2012, Q1, P8

⊙ **A9586** Florbetapir F18, diagnostic, per study dose, up to 10 millicuries Ⓑ Qp Qh   N1 N

* **A9587** Gallium Ga-68, dotatate, diagnostic, 0.1 millicurie Qp Qh   K2 G

    Coding Clinic: 2017, Q1, P9

* **A9589** Instillation, hexaminolevulinate hydrochloride, 100 mg   N1 N

* **A9588** Fluciclovine F-18, diagnostic, 1 millicurie Qp Qh   K2 G

    Coding Clinic: 2017, Q1, P9

* **A9590** Iodine I-131, iobenguane, 1 millicurie   N

* **A9591** Fluoroestradiol F 18, diagnostic, 1 millicurie   K2 G

   🔬 **MIPS**   Qp **Quantity Physician**   Qh **Quantity Hospital**   ♀ **Female only**

   ♂ **Male only**   A **Age**   ♿ **DMEPOS**   A2-Z3 **ASC Payment Indicator**   A-Y **ASC Status Indicator**   *Coding Clinic*

✳ **A9592** Copper cu-64, dotatate, diagnostic, 1 millicurie   K2 G

✳ **A9593** Gallium ga-68 psma-11, diagnostic, (ucsf), 1 millicurie   K2 G

✳ **A9594** Gallium ga-68 psma-11, diagnostic, (ucla), 1 millicurie   K2 G

✳ **A9595** Piflufolastat f-18, diagnostic, 1 millicurie   K2 G

A9596 Gallium GA-68 gozetotide, diagnostic, (illuccix), 1 millicurie   G

✳ **A9597** Positron emission tomography radiopharmaceutical, diagnostic, for tumor identification, not otherwise classified   N1 N

Coding Clinic: 2017, Q1, P8-9

✳ **A9598** Positron emission tomography radiopharmaceutical, diagnostic, for non-tumor identification, not otherwise classified   N1 N

Coding Clinic: 2017, Q1, P8-9

✳ **A9600** Strontium Sr-89 chloride, therapeutic, per millicurie ⑧ Qp Qh   K

A9601 Flortaucipir F 18 injection, diagnostic, 1 millicurie   K5 E1

A9602 Fluorodopa F-18, diagnostic, per millicurie   K2 G

▶ **A9603** Injection, pafolacianine, 0.1 mg   N1

✳ **A9604** Samarium SM-153 lexidronam, therapeutic, per treatment dose, up to 150 millicuries ⑧ Qp Qh   K

✳ **A9606** Radium Ra-223 dichloride, therapeutic, per microcurie Qp Qh   K

A9607 Lutetium LU 177 vipivotide tetraxetan, therapeutic, 1 millicurie   G

▶ **A9697** Injection, carboxydextran-coated superparamagnetic iron oxide, per study dose   N1

☺ **A9698** Non-radioactive contrast imaging material, not otherwise classified, per study ⑧   N1 N

IOM: 100-04, 12, 70; 100-04, 13, 20

Coding Clinic: 2017, Q1, P8

✳ **A9699** Radiopharmaceutical, therapeutic, not otherwise classified ⑧   N

☺ **A9700** Supply of injectable contrast material for use in echocardiography, per study ⑧ Qp Qh   N1 N

IOM: 100-04, 12, 30.4

Coding Clinic: 2017, Q1, P8

A9800 Gallium GA-68 gozetotide, diagnostic, (locametz), 1 millicurie   K2 G

Miscellaneous Service Component

✳ **A9900** Miscellaneous DME supply, accessory, and/or service component of another HCPCS code ⑧ ⑥   Y

On DMEPOS fee schedule as a payable replacement for miscellaneous implanted or non-implanted items.

✳ **A9901** DME delivery, set up, and/or dispensing service component of another HCPCS code ⑥   A

✳ **A9999** Miscellaneous DME supply or accessory, not otherwise specified ⑧ ⑥   Y

On DMEPOS fee schedule as a payable replacement for miscellaneous implanted or non-implanted items.

▶ **New**   ↻ **Revised**   ✔ **Reinstated**   ~~deleted~~ **Deleted**   ⊘ **Not covered or valid by Medicare**
☺ **Special coverage instructions**   ✳ **Carrier discretion**   ⑧ **Bill Part B MAC**   ⑥ **Bill DME MAC**

A9592 – A9999   ADMINISTRATIVE, MISCELLANEOUS, AND INVESTIGATIONAL

ENTERAL AND PARENTERAL THERAPY
(B4000-B9999)

Enteral Feeding Supplies

⚙ **B4034** Enteral feeding supply kit; syringe fed, per day, includes but not limited to feeding/flushing syringe, administration set tubing, dressings, tape Ⓑ Qh   Y

Dressings used with gastrostomy tubes for enteral nutrition (covered under the prosthetic device benefit) are included in the payment.

IOM: 100-02, 15, 120; 100-03, 3, 180.2; 100-04, 20, 100.2.2

PEN: On Fee Schedule

⚙ **B4035** Enteral feeding supply kit; pump fed, per day, includes but not limited to feeding/flushing syringe, administration set tubing, dressings, tape Ⓖ Qh   Y

IOM: 100-02, 15, 120; 100-03, 3, 180.2; 100-04, 20, 100.2.2

PEN: On Fee Schedule

⚙ **B4036** Enteral feeding supply kit; gravity fed, per day, includes but not limited to feeding/flushing syringe, administration set tubing, dressings, tape Ⓖ Qh   Y

IOM: 100-02, 15, 120; 100-03, 3, 180.2; 100-04, 20, 100.2.2

PEN: On Fee Schedule

⚙ **B4081** Nasogastric tubing with stylet Ⓑ Qp Qh   Y

More than 3 nasogastric tubes (B4081-B4083), or 1 gastrostomy/jejunostomy tube (B4087-B4088) every three months is rarely medically necessary.

IOM: 100-02, 15, 120; 100-03, 3, 180.2; 100-04, 20, 100.2.2

PEN: On Fee Schedule

⚙ **B4082** Nasogastric tubing without stylet Ⓖ Qp Qh   Y

IOM: 100-02, 15, 120; 100-03, 3, 180.2; 100-04, 20, 100.2.2

PEN: On Fee Schedule

⚙ **B4083** Stomach tube - Levine type Ⓖ Qp Qh   Y

IOM: 100-02, 15, 120; 100-03, 3, 180.2; 100-04, 20, 100.2.2

PEN: On Fee Schedule

✳ **B4087** Gastrostomy/jejunostomy tube, standard, any material, any type, each Ⓑ Qp Qh   A

PEN: On Fee Schedule

✳ **B4088** Gastrostomy/jejunostomy tube, low-profile, any material, any type, each Ⓑ Qp Qh   A

PEN: On Fee Schedule

Enteral Formulas and Additives

⊘ **B4100** Food thickener, administered orally, per ounce Ⓑ   E1

⚙ **B4102** Enteral formula, for adults, used to replace fluids and electrolytes (e.g., clear liquids), 500 ml = 1 unit Ⓑ Ⓐ   Y

IOM: 100-03, 3, 180.2

⚙ **B4103** Enteral formula, for pediatrics, used to replace fluids and electrolytes (e.g., clear liquids), 500 ml = 1 unit Ⓑ Ⓐ   Y

IOM: 100-03, 3, 180.2

⚙ **B4104** Additive for enteral formula (e.g., fiber) Ⓑ   E1

IOM: 100-03, 3, 180.2

⚙ **B4105** In-line cartridge containing digestive enzyme(s) for enteral feeding, each   Y

Cross Reference Q9994

▶ **B4148** Enteral feeding supply kit; elastomeric control fed, per day, includes but not limited to feeding/flushing syringe, administration set tubing, dressings, tape

⚙ **B4149** Enteral formula, manufactured blenderized natural foods with intact nutrients, includes proteins, fats, carbohydrates, vitamins and minerals, may include fiber, administered through an enteral feeding tube, 100 calories = 1 unit Ⓑ Qp Qh   Y

Produced to meet unique nutrient needs for specific disease conditions; medical record must document specific condition and need for special nutrient.

IOM: 100-02, 15, 120; 100-03, 3, 180.2; 100-04, 20, 100.2.2

PEN: On Fee Schedule

ENTERAL AND PARENTERAL THERAPY   B4034 — B4149

⊗ **B4150** Enteral formulae, nutritionally complete with intact nutrients, includes proteins, fats, carbohydrates, vitamins, and minerals, may include fiber, administered through an enteral feeding tube, 100 calories = 1 unit Ⓓ Qh   Y

IOM: 100-02, 15, 120; 100-03, 3, 180.2; 100-04, 20, 100.2.2

PEN: On Fee Schedule

⊗ **B4152** Enteral formula, nutritionally complete, calorically dense (equal to or greater than 1.5 kcal/ml) with intact nutrients, includes proteins, fats, carbohydrates, vitamins and minerals, may include fiber, administered through an enteral feeding tube, 100 calories = 1 unit Ⓓ Qh   Y

IOM: 100-02, 15, 120; 100-03, 3, 180.2; 100-04, 20, 100.2.2

PEN: On Fee Schedule

⊗ **B4153** Enteral formula, nutritionally complete, hydrolyzed proteins (amino acids and peptide chain), includes fats, carbohydrates, vitamins and minerals, may include fiber, administered through an enteral feeding tube, 100 calories = 1 unit Ⓑ Qp Qh   Y

If 2 enteral nutrition products described by same HCPCS code and provided at same time billed on single claim line with units of service reflecting total calories of both nutrients

IOM: 100-02, 15, 120; 100-03, 3, 180.2; 100-04, 20, 100.2.2

PEN: On Fee Schedule

⊗ **B4154** Enteral formula, nutritionally complete, for special metabolic needs, excludes inherited disease of metabolism, includes altered composition of proteins, fats, carbohydrates, vitamins and/or minerals, may include fiber, administered through an enteral feeding tube, 100 calories = 1 unit Ⓓ Qh   Y

IOM: 100-02, 15, 120; 100-03, 3, 180.2; 100-04, 20, 100.2.2

PEN: On Fee Schedule

⊗ **B4155** Enteral formula, nutritionally incomplete/modular nutrients, includes specific nutrients, carbohydrates (e.g., glucose polymers), proteins/amino acids (e.g., glutamine, arginine), fat (e.g., medium chain triglycerides) or combination, administered through an enteral feeding tube, 100 calories = 1 unit Ⓑ Qh   Y

IOM: 100-02, 15, 120; 100-03, 3, 180.2; 100-04, 20, 100.2.2

PEN: On Fee Schedule

⊗ **B4157** Enteral formula, nutritionally complete, for special metabolic needs for inherited disease of metabolism, includes proteins, fats, carbohydrates, vitamins and minerals, may include fiber, administered through an enteral feeding tube, 100 calories = 1 unit Ⓑ Qp Qh   Y

IOM: 100-03, 3, 180.2

⊗ **B4158** Enteral formula, for pediatrics, nutritionally complete with intact nutrients, includes proteins, fats, carbohydrates, vitamins and minerals, may include fiber and/or iron, administered through an enteral feeding tube, 100 calories = 1 unit Ⓑ Qh A   Y

IOM: 100-03, 3, 180.2

⊗ **B4159** Enteral formula, for pediatrics, nutritionally complete soy based with intact nutrients, includes proteins, fats, carbohydrates, vitamins and minerals, may include fiber and/or iron, administered through an enteral feeding tube, 100 calories = 1 unit Ⓑ Qh A   Y

IOM: 100-03, 3, 180.2

⊗ **B4160** Enteral formula, for pediatrics, nutritionally complete calorically dense (equal to or greater than 0.7 kcal/ml) with intact nutrients, includes proteins, fats, carbohydrates, vitamins and minerals, may include fiber, administered through an enteral feeding tube, 100 calories = 1 unit Ⓑ Qp Qh A   Y

IOM: 100-03, 3, 180.2

⊗ **B4161** Enteral formula, for pediatrics, hydrolyzed/amino acids and peptide chain proteins, includes fats, carbohydrates, vitamins and minerals, may include fiber, administered through an enteral feeding tube, 100 calories = 1 unit Ⓑ Qh A   Y

IOM: 100-03, 3, 180.2

▶ **New**   ↻ **Revised**   ✔ **Reinstated**   ̶d̶e̶l̶e̶t̶e̶d̶ **Deleted**   ⊘ **Not covered or valid by Medicare**
⊗ **Special coverage instructions**   ✳ **Carrier discretion**   Ⓑ **Bill Part B MAC**   Ⓓ **Bill DME MAC**

Figure 8 Total Parenteral Nutrition (TPN) involves percutaneous placement of central venous catheter into vena cava or right atrium.

○ **B4162** Enteral formula, for pediatrics, special metabolic needs for inherited disease of metabolism, includes proteins, fats, carbohydrates, vitamins and minerals, may include fiber, administered through an enteral feeding tube, 100 calories = 1 unit ⓑ Qh A   Y

IOM: 100-03, 3, 180.2

Parenteral Nutritional Solutions and Supplies

○ **B4164** Parenteral nutrition solution: carbohydrates (dextrose), 50% or less (500 ml = 1 unit) - home mix ⓑ Qp Qh   Y

IOM: 100-02, 15, 120; 100-03, 3, 180.2; 100-04, 20, 100.2.2

PEN: On Fee Schedule

○ **B4168** Parenteral nutrition solution; amino acid, 3.5%, (500 ml = 1 unit) - home mix ⓑ Qp Qh   Y

IOM: 100-02, 15, 120; 100-03, 3, 180.2; 100-04, 20, 100.2.2

PEN: On Fee Schedule

○ **B4172** Parenteral nutrition solution; amino acid, 5.5% through 7%, (500 ml = 1 unit) - home mix ⓑ Qp Qh   Y

IOM: 100-02, 15, 120; 100-03, 3, 180.2; 100-04, 20, 100.2.2

○ **B4176** Parenteral nutrition solution; amino acid, 7% through 8.5%, (500 ml = 1 unit) - home mix ⓑ Qp Qh   Y

IOM: 100-02, 15, 120; 100-03, 3, 180.2; 100-04, 20, 100.2.2

PEN: On Fee Schedule

○ **B4178** Parenteral nutrition solution: amino acid, greater than 8.5% (500 ml = 1 unit) - home mix ⓑ Qp Qh   Y

IOM: 100-02, 15, 120; 100-03, 3, 180.2; 100-04, 20, 100.2.2

PEN: On Fee Schedule

○ **B4180** Parenteral nutrition solution; carbohydrates (dextrose), greater than 50% (500 ml = 1 unit) - home mix ⓑ Qp Qh   Y

IOM: 100-02, 15, 120; 100-03, 3, 180.2; 100-04, 20, 100.2.2

PEN: On Fee Schedule

○ **B4185** Parenteral nutrition solution, not otherwise specified, 10 grams lipids ⓑ   B

PEN: On Fee Schedule

○ **B4187** Omegaven, 10 grams lipids   Y

○ **B4189** Parenteral nutrition solution; compounded amino acid and carbohydrates with electrolytes, trace elements, and vitamins, including preparation, any strength, 10 to 51 grams of protein - premix ⓑ Qp Qh   Y

IOM: 100-02, 15, 120; 100-03, 3, 180.2; 100-04, 20, 100.2.2

PEN: On Fee Schedule

○ **B4193** Parenteral nutrition solution; compounded amino acid and carbohydrates with electrolytes, trace elements, and vitamins, including preparation, any strength, 52 to 73 grams of protein - premix ⓑ Qh   Y

IOM: 100-02, 15, 120; 100-03, 3, 180.2; 100-04, 20, 100.2.2

PEN: On Fee Schedule

○ **B4197** Parenteral nutrition solution; compounded amino acid and carbohydrates with electrolytes, trace elements and vitamins, including preparation, any strength, 74 to 100 grams of protein - premix ⓑ Qh   Y

IOM: 100-02, 15, 120; 100-03, 3, 180.2; 100-04, 20, 100.2.2

PEN: On Fee Schedule

ENTERAL AND PARENTERAL THERAPY   B4162 — B4197

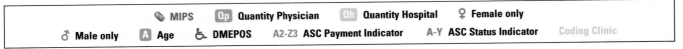

🐾 MIPS   Qp **Quantity Physician**   Qh **Quantity Hospital**   ♀ **Female only**
♂ **Male only**   A **Age**   & **DMEPOS**   A2-Z3 **ASC Payment Indicator**   A-Y **ASC Status Indicator**   Coding Clinic

⊗ **B4199** Parenteral nutrition solution; compounded amino acid and carbohydrates with electrolytes, trace elements and vitamins, including preparation, any strength, over 100 grams of protein - premix ⑧ Qp Qh   Y

IOM: 100-02, 15, 120; 100-03, 3, 180.2; 100-04, 20, 100.2.2

PEN: On Fee Schedule

⊗ **B4216** Parenteral nutrition; additives (vitamins, trace elements, heparin, electrolytes) home mix per day ⑧ Qh   Y

IOM: 100-02, 15, 120; 100-03, 3, 180.2; 100-04, 20, 100.2.2

PEN: On Fee Schedule

⊗ **B4220** Parenteral nutrition supply kit; premix, per day ⑧ Qh   Y

IOM: 100-02, 15, 120; 100-03, 3, 180.2; 100-04, 20, 100.2.2

PEN: On Fee Schedule

⊗ **B4222** Parenteral nutrition supply kit; home mix, per day ⑧ Qh   Y

IOM: 100-02, 15, 120; 100-03, 3, 180.2; 100-04, 20, 100.2.2

PEN: On Fee Schedule

⊗ **B4224** Parenteral nutrition administration kit, per day ⑧ Qh   Y

Dressings used with parenteral nutrition (covered under the prosthetic device benefit) are included in the payment. (www.cms.gov/medicare-coverage-database/)

IOM: 100-02, 15, 120; 100-03, 3, 180.2; 100-04, 20, 100.2.2

PEN: On Fee Schedule

⊗ **B5000** Parenteral nutrition solution compounded amino acid and carbohydrates with electrolytes, trace elements, and vitamins, including preparation, any strength, renal - Aminosyn-RF, NephrAmine, RenAmine - premix ⑧ Qp Qh   Y

IOM: 100-02, 15, 120; 100-03, 3, 180.2; 100-04, 20, 100.2.2

PEN: On Fee Schedule

⊗ **B5100** Parenteral nutrition solution compounded amino acid and carbohydrates with electrolytes, trace elements, and vitamins, including preparation, any strength, hepatic, HepatAmine - premix ⑧ Qp Qh   Y

IOM: 100-02, 15, 120; 100-03, 3, 180.2; 100-04, 20, 100.2.2

PEN: On Fee Schedule

⊗ **B5200** Parenteral nutrition solution compounded amino acid and carbohydrates with electrolytes, trace elements, and vitamins, including preparation, any strength, stress-branch chain amino acids-FreAmine-HBC - premix ⑧ Qp Qh   Y

IOM: 100-02, 15, 120; 100-03, 3, 180.2; 100-04, 20, 100.2.2

Enteral and Parenteral Pumps

⊗ **B9002** Enteral nutrition infusion pump, any type ⑧ Qh   Y

IOM: 100-02, 15, 120; 100-03, 3, 180.2; 100-04, 20, 100.2.2

PEN: On Fee Schedule

⊗ **B9004** Parenteral nutrition infusion pump, portable ⑧ Qh   Y

IOM: 100-02, 15, 120; 100-03, 3, 180.2; 100-04, 20, 100.2.2

PEN: On Fee Schedule

⊗ **B9006** Parenteral nutrition infusion pump, stationary ⑧ Qh   Y

IOM: 100-02, 15, 120; 100-03, 3, 180.2; 100-04, 20, 100.2.2

PEN: On Fee Schedule

⊗ **B9998** NOC for enteral supplies ⑧   Y

IOM: 100-02, 15, 120; 100-03, 3, 180.2; 100-04, 20, 100.2.2

⊗ **B9999** NOC for parenteral supplies ⑧   Y

Determine if an alternative HCPCS Level II or a CPT code better describes the service being reported. This code should be reported only if a more specific code is unavailable.

IOM: 100-02, 15, 120; 100-03, 3, 180.2; 100-04, 20, 100.2.2

CMS HOSPITAL OUTPATIENT PAYMENT SYSTEM (C1000-C9999)

NOTE: C-codes are used on Medicare Ambulatory Surgical Center (ASC) and Hospital Outpatient Prospective Payment System (OPPS) claims, but may also be recognized on claims from other providers or by other payment systems. As of 10/01/2006, the following non-OPPS providers have been able to bill Medicare using the C-codes, or an appropriate CPT code on Types of Bill (TOBs) 12X, 13X, or 85X:

- Critical Access Hospitals (CAHs);
- Indian Health Service Hospitals (IHS);
- Hospitals located in American Samoa, Guam, Saipan or the Virgin Islands; and
- Maryland waiver hospitals.

The billing of C-codes by Method I and Method II Critical Access Hospitals (CAHs) is limited to the billing for facility (technical) services. The C-codes shall not be billed by Method II CAHs for professional services with revenue codes (RCs) 96X, 97X, or 98X.

C codes are updated quarterly by the Centers for Medicare and Medicaid Services (CMS).

Devices and Supplies

- **C1052** Hemostatic agent, gastrointestinal, topical   **J7 H**
- **C1062** Intravertebral body fracture augmentation with implant (e.g., metal, polymer)   **J7 H**
- **C1713** Anchor/Screw for opposing bone-to-bone or soft tissue-to-bone (implantable) **Qh**   **N1 N**

  Medicare Statute 1833(t)

  Coding Clinic: 2022, Q4, P13; 2022, Q3, P9; 2021, Q1, P9-10; 2020, Q4, P7-8; 2018, Q2, P5; Q1, P4; 2016, Q3, P16; 2015, Q3, P2; 2010, Q2, P3

- **C1714** Catheter, transluminal atherectomy, directional **Qh**   **N1 N**

  Medicare Statute 1833(t)

- **C1715** Brachytherapy needle **Qh**   **N1 N**

  Medicare Statute 1833(t)

Brachytherapy Sources

- **C1716** Brachytherapy source, non-stranded, gold-198, per source **Qp** **Qh**   **H2 U**

  Medicare Statute 1833(t)

Figure 9 (A) Brachytherapy device, (B) Brachytherapy device inserted.

- **C1717** Brachytherapy source, non-stranded, high dose rate iridium 192, per source **Qp** **Qh**   **H2 U**

  Medicare Statute 1833(t)

- **C1719** Brachytherapy source, non-stranded, non-high dose rate iridium-192, per source **Qp** **Qh**   **H2 U**

  Medicare Statute 1833(t)

Cardioverter-Defibrilators

- **C1721** Cardioverter-defibrillator, dual chamber (implantable) **Qp** **Qh**   **N1 N**

  Related CPT codes: 33224, 33240, 33249.

  Medicare Statute 1833(t)

- **C1722** Cardioverter-defibrillator, single chamber (implantable) **Qp** **Qh**   **N1 N**

  Related CPT codes: 33240, 33249.

  Medicare Statute 1833(t)

  Coding Clinic: 2017, Q2, P5; 2006, Q2, P9

Catheters

- **C1724** Catheter, transluminal atherectomy, rotational **Qh**   **N1 N**

  Medicare Statute 1833(t)

  Coding Clinic; 2016, Q3, P9

- **C1725** Catheter, transluminal angioplasty, non-laser (may include guidance, infusion/perfusion capability) **Qh**   **N1 N**

  Medicare Statute 1833(t)

  Coding Clinic: 2016, Q3, P16, P19

- **C1726** Catheter, balloon dilatation, non-vascular **Qh**   **N1 N**

  Medicare Statute 1833(t)

  Coding Clinic: 2016, Q3, P16, P19

- **C1727** Catheter, balloon tissue dissector, non-vascular (insertable) **Qh**   **N1 N**

  Medicare Statute 1833(t)

  Coding Clinic: 2016, Q3, P16

🐾 MIPS	**Qp** Quantity Physician	**Qh** Quantity Hospital	♀ Female only
♂ Male only	**A** Age	♿ DMEPOS	A2-Z3 ASC Payment Indicator A-Y ASC Status Indicator Coding Clinic

○ **C1728** Catheter, brachytherapy seed administration [Qh] N1 N

Medicare Statute 1833(t)

○ **C1729** Catheter, drainage [Qh] N1 N

Medicare Statute 1833(t)

Coding Clinic: 2016, Q3, P17

○ **C1730** Catheter, electrophysiology, diagnostic, other than 3D mapping (19 or fewer electrodes) [Qp] [Qh] N1 N

Medicare Statute 1833(t)

Coding Clinic: 2016, Q3, P17

○ **C1731** Catheter, electrophysiology, diagnostic, other than 3D mapping (20 or more electrodes) [Qp] [Qh] N1 N

Medicare Statute 1833(t)

Coding Clinic: 2016, Q3, P17

○ **C1732** Catheter, electrophysiology, diagnostic/ablation, 3D or vector mapping [Qp] [Qh] N1 N

Medicare Statute 1833(t)

Coding Clinic: 2016, Q3, P15, P17, P19

○ **C1733** Catheter, electrophysiology, diagnostic/ablation, other than 3D or vector mapping, other than cool-tip [Qp] [Qh] N1 N

Medicare Statute 1833(t)

Coding Clinic: 2016, Q3, P17

○ **C1734** Orthopedic/device/drug matrix for opposing bone-to-bone or soft tissue-to-bone (implantable) N1

C1747 Endoscope, single-use (i.e. disposable), urinary tract, imaging/illumination device (insertable) J7 H

○ **C1748** Endoscope, single-use (i.e. disposable), upper gi, imaging/illumination device (insertable) J7 H

○ **C1749** Endoscope, retrograde imaging/ illumination colonoscope device (implantable) [Qp] [Qh] N1 N

Medicare Statute 1833(t)

○ **C1750** Catheter, hemodialysis/peritoneal, long-term [Qh] N1 N

Medicare Statute 1833(t)

Coding Clinic: 2015, Q4, P6

○ **C1751** Catheter, infusion, inserted peripherally, centrally, or midline (other than hemodialysis) [Qh] N1 N

Medicare Statute 1833(t)

○ **C1752** Catheter, hemodialysis/peritoneal, short-term [Qh] N1 N

Medicare Statute 1833(t)

○ **C1753** Catheter, intravascular ultrasound [Qh] N1 N

Medicare Statute 1833(t)

○ **C1754** Catheter, intradiscal [Qh] N1 N

Medicare Statute 1833(t)

○ **C1755** Catheter, instraspinal [Qh] N1 N

Medicare Statute 1833(t)

○ **C1756** Catheter, pacing, transesophageal [Qh] N1 N

Medicare Statute 1833(t)

○ **C1757** Catheter, thrombectomy/ embolectomy [Qh] N1 N

Medicare Statute 1833(t)

○ **C1758** Catheter, ureteral [Qh] N1 N

Medicare Statute 1833(t)

○ **C1759** Catheter, intracardiac echocardiography [Qh] N1 N

Medicare Statute 1833(t)

Devices

○ **C1760** Closure device, vascular (implantable/ insertable) [Qh] N1 N

Medicare Statute 1833(t)

Coding Clinic: 2016, Q3, P19

Figure 10 (A) Single pacemaker, (B) Dual pacemaker, (C) Biventricular pacemaker.

▶ New   ↻ Revised   ✔ Reinstated   ~~deleted~~ Deleted   ⊘ Not covered or valid by Medicare
○ Special coverage instructions   ✳ Carrier discretion   Ⓑ Bill Part B MAC   Ⓑ Bill DME MAC

⚙ **C1761** Catheter, transluminal intravascular
lithotripsy, coronary   J7

Coding Clinic: 2023, Q2, P19

⚙ **C1762** Connective tissue, human (includes
fascia lata) `Qh`   N1 N

Medicare Statute 1833(t)

Coding Clinic: 2016, Q3, P9, P16, P19; 2015, Q3, P2;
2003, Q3, P12

⚙ **C1763** Connective tissue, non-human
(includes synthetic) `Qh`   N1 N

Medicare Statute 1833(t)

Coding Clinic: 2016, Q3, P9, P17, P19; 2010, Q4, P3;
Q2, P3; 2003, Q3, P12

⚙ **C1764** Event recorder, cardiac
(implantable) `Qp` `Qh`   N1 N

Medicare Statute 1833(t)

Coding Clinic: 2015, Q2, P8

⚙ **C1765** Adhesion barrier `Qh`   N1 N

Medicare Statute 1833(t)

Coding Clinic: 2016, Q3, P16

⚙ **C1766** Introducer/sheath, guiding, intracardiac
electrophysiological, steerable, other
than peel-away `Qh`   N1 N

Medicare Statute 1833(t)

⚙ **C1767** Generator, neurostimulator
(implantable),
nonrechargeable `Qp` `Qh`   N1 N

Related CPT codes: 61885, 61886,
63685, 64590.

Medicare Statute 1833(t)

Coding Clinic: 2021, Q1, P8; 2007, Q1, P8

⚙ **C1768** Graft, vascular `Qh`   N1 N

Medicare Statute 1833(t)

⚙ **C1769** Guide wire `Qh`   N1 N

Medicare Statute 1833(t)

Coding Clinic: 2019, Q3, P10; 2016, Q3, P3;
2007, Q2, P7-8

⚙ **C1770** Imaging coil, magnetic reasonance
(insertable) `Qh`   N1 N

Medicare Statute 1833(t)

⚙ **C1771** Repair device, urinary, incontinence,
with sling graft `Qp` `Qh`   N1 N

Medicare Statute 1833(t)

Coding Clinic: 2016, Q3, P19; 2008, Q3, P7

⚙ **C1772** Infusion pump, programmable
(implantable) `Qp` `Qh`   N1 N

Medicare Statute 1833(t)

⚙ **C1773** Retrieval device, insertable (used
to retrieve fractured medical
devices) `Qh`   N1 N

Medicare Statute 1833(t)

Coding Clinic: 2016, Q3, P19

⚙ **C1776** Joint device (implantable) `Qp` `Qh` N1 N

Medicare Statute 1833(t)

Coding Clinic: 2020, Q1, P16; 2018, Q3, P6; 2016, Q3,
P3, P18; 2010, Q3, P6; 2008, Q4, P10

⚙ **C1777** Lead, cardioverter-defibrillator,
endocardial single coil
(implantable) `Qh`   N1 N

Related CPT codes: 33216, 33217, 33249.

Medicare Statute 1833(t)

Coding Clinic: 2017, Q2, P5; 2006, Q2, P9

⚙ **C1778** Lead, neurostimulator
(implantable) `Qp` `Qh`   N1 N

Related CPT codes: 43647, 63650,
63655, 63663, 63664, 64553, 64555,
64560, 64561, 64565, 64573, 64575,
64577, 64580, 64581.

Medicare Statute 1833(t)

Coding Clinic: 2022, Q4, P16; 2021, Q1, P8; 2019, Q1,
P5; 2007, Q1, P8

⚙ **C1779** Lead, pacemaker, trasvenous VDD
single pass `Qh`   N1 N

Related CPT codes: 33206, 33207,
33208, 33210, 33211, 33214, 33216,
33217, 33249.

Medicare Statute 1833(t)

Coding Clinic: 2016, Q3, P19

⚙ **C1780** Lens, intraocular (new
technology) `Qh`   N1 N

Medicare Statute 1833(t)

Coding Clinic: 2016, Q3, P18

⚙ **C1781** Mesh (implantable) `Qh`   N1 N

Medicare Statute 1833(t)

Coding Clinic: 2022, Q4, P16-17; 2019, Q1, P5; 2016,
Q3, P18-19; 2012, Q2, P3; 2010, Q2, P2-3

⚙ **C1782** Morcellator `Qp` `Qh`   N1 N

Medicare Statute 1833(t)

Coding Clinic: 2016, Q3, P18

⚙ **C1783** Ocular implant, aqueous drainage
assist device `Qh`   N1 N

Medicare Statute 1833(t)

Coding Clinic: 2017, Q1, P5

⚙ **C1784** Ocular device, intraoperative, detached
retina `Qh`   N1 N

Medicare Statute 1833(t)

Coding Clinic: 2016, Q3, P18

🐍 MIPS   `Qp` **Quantity Physician**   `Qh` **Quantity Hospital**   ♀ **Female only**

♂ **Male only**   `A` **Age**   � **DMEPOS**   A2-Z3 **ASC Payment Indicator**   A-Y **ASC Status Indicator**   Coding Clinic

⊛ **C1785** Pacemaker, dual chamber, rate-responsive (implantable) `Qp` `Qh` N1 N

Related CPT codes: 33206, 33207, 33208, 33213, 33214, 33224.

Medicare Statute 1833(t)

⊛ **C1786** Pacemaker, single chamber, rate-responsive (implantable) `Qp` `Qh` N1 N

Related CPT codes: 33206, 33207, 33212.

Medicare Statute 1833(t)

⊛ **C1787** Patient programmer, neurostimulator `Qh` N1 N

Medicare Statute 1833(t)

Coding Clinic: 2016, Q3, P19

⊛ **C1788** Port, indwelling (implantable) `Qh` N1 N

Medicare Statute 1833(t)

⊛ **C1789** Prosthesis, breast (implantable) `Qh` N1 N

Medicare Statute 1833(t)

⊛ **C1813** Prosthesis, penile, inflatable `Qp` `Qh` ♂ N1 N

Medicare Statute 1833(t)

⊛ **C1814** Retinal tamponade device, silicone oil `Qh` N1 N

Medicare Statute 1833(t)

Coding Clinic: 2016, Q3, P19; 2006, Q2, P9

⊛ **C1815** Prosthesis, urinary sphincter (implantable) `Qp` `Qh` N1 N

Medicare Statute 1833(t)

⊛ **C1816** Receiver and/or transmitter, neurostimulator (implantable) `Qh` N1 N

Medicare Statute 1833(t)

Coding Clinic: 2022, Q4, P16

⊛ **C1817** Septal defect implant system, intracardiac `Qp` `Qh` N1 N

Medicare Statute 1833(t)

Coding Clinic: 2016, Q3, P19

⊛ **C1818** Integrated keratoprosthesic `Qh` N1 N

Medicare Statute 1833(t)

Coding Clinic: 2016, Q3, P18

⊛ **C1819** Surgical tissue localization and excision device (implantable) `Qh` N1 N

Medicare Statute 1833(t)

⊛ **C1820** Generator, neurostimulator (implantable), with rechargeable battery and charging system `Qp` `Qh` N1 N

Related CPT codes: 61885, 61886, 63685, 64590.

Medicare Statute 1833(t)

Coding Clinic: 2016, Q2, P7

⊛ **C1821** Interspinous process distraction device (implantable) `Qh` N1 N

Medicare Statute 1833(t)

⊛ **C1822** Generator, neurostimulator (implantable), high frequency, with rechargeable battery and charging system `Qp` `Qh` N1 N

Medicare Statute 1833(T)

Coding Clinic: 2016, Q2, P7

⊛ **C1823** Generator, neurostimulator (implantable), non-rechargeable, with transvenous sensing and stimulation leads H

Medicare Statute 1833(t)

⊛ **C1824** Generator, cardiac contractility modulation (implantable) N1

⊛ **C1825** Generator, neurostimulator (implantable), non-rechargeable with carotid sinus baroreceptor stimulation lead(s) J7 H

⊛ **C1826** Generator, neurostimulator (implantable), includes closed feedback loop leads and all implantable components, with rechargeable battery and charging system J7 H

⊛ **C1827** Generator, neurostimulator (implantable), non-rechargeable, with implantable stimulation lead and external paired stimulation controller J7 H

⊛ **C1830** Powered bone marrow biopsy needle `Qp` `Qh` N1 N

Medicare Statute 1833(t)

⊛ **C1831** Interbody cage, anterior, lateral or posterior, personalized (implantable) J7 H

⊛ **C1832** Autograft suspension, including cell processing and application, and all system components J7 H

⊛ **C1833** Monitor, cardiac, including intracardiac lead and all system components (implantable) J7 H

~~C1834~~ ~~Pressure sensor system, includes all components (e.g., introducer, sensor), intramuscular (implantable), excludes mobile (wireless) software application~~ ~~J7~~ ~~H~~

⊛ **C1839** Iris prosthesis N1

⊛ **C1840** Lens, intraocular (telescopic) `Qp` `Qh` N1 N

Medicare Statute 1833(t)

Coding Clinic: 2012, Q3, P10

⊛ **C1874** Stent, coated/covered, with delivery system `Qh` N1 N

Medicare Statute 1833(t)

Coding Clinic: 2023, Q2, P17,19; 2016, Q3, P16-17, P19

▶ New   ↻ Revised   ✔ Reinstated   ~~deleted~~ Deleted   ⊘ Not covered or valid by Medicare

⊛ Special coverage instructions   ✳ Carrier discretion   Ⓑ Bill Part B MAC   Ⓓ Bill DME MAC

C1875 Stent, coated/covered, without delivery system `Qh` N1 N

Medicare Statute 1833(t)

Coding Clinic: 2023, Q2, P17; 2020, Q2, P9; 2016, Q3, P16-17

C1876 Stent, non-coated/non-covered, with delivery system `Qh` N1 N

Medicare Statute 1833(t)

Coding Clinic: 2016, Q3, P19

C1877 Stent, non-coated/non-covered, without delivery system `Qh` N1 N

Medicare Statute 1833(t)

C1878 Material for vocal cord medialization, synthetic (implantable) `Qh` N1 N

Medicare Statute 1833(t)

Coding Clinic: 2016, Q3, P18

C1880 Vena cava filter `Qh` N1 N

Medicare Statute 1833(t)

C1881 Dialysis access system (implantable) `Qh` N1 N

Medicare Statute 1833(t)

C1882 Cardioverter-defibrillator, other than single or dual chamber (implantable) `Qp` `Qh` N1 N

Related CPT codes: 33224, 33240, 33249.

Medicare Statute 1833(t)

Coding Clinic: 2016, Q3, P16; 2012, Q2, P9; 2006, Q2, P9

C1883 Adapter/Extension, pacing lead or neurostimulator lead (implantable) `Qh` N1 N

Medicare Statute 1833(t)

Coding Clinic: 2016, Q3, P15, P17; 2007, Q1, P8

C1884 Embolization protective system `Qh` N1 N

Medicare Statute 1833(t)

Coding Clinic: 2016, Q3, P17

C1885 Catheter, transluminal angioplasty, laser `Qh` N1 N

Medicare Statute 1833(t)

Coding Clinic: 2016, Q3, p16, Q1, P5

C1886 Catheter, extravascular tissue ablation, any modality (insertable) `Qp` `Qh` N1 N

Medicare Statute 1833(t)

C1887 Catheter, guiding (may include infusion/perfusion capability) `Qh` N1 N

Medicare Statute 1833(t)

Coding Clinic: 2016, Q3, P17

C1888 Catheter, ablation, non-cardiac, endovascular (implantable) `Qh` N1 N

Medicare Statute 1833(t)

Coding Clinic: 2016, Q3, P16

C1889 Implantable/insertable device, not otherwise classified N1 N

Medicare Statute 1833(T)

C1891 Infusion pump, non-programmable, permanent (implantable) `Qp` `Qh` N1 N

Medicare Statute 1833(t)

C1892 Introducer/sheath, guiding, intracardiac electrophysiological, fixed-curve, peel-away `Qh` N1 N

Medicare Statute 1833(t)

Coding Clinic: 2016, Q3, P19

C1893 Introducer/sheath, guiding, intracardiac electrophysiological, fixed-curve, other than peel-away `Qh` N1 N

Medicare Statute 1833(t)

C1894 Introducer/sheath, other than guiding, other than intracardiac electrophysiological, non-laser `Qh` N1 N

Medicare Statute 1833(t)

C1895 Lead, cardioverter-defibrillator, endocardial dual coil (implantable) `Qh` N1 N

Related CPT codes: 33216, 33217, 33249.

Medicare Statute 1833(t)

Coding Clinic: 2006, Q2, P9

C1896 Lead, cardioverter-defibrillator, other than endocardial single or dual coil (implantable) `Qh` N1 N

Related CPT codes: 33216, 33217, 33249.

Medicare Statute 1833(t)

C1897 Lead, neurostimulator test kit (implantable) `Qh` N1 N

Related CPT codes: 43647, 63650, 63655, 63663, 63664, 64553, 64555, 64560, 64561, 64565, 64575, 64577, 64580, 64581.

Medicare Statute 1833(t)

Coding Clinic: 2007, Q1, P8

C1898 Lead, pacemaker, other than transvenous VDD single pass `Qh` N1 N

Related CPT codes: 33206, 33207, 33208, 33210, 33211, 33214, 33216, 33217, 33249.

Medicare Statute 1833(t)

Coding Clinic: 2002, Q3, P8

🐾 MIPS `Qp` Quantity Physician `Qh` Quantity Hospital ♀ Female only
♂ Male only `A` Age ♿ DMEPOS A2-Z3 ASC Payment Indicator A-Y ASC Status Indicator Coding Clinic

CMS HOSPITAL OUTPATIENT PAYMENT SYSTEM C1875 — C1898

151

⊛ **C1899** Lead, pacemaker/cardioverter-defibrillator combination (implantable) Qh   N1 N

Related CPT codes: 33216, 33217, 33249.

Medicare Statute 1833(t)

⊛ **C1900** Lead, left ventricular coronary venous system Qp Qh   N1 N

Related CPT codes: 33224, 33225.

Medicare Statute 1833(t)

Coding Clinic: 2016, Q3, P18

⊛ **C1982** Catheter, pressure-generating, one-way valve, intermittently occlusive   N1

⊛ **C2596** Probe, image-guided, robotic, waterjet ablation   N1 H

⊛ **C2613** Lung biopsy plug with delivery system Qp Qh   N1 H

Medicare Statute 1833(t)

Coding Clinic: 2015, Q2, P11

⊛ **C2614** Probe, percutaneous lumbar discectomy Qh   N1 N

Medicare Statute 1833(t)

⊛ **C2615** Sealant, pulmonary, liquid Qh   N1 N

Medicare Statute 1833(t)

Coding Clinic: 2016, Q3, P18

Brachytherapy Source

⊛ **C2616** Brachytherapy source, non-stranded, yttrium-90, per source Qp Qh   H2 U

Medicare Statute 1833(t)

Cardiovascular and Genitourinary Devices

⊛ **C2617** Stent, non-coronary, temporary, without delivery system Qh   N1 N

Medicare Statute 1833(t)

Coding Clinic: 2018, Q1, P4; 2016, Q3, P3, P19

⊛ **C2618** Probe/needle, cryoablation Qh   N1 N

Medicare Statute 1833(t)

⊛ **C2619** Pacemaker, dual chamber, non rate-responsive (implantable) Qp Qh   N1 N

Related CPT codes: 33206, 33207, 33208, 33213, 33214, 33224.

Medicare Statute 1833(t)

⊛ **C2620** Pacemaker, single chamber, non rate-responsive (implantable) Qp Qh   N1 N

Related CPT codes: 33206, 33207, 33212, 33224.

Medicare Statute 1833(t)

⊛ **C2621** Pacemaker, other than single or dual chamber (implantable) Qp Qh   N1 N

Related CPT codes: 33206, 33207, 33208, 33212, 33213, 33214, 33224.

Medicare Statute 1833(t)

Coding Clinic: 2016, Q3, P18; 2002, Q3, P8

⊛ **C2622** Prosthesis, penile, non-inflatable Qp Qh ♂   N1 N

Medicare Statute 1833(t)

⊛ **C2623** Catheter, transluminal angioplasty, drug-coated, non-laser Qp Qh   N1 N

Medicare Statute 1833(t)

⊛ **C2624** Implantable wireless pulmonary artery pressure sensor with delivery catheter, including all system components Qp Qh   N1 N

Medicare Statute 1833(t)

Coding Clinic: 2015, Q3, P2

⊛ **C2625** Stent, non-coronary, temporary, with delivery system Qh   N1 N

Medicare Statute 1833(t)

Coding Clinic: 2016, Q3, P19; 2015, Q2, P9

⊛ **C2626** Infusion pump, non-programmable, temporary (implantable) Qp Qh   N1 N

Medicare Statute 1833(t)

Coding Clinic: 2016, Q3, P18

⊛ **C2627** Catheter, suprapubic/cystoscopic Qh   N1 N

Medicare Statute 1833(t)

⊛ **C2628** Catheter, occlusion Qh   N1 N

Medicare Statute 1833(t)

⊛ **C2629** Introducer/Sheath, other than guiding, other than intracardiac electrophysiological, laser Qh   N1 N

Medicare Statute 1833(t)

⊛ **C2630** Catheter, electrophysiology, diagnostic/ablation, other than 3D or vector mapping, cool-tip Qp Qh   N1 N

Medicare Statute 1833(t)

Coding Clinic: 2016, Q3, P17

⊛ **C2631** Repair device, urinary, incontinence, without sling graft Qp Qh   N1 N

Medicare Statute 1833(t)

▶ **New**   ⟳ **Revised**   ✔ **Reinstated**   ~~deleted~~ **Deleted**   ⊘ **Not covered or valid by Medicare**
⊛ **Special coverage instructions**   ✳ **Carrier discretion**   Ⓑ **Bill Part B MAC**   Ⓓ **Bill DME MAC**

Brachytherapy Sources

⊙ **C2634** Brachytherapy source, non-stranded, high activity, iodine-125, greater than 1.01 mci (NIST), per source `Qp` `Qh`　　　H2 U

Medicare Statute 1833(t)

⊙ **C2635** Brachytherapy source, non-stranded, high activity, palladium-103, greater than 2.2 mci (NIST), per source `Qp` `Qh`　　　H2 U

Medicare Statute 1833(t)

⊙ **C2636** Brachytherapy linear source, non-stranded, palladium-103, per 1 mm `Qp` `Qh`　　　H2 U

⊙ **C2637** Brachytherapy source, non-stranded, Ytterbium-169, per source `Qp` `Qh`　　　B

Medicare Statute 1833(t)

⊙ **C2638** Brachytherapy source, stranded, iodine-125, per source `Qp` `Qh`　　　H2 U

Medicare Statute 1833(t)(2)

⊙ **C2639** Brachytherapy source, non-stranded, iodine-125, per source `Qp` `Qh`　　　H2 U

Medicare Statute 1833(t)(2)

⊙ **C2640** Brachytherapy source, stranded, palladium-103, per source `Qp` `Qh` H2 U

Medicare Statute 1833(t)(2)

⊙ **C2641** Brachytherapy source, non-stranded, palladium-103, per source `Qp` `Qh` H2 U

Medicare Statute 1833(t)(2)

⊙ **C2642** Brachytherapy source, stranded, cesium-131, per source `Qp` `Qh`　　　H2 U

Medicare Statute 1833(t)(2)

⊙ **C2643** Brachytherapy source, non-stranded, cesium-131, per source `Qp` `Qh`　　　H2 U

Medicare Statute 1833(t)(2)

⊙ **C2644** Brachytherapy source, Cesium-131 chloride solution, per millicurie `Qp` `Qh`　　　H2 U

Medicare Statute 1833(t)

⊙ **C2645** Brachytherapy planar source, palladium-103, per square millimeter `Qp` `Qh`　　　H2 U

Medicare Statute 1833(T)

⊙ **C2698** Brachytherapy source, stranded, not otherwise specified, per source　　　H2 U

Medicare Statute 1833(t)(2)

⊙ **C2699** Brachytherapy source, non-stranded, not otherwise specified, per source H2 U

Medicare Statute 1833(t)(2)

Skin Substitute Graft Application

⊙ **C5271** Application of low cost skin substitute graft to trunk, arms, legs, total wound surface area up to 100 sq cm; first 25 sq cm or less wound surface area `Qp` `Qh`　　　T

Medicare Statute 1833(t)

⊙ **C5272** Application of low cost skin substitute graft to trunk, arms, legs, total wound surface area up to 100 sq cm; each additional 25 sq cm wound surface area, or part thereof (list separately in addition to code for primary procedure) `Qp` `Qh`　　　N

Medicare Statute 1833(t)

⊙ **C5273** Application of low cost skin substitute graft to trunk, arms, legs, total wound surface area greater than or equal to 100 sq cm; first 100 sq cm wound surface area, or 1% of body area of infants and children `Qp` `Qh` `A`　　　T

Medicare Statute 1833(t)

⊙ **C5274** Application of low cost skin substitute graft to trunk, arms, legs, total wound surface area greater than or equal to 100 sq cm; each additional 100 sq cm wound surface area, or part thereof, or each additional 1% of body area of infants and children, or part thereof (list separately in addition to code for primary procedure) `Qp` `Qh` `A`　　　N

Medicare Statute 1833(t)

⊙ **C5275** Application of low cost skin substitute graft to face, scalp, eyelids, mouth, neck, ears, orbits, genitalia, hands, feet, and/or multiple digits, total wound surface area up to 100 sq cm; first 25 sq cm or less wound surface area `Qp` `Qh`　　　T

Medicare Statute 1833(t)

⊙ **C5276** Application of low cost skin substitute graft to face, scalp, eyelids, mouth, neck, ears, orbits, genitalia, hands, feet, and/or multiple digits, total wound surface area up to 100 sq cm; each additional 25 sq cm wound surface area, or part thereof (list separately in addition to code for primary procedure) `Qp` `Qh`　　　N

Medicare Statute 1833(t)

⊙ **C5277** Application of low cost skin substitute graft to face, scalp, eyelids, mouth, neck, ears, orbits, genitalia, hands, feet, and/or multiple digits, total wound surface area greater than or equal to 100 sq cm; first 100 sq cm wound surface area, or 1% of body area of infants and children `Qp` `Qh` `A`　　　T

Medicare Statute 1833(t)

⊚ **C5278** Application of low cost skin substitute graft to face, scalp, eyelids, mouth, neck, ears, orbits, genitalia, hands, feet, and/or multiple digits, total wound surface area greater than or equal to 100 sq cm; each additional 100 sq cm wound surface area, or part thereof, or each additional 1% of body area of infants and children, or part thereof (list separately in addition to code for primary procedure) **Qp Qh A**   N

Medicare Statute 1833(t)

C7500 Debridement, bone including epidermis, dermis, subcutaneous tissue, muscle and/or fascia, if performed, first 20 sq cm or less with manual preparation and insertion of deep (eg, subfacial) drug-delivery device(s) ⑧   E1

C7501 Percutaneous breast biopsies using stereotactic guidance, with placement of breast localization device(s) (eg, clip, metallic pellet), when performed, and imaging of the biopsy specimen, when performed, all lesions unilateral and bilateral (for single lesion biopsy, use appropriate code) ⑧   E1

C7502 Percutaneous breast biopsies using magnetic resonance guidance, with placement of breast localization device(s) (eg, clip, metallic pellet), when performed, and imaging of the biopsy specimen, when performed, all lesions unilateral or bilateral (for single lesion biopsy, use appropriate code) ⑧   E1

C7503 Open biopsy or excision of deep cervical node(s) with intraoperative identification (eg, mapping) of sentinel lymph node(s) including injection of non-radioactive dye when performed ⑧   E1

C7504 Percutaneous vertebroplasties (bone biopsies included when performed), first cervicothoracic and any additional cervicothoracic or lumbosacral vertebral bodies, unilateral or bilateral injection, inclusive of all imaging guidance ⑧   E1

C7505 Percutaneous vertebroplasties (bone biopsies included when performed), first lumbosacral and any additional cervicothoracic or lumbosacral vertebral bodies, unilateral or bilateral injection, inclusive of all imaging guidance ⑧   E1

C7506 Arthrodesis, interphalangeal joints, with or without internal fixation ⑧   E1

C7507 Percutaneous vertebral augmentations, first thoracic and any additional thoracic or lumbar vertebral bodies, including cavity creations (fracture reductions and bone biopsies included when performed) using mechanical device (eg, kyphoplasty), unilateral or bilateral cannulations, inclusive of all imaging guidance ⑧   E1

C7508 Percutaneous vertebral augmentations, first lumbar and any additional thoracic or lumbar vertebral bodies, including cavity creations (fracture reductions and bone biopsies included when performed) using mechanical device (eg, kyphoplasty), unilateral or bilateral cannulations, inclusive of all imaging guidance ⑧   E1

C7509 Bronchoscopy, rigid or flexible, diagnostic with cell washing(s) when performed, with computer-assisted image-guided navigation, including fluoroscopic guidance when performed ⑧   E1

C7510 Bronchoscopy, rigid or flexible, with bronchial alveolar lavage(s), with computer-assisted image-guided navigation, including fluoroscopic guidance when performed ⑧   E1

C7511 Bronchoscopy, rigid or flexible, with single or multiple bronchial or endobronchial biopsy(ies), single or multiple sites, with computer-assisted image-guided navigation, including fluoroscopic guidance when performed ⑧   E1

C7512 Bronchoscopy, rigid or flexible, with single or multiple bronchial or endobronchial biopsy(ies), single or multiple sites, with transendoscopic endobronchial ultrasound (EBUS) during bronchoscopic diagnostic or therapeutic intervention(s) for peripheral lesion(s), including fluoroscopic guidance when performed ⑧   E1

▶ **New**   ⟲ **Revised**   ✔ **Reinstated**   ~~deleted~~ **Deleted**   ⊘ **Not covered or valid by Medicare**
⊛ **Special coverage instructions**   ✳ **Carrier discretion**   ⑧ **Bill Part B MAC**   ⑥ **Bill DME MAC**

C7513 Dialysis circuit, introduction of needle(s) and/or catheter(s), with diagnostic angiography of the dialysis circuit, including all direct puncture(s) and catheter placement(s), injection(s) of contrast, all necessary imaging from the arterial anastomosis and adjacent artery through entire venous outflow including the inferior or superior vena cava, fluoroscopic guidance, with transluminal balloon angioplasty of central dialysis segment, performed through dialysis circuit, including all required imaging, radiological supervision and interpretation, image documentation and report ⒷⒼ   E1

C7514 Dialysis circuit, introduction of needle(s) and/or catheter(s), with diagnostic angiography of the dialysis circuit, including all direct puncture(s) and catheter placement(s), injection(s) of contrast, all necessary imaging from the arterial anastomosis and adjacent artery through entire venous outflow including the inferior or superior vena cava, fluoroscopic guidance, with all angioplasty in the central dialysis segment, and transcatheter placement of intravascular stent(s), central dialysis segment, performed through dialysis circuit, including all required imaging, radiological supervision and interpretation, image documentation and report ⒷⒼ   E1

C7515 Dialysis circuit, introduction of needle(s) and/or catheter(s), with diagnostic angiography of the dialysis circuit, including all direct puncture(s) and catheter placement(s), injection(s) of contrast, all necessary imaging from the arterial anastomosis and adjacent artery through entire venous outflow including the inferior or superior vena cava, fluoroscopic guidance, with dialysis circuit permanent endovascular embolization or occlusion of main circuit or any accessory veins, including all required imaging, radiological supervision and interpretation, image documentation and report ⒷⒼ   E1

C7516 Catheter placement in coronary artery(s) for coronary angiography, including intraprocedural injection(s) for coronary angiography, with endoluminal imaging of initial coronary vessel or graft using intravascular ultrasound (IVUS) or optical coherence tomography (OCT) during diagnostic evaluation and/or therapeutic intervention including imaging supervision, interpretation and report ⒷⒼ   E1

C7517 Catheter placement in coronary artery(s) for coronary angiography, including intraprocedural injection(s) for coronary angiography, with iliac and/or femoral artery angiography, non-selective, bilateral or ipsilateral to catheter insertion, performed at the same time as cardiac catheterization and/or coronary angiography, includes positioning or placement of the catheter in the distal aorta or ipsilateral femoral or iliac artery, injection of dye, production of permanent images, and radiologic supervision and interpretation ⒷⒼ   E1

C7518 Catheter placement in coronary artery(ies) for coronary angiography, including intraprocedural injection(s) for coronary angiography, imaging supervision and interpretation, with catheter placement(s) in bypass graft(s) (internal mammary, free arterial, venous grafts) including intraprocedural injection(s) for bypass graft angiography with endoluminal imaging of initial coronary vessel or graft using intravascular ultrasound (IVUS) or optical coherence tomography (OCT) during diagnostic evaluation and/or therapeutic intervention including imaging, supervision, interpretation and report ⒷⒼ   E1

C7519 Catheter placement in coronary artery(ies) for coronary angiography, including intraprocedural injection(s) for coronary angiography, imaging supervision and interpretation, with catheter placement(s) in bypass graft(s) (internal mammary, free arterial, venous grafts) including intraprocedural injection(s) for bypass graft angiography with intravascular doppler velocity and/or pressure derived coronary flow reserve measurement (initial coronary vessel or graft) during coronary angiography including pharmacologically induced stress ⒷⒼ   E1

🔊 MIPS	Ⓠⓟ Quantity Physician	Ⓠⓗ Quantity Hospital	♀ Female only
♂ Male only	Ⓐ Age	♿ DMEPOS A2-Z3 ASC Payment Indicator	A-Y ASC Status Indicator Coding Clinic

CMS HOSPITAL OUTPATIENT PAYMENT SYSTEM   C7513 — C7519

155

C7520 Catheter placement in coronary artery(ies) for coronary angiography, including intraprocedural injection(s) for coronary angiography, imaging supervision and interpretation, with catheter placement(s) in bypass graft(s) (internal mammary, free arterial, venous grafts) includes intraprocedural injection(s) for bypass graft angiography with iliac and/or femoral artery angiography, non-selective, bilateral or ipsilateral to catheter insertion, performed at the same time as cardiac catheterization and/or coronary angiography, includes positioning or placement of the catheter in the distal aorta or ipsilateral femoral or iliac artery, injection of dye, production of permanent images, and radiologic supervision and interpretation Ⓑ   E1

C7521 Catheter placement in coronary artery(ies) for coronary angiography, including intraprocedural injection(s) for coronary angiography with right heart catheterization with endoluminal imaging of initial coronary vessel or graft using intravascular ultrasound (IVUS) or optical coherence tomography (OCT) during diagnostic evaluation and/or therapeutic intervention including imaging supervision, interpretation and report Ⓑ   E1

C7522 Catheter placement in coronary artery(ies) for coronary angiography, including intraprocedural injection(s) for coronary angiography, imaging supervision and interpretation with right heart catheterization, with intravascular doppler velocity and/or pressure derived coronary flow reserve measurement (initial coronary vessel or graft) during coronary angiography including pharmacologically induced stress Ⓑ   E1

C7523 Catheter placement in coronary artery(ies) for coronary angiography, including intraprocedural injection(s) for coronary angiography, imaging supervision and interpretation, with left heart catheterization including intraprocedural injection(s) for left ventriculography, when performed, with endoluminal imaging of initial coronary vessel or graft using intravascular ultrasound (IVUS) or optical coherence tomography (OCT) during diagnostic evaluation and/or therapeutic intervention including imaging supervision, interpretation and report Ⓑ   E1

C7524 Catheter placement in coronary artery(ies) for coronary angiography, including intraprocedural injection(s) for coronary angiography, imaging supervision and interpretation, with left heart catheterization including intraprocedural injection(s) for left ventriculography, when performed, with intravascular doppler velocity and/or pressure derived coronary flow reserve measurement (initial coronary vessel or graft) during coronary angiography including pharmacologically induced stress Ⓑ E1

C7525 Catheter placement in coronary artery(ies) for coronary angiography, including intraprocedural injection(s) for coronary angiography, imaging supervision and interpretation, with left heart catheterization including intraprocedural injection(s) for left ventriculography, when performed, catheter placement(s) in bypass graft(s) (internal mammary, free arterial, venous grafts) with bypass graft angiography with endoluminal imaging of initial coronary vessel or graft using intravascular ultrasound (IVUS) or optical coherence tomography (OCT) during diagnostic evaluation and/or therapeutic intervention including imaging supervision, interpretation and report Ⓑ   E1

▶ New   ↻ Revised   ✔ Reinstated   deleted Deleted   ⊘ Not covered or valid by Medicare

✵ Special coverage instructions   ✳ Carrier discretion   Ⓑ Bill Part B MAC   Ⓑ Bill DME MAC

C7526 Catheter placement in coronary artery(ies) for coronary angiography, including intraprocedural injection(s) for coronary angiography, imaging supervision and interpretation, with left heart catheterization including intraprocedural injection(s) for left ventriculography, when performed, catheter placement(s) in bypass graft(s) (internal mammary, free arterial, venous grafts) with bypass graft angiography with intravascular doppler velocity and/or pressure derived coronary flow reserve measurement (initial coronary vessel or graft) during coronary angiography including pharmacologically induced stress ⑧ E1

C7527 Catheter placement in coronary artery(ies) for coronary angiography, including intraprocedural injection(s) for coronary angiography, imaging supervision and interpretation, with right and left heart catheterization including intraprocedural injection(s) for left ventriculography, when performed, with endoluminal imaging of initial coronary vessel or graft using intravascular ultrasound (IVUS) or optical coherence tomography (OCT) during diagnostic evaluation and/or therapeutic intervention including imaging supervision, interpretation and report ⑧ E1

C7528 Catheter placement in coronary artery(ies) for coronary angiography, including intraprocedural injection(s) for coronary angiography, imaging supervision and interpretation, with right and left heart catheterization including intraprocedural injection(s) for left ventriculography, when performed, with intravascular doppler velocity and/or pressure derived coronary flow reserve measurement (initial coronary vessel or graft) during coronary angiography including pharmacologically induced stress ⑧ E1

C7529 Catheter placement in coronary artery(ies) for coronary angiography, including intraprocedural injection(s) for coronary angiography, imaging supervision and interpretation, with right and left heart catheterization including intraprocedural injection(s) for left ventriculography, when performed, catheter placement(s) in bypass graft(s) (internal mammary, free arterial, venous grafts) with bypass graft angiography with intravascular doppler velocity and/or pressure derived coronary flow reserve measurement (initial coronary vessel or graft) during coronary angiography including pharmacologically induced stress ⑧ E1

C7530 Dialysis circuit, introduction of needle(s) and/or catheter(s), with diagnostic angiography of the dialysis circuit, including all direct puncture(s) and catheter placement(s), injection(s) of contrast, all necessary imaging from the arterial anastomosis and adjacent artery through entire venous outflow including the inferior or superior vena cava, fluoroscopic guidance, with transluminal balloon angioplasty, peripheral dialysis segment, including all imaging and radiological supervision and interpretation necessary to perform the angioplasty and all angioplasty in the central dialysis segment, with transcatheter placement of intravascular stent(s), central dialysis segment, performed through dialysis circuit, including all imaging, radiological supervision and interpretation, documentation and report ⑧ E1

C7531 Revascularization, endovascular, open or percutaneous, femoral, popliteal artery(ies), unilateral, with transluminal angioplasty with intravascular ultrasound (initial noncoronary vessel) during diagnostic evaluation and/or therapeutic intervention, including radiological supervision and interpretation ⑧ E1

C7532 Transluminal balloon angioplasty (except lower extremity artery(ies) for occlusive disease, intracranial, coronary, pulmonary, or dialysis circuit), initial artery, open or percutaneous, including all imaging and radiological supervision and interpretation necessary to perform the angioplasty within the same artery, with intravascular ultrasound (initial noncoronary vessel) during diagnostic evaluation and/or therapeutic intervention, including radiological supervision and interpretation Ⓑ   E1

C7533 Percutaneous transluminal coronary angioplasty, single major coronary artery or branch with transcatheter placement of radiation delivery device for subsequent coronary intravascular brachytherapy Ⓑ   E1

C7534 Revascularization, endovascular, open or percutaneous, femoral, popliteal artery(ies), unilateral, with atherectomy, includes angioplasty within the same vessel, when performed with intravascular ultrasound (initial noncoronary vessel) during diagnostic evaluation and/or therapeutic intervention, including radiological supervision and interpretation Ⓑ   E1

C7535 Revascularization, endovascular, open or percutaneous, femoral, popliteal artery(ies), unilateral, with transluminal stent placement(s), includes angioplasty within the same vessel, when performed, with intravascular ultrasound (initial noncoronary vessel) during diagnostic evaluation and/or therapeutic intervention, including radiological supervision and interpretation Ⓑ   E1

C7537 Insertion of new or replacement of permanent pacemaker with atrial transvenous electrode(s), with insertion of pacing electrode, cardiac venous system, for left ventricular pacing, at time of insertion of implantable debribrillator or pacemake pulse generator (eg, for upgrade to dual chamber system) Ⓑ   E1

C7538 Insertion of new or replacement of permanent pacemaker with ventricular transvenous electrode(s), with insertion of pacing electrode, cardiac venous system, for left ventricular pacing, at time of insertion of implantable defibrillator or pacemaker pulse generator (eg, for upgrade to dual chamber system) Ⓑ   E1

C7539 Insertion of new or replacement of permanent pacemaker with atrial and ventricular transvenous electrode(s), with insertion of pacing electrode, cardiac venous system, for left ventricular pacing, at time of insertion of implantable defibrillator or pacemaker pulse generator (eg, for upgrade to dual chamber system) Ⓑ   E1

C7540 Removal of permanent pacemaker pulse generator with replacement of pacemaker pulse generator, dual lead system, with insertion of pacing electrode, cardiac venous system, for left ventricular pacing, at time of insertion of implantable defibrillator or pacemaker pulse generator (eg, for upgrade to dual chamber system) Ⓑ   E1

C7541 Diagnostic endoscopic retrograde cholangiopancreatography (ERCP), including collection of specimen(s) by brushing or washing, when performed, with endoscopic cannulation of papilla with direct visualization of pancreatic/common bile ducts(s) Ⓑ   E1

C7542 Endoscopic retrograde cholangiopancreatography (ercp) with biopsy, single or multiple, with endoscopic cannulation of papilla with direct visualization of pancreatic/common bile ducts(s) Ⓑ   E1

C7543 Endoscopic retrograde cholangiopancreatography (ERCP) with sphincterotomy/papillotomy, with endoscopic cannulation of papilla with direct visualization of pancreatic/common bile ducts(s) Ⓑ   E1

C7544 Endoscopic retrograde cholangiopancreatography (ERCP) with removal of calculi/debris from biliary/pancreatic duct(s), with endoscopic cannulation of papilla with direct visualization of pancreatic/common bile ducts(s) Ⓑ   E1

C7545 Percutaneous exchange of biliary drainage catheter (eg, external, internal-external, or conversion of internal-external to external only), with removal of calculi/debris from biliary duct(s) and/or gallbladder, including destruction of calculi by any method (eg, mechanical, electrohydraulic, lithotripsy) when performed, including diagnostic cholangiography(ies) when performed, imaging guidance (eg, fluoroscopy), and all associated radiological supervision and interpretation Ⓑ   E1

▶ **New**   ⟳ **Revised**   ✔ **Reinstated**   ~~deleted~~ **Deleted**   ⊘ **Not covered or valid by Medicare**

⊛ **Special coverage instructions**   ✳ **Carrier discretion**   Ⓑ **Bill Part B MAC**   Ⓓ **Bill DME MAC**

C7546 Removal and replacement of externally accessible nephroureteral catheter (eg, external/internal stent) requiring fluoroscopic guidance, with ureteral stricture balloon dilation, including imaging guidance and all associated radiological supervision and interpretation ⑬ E1

C7547 Convert nephrostomy catheter to nephroureteral catheter, percutaneous via pre-existing nephrostomy tract, with ureteral stricture balloon dialation, including diagnostic nephrostogram and/or ureterogram when performed, imaging guidance (eg, ultrasound and/or fluoroscopy) and all associated radiological supervision and interpretation ⑬ E1

C7548 Exchange nephrostomy catheter, percutaneous, with ureteral stricture balloon dilation, including diagnostic nephrostogram and/or ureterogram when performed, imaging guidance (eg, ultrasound and/or fluoroscopy) and all associated radiological supervision and interpretation ⑬ E1

C7549 Change of ureterostomy tube or externally accessible ureteral stent via ileal conduit with ureteral stricture balloon dilation, including imaging guidance (eg, ultrasound and/or fluoroscopy) and all associated radiological supervision and interpretation ⑬ E1

C7550 Cystourethroscopy, with biopsy(ies) with adjuctive blue light cystoscopy with fluorescent imaging agent ⑬ E1

C7551 Excision of major peripheral nerve neuroma, except sciatic, with implantation of nerve end into bone or muscle ⑬ E1

C7552 Catheter placement in coronary artery(s) for coronary angiography, including intraprocedural injection(s) for coronary angiography, imaging supervision and interpretation; with catheter placement(s) in bypass graft(s) (internal mammary, free arterial, venous grafts) including intraprocedural injection(s) for bypass graft angiography and right heart catheterization with intravascular doppler velocity and/or pressure derived coronary flow reserve measurement (coronary vessel or graft) during coronary angiography including pharmacologically induced stress, initial vessel ⑬ E1

C7553 Catheter placement in coronary artery(s) for coronary angiography, including intraprocedural injection(s) for coronary angiography, imaging supervision and interpretation; with right and left heart catheterization including intraprocedural injection(s) for left ventriculography, when performed, catheter placement(s) in bypass graft(s) (internal mammary, free arterial, venous grafts) with bypass graft angiography with pharmacologic agent administration (eg, inhaled nitric oxide, intravenous infusion of nitroprusside, dobutamine, milrinone, or other agent) including assessing hemodynamic measurements before, during, after and repeat pharmacologic agent administration, when performed ⑬ E1

C7554 Cystourethroscopy with adjunctive blue light cystoscopy with fluorescent imaging agent ⑬ E1

C7555 Thyroidectomy, total or complete with parathyroid autotransplantation ⑬ E1

C7900 Service for diagnosis, evaluation, or treatment of a mental health or substance use disorder, initial 15-29 minutes, provided remotely by hospital staff who are licensed to provide mental health services under applicable state law(s), when the patient is in their home, and there is no associated professional service ⑬ S

C7901 Service for diagnosis, evaluation, or treatment of a mental health or substance use disorder, initial 30-60 minutes, provided remotely by hospital staff who are licensed to provided mental health services under applicable state law(s), when the patient is in their home, and there is no associated professional service ⑬ S

C7902 Service for diagnosis, evaluation, or treatment of a mental health or substance use disorder, each additional 15 minutes, provided remotely by hospital staff who are licensed to provide mental health services under applicable state law(s), when the patient is in their home, and there is no associated professional service (list separately in addition to code for primary service) ⑬ N

🖐 MIPS   Qp Quantity Physician   Qh Quantity Hospital   ♀ Female only
♂ Male only   A Age   & DMEPOS   A2-Z3 ASC Payment Indicator   A-Y ASC Status Indicator   Coding Clinic

Magnetic Resonance Angiography: Trunk and Lower Extremities

⊛ **C8900**   Magnetic resonance angiography with contrast, abdomen **Qp** **Qh**   Z2 Q3

Medicare Statute 1833(t)(2)

⊛ **C8901**   Magnetic resonance angiography without contrast, abdomen **Qp** **Qh**   Z2 Q3

Medicare Statute 1833(t)(2)

⊛ **C8902**   Magnetic resonance angiography without contrast followed by with contrast, abdomen **Qp** **Qh**   Z2 Q3

Medicare Statute 1833(t)(2)

⊛ **C8903**   Magnetic resonance imaging with contrast, breast; unilateral **Qp** **Qh** Z2 Q3

Medicare Statute 1833(t)(2)

⊛ **C8905**   Magnetic resonance imaging without contrast followed by with contrast, breast; unilateral **Qp** **Qh**   Z2 Q3

Medicare Statute 1833(t)(2)

⊛ **C8906**   Magnetic resonance imaging with contrast, breast; bilateral **Qp** **Qh** Z2 Q3

Medicare Statute 1833(t)(2)

⊛ **C8908**   Magnetic resonance imaging without contrast followed by with contrast, breast; bilateral **Qp** **Qh**   Z2 Q3

Medicare Statute 1833(t)(2)

⊛ **C8909**   Magnetic resonance angiography with contrast, chest (excluding myocardium) **Qp** **Qh**   Z2 Q3

Medicare Statute 1833(t)(2)

⊛ **C8910**   Magnetic resonance angiography without contrast, chest (excluding myocardium) **Qp** **Qh**   Z2 Q3

Medicare Statute 1833(t)(2)

⊛ **C8911**   Magnetic resonance angiography without contrast followed by with contrast, chest (excluding myocardium) **Qp** **Qh**   Z2 Q3

Medicare Statute 1833(t)(2)

⊛ **C8912**   Magnetic resonance angiography with contrast, lower extremity **Qp** **Qh**   Z2 Q3

Medicare Statute 1833(t)(2)

⊛ **C8913**   Magnetic resonance angiography without contrast, lower extremity **Qp** **Qh**   Z2 Q3

Medicare Statute 1833(t)(2)

⊛ **C8914**   Magnetic resonance angiography without contrast followed by with contrast, lower extremity **Qp** **Qh**   Z2 Q3

Medicare Statute 1833(t)(2)

⊛ **C8918**   Magnetic resonance angiography with contrast, pelvis **Qp** **Qh**   Z2 Q3

Medicare Statute 1833(t)(2)

⊛ **C8919**   Magnetic resonance angiography without contrast, pelvis **Qp** **Qh**   Z2 Q3

Medicare Statute 1833(t)(2)

⊛ **C8920**   Magnetic resonance angiography without contrast followed by with contrast, pelvis **Qp** **Qh**   Z2 Q3

Medicare Statute 1833(t)(2)

Transthoracic and Transesophageal Echocardiography

⊛ **C8921**   Transthoracic echocardiography with contrast, or without contrast followed by with contrast, for congenital cardiac anomalies; complete **Qp** **Qh**   S

Medicare Statute 1833(t)(2)

Coding Clinic: 2012, Q3, P8

⊛ **C8922**   Transthoracic echocardiography with contrast, or without contrast followed by with contrast, for congenital cardiac anomalies; follow-up or limited study **Qp** **Qh**   S

Medicare Statute 1833(t)(2)

Coding Clinic: 2012, Q3, P8

⊛ **C8923**   Transthoracic echocardiography with contrast, or without contrast followed by with contrast, real-time with image documentation (2D), includes M-mode recording, when performed, complete, without spectral or color Doppler echocardiography **Qp** **Qh**   S

Medicare Statute 1833(t)(2)

Coding Clinic: 2012, Q3, P8

⊛ **C8924**   Transthoracic echocardiography with contrast, or without contrast followed by with contrast, real-time with image documentation (2D), includes M-mode recording, when performed, follow-up or limited study **Qp** **Qh**   S

Medicare Statute 1833(t)(2)

Coding Clinic: 2012, Q3, P8

⊛ **C8925**   Transesophageal echocardiography (TEE) with contrast, or without contrast followed by with contrast, real time with image documentation (2D) (with or without M-mode recording); including probe placement, image acquisition, interpretation and report **Qp** **Qh**   S

Medicare Statute 1833(t)(2)

Coding Clinic: 2012, Q3, P8

▶ New   ↻ Revised   ✓ Reinstated   ~~deleted~~ Deleted   ⊘ Not covered or valid by Medicare
⊛ Special coverage instructions   ✳ Carrier discretion   Ⓑ Bill Part B MAC   Ⓑ Bill DME MAC

⊘ **C8926** Transesophageal echocardiography (TEE) with contrast, or without contrast followed by with contrast, for congenital cardiac anomalies; including probe placement, image acquisition, interpretation and report `Qp` `Qh` S

Medicare Statute 1833(t)(2)

Coding Clinic: 2012, Q3, P8

⊘ **C8927** Transesophageal echocardiography (TEE) with contrast, or without contrast followed by with contrast, for monitoring purposes, including probe placement, real time 2-dimensional image acquisition and interpretation leading to ongoing (continuous) assessment of (dynamically changing) cardiac pumping function and to therapeutic measures on an immediate time basis `Qp` `Qh` S

Medicare Statute 1833(t)(2)

Coding Clinic: 2012, Q3, P8

⊘ **C8928** Transthoracic echocardiography with contrast, or without contrast followed by with contrast, real-time with image documentation (2D), includes M-mode recording, when performed, during rest and cardiovascular stress test using treadmill, bicycle exercise and/or pharmacologically induced stress, with interpretation and report `Qp` `Qh` S

Medicare Statute 1833(t)(2)

Coding Clinic: 2012, Q3, P8

⊘ **C8929** Transthoracic echocardiography with contrast, or without contrast followed by with contrast, real-time with image documentation (2D), includes M-mode recording, when performed, complete, with spectral Doppler echocardiography, and with color flow Doppler echocardiography `Qp` `Qh` S

Medicare Statute 1833(t)(2)

Coding Clinic: 2012, Q3, P8

⊘ **C8930** Transthoracic echocardiography, with contrast, or without contrast followed by with contrast, real-time with image documentation (2D), includes M-mode recording, when performed, during rest and cardiovascular stress test using treadmill, bicycle exercise and/or pharmacologically induced stress, with interpretation and report; including performance of continuous electrocardiographic monitoring, with physician supervision `Qp` `Qh` S

Medicare Statute 1833(t)(2)

Coding Clinic: 2012, Q3, P8

Magnetic Resonance Angiography: Spine and Upper Extremities

⊘ **C8931** Magnetic resonance angiography with contrast, spinal canal and contents `Qp` `Qh` Z2 Q3

Medicare Statute 1833(t)

⊘ **C8932** Magnetic resonance angiography without contrast, spinal canal and contents `Qp` `Qh` Z2 Q3

Medicare Statute 1833(t)

⊘ **C8933** Magnetic resonance angiography without contrast followed by with contrast, spinal canal and contents `Qp` `Qh` Z2 Q3

Medicare Statute 1833(t)

⊘ **C8934** Magnetic resonance angiography with contrast, upper extremity `Qh` Z2 Q3

Medicare Statute 1833(t)

⊘ **C8935** Magnetic resonance angiography without contrast, upper extremity `Qh` Z2 Q3

Medicare Statute 1833(t)

⊘ **C8936** Magnetic resonance angiography without contrast followed by with contrast, upper extremity `Qh` Z2 Q3

Medicare Statute 1833(t)

⊘ **C8937** Computer-aided detection, including computer algorithm analysis of breast MRI image data for lesion detection/characterization, pharmacokinetic analysis, with further physician review for interpretation (list separately in addition to code for primary procedure) N

Medicare Statute 1833(t)

Drugs and Biologicals

⊘ **C8957** Intravenous infusion for therapy/diagnosis; initiation of prolonged infusion (more than 8 hours), requiring use of portable or implantable pump `Qp` `Qh` S

Medicare Statute 1833(t)

Coding Clinic: 2008, Q3, P8

⊘ **C9034** Injection, dexamethasone 9%, intraocular, 1 mcg G

Medicare Statute 1833(t)

⊘ **C9046** Cocaine hydrochloride nasal solution for topical administration, 1 mg K2 N

⊘ **C9047** Injection, caplacizumab-yhdp, 1 mg K2 K

⊘ **C9061** Injection, teprotumumab-trbw, 10 mg

⊘ **C9063** Injection, eptinezumab-jjmr, 1 mg

🐾 MIPS   `Qp` **Quantity Physician**   `Qh` **Quantity Hospital**   ♀ **Female only**

♂ **Male only**   `A` **Age**   👤 **DMEPOS**   **A2-Z3** **ASC Payment Indicator**   **A-Y** **ASC Status Indicator**   Coding Clinic

⊜ **C9067** Gallium ga-68, dotatoc, diagnostic, 0.01 mci   K2 G

⊜ **C9084** injection, loncastuximab tesirine-lpyl, 0.1 mg   K2 D

⊜ **C9085** Injection, avalglucosidase alfa-ngpt, 4 mg   K2 G

⊜ **C9086** Injection, anifrolumab-fnia, 1 mg   K2 G

⊜ **C9087** Injection, cyclophosphamide, (auromedics), 10 mg   K2 G

⊜ **C9088** Instillation, bupivacaine and meloxicam, 1 mg/0.03 mg   K2 N

⊜ **C9089** Bupivacaine, collagen-matrix implant, 1 mg   K2 N

✳ **C9101** Injection, oliceridine, 0.1 mg   K2 G

⊜ **C9113** Injection, pantoprazole sodium, per vial Qp Qh   N1 N

Medicare Statute 1833(t)

✳ **C9143** Cocaine hydrochloride nasal solution (numbrino), 1 mg   N

✳ **C9144** Injection, bupivacaine (posimir), 1 mg   K2 N

⊜ **C9248** Injection, clevidipine butyrate, 1 mg Qp Qh   N1 K

Medicare Statute 1833(t)

⊜ **C9250** Human plasma fibrin sealant, vapor-heated, solvent-detergent (ARTISS), 2 ml Qp Qh   K2 K

Example of diagnosis codes to be reported with C9250: T20.00-T25.799.

Medicare Statute 621MMA

▶ ⊜ **C9150** Xenon xe-129 hyperpolarized gas, diagnostic, per study dose

▶ ⊜ **C9152** Injection, aripiprazole, (abilify asimtufii), 1 mg

▶ ⊜ **C9153** Injection, amisulpride, 1 mg

▶ ⊜ **C9154** Injection, buprenorphine extended-release (brixadi), 1 mg

▶ ⊜ **C9155** Injection, epcoritamab-bysp, 0.16 mg

▶ ⊜ **C9156** Flotufolastat F18, diagnostic, 1 millicurie

▶ ⊜ **C9157** Injection, tofersen, 1 mg

▶ ⊜ **C9158** Injection, risperidone, (uzedy), 1 mg

⊜ **C9254** Injection, lacosamide, 1 mg Qp Qh N1 N

Medicare Statute 621MMA

⊜ **C9257** injection, bevacizumab, 0.25 mg Qp Qh   K2 K

Medicare Statute 1833(t)

⊜ **C9285** Lidocaine 70 mg/tetracaine 70 mg, per patch Qp Qh   N1 N

Medicare Statute 1833(t)

Coding Clinic: 2011, Q3, P9

⊜ **C9290** Injection, bupivacine liposome, 1 mg Qp Qh   N1 N

Medicare Statute 1833(t)

Coding Clinic: 2023, Q1, P23

⊜ **C9293** Injection, glucarpidase, 10 units Qp Qh   K2 K

Medicare Statute 1833(t)

⊜ **C9352** Microporous collagen implantable tube (NeuraGen Nerve Guide), per centimeter length Qp Qh   N1 N

Medicare Statute 621MMA

⊜ **C9353** Microporous collagen implantable slit tube (NeuraWrap Nerve Protector), per centimeter length Qp Qh   N1 N

Medicare Statute 621MMA

⊜ **C9354** Acellular pericardial tissue matrix of non-human origin (Veritas), per square centimeter Qp Qh   N1 N

Medicare Statute 621MMA

⊜ **C9355** Collagen nerve cuff (NeuroMatrix), per 0.5 centimeter length Qp Qh   N1 N

Medicare Statute 621MMA

⊜ **C9356** Tendon, porous matrix of cross-linked collagen and glycosaminoglycan matrix (TenoGlide Tendon Protector Sheet), per square centimeter Qp Qh   N1 N

Medicare Statute 621MMA

⊜ **C9358** Dermal substitute, native, non-denatured collagen, fetal bovine origin (SurgiMend Collagen Matrix), per 0.5 square centimeters Qp Qh   N1 N

Medicare Statute 621MMA

Coding Clinic: 2013, Q3, P9; 2012, Q2, P7

⊜ **C9359** Porous purified collagen matrix bone void filler (Integra Mozaik Osteoconductive Scaffold Putty, Integra OS Osteoconductive Scaffold Putty), per 0.5 cc Qp Qh   N1 N

Medicare Statute 1833(t)

Coding Clinic: 2015, Q3, P2

⊜ **C9360** Dermal substitute, native, non-denatured collagen, neonatal bovine origin (SurgiMend Collagen Matrix), per 0.5 square centimeters Qp Qh   N1 N

Medicare Statute 621MMA

Coding Clinic: 2012, Q2, P7

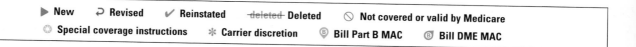

▶ New   ↻ Revised   ✔ Reinstated   ~~deleted~~ Deleted   ⊘ Not covered or valid by Medicare
⊜ Special coverage instructions   ✳ Carrier discretion   Ⓑ Bill Part B MAC   Ⓑ Bill DME MAC

C9361   Collagen matrix nerve wrap (NeuroMend Collagen Nerve Wrap), per 0.5 centimeter length **Qp** **Qh**   N1 N

Medicare Statute 621MMA

C9362   Porous purified collagen matrix bone void filler (Integra Mozaik Osteoconductive Scaffold Strip), per 0.5 cc **Qp** **Qh**   N1 N

Medicare Statute 621MMA

Coding Clinic: 2010, Q2, P8

C9363   Skin substitute, Integra Meshed Bilayer Wound Matrix, per square centimeter **Qp** **Qh**   N1 N

Medicare Statute 621MMA

Coding Clinic: 2012, Q2, P7; 2010, Q2, P8

C9364   Porcine implant, Permacol, per square centimeter **Qp** **Qh**   N1 N

Medicare Statute 621MMA

C9399   Unclassified drugs or biologicals   K7 A

Medicare Statute 621MMA

Coding Clinic: 2017, Q1, P1-3, P8; 2016, Q4, P10; 2014, Q2, P8; 2013, Q2, P3; 2010, Q3, P8

C9460   Injection, cangrelor, 1 mg **Qp** **Qh**   K2 G

Medicare Statute 1833(t)

C9462   Injection, delafloxacin, 1 mg   K2 E2

Medicare Statute 1833(t)

C9482   Injection, sotalol hydrochloride, 1 mg **Qp** **Qh**   K2 G

Medicare Statute 1833(t)

Coding Clinic: 2016, Q4, P9

C9488   Injection, conivaptan hydrochloride, 1 mg   K2 G

Medicare Statute 1833(t)

C9507   Plasma, high titer covid-19 convalescent, each unit   R

Percutaneous Transcatheter and Transluminal Coronary Procedures

C9600   Percutaneous transcatheter placement of drug-eluting intracoronary stent(s), with coronary angioplasty when performed; a single major coronary artery or branch **Qp** **Qh**   J1

Medicare Statute 1833(t)

Coding Clinic: 2023, Q2, P18-19

C9601   Percutaneous transcatheter placement of drug-eluting intracoronary stent(s), with coronary angioplasty when performed; each additional branch of a major coronary artery (list separately in addition to code for primary procedure) **Qp** **Qh**   N

Medicare Statute 1833(t)

Coding Clinic: 2023, Q2, P18-19

C9602   Percutaneous transluminal coronary atherectomy, with drug-eluting intracoronary stent, with coronary angioplasty when performed; a single major coronary artery or branch **Qp** **Qh**   J1

Medicare Statute 1833(t)

Coding Clinic: 2023, Q2, P18-19

C9603   Percutaneous transluminal coronary atherectomy, with drug-eluting intracoronary stent, with coronary angioplasty when performed; each additional branch of a major coronary artery (list separately in addition to code for primary procedure) **Qp** **Qh**   N

Medicare Statute 1833(t)

Coding Clinic: 2023, Q2, P18-19

C9604   Percutaneous transluminal revascularization of or through coronary artery bypass graft (internal mammary, free arterial, venous), any combination of drug-eluting intracoronary stent, atherectomy and angioplasty, including distal protection when performed; a single vessel **Qp** **Qh**   J1

Coding Clinic: 2023, Q2, P18-19

C9605   Percutaneous transluminal revascularization of or through coronary artery bypass graft (internal mammary, free arterial, venous), any combination of drug-eluting intracoronary stent, atherectomy and angioplasty, including distal protection when performed; each additional branch subtended by the bypass graft (list separately in addition to code for primary procedure) **Qp** **Qh**   N

Medicare Statute 1833(t)

Coding Clinic: 2023, Q2, P18-19

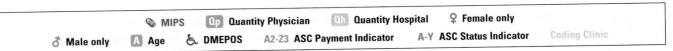

⊘ **C9606** Percutaneous transluminal revascularization of acute total/subtotal occlusion during acute myocardial infarction, coronary artery or coronary artery bypass graft, any combination of drug-eluting intracoronary stent, atherectomy and angioplasty, including aspiration thrombectomy when performed, single vessel **Qp** **Qh** J1

Medicare Statute 1833(t)

Coding Clinic: 2023, Q2, P18-19

⊘ **C9607** Percutaneous transluminal revascularization of chronic total occlusion, coronary artery, coronary artery branch, or coronary artery bypass graft, any combination of drug-eluting intracoronary stent, atherectomy and angioplasty; single vessel **Qp** **Qh** J1

Medicare Statute 1833(t)

Coding Clinic: 2023, Q2, P18-19

⊘ **C9608** Percutaneous transluminal revascularization of chronic total occlusion, coronary artery, coronary artery branch, or coronary artery bypass graft, any combination of drug-eluting intracoronary stent, atherectomy and angioplasty; each additional coronary artery, coronary artery branch, or bypass graft (list separately in addition to code for primary procedure) **Qp** **Qh** N

Medicare Statute 1833(t)

Coding Clinic: 2023, Q2, P18-19

Therapeutic Services and Supplies

⊘ **C9725** Placement of endorectal intracavitary applicator for high intensity brachytherapy **Qp** **Qh** T

Medicare Statute 1833(t)

⊘ **C9726** Placement and removal (if performed) of applicator into breast for intraoperative radiation therapy, add-on to primary breast procedure **Qh** N

Medicare Statute 1833(t)

⊘ **C9727** Insertion of implants into the soft palate; minimum of three implants **Qp** **Qh** T

Medicare Statute 1833(t)

⊘ **C9728** Placement of interstitial device(s) for radiation therapy/surgery guidance (e.g., fiducial markers, dosimeter), for other than the following sites (any approach): abdomen, pelvis, prostate, retroperitoneum, thorax, single or multiple **Qp** **Qh** S

Medicare Statute 1833(t)

Coding Clinic: 2018, Q2, P4

⊘ **C9733** Non-ophthalmic fluorescent vascular angiography **Qp** **Qh** Q2

Medicare Statute 1833(t)

Coding Clinic: 2023, Q1, P22; 2012, Q1, P7

⊘ **C9734** Focused ultrasound ablation/ therapeutic intervention, other than uterine leiomyomata, with magnetic resonance (MR) guidance **Qp** **Qh** J1

Medicare Statute 1833(t)

⊘ **C9738** Adjunctive blue light cystoscopy with fluorescent imaging agent (list separately in addition to code for primary procedure) N1 N

Medicare Statute 1833(t)

⊘ **C9739** Cystourethroscopy, with insertion of transprostatic implant; 1 to 3 implants **Qp** **Qh** J1

Medicare Statute 1833(t)

Coding Clinic: 2014, Q2, P6

⊘ **C9740** Cystourethroscopy, with insertion of transprostatic implant; 4 or more implants **Qp** **Qh** J1

Medicare Statute 1833(t)

Coding Clinic: 2014, Q2, P6

⊘ **C9751** Bronchoscopy, rigid or flexible, transbronchial ablation of lesion(s) by microwave energy, including fluoroscopic guidance, when performed, with computed tomography acquisition(s) and 3-D rendering, computer-assisted, image-guided navigation, and endobronchial ultrasound (EBUS) guided transtracheal and/or transbronchial sampling (e.g., aspiration[s]/biopsy[ies]) and all mediastinal and/or hilar lymph node stations or structures and therapeutic intervention(s) T

Medicare Statute 1833(t)

⊘ **C9756** Intraoperative near-infrared fluorescence lymphatic mapping of lymph node(s) (sentinel or tumor draining) with administration of indocyanine green (ICG) (list separately in addition to code for primary procedure) N

Coding Clinic: 2021, Q1, P9

▶ New ↻ Revised ✔ Reinstated ~~deleted~~ Deleted ⊘ Not covered or valid by Medicare
⊘ Special coverage instructions ✳ Carrier discretion ⑧ Bill Part B MAC ⑧ Bill DME MAC

○ **C9757** Laminotomy (hemilaminectomy), with decompression of nerve root(s), including partial facetectomy, foraminotomy and excision of herniated intervertebral disc, and repair of annular defect with implantation of bone anchored annular closure device, including annular defect measurement, alignment and sizing assessment, and image guidance; 1 interspace, lumbar   **J1**

○ **C9758** Blinded procedure for NYHA class III/IV heart failure; transcatheter implantation of interatrial shunt or placebo control, including right heart catheterization, trans-esophageal echocardiography (TEE)/intracardiac echocardiography (ICE), and all imaging with or without guidance (e.g., ultrasound, fluoroscopy), performed in an approved investigational device exemption (IDE) study   **T**

○ **C9759** Transcatheter intraoperative blood vessel microinfusion(s) (e.g., intraluminal, vascular wall and/or perivascular) therapy, any vessel, including radiological supervision and interpretation, when performed   **N**

○ **C9760** Non-randomized, non-blinded procedure for NYHA class ii, iii, iv heart failure; transcatheter implantation of interatrial shunt, including right and left heart catheterization, transeptal puncture, trans-esophageal echocardiography (tee)/intracardiac echocardiography (ice), and all imaging with or without guidance (e.g., ultrasound, fluoroscopy), performed in an approved investigational device exemption (ide) study   **T**

○ **C9761** Cystourethroscopy, with ureteroscopy and/or pyeloscopy, with lithotripsy, and ureteral catheterization for steerable vacuum aspiration of the kidney, collecting system, ureter, bladder, and urethra if applicable (must use a steerable ureteral catheter)   **J1**

○ **C9762** Cardiac magnetic resonance imaging for morphology and function, quantification of segmental dysfunction; with strain imaging   **Z2 Q3**

○ **C9763** Cardiac magnetic resonance imaging for morphology and function, quantification of segmental dysfunction; with stress imaging   **Z2 Q3**

○ **C9764** Revascularization, endovascular, open or percutaneous, any vessel(s); with intravascular lithotripsy, includes angioplasty within the same vessel(s), when performed   **J1**

○ **C9765** Revascularization, endovascular, open or percutaneous, any vessel(s); with intravascular lithotripsy, and transluminal stent placement(s), includes angioplasty within the same vessel(s), when performed   **J1**

○ **C9766** Revascularization, endovascular, open or percutaneous, any vessel(s); with intravascular lithotripsy and atherectomy, includes angioplasty within the same vessel(s), when performed

○ **C9767** Revascularization, endovascular, open or percutaneous, any vessel(s); with intravascular lithotripsy and transluminal stent placement(s), and atherectomy, includes angioplasty within the same vessel(s), when performed   **J1**

○ **C9768** Endoscopic ultrasound-guided direct measurement of hepatic portosystemic pressure gradient by any method (list separately in addition to code for primary procedure)   **N**

○ **C9769** Cystourethroscopy, with insertion of temporary prostatic implant/stent with fixation/anchor and incisional struts   **N**

○ **C9770** Vitrectomy, mechanical, pars plana approach, with subretinal injection of pharmacologic/biologic agent   **T**

○ **C9771** Nasal/sinus endoscopy, cryoablation nasal tissue(s) and/or nerve(s), unilateral or bilateral   **J1**

○ **C9772** Revascularization, endovascular, open or percutaneous, tibial/peroneal artery(ies), with intravascular lithotripsy, includes angioplasty within the same vessel(s), when performed   **J1**

○ **C9973** Revascularization, endovascular, open or percutaneous, tibial/peroneal artery(ies); with intravascular lithotripsy, and transluminal stent placement(s), includes angioplasty within the same vessel(s), when performed   **J1**

○ **C9774** Revascularization, endovascular, open or percutaneous, tibial/peroneal artery(ies); with intravascular lithotripsy and atherectomy, includes angioplasty within the same vessel(s), when performed   **J1**

🖥 **MIPS**   **Qp** Quantity Physician   **Qh** Quantity Hospital   ♀ **Female only**

♂ **Male only**   **A** Age   ♿ **DMEPOS**   A2-Z3 **ASC Payment Indicator**   A-Y **ASC Status Indicator**   Coding Clinic

⚙ **C9775** Revascularization, endovascular, open or percutaneous, tibial/peroneal artery(ies); with intravascular lithotripsy and transluminal stent placement(s), and atherectomy, includes angioplasty within the same vessel(s), when performed   J1

⚙ **C9776** Intraoperative near-infrared fluorescence imaging of major extra-hepatic bile duct(s) (e.g., cystic duct, common bile duct and common hepatic duct) with intravenous administration of indocyanine green (icg) (list separately in addition to code for primary procedure)

Coding Clinic: 2023, Q2, P19

⚙ **C9777** Esophageal mucosal integrity testing by electrical impedance, transoral, includes esophagoscopy or esophagogastroduodenoscopy

⚙ **C9778** Colpopexy, vaginal; minimally invasive extra-peritoneal approach (sacrospinous)

⚙ **C9779** Endoscopic submucosal dissection (esd), including endoscopy or colonoscopy, mucosal closure, when performed   J1

Coding Clinic: 2023, Q3, P9-10

⚙ **C9780** Insertion of central venous catheter through central venous occlusion via inferior and superior approaches (e.g., inside-out technique), including imaging guidance   S

C9781 Arthroscopy, shoulder, surgical; with implantation of subacromial spacer (e.g., balloon), includes debridement (e.g., limited or extensive), subacromial decompression, acromioplasty, and biceps tenodesis when performed   J1

C9782 Blinded procedure for New York heart association (NYHA) class ii or iii heart failure, or Canadian cardiovascular society (ccs) class iii or iv chronic refractory angina; transcatheter intramyocardial transplantation of autologous bone marrow cells (e.g., mononuclear) or placebo control, autologous bone marrow harvesting and preparation for transplantation, left heart catheterization including ventriculography, all laboratory services, and all imaging with or without guidance (e.g., transthoracic echocardiography, ultrasound, fluoroscopy), performed in an approved investigational device exemption (IDE) study   T

C9783 Blinded procedure for transcatheter implantation of coronary sinus reduction device or placebo control, including vascular access and closure, right heart catherization, venous and coronary sinus angiography, imaging guidance and supervision and interpretation when performed in an approved investigational device exemption (IDE) study   J1

▶ ⚙ **C9784** Gastric restrictive procedure, endoscopic sleeve gastroplasty, with esophagogastroduodenoscopy and intraluminal tube insertion, if performed, including all system and tissue anchoring components

▶ ⚙ **C9785** Endoscopic outlet reduction, gastric pouch application, with endoscopy and intraluminal tube insertion, if performed, including all system and tissue anchoring components

▶ ⚙ **C9786** Echocardiography image post processing for computer aided detection of heart failure with preserved ejection fraction, including interpretation and report

▶ ⚙ **C9787** Gastric electrophysiology mapping with simultaneous patient symptom profiling

▶ ⚙ **C9788** Opto-acoustic imaging, breast (including axilla when performed), unilateral, with image documentation, analysis and report, obtained with ultrasound examination

▶ ⚙ **C9789** Instillation of anti-neoplastic pharmacologic/biologic agent into renal pelvis, any method, including all imaging guidance, including volumetric measurement if performed

▶ ⚙ **C9790** Histotripsy (ie, non-thermal ablation via acoustic energy delivery) of malignant renal tissue, including image guidance

▶ ⚙ **C9791** Magnetic resonance imaging with inhaled hyperpolarized xenon-129 contrast agent, chest, including preparation and administration of agent

▶ ⚙ **C9792** Blinded or nonblinded procedure for symptomatic new york heart association (nyha) class ii, iii, iva heart failure; transcatheter implantation of left atrial to coronary sinus shunt using jugular vein access, including all imaging necessary to intra procedurally map the coronary sinus for optimal shunt placement (e.g., tee or ice ultrasound, fluoroscopy), performed under general anesthesia in an approved investigational device exemption (ide) study

---

▶ New   ↻ Revised   ✔ Reinstated   ~~deleted~~ Deleted   ⊘ Not covered or valid by Medicare
⚙ Special coverage instructions   ✳ Carrier discretion   ⑧ Bill Part B MAC   ⑧ Bill DME MAC

◎ **C9803** Hospital outpatient clinic visit specimen collection for severe acute respiratory syndrome coronavirus 2 (SARS-CoV-2) (coronavirus disease [COVID-19]), any specimen source   Q1

◎ **C9898** Radiolabeled product provided during a hospital inpatient stay Qh   N

◎ **C9899** Implanted prosthetic device, payable only for inpatients who do not have inpatient coverage   A

Medicare Statute 1833(t)

DENTAL PROCEDURES (D0000-D9999)

Diagnostic (D0120-D0999)
Clinical Oral Evaluations

D0120   Periodic oral evaluation - established patient ⓑ   B

An evaluation performed on a patient of record to determine any changes in the patient's dental and medical health status since a previous comprehensive or periodic evaluation. This includes an oral cancer evaluation, periodontal screening where indicated, and may require interpretation of information acquired through additional diagnostic procedures. The findings are discussed with the patient. Report additional diagnostic procedures separately.

D0140   Limited oral evaluation - problem focused ⓑ   B

An evaluation limited to a specific oral health problem or complaint. This may require interpretation of information acquired through additional diagnostic procedures. Report additional diagnostic procedures separately. Definitive procedures may be required on the same date as the evaluation. Typically, patients receiving this type of evaluation present with a specific problem and/or dental emergencies, trauma, acute infections, etc.

D0145   Oral evaluation for a patient under three years of age and counseling with primary caregiver ⓑ Ⓐ   B

Diagnostic services performed for a child under the age of three, preferably within the first six months of the eruption of the first primary tooth, including recording the oral and physical health history, evaluation of caries susceptibility, development of an appropriate preventive oral health regimen and communication with and counseling of the child's parent, legal guardian and/or primary caregiver.

D0150   Comprehensive oral evaluation - new or established patient ⓑ   S

Used by a general dentist and/or a specialist when evaluating a patient comprehensively. This applies to new patients; established patients who have had a significant change in health conditions or other unusual circumstances, by report, or established patients who have been absent from active treatment for three or more years. It is a thorough evaluation and recording of the extraoral and intraoral hard and soft tissues. It may require interpretation of information acquired through additional diagnostic procedures. Additional diagnostic procedures should be reported separately. This includes an evaluation for oral cancer, the evaluation and recording of the patient's dental and medical history and a general health assessment. It may include the evaluation and recording of dental caries, missing or unerupted teeth, restorations, existing prostheses, occlusal relationships, periodontal conditions (including periodontal screening and/or charting), hard and soft tissue anomalies, etc.

D0160   Detailed and extensive oral evaluation - problem focused, by report ⓑ   B

A detailed and extensive problem focused evaluation entails extensive diagnostic and cognitive modalities based on the findings of a comprehensive oral evaluation. Integration of more extensive diagnostic modalities to develop a treatment plan for a specific problem is required. The condition requiring this type of evaluation should be described and documented. Examples of conditions requiring this type of evaluation may include dentofacial anomalies, complicated perio-prosthetic conditions, complex temporomandibular dysfunction, facial pain of unknown origin, conditions requiring multi-disciplinary consultation, etc.

▶ **New**   ↻ **Revised**   ✔ **Reinstated**   ~~deleted~~ **Deleted**   ⊘ **Not covered or valid by Medicare**
⊚ **Special coverage instructions**   ✳ **Carrier discretion**   ⓑ **Bill Part B MAC**   ⓖ **Bill DME MAC**

D0170 Re-evaluation - limited, problem focused (established patient; not post-operative visit) ⒷB

Assessing the status of a previously existing condition. For example: a traumatic injury where no treatment was rendered but patient needs follow-up monitoring; evaluation for undiagnosed continuing pain; soft tissue lesion requiring follow-up evaluation.

D0171 Re-evaluation - post-operative office visit ⒷB

D0180 Comprehensive periodontal evaluation - new or established patient ⒷB

This procedure is indicated for patients showing signs or symptoms of periodontal disease and for patients with risk factors such as smoking or diabetes. It includes evaluation of periodontal conditions, probing and charting, an evaluation for oral cancer, the evaluation and recording of the patient's dental and medical history and general health assessment. It may include the evaluation and recording of dental caries, missing or unerupted teeth, restorations, and occlusal relationships.

Pre-Diagnostic Services

D0190 Screening of a patient ⒷB

A screening, including state or federally mandated screenings, to determine an individual's need to be seen by a dentist for diagnosis.

D0191 Assessment of a patient ⒷB

A limited clinical inspection that is performed to identify possible signs of oral or systemic disease, malformation, or injury, and the potential need for referral for diagnosis and treatment.

Diagnostic Imaging

D0210 Intraoral - complete series of radiographic images ⒷB

A radiographic survey of the whole mouth, intended to display the crowns and roots of all teeth, periapical areas, interproximal areas and alveolar bone including edentulous areas.

Cross Reference 70320

D0220 Intraoral - periapical first radiographic image ⒷB

Cross Reference 70300

D0230 Intraoral - periapical each additional radiographic image ⒷB

Cross Reference 70310

D0240 Intraoral - occlusal radiographic image ⒷS

D0250 Extra-oral — 2D projection radiographic image created using a stationary radiation source, detector ⒷS

These images include, but are not limited to: Lateral Skull; Posterior-Anterior Skull; Submentovertex; Waters; Reverse Tomes; Oblique Mandibular Body; Lateral Ramus.

D0251 Extra-oral posterior dental radiographic image ⒷQ1

Image limited to exposure of complete posterior teeth in both dental arches. This is a unique image that is not derived from another image.

D0270 Bitewing - single radiographic image ⒷS

D0272 Bitewings - two radiographic images ⒷS

D0273 Bitewings - three radiographic images ⒷB

D0274 Bitewings - four radiographic images ⒷS

D0277 Vertical bitewings - 7 to 8 radiographic images ⒷS

This does not constitute a full mouth intraoral radiographic series.

D0310 Sialography ⒷB

Cross Reference 70390

D0320 Temporomandibular joint arthrogram, including injection ⒷB

Cross Reference 70332

D0321 Other temporomandibular joint radiographic image, by report ⒷB

Cross Reference 76499

D0322 Tomographic survey ⒷB

D0330 Panoramic radiographic image ⒷB

Cross Reference 70320

D0340 2D cephalometric radiographic image - acquisition, measurement and analysis ⒷB

Image of the head made using a cephalostat to standardize anatomic positioning, and with reproducible x-ray beam geometry.

Cross Reference 70350

D0350 2D oral/facial photographic image obtained intra-orally or extra-orally Ⓑ   B

D0364 Cone beam CT capture and interpretation with limited field of view - less than one whole jaw Ⓑ   B

D0365 Cone beam CT capture and interpretation with field of view of one full dental arch - mandible Ⓑ   B

D0366 Cone beam CT capture and interpretation with field of view of one full dental arch - maxilla, with or without cranium Ⓑ   B

D0367 Cone beam CT capture and interpretation with field of view of both jaws, with or without cranium Ⓑ   B

D0368 Cone beam CT capture and interpretation for TMJ series including two or more exposures Ⓑ   B

D0369 Maxillofacial MRI capture and interpretation Ⓑ   B

D0370 Maxillofacial ultrasound capture and interpretation Ⓑ   B

D0371 Sialoendoscopy capture and interpretation Ⓑ   B

D0372 Intraoral tomosynthesis – comprehensive series of radiographic images Ⓑ   B

A radiographic survey of the whole mouth intended to display the crowns and roots of all teeth, periapical areas, interproximal areas and alveolar bone including edentulous areas.

D0373 Intraoral tomosynthesis – bitewing radiographic image Ⓑ   B

D0374 Intraoral tomosynthesis – periapical radiographic image Ⓑ   B

D0380 Cone beam CT image capture with limited field of view - less than one whole jaw Ⓑ   B

D0381 Cone beam CT image capture with field of view of one full dental arch - mandible Ⓑ   B

D0382 Cone beam CT image capture with field of view of one full dental arch - maxilla, with or without cranium Ⓑ   B

D0383 Cone beam CT image capture with field of view of both jaws, with or without cranium Ⓑ   B

D0384 Cone beam CT image capture for TMJ series including two or more exposures Ⓑ   B

D0385 Maxillofacial MRI image capture Ⓑ   B

D0386 Maxillofacial ultrasound image capture Ⓑ   B

D0387 Intraoral tomosynthesis – comprehensive series of radiographic images – image capture only Ⓑ   B

A radiographic survey of the whole mouth intended to display the crowns and roots of all teeth, periapical areas, interproximal areas and alveolar bone including edentulous areas.

D0388 Intraoral tomosynthesis – bitewing radiographic image – image capture only Ⓑ   B

D0389 Intraoral tomosynthesis – periapical radiographic image – image capture only Ⓑ   B

D0391 Interpretation of diagnostic image by a practitioner not associated with capture of the image, including report Ⓑ   B

D0393 Virtual treatment simulation using 3D image volume or surface scan Ⓑ   B

Virtual simulation of treatment including, but not limited to, dental implant placement, prosthetic reconstruction, orthognathic surgery and orthodontic tooth movement.

D0394 Digital subtraction of two or more images or image volumes of the same modality Ⓑ   B

To demonstrate changes that have occurred over time.

D0395 Fusion of two or more 3D image volumes of one or more modalities Ⓑ   B

▶ **D0396** 3D printing of a 3D dental surface scan

3D printing of a 3D dental surface scan to obtain a physical model.

Tests and Examinations

D0411 HbA1c in-office point of service testing Ⓑ   B

D0412 Blood glucose level test - in-office using a glucose meter Ⓑ   B

D0414 Laboratory processing of microbial specimen to include culture and sensitivity studies, preparation and transmission of written report Ⓑ   B

D0415 Collection of microorganisms for culture and sensitivity Ⓑ   B

Cross Reference D0410

D0416 Viral culture Ⓑ   B

A diagnostic test to identify viral organisms, most often herpes virus.

D0417 Collection and preparation of saliva sample for laboratory diagnostic testing Ⓑ   B

▶ New   ↻ Revised   ✔ Reinstated   ~~deleted~~ Deleted   ⊘ Not covered or valid by Medicare
✿ Special coverage instructions   ✳ Carrier discretion   Ⓑ Bill Part B MAC   Ⓑ Bill DME MAC

D0418 Analysis of saliva sample Ⓑ   B

Chemical or biological analysis of saliva sample for diagnostic purposes.

D0419 Assessment of salivary flow by measurement   B

D0422 Collection and preparation of genetic sample material for laboratory analysis and report Ⓑ   B

D0423 Genetic test for susceptibility to diseases - specimen analysis Ⓑ   B

Certified laboratory analysis to detect specific genetic variations associated with increased susceptibility for diseases.

D0425 Caries susceptibility tests Ⓑ   B

Not to be used for carious dentin staining.

D0431 Adjunctive pre-diagnostic test that aids in detection of mucosal abnormalities including premalignant and malignant lesions, not to include cytology or biopsy procedures Ⓑ   B

D0460 Pulp vitality tests Ⓑ   S

Includes multiple teeth and contra-lateral comparison(s), as indicated.

D0470 Diagnostic casts Ⓑ   B

Also known as diagnostic models or study models.

Oral Pathology Laboratory (Use Codes D0472 – D0502)

D0472 Accession of tissue, gross examination, preparation and transmission of written report Ⓑ   B

To be used in reporting architecturally intact tissue obtained by invasive means.

D0473 Accession of tissue, gross and microscopic examination, preparation and transmission of written report Ⓑ   B

To be used in reporting architecturally intact tissue obtained by invasive means.

D0474 Accession of tissue, gross and microscopic examination, including assessment of surgical margins for presence of disease, preparation and transmission of written report Ⓑ   B

To be used in reporting architecturally intact tissue obtained by invasive means.

D0475 Decalcification procedure Ⓑ   B

Procedure in which hard tissue is processed in order to allow sectioning and subsequent microscopic examination.

D0476 Special stains for microorganisms Ⓑ   B

Procedure in which additional stains are applied to biopsy or surgical specimen in order to identify microorganisms.

D0477 Special stains, not for microorganisms Ⓑ   B

Procedure in which additional stains are applied to a biopsy or surgical specimen in order to identify such things as melanin, mucin, iron, glycogen, etc.

D0478 Immunohistochemical stains Ⓑ   B

A procedure in which specific antibody based reagents are applied to tissue samples in order to facilitate diagnosis.

D0479 Tissue in-situ hybridization, including interpretation Ⓑ   B

A procedure which allows for the identification of nucleic acids, DNA and RNA, in the tissue sample in order to aid in the diagnosis of microorganisms and tumors.

D0480 Accession of exfoliative cytologic smears, microscopic examination, preparation and transmission of written report Ⓑ   B

To be used in reporting disaggregated, non-transepithelial cell cytology sample via mild scraping of the oral mucosa.

D0481 Electron microscopy Ⓑ   B

D0482 Direct immunofluorescence Ⓑ   B

A technique used to identify immunoreactants which are localized to the patient's skin or mucous membranes.

D0483 Indirect immunofluorescence Ⓑ   B

A technique used to identify circulating immunoreactants.

D0484 Consultation on slides prepared elsewhere Ⓑ   B

A service provided in which microscopic slides of a biopsy specimen prepared at another laboratory are evaluated to aid in the diagnosis of a difficult case or to offer a consultative opinion at the patient's request. The findings are delivered by written report.

D0485 Consultation, including preparation of slides from biopsy material supplied by referring source Ⓑ B

A service that requires the consulting pathologist to prepare the slides as well as render a written report. The slides are evaluated to aid in the diagnosis of a difficult case or to offer a consultative opinion at the patient's request.

D0486 Laboratory accession of transepithelial cytologic sample, microscopic examination, preparation and transmission of written report Ⓑ B

Analysis, and written report of findings, of cytologic sample of disaggregated transepithelial cells.

D0502 Other oral pathology procedures, by report Ⓑ B

Tests and Examinations

D0600 Non-ionizing diagnostic procedure capable of quantifying, monitoring, and recording changes in structure of enamel, dentin, and cementum Ⓑ S

D0601 Caries risk assessment and documentation, with a finding of low risk Ⓑ B

Using recognized assessment tools.

D0602 Caries risk assessment and documentation, with a finding of moderate risk Ⓑ B

Using recognized assessment tools.

D0603 Caries risk assessment and documentation, with a finding of high risk Ⓑ B

Using recognized assessment tools.

D0604 Antigen testing for public health related pathogen, including coronavirus B

D0605 Antibody testing for public health related pathogen, including coronavirus B

D0701 Panoramic radiographic image – image capture only B

D0702 2-D cephalometric radiographic image – image capture only B

D0703 2-D oral/facial photographic image obtained intra-orally or extra-orally – image capture only B

D0705 Extra-oral posterior dental radiographic image – image capture only B

Image limited to exposure of complete posterior teeth in both dental arches.

This is a unique image that is not derived from another image.

D0706 Intraoral – occlusal radiographic image – image capture only B

D0707 Intraoral – periapical radiographic image – image capture only B

D0708 Intraoral – bitewing radiographic image – image capture only B

Image axis may be horizontal or vertical.

D0709 Intraoral – complete series of radiographic images – image capture only B

A radiographic survey of the whole mouth intended to display the crowns and roots of all teeth, periapical areas, interproximal areas and alveolar bone including edentulous areas.

3D Scan

D0801 3D dental surface scan – direct B
D0802 3D dental surface scan – indirect B

A surface scan of a diagnostic cast.

D0803 3D facial surface scan – direct B
D0804 3D facial surface scan – indirect B

A surface scan of constructed facial features.

None

D0999 Unspecified diagnostic procedure, by report Ⓑ B

Used for procedure that is not adequately described by a code. Describe procedure.

Preventative (D1110-D1999)
Dental Prophylaxis

D1110 Prophylaxis - adult Ⓑ Ⓐ B

Removal of plaque, calculus and stains from the tooth structures and implants in the permanent and transitional dentition. It is intended to control local irritational factors.

D1120 Prophylaxis - child Ⓑ Ⓐ B

Removal of plaque, calculus and stains from the tooth structures and implants in the primary and transitional dentition. It is intended to control local irritational factors.

Topical Fluoride Treatment (Office Procedure)

D1206 Topical application of fluoride varnish Ⓑ   B

D1208 Topical application of fluoride — excluding varnish Ⓑ   B

Other Preventative Services

▶ **D1301** Immunization counseling   B

A review of a patient's vaccine and medical history, and discussion of the vaccine benefits, risks, and consequences of not obtaining the vaccine. Counseling also includes a discussion of questions and concerns the patient, family, or caregiver may have and suggestions on where the patient can obtain the vaccine.

D1310 Nutritional counseling for the control of dental disease Ⓑ   B

Counseling on food selection and dietary habits as a part of treatment and control of periodontal disease and caries.

D1320 Tobacco counseling for the control and prevention of oral disease Ⓑ   B

Tobacco prevention and cessation services reduce patient risks of developing tobacco-related oral diseases and conditions and improves prognosis for certain dental therapies.

D1321 Counseling for the control and prevention of adverse oral, behavioral, and systemic health effects associated with high-risk substance use   B

Counseling services may include patient education about adverse oral, behavioral, and systemic effects associated with high-risk substance use and administration routes. This includes ingesting, injecting, inhaling and vaping. Substances used in a high-risk manner may include but are not limited to alcohol, opioids, nicotine, cannabis, methamphetamine and other pharmaceuticals or chemicals.

D1330 Oral hygiene instruction Ⓑ   B

This may include instructions for home care. Examples include tooth brushing technique, flossing, use of special oral hygiene aids.

D1351 Sealant - per tooth Ⓑ   B

Mechanically and/or chemically prepared enamel surface sealed to prevent decay.

D1352 Preventive resin restoration in a moderate to high caries risk patient — permanent tooth Ⓑ   B

Conservative restoration of an active cavitated lesion in a pit or fissure that does not extend into dentin; includes placement of a sealant in any radiating non-carious fissures or pits.

D1353 Sealant repair — per tooth Ⓑ   B

D1354 Application of caries arresting medicament — per tooth Ⓑ   B

Conservative treatment of an active, non-symptomatic carious lesion by topical application of a caries arresting or inhibiting medicament and without mechanical removal of sound tooth structure.

D1355 Caries preventive medicament application – per tooth   B

For primary prevention or remineralization. Medicaments applied do not include topical fluorides.

Space Maintenance (Passive Appliances)

D1510 Space maintainer - fixed - unilateral - per quadrant Ⓑ   S

Excludes a distal shoe space maintainer.

D1516 Space Maintainer - fixed - bilateral, maxillary Ⓑ   S

D1517 Space Maintainer - fixed - bilateral, mandibular Ⓑ   S

D1520 Space maintainer - removable - unilateral - per quadrant Ⓑ   S

D1526 Space maintainer - removable - bilateral, maxillary Ⓑ   S

D1527 Space maintainer - removable - bilateral, mandibular Ⓑ   S

D1551 Re-cement or re-bond bilateral space maintainer - maxillary   S

D1552 Re-cement or re-bond bilateral space maintainer - mandibular   S

D1553 Re-cement or re-bond unilateral space maintainer - per quadrant   S

D1556 Removal of fixed unilateral space maintainer - per quadrant   B

D1557 Removal of fixed bilateral space maintainer - maxillary   B

D1558 Removal of fixed bilateral space maintainer - mandibular   B

🐾 MIPS   Ⓠⓟ **Quantity Physician**   Ⓠⓗ **Quantity Hospital**   ♀ **Female only**   ♂ **Male only**   Ⓐ **Age**   & **DMEPOS**   A2-Z3 **ASC Payment Indicator**   A-Y **ASC Status Indicator**   Coding Clinic

173

Space Maintainers

D1575 Distal shoe space maintainer - fixed - unilateral - per quadrant Ⓑ   S

Fabrication and delivery of fixed appliance extending subgingivally and distally to guide the eruption of the first permanent molar. Does not include ongoing follow-up or adjustments, or replacement appliances, once the tooth has erupted.

Vaccine administration

D1781 Vaccine administration – human papillomavirus – Dose 1   E1

Gardasil 9 0.5mL intramuscular vaccine injection.

D1782 Vaccine administration – human papillomavirus – Dose 2   E1

Gardasil 9 0.5mL intramuscular vaccine injection.

D1783 Vaccine administration – human papillomavirus – Dose 3   E1

Gardasil 9 0.5mL intramuscular vaccine injection.

None

D1999 Unspecified preventive procedure, by report Ⓑ   B

Used for procedure that is not adequately described by another CDT Code. Describe procedure.

Restorative (D2140-D2999)
Amalgam Restorations (Including Polishing)

D2140 Amalgam - one surface, primary or permanent Ⓑ   B

D2150 Amalgam - two surfaces, primary or permanent Ⓑ   B

D2160 Amalgam - three surfaces, primary or permanent Ⓑ   B

D2161 Amalgam - four or more surfaces, primary or permanent Ⓑ   B

Resin-Based Composite Restorations – Direct

D2330 Resin-based composite - one surface, anterior Ⓑ   B

D2331 Resin-based composite - two surfaces, anterior Ⓑ   B

D2332 Resin-based composite - three surfaces, anterior Ⓑ   B

↻ **D2335** Resin-based composite - four or more surfaces (anterior) Ⓑ   B

A band, typically cemented around a molar tooth after a multi-surface restoration is placed, to add support and resistance to fracture until a patient is ready for the full cuspal coverage restoration.

D2390 Resin-based composite crown, anterior Ⓑ   B

Full resin-based composite coverage of tooth.

D2391 Resin-based composite - one surface, posterior Ⓑ   B

Used to restore a carious lesion into the dentin or a deeply eroded area into the dentin. Not a preventive procedure.

D2392 Resin-based composite - two surfaces, posterior Ⓑ   B

D2393 Resin-based composite - three surfaces, posterior Ⓑ   B

D2394 Resin-based composite - four or more surfaces, posterior Ⓑ   B

Gold Foil Restorations

D2410 Gold foil - one surface Ⓑ   B

D2420 Gold foil - two surfaces Ⓑ   B

D2430 Gold foil - three surfaces Ⓑ   B

Inlay/Onlay Restorations

D2510 Inlay - metallic - one surface Ⓑ   B

D2520 Inlay - metallic - two surfaces Ⓑ   B

D2530 Inlay - metallic - three or more surfaces Ⓑ   B

D2542 Onlay - metallic - two surfaces Ⓑ   B

D2543 Onlay - metallic - three surfaces Ⓑ   B

D2544 Onlay - metallic - four or more surfaces Ⓑ   B

D2610 Inlay - porcelain/ceramic - one surface Ⓑ   B

D2620 Inlay - porcelain/ceramic - two surfaces Ⓑ   B

D2630 Inlay - porcelain/ceramic - three or more surfaces Ⓑ   B

D2642 Onlay - porcelain/ceramic - two surfaces Ⓑ   B

D2643 Onlay - porcelain/ceramic - three surfaces Ⓑ   B

D2644 Onlay - porcelain/ceramic - four or more surfaces Ⓑ   B

D2650 Inlay - resin-based composite - one surface Ⓑ   B

▶ New   ↻ Revised   ✔ Reinstated   ~~deleted~~ Deleted   ⊘ Not covered or valid by Medicare

✿ Special coverage instructions   ✳ Carrier discretion   Ⓑ Bill Part B MAC   Ⓓ Bill DME MAC

D2651 Inlay - resin-based composite - two surfaces Ⓑ   B

D2652 Inlay - resin-based composite - three or more surfaces Ⓑ   B

D2662 Onlay - resin-based composite - two surfaces Ⓑ   B

D2663 Onlay - resin-based composite - three surfaces Ⓑ   B

D2664 Onlay - resin-based composite - four or more surfaces Ⓑ   B

Crowns – Single Restoration Only

D2710 Crown - resin-based composite (indirect) Ⓑ   B

D2712 Crown - 3/4 resin-based composite (indirect) Ⓑ   B

This procedure does not include facial veneers.

D2720 Crown - resin with high noble metal Ⓑ   B

D2721 Crown - resin with predominantly base metal Ⓑ   B

D2722 Crown - resin with noble metal Ⓑ   B

D2740 Crown - porcelain/ceramic Ⓑ   B

D2750 Crown - porcelain fused to high noble metal Ⓑ   B

D2751 Crown - porcelain fused to predominantly base metal Ⓑ   B

D2752 Crown - porcelain fused to noble metal Ⓑ   B

D2753 Crown - porcelain fused to titanium and titanium alloys   B

D2780 Crown - 3/4 cast high noble metal Ⓑ   B

D2781 Crown - 3/4 cast predominantly base metal Ⓑ   B

D2782 Crown - 3/4 cast noble metal Ⓑ   B

D2783 Crown - 3/4 porcelain/ceramic Ⓑ   B

This procedure does not include facial veneers.

D2790 Crown - full cast high noble metal Ⓑ B   B

D2791 Crown - full cast predominantly base metal Ⓑ   B

D2792 Crown - full cast noble metal Ⓑ   B

D2794 Crown - titanium and titanium alloys Ⓑ   B

D2799 Interim crown - further treatment or completion of diagnosis necessary prior to final impression Ⓑ   B

Not to be used as a temporary crown for a routine prosthetic restoration.

Other Restorative Services

D2910 Re-cement or re-bond inlay, onlay, veneer or partial coverage restoration Ⓑ   B

D2915 Re-cement or re-bond indirectly fabricated cast or prefabricated post and core Ⓑ   B

D2920 Re-cement or re-bond crown Ⓑ   B

D2921 Reattachment of tooth fragment, incisal edge or cusp Ⓑ   B

D2928 Prefabricated porcelain/ceramic crown – permanent tooth

D2929 Prefabricated porcelain/ceramic crown - primary tooth Ⓑ   B

D2930 Prefabricated stainless steel crown - primary tooth Ⓑ   B

D2931 Prefabricated stainless steel crown - permanent tooth Ⓑ   B

D2932 Prefabricated resin crown Ⓑ   B

D2933 Prefabricated stainless steel crown with resin window Ⓑ   B

Open-face stainless steel crown with aesthetic resin facing or veneer.

D2934 Prefabricated esthetic coated stainless steel crown - primary tooth Ⓑ   B

Stainless steel primary crown with exterior esthetic coating.

D2940 Protective restoration Ⓑ   B

Direct placement of a restorative material to protect tooth and/or tissue form. This procedure may be used to relieve pain, promote healing, or prevent further deterioration. Not to be used for endodontic access closure, or as a base or liner under a restoration.

D2941 Interim therapeutic restoration - primary dentition Ⓑ   B

Placement of an adhesive restorative material following caries debridement by hand or other method for the management of early childhood caries. Not considered a definitive restoration.

D2949 Restorative foundation for an indirect restoration Ⓑ   B

Placement of restorative material to yield a more ideal form, including elimination of undercuts.

D2950 Core build-up, including any pins when required Ⓑ   B

Refers to building up of coronal structure when there is insufficient retention for a separate extracoronal restorative procedure. A core build-up is not a filler to eliminate any undercut, box form, or concave irregularity in a preparation.

D2951 Pin retention - per tooth, in addition to restoration Ⓑ   B

D2952 Post and core in addition to crown, indirectly fabricated Ⓑ   B

Post and core are custom fabricated as a single unit.

D2953 Each additional indirectly fabricated post - same tooth Ⓑ   B

To be used with D2952.

D2954 Prefabricated post and core in addition to crown Ⓑ   B

Core is built around a prefabricated post. This procedure includes the core material.

D2955 Post removal Ⓑ   B

D2957 Each additional prefabricated post - same tooth Ⓑ   B

To be used with D2954.

D2960 Labial veneer (laminate) - direct Ⓑ   B

Refers to labial/facial direct resin bonded veneers.

D2961 Labial veneer (resin laminate) - indirect Ⓑ   B

Refers to labial/facial indirect resin bonded veneers.

D2962 Labial veneer (porcelain laminate) - indirect Ⓑ   B

Refers also to facial veneers that extend interproximally and/or cover the incisal edge. Porcelain/ceramic veneers presently include all ceramic and porcelain veneers.

D2971 Additional procedures to customize a crown to fit under existing partial denture framework Ⓑ   B

This procedure is in addition to the separate crown procedure documented with its own code.

D2975 Coping Ⓑ   B

A thin covering of the coronal portion of a tooth, usually devoid of anatomic contour, that can be used as a definitive restoration.

▶ **D2976** Band stabilization – per tooth   B

A band, typically cemented around a molar tooth after a multi-surface restoration is placed, to add support and resistance to fracture until a patient is ready for the full cuspal coverage restoration.

D2980 Crown repair, necessitated by restorative material failure Ⓑ   B

D2981 Inlay repair necessitated by restorative material failure Ⓑ   B

D2982 Onlay repair necessitated by restorative material failure Ⓑ   B

D2983 Veneer repair necessitated by restorative material failure Ⓑ   B

▶ **D2989** Excavation of a tooth resulting in the determination of non-restorability

D2990 Resin infiltration of incipient smooth surface lesions Ⓑ   B

Placement of an infiltrating resin restoration for strengthening, stabilizing and/or limiting the progression of the lesion.

▶ **D2991** Excavation of a tooth resulting in the determination of non-restorability

Preparation of tooth surfaces and topical application of a scaffold to guide hydroxyapatite regeneration.

None

D2999 Unspecified restorative procedure, by report Ⓑ   S

Use for procedure that is not adequately described by a code. Describe procedure.

Endodontics (D3110-D3999)
Pulp Capping

D3110 Pulp cap - direct (excluding final restoration) Ⓑ   B

Procedure in which the exposed pulp is covered with a dressing or cement that protects the pulp and promotes healing and repair.

D3120 Pulp cap - indirect (excluding final restoration) Ⓑ   B

Procedure in which the nearly exposed pulp is covered with a protective dressing to protect the pulp from additional injury and to promote healing and repair via formation of secondary dentin. This code is not to be used for bases and liners when all caries has been removed.

▶ New   ↻ Revised   ✔ Reinstated   deleted Deleted   ⊘ Not covered or valid by Medicare
✿ Special coverage instructions   ✳ Carrier discretion   Ⓑ Bill Part B MAC   Ⓓ Bill DME MAC

Pulpotomy

D3220 Therapeutic pulpotomy (excluding final restoration) removal of pulp coronal to the dentinocemental junction and application of medicament Ⓑ   B

Pulpotomy is the surgical removal of a portion of the pulp with the aim of maintaining the vitality of the remaining portion by means of an adequate dressing.

– To be performed on primary or permanent teeth.

– This is not to be construed as the first stage of root canal therapy.

– Not to be used for apexogenesis.

D3221 Pulpal debridement, primary and permanent teeth Ⓑ   B

Pulpal debridement for the relief of acute pain prior to conventional root canal therapy. This procedure is not to be used when endodontic treatment is completed on the same day.

D3222 Partial pulpotomy for apexogenesis - permanent tooth with incomplete root development Ⓑ   B

Removal of a portion of the pulp and application of a medicament with the aim of maintaining the vitality of the remaining portion to encourage continued physiological development and formation of the root. This procedure is not to be construed as the first stage of root canal therapy.

Endodontic Therapy on Primary Teeth

D3230 Pulpal therapy (resorbable filling) - anterior, primary tooth (excluding final restoration) Ⓑ   B

Primary incisors and cuspids.

D3240 Pulpal therapy (resorbable filling) - posterior, primary tooth (excluding final restoration) Ⓑ   B

Primary first and second molars.

Endodontic Therapy (Including Treatment Plan, Clinical Procedures and Follow-Up Care)

D3310 Endodontic therapy, anterior tooth (excluding final restoration) Ⓑ   B

D3320 Endodontic therapy, premolar tooth (excluding final restoration) Ⓑ   B

D3330 Endodontic therapy, molar (excluding final restoration) Ⓑ   B

D3331 Treatment of root canal obstruction; non-surgical access Ⓑ   B

In lieu of surgery, the formation of a pathway to achieve an apical seal without surgical intervention because of a non-negotiable root canal blocked by foreign bodies, including but not limited to separated instruments, broken posts or calcification of 50% or more of the length of the tooth root.

D3332 Incomplete endodontic therapy; inoperable, unrestorable or fractured tooth Ⓑ   B

Considerable time is necessary to determine diagnosis and/or provide initial treatment before the fracture makes the tooth unretainable.

D3333 Internal root repair of perforation defects Ⓑ   B

Non-surgical seal of perforation caused by resorption and/or decay but not iatrogenic by provider filing claim.

Endodontic Retreatment

D3346 Retreatment of previous root canal therapy - anterior Ⓑ   B

D3347 Retreatment of previous root canal therapy - premolar Ⓑ   B

D3348 Retreatment of previous root canal therapy - molar Ⓑ   B

Apexification/Recalcification

D3351 Apexification/recalcification - initial visit (apical closure/calcific repair of perforations, root resorption, etc.) Ⓑ   B

Includes opening tooth, preparation of canal spaces, first placement of medication and necessary radiographs. (This procedure may include first phase of complete root canal therapy.)

D3352 Apexification/recalcification - interim medication replacement (apical closure/ calcific repair of perforations, root resorption, pulp space disinfection, etc.) Ⓑ   B

For visits in which the intra-canal medication is replaced with new medication. Includes any necessary radiographs.

D3353 Apexification/recalcification - final visit (includes completed root canal therapy - apical closure/calcific repair of perforations, root resorption, etc.) Ⓑ   B

Includes removal of intra-canal medication and procedures necessary to place final root canal filling material including necessary radiographs. (This procedure includes last phase of complete root canal therapy.)

Pulpal Regeneration

D3355 Pulpal regeneration - initial visit Ⓑ   B

Includes opening tooth, preparation of canal spaces, placement of medication.

D3356 Pulpal regeneration - interim medication replacement Ⓑ   B

D3357 Pulpal regeneration - completion of treatment Ⓑ   B

Does not include final restoration.

Apicoectomy/Periradicular Services

D3410 Apicoectomy - anterior Ⓑ   B

For surgery on root of anterior tooth. Does not include placement of retrograde filling material.

D3421 Apicoectomy - premolar (first root) Ⓑ B

For surgery on one root of a premolar. Does not include placement of retrograde filling material. If more than one root is treated, see D3426.

D3425 Apicoectomy - molar (first root) Ⓑ   B

For surgery on one root of a molar tooth. Does not include placement of retrograde filling material. If more than one root is treated, see D3426.

D3426 Apicoectomy (each additional root) Ⓑ B

Typically used for premolar and molar surgeries when more than one root is treated during the same procedure. This does not include retrograde filling material placement.

D3428 Bone graft in conjunction with periradicular surgery - per tooth, single site Ⓑ   B

Includes non-autogenous graft material.

D3429 Bone graft in conjunction with periradicular surgery - each additional contiguous tooth in the same surgical site Ⓑ   B

Includes non-autogenous graft material.

D3430 Retrograde filling - per root Ⓑ   B

For placement of retrograde filling material during periradicular surgery procedures. If more than one filling is placed in one root - report as D3999 and describe.

D3431 Biologic materials to aid in soft and osseous tissue regeneration in conjunction with periradicular surgery Ⓑ   B

D3432 Guided tissue regeneration, resorbable barrier, per site, in conjunction with periradicular surgery Ⓑ   B

D3450 Root amputation - per root Ⓑ   B

Root resection of a multi-rooted tooth while leaving the crown. If the crown is sectioned, see D3920.

D3460 Endodontic endosseous implant Ⓑ   S

Placement of implant material, which extends from a pulpal space into the bone beyond the end of the root.

D3470 Intentional replantation (including necessary splinting) Ⓑ   B

For the intentional removal, inspection and treatment of the root and replacement of a tooth into its own socket. This does not include necessary retrograde filling material placement.

D3471 Surgical repair of root resorption – anterior   B

For surgery on root of anterior tooth. Does not include placement of restoration.

D3472 Surgical repair of root resorption – premolar   B

For surgery on root of premolar tooth. Does not include placement of restoration.

D3473 Surgical repair of root resorption – molar   B

For surgery on root of molar tooth. Does not include placement of restoration.

D3501 Surgical exposure of root surface without apicoectomy or repair of root resorption – anterior B

Exposure of root surface followed by observation and surgical closure of the exposed area. Not to be used for or in conjunction with apicoectomy or repair of root resorption.

D3502 Surgical exposure of root surface without apicoectomy or repair of root resorption – premolar B

Exposure of root surface followed by observation and surgical closure of the exposed area. Not to be used for or in conjunction with apicoectomy or repair of root resorption.

D3503 Surgical exposure of root surface without apicoectomy or repair of root resorption – molar B

Exposure of root surface followed by observation and surgical closure of the exposed area. Not to be used for or in conjunction with apicoectomy or repair of root resorption.

Other Endodontic Procedures

D3910 Surgical procedure for isolation of tooth with rubber dam ⑧ B

D3911 Intraorifice barrier B

Not to be used as a final restoration.

D3920 Hemisection (including any root removal), not including root canal therapy ⑧ B

Includes separation of a multi-rooted tooth into separate sections containing the root and the overlying portion of the crown. It may also include the removal of one or more of those sections.

D3921 Decoronation or submergence of an erupted tooth

Intentional removal of coronal tooth structure for preservation of the root and surrounding bone.

D3950 Canal preparation and fitting of preformed dowel or post ⑧ B

Should not be reported in conjunction with D2952, D2953, D2954 or D2957 by the same practitioner.

None

D3999 Unspecified endodontic procedure, by report ⑧ S

Used for procedure that is not adequately described by a code. Describe procedure.

Periodontics (D4210-D4999)
Surgical Services (Including Usual Postoperative Care)

D4210 Gingivectomy or gingivoplasty - four or more contiguous teeth or tooth bounded spaces per quadrant ⑧ B

It is performed to eliminate suprabony pockets or to restore normal architecture when gingival enlargements or asymmetrical or unaesthetic topography is evident with normal bony configuration.

Cross Reference 41820

D4211 Gingivectomy or gingivoplasty - one to three contiguous teeth or tooth bounded spaces per quadrant ⑧ B

It is performed to eliminate suprabony pockets or to restore normal architecture when gingival enlargements or asymmetrical or unaesthetic topography is evident with normal bony configuration.

D4212 Gingivectomy or gingivoplasty to allow access for restorative procedure, per tooth ⑧ B

D4230 Anatomical crown exposure - four or more contiguous teeth or bounded tooth spaces per quadrant ⑧ B

This procedure is utilized in an otherwise periodontally healthy area to remove enlarged gingival tissue and supporting bone (ostectomy) to provide an anatomically correct gingival relationship.

D4231 Anatomical crown exposure - one to three teeth or bounded tooth spaces per quadrant ⑧ B

This procedure is utilized in an otherwise periodontally healthy area to remove enlarged gingival tissue and supporting bone (ostectomy) to provide an anatomically correct gingival relationship.

D4240 Gingival flap procedure, including root planing - four or more contiguous teeth or tooth bounded spaces per quadrant Ⓑ **B**

A soft tissue flap is reflected or resected to allow debridement of the root surface and the removal of granulation tissue. Osseous recontouring is not accomplished in conjunction with this procedure. May include open flap curettage, reverse bevel flap surgery, modified Kirkland flap procedure, and modified Widman surgery. This procedure is performed in the presence of moderate to deep probing depths, loss of attachment, need to maintain esthetics, need for increased access to the root surface and alveolar bone, or to determine the presence of a cracked tooth, fractured root, or external root resorption. Other procedures may be required concurrent to D4240 and should be reported separately using their own unique codes.

D4241 Gingival flap procedure, including root planing - one to three contiguous teeth or tooth bounded spaces per quadrant Ⓑ **B**

A soft tissue flap is reflected or resected to allow debridement of the root surface and the removal of granulation tissue. Osseous recontouring is not accomplished in conjunction with this procedure. May include open flap curettage, reverse bevel flap surgery, modified Kirkland flap procedure, and modified Widman surgery. This procedure is performed in the presence of moderate to deep probing depths, loss of attachment, need to maintain esthetics, need for increased access to the root surface and alveolar bone, or to determine the presence of a cracked tooth, fractured root, or external root resorption. Other procedures may be required concurrent to D4241 and should be reported separately using their own unique codes.

D4245 Apically positioned flap Ⓑ **B**

Procedure is used to preserve keratinized gingiva in conjunction with osseous resection and second stage implant procedure. Procedure may also be used to preserve keratinized/attached gingiva during surgical exposure of labially impacted teeth, and may be used during treatment of peri-implantitis.

D4249 Clinical crown lengthening - hard tissue Ⓑ **B**

This procedure is employed to allow a restorative procedure on a tooth with little or no tooth structure exposed to the oral cavity. Crown lengthening requires reflection of a full thickness flap and removal of bone, altering the crown to root ratio. It is performed in a healthy periodontal environment, as opposed to osseous surgery, which is performed in the presence of periodontal disease.

D4260 Osseous surgery (including elevation of a full thickness flap and closure) - four or more contiguous teeth or tooth bounded spaces per quadrant Ⓑ **S**

This procedure modifies the bony support of the teeth by reshaping the alveolar process to achieve a more physiologic form during the surgical procedure. This must include the removal of supporting bone (ostectomy) and/or non-supporting bone (osteoplasty). Other procedures may be required concurrent to D4260 and should be reported using their own unique codes.

D4261 Osseous surgery (including elevation of a full thickness flap and closure) - one to three contiguous teeth or tooth bounded spaces per quadrant Ⓑ **B**

This procedure modifies the bony support of the teeth by reshaping the alveolar process to achieve a more physiologic form during the surgical procedure. This must include the removal of supporting bone (ostectomy) and/or non-supporting bone (osteoplasty). Other procedures may be required concurrent to D4261 and should be reported using their own unique codes.

D4263 Bone replacement graft - retained natural tooth - first site in quadrant Ⓑ **S**

This procedure involves the use of grafts to stimulate periodontal regeneration when the disease process has led to a deformity of the bone. This procedure does not include flap entry and closure, wound debridement, osseous contouring, or the placement of biologic materials to aid in osseous tissue regeneration or barrier membranes. Other separate procedures delivered concurrently are documented with their own codes. Not to be reported for an edentulous space or an extraction site.

D4264 Bone replacement graft - retained natural tooth - each additional site in quadrant Ⓑ S

This procedure involves the use of grafts to stimulate periodontal regeneration when the disease process has led to a deformity of the bone. This procedure does not include flap entry and closure, wound debridement, osseous contouring, or the placement of biologic materials to aid in osseous tissue regeneration or barrier membranes. This procedure is performed concurrently with one or more bone replacement grafts to document the number of sites involved. Not to be reported for an edentulous space or an extraction site.

D4265 Biologic materials to aid in soft and osseous tissue regeneration, per site Ⓑ B

Biologic materials may be used alone or with other regenerative substrates such as bone and barrier membranes, depending upon their formulation and the presentation of the periodontal defect. This procedure does not include surgical entry and closure, wound debridement, osseous contouring, or the placement of graft materials and/or barrier membranes. Other separate procedures may be required concurrent to D4265 and should be reported using their own unique codes.

D4266 Guided tissue regeneration - resorbable barrier, per site Ⓑ B

This procedure does not include flap entry and closure, or, when indicated, wound debridement, osseous contouring, bone replacement grafts, and placement of biologic materials to aid in osseous regeneration. This procedure can be used for periodontal defects around natural teeth.

D4267 Guided tissue regeneration - nonresorbable barrier, per site, (includes membrane removal) Ⓑ B

This procedure does not include flap entry and closure, or, when indicated, wound debridement, osseous contouring, bone replacement grafts, and placement of biologic materials to aid in osseous regeneration. This procedure can be used for periodontal defects around natural teeth.

D4268 Surgical revision procedure, per tooth Ⓑ S

This procedure is to refine the results of a previously provided surgical procedure. This may require a surgical procedure to modify the irregular contours of hard or soft tissue. A mucoperiosteal flap may be elevated to allow access to reshape alveolar bone. The flaps are replaced or repositioned and sutured.

D4270 Pedicle soft tissue graft procedure Ⓑ S

A pedicle flap of gingiva can be raised from an edentulous ridge, adjacent teeth, or from the existing gingiva on the tooth and moved laterally or coronally to replace alveolar mucosa as marginal tissue. The procedure can be used to cover an exposed root or to eliminate a gingival defect if the root is not too prominent in the arch.

D4273 Autogenous connective tissue graft procedure (including donor and recipient surgical sites) first tooth, implant, or edentulous tooth position in graft Ⓑ S

There are two surgical sites. The recipient site utilizes a split thickness incision, retaining the overlapping flap of gingiva and/or mucosa. The connective tissue is dissected from a separate donor site leaving an epithelialized flap for closure.

D4274 Mesial/distal wedge procedure, single tooth (when not performed in conjuction with surgical procedures in the same anatomical area) Ⓑ B

This procedure is performed in an edentulous area adjacent to a tooth, allowing removal of a tissue wedge to gain access for debridement, permit close flap adaptation, and reduce pocket depths.

D4275 Non-autogenous connective tissue graft (including recipient site and donor material) first tooth, implant, or edentulous tooth position in graft Ⓑ B

There is only a recipient surgical site utilizing split thickness incision, retaining the overlaying flap of gingiva and/or mucosa. A donor surgical site is not present.

D4276 Combined connective tissue and pedicle graft, per tooth Ⓑ B

Advanced gingival recession often cannot be corrected with a single procedure. Combined tissue grafting procedures are needed to achieve the desired outcome.

D4277 Free soft tissue graft procedure (including recipient and donor surgical sites) first tooth, implant or edentulous tooth position in graft Ⓑ B

🔧 MIPS	Qp Quantity Physician	Qh Quantity Hospital	♀ Female only
♂ Male only	A Age	⅙ DMEPOS	A2-Z3 ASC Payment Indicator	A-Y ASC Status Indicator	Coding Clinic

DENTAL PROCEDURES D4264 — D4277

181

D4278 Free soft tissue graft procedure (including recipient and donor surgical sites) each additional contiguous tooth, implant or edentulous tooth position in same graft site ⑧   B

Used in conjunction with D4277.

D4283 Autogenous connective tissue graft procedure (including donor and recipient surgical sites) - each additional contiguous tooth, implant or edentulous tooth position in same graft site ⑧   B

Used in conjunction with D4273.

D4285 Non-autogenous connective tissue graft procedure (including recipient surgical site and donor material) - each additional contiguous tooth, implant or edentulous tooth position in same graft site ⑧   B

Used in conjunction with D4275.

D4286 Removal of non-resorbable barrier ⑧   B

Non-Surgical Periodontal Services

D4322 Splint – intra-coronal; natural teeth or prosthetic crowns   B

Additional procedure that physically links individual teeth or prosthetic crowns to provide stabilization and additional strength.

D4323 Splint – extra-coronal; natural teeth or prosthetic crowns   B

Additional procedure that physically links individual teeth or prosthetic crowns to provide stabilization and additional strength.

D4341 Periodontal scaling and root planing - four or more teeth per quadrant ⑧   B

This procedure involves instrumentation of the crown and root surfaces of the teeth to remove plaque and calculus from these surfaces. It is indicated for patients with periodontal disease and is therapeutic, not prophylactic, in nature. Root planing is the definitive procedure designed for the removal of cementum and dentin that is rough, and/or permeated by calculus or contaminated with toxins or microorganisms. Some soft tissue removal occurs. This procedure may be used as a definitive treatment in some stages of periodontal disease and/or as a part of pre-surgical procedures in others.

D4342 Periodontal scaling and root planing - one to three teeth, per quadrant ⑧   B

This procedure involves instrumentation of the crown and root surfaces of the teeth to remove plaque and calculus from these surfaces. It is indicated for patients with periodontal disease and is therapeutic, not prophylactic, in nature. Root planing is the definitive procedure designed for the removal of cementum and dentin that is rough, and/or permeated by calculus or contaminated with toxins or microorganisms. Some soft tissue removal occurs. This procedure may be used as a definitive treatment in some stages of periodontal disease and/or as a part of pre-surgical procedures in others.

D4346 Scaling in presence of generalized moderate or severe gingival inflammation - full mouth, after oral evaluation ⑧   B

The removal of plaque, calculus and stains from supra- and sub-gingival tooth surfaces when there is generalized moderate or severe gingival inflammation in the absence of periodontitis. It is indicated for patients who have swollen, inflamed gingiva, generalized suprabony pockets, and moderate to severe bleeding on probing. Should not be reported in conjunction with prophylaxis, scaling and root planing, or debridement procedures.

D4355 Full mouth debridement to enable a comprehensive periodontal evaluation and diagnosis on a subsequent visit ⑧ S

Full mouth debridement involves the preliminary removal of plaque and calculus that interferes with the ability of the dentist to perform a comprehensive oral evaluation. Not to be completed on the same day as D0150, D0160, or D0180.

D4381 Localized delivery of antimicrobial agents via a controlled release vehicle into diseased crevicular tissue, per tooth ⑧   S

FDA approved subgingival delivery devices containing antimicrobial medication(s) are inserted into periodontal pockets to suppress the pathogenic microbiota. These devices slowly release the pharmacological agents so they can remain at the intended site of action in a therapeutic concentration for a sufficient length of time.

▶ New   ↩ Revised   ✔ Reinstated   ~~deleted~~ Deleted   ⊘ Not covered or valid by Medicare

✿ Special coverage instructions   ✳ Carrier discretion   ⑧ Bill Part B MAC   ⑩ Bill DME MAC

Other Periodontal Services

D4910 Periodontal maintenance ⓑ   B

This procedure is instituted following periodontal therapy and continues at varying intervals, determined by the clinical evaluation of the dentist, for the life of the dentition or any implant replacements. It includes removal of the bacterial plaque and calculus from supragingival and subgingival regions, site specific scaling and root planing where indicated, and polishing the teeth. If new or recurring periodontal disease appears, additional diagnostic and treatment procedures must be considered.

D4920 Unscheduled dressing change (by someone other than treating dentist or their staff) ⓑ   B

D4921 Gingival irrigation with a medicinal agent - per quadrant ⓑ   B

Irrigation of gingival pockets with medicinal agent. Not to be used to report use of mouth rinses or non-invasive chemical debridement.

None

D4999 Unspecified periodontal procedure, by report ⓑ   B

Use for procedure that is not adequately described by a code. Describe procedure.

Prosthodontics (removable)
Complete Dentures (Including Routine Post-Delivery Care)

D5110 Complete denture - maxillary ⓑ   B

D5120 Complete denture - mandibular ⓑ   B

D5130 Immediate denture - maxillary ⓑ   B

Includes limited follow-up care only; does not include required future rebasing/relining procedure(s).

D5140 Immediate denture - mandibular ⓑ   B

Includes limited follow-up care only; does not include required future rebasing/relining procedure(s).

Partial Dentures (Including Routine Post-Delivery Care)

D5211 Maxillary partial denture-resin base (including retentive/clasping materials, rests and teeth) ⓑ   B

Includes acrylic resin base denture with resin or wrought wire clasps.

D5212 Mandibular partial denture-resin base (including, retentive/clasping materials, rests and teeth) ⓑ   B

Includes acrylic resin base denture with resin or wrought wire clasps.

D5213 Maxillary partial denture - cast metal framework with resin denture bases (including retentive/clasping materials, rests and teeth) ⓑ

D5214 Mandibular partial denture - cast metal framework with resin denture bases (including retentive/clasping materials, rests and teeth) ⓑ   B

D5221 Immediate maxillary partial denture - resin base (including retentive/clasping materials, rests and teeth) ⓑ   B

Includes limited follow-up care only; does not include future rebasing/relining procedure(s).

D5222 Immediate mandibular partial denture - resin base (including retentive/clasping materials, rests and teeth) ⓑ   B

Includes limited follow-up care only; does not include future rebasing/relining procedure(s).

D5223 Immediate maxillary partial denture - cast metal framework with resin denture bases (including retentive/clasping materials, rests and teeth) ⓑ   B

Includes limited follow-up care only; does not include future rebasing/relining procedure(s).

D5224 Immediate mandibular partial denture - cast metal framework with resin denture bases (including retentive/clasping materials, rests and teeth) ⓑ   B

Includes limited follow-up care only; does not include future rebasing/relining procedure(s).

D5225 Maxillary partial denture - flexible base (including retentive/clasping materials, rests and teeth) ⓑ   B

D5226 Mandibular partial denture - flexible base (including retentive/clasping materials, rests and teeth) ⓑ   B

D5227 Immediate maxillary partial denture - flexible base (including any clasps, rests and teeth)   B

D5228 Immediate mandibular partial denture - flexible base (including any clasps, rests and teeth)   B

D5282 Removable unilateral partial denture - one piece cast metal (including retentive/clasping materials, and teeth), maxillary ⓑ   B

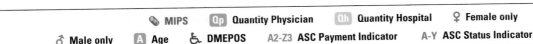

D5283 Removable unilateral partial denture - one piece cast metal (including retentive/clasping materials, rests, and teeth), mandibular Ⓑ   B

D5284 Removable unilateral partial denture - one piece flexible base (including retentive/clasping materials, rests, rests, and teeth) - per quadrant   B

D5286 Removable unilateral partial denture - one piece resin (including retentive/clasping materials, rests, and teeth) - per quadrant   B

Adjustment to Dentures

D5410 Adjust complete denture - maxillary Ⓑ   B

D5411 Adjust complete denture - mandibular Ⓑ   B

D5421 Adjust partial denture - maxillary Ⓑ   B

D5422 Adjust partial denture - mandibular Ⓑ   B

Repairs to Complete Dentures

D5511 Repair broken complete denture base, mandibular Ⓑ   B

D5512 Repair broken complete denture base, maxillary Ⓑ   B

D5520 Replace missing or broken teeth- complete denture (each tooth) Ⓑ   B

Repairs to Partial Dentures

D5611 Repair resin partial denture base, mandibular Ⓑ   B

D5612 Repair resin partial denture base, maxillary Ⓑ   B

D5621 Repair cast partial framework, mandibular Ⓑ   B

D5622 Repair cast partial framework, maxillary Ⓑ   B

D5630 Repair or replace broken, retentive clasping materials - per tooth Ⓑ   B

D5640 Replace broken teeth - per tooth Ⓑ   B

D5650 Add tooth to existing partial denture Ⓑ   B

D5660 Add clasp to existing partial denture - per tooth Ⓑ   B

D5670 Replace all teeth and acrylic on cast metal framework (maxillary) Ⓑ   B

D5671 Replace all teeth and acrylic on cast metal framework (mandibular) Ⓑ   B

Denture Rebase Procedures

D5710 Rebase complete maxillary denture Ⓑ   B

D5711 Rebase complete mandibular denture Ⓑ   B

D5720 Rebase maxillary partial denture Ⓑ   B

D5721 Rebase mandibular partial denture Ⓑ   B

D5725 Rebase hybrid prosthesis   B

Replacing the base material connected to the framework.

Denture Reline Procedures

D5730 Reline complete maxillary denture (direct) Ⓑ   B

D5731 Reline lower complete mandibular denture (direct) Ⓑ   B

D5740 Reline maxillary partial denture (direct) Ⓑ   B

D5741 Reline mandibular partial denture (direct) Ⓑ   B

D5750 Reline complete maxillary denture (indirect) Ⓑ   B

D5751 Reline complete mandibular denture (indirect) Ⓑ   B

D5760 Reline maxillary partial denture (indirect) Ⓑ   B

D5761 Reline mandibular partial denture (indirect) Ⓑ   B

D5765 Soft liner for complete or partial removable denture – indirect   B

A discrete procedure provided when the dentist determines placement of the soft liner is clinically indicated.

Interim Prosthesis

D5810 Interim complete denture (maxillary) Ⓑ   B

D5811 Interim complete denture (mandibular) Ⓑ   B

D5820 Interim partial denture (including retentive/clasping materials, rests, and teeth), maxillary Ⓑ   B

D5821 Interim partial denture (including retentive/clasping materials, rests, and teeth), mandibular Ⓑ   B

▶ New   ↻ Revised   ✔ Reinstated   deleted Deleted   ⊘ Not covered or valid by Medicare

⊛ Special coverage instructions   ✳ Carrier discretion   Ⓑ Bill Part B MAC   Ⓑ Bill DME MAC

Other Removable Prosthetic Services

D5850 Tissue conditioning, maxillary Ⓑ   B

Treatment reline using materials designed to heal unhealthy ridges prior to more definitive final restoration.

D5851 Tissue conditioning, mandibular Ⓑ   B

Treatment reline using materials designed to heal unhealthy ridges prior to more definitive final restoration.

D5862 Precision attachment, by report Ⓑ   B

Each pair of components is one precision attachment. Describe the type of attachment used.

D5863 Overdenture - complete maxillary Ⓑ   B

D5864 Overdenture - partial maxillary Ⓑ   B

D5865 Overdenture - complete mandibular Ⓑ   B

D5866 Overdenture - partial mandibular Ⓑ   B

D5867 Replacement of replaceable part of semi-precision or precision attachment, per attachment Ⓑ   B

D5875 Modification of removable prosthesis following implant surgery Ⓑ   B

Attachment assemblies are reported using separate codes.

↻ **D5876** Add metal substructure to acrylic full denture (per arch) Ⓑ   B

Use of metal substructure in removable complete dentures without a framework.

None

D5899 Unspecified removable prosthodontic procedure, by report Ⓑ   B

Use for a procedure that is not adequately described by a code. Describe procedure.

Maxillofacial Prosthetics

D5911 Facial moulage (sectional) Ⓑ   S

A sectional facial moulage impression is a procedure used to record the soft tissue contours of a portion of the face. Occasionally several separate sectional impressions are made, then reassembled to provide a full facial contour cast. The impression is utilized to create a partial facial moulage and generally is not reusable.

D5912 Facial moulage (complete) Ⓑ   S

Synonymous terminology: facial impression, face mask impression. A complete facial moulage impression is a procedure used to record the soft tissue contours of the whole face. The impression is utilized to create a facial moulage and generally is not reusable.

D5913 Nasal prosthesis Ⓑ   B

Synonymous terminology: artificial nose. A removable prosthesis attached to the skin, which artificially restores part or all of the nose. Fabrication of a nasal prosthesis requires creation of an original mold. Additional prostheses usually can be made from the same mold, and assuming no further tissue changes occur, the same mold can be utilized for extended periods of time. When a new prosthesis is made from the existing mold, this procedure is termed a nasal prosthesis replacement.

Cross Reference 21087

D5914 Auricular prosthesis Ⓑ   B

Synonymous terminology: artificial ear, ear prosthesis. A removable prosthesis, which artificially restores part or all of the natural ear. Usually, replacement prostheses can be made from the original mold if tissue bed changes have not occurred. Creation of an auricular prosthesis requires fabrication of a mold, from which additional prostheses usually can be made, as needed later (auricular prosthesis, replacement).

Cross Reference 21086

D5915 Orbital prosthesis Ⓑ   B

A prosthesis, which artificially restores the eye, eyelids, and adjacent hard and soft tissue, lost as a result of trauma or surgery. Fabrication of an orbital prosthesis requires creation of an original mold. Additional prostheses usually can be made from the same mold, and assuming no further tissue changes occur, the same mold can be utilized for extended periods of time. When a new prosthesis is made from the existing mold, this procedure is termed an orbital prosthesis replacement.

Cross Reference L8611

🐾 MIPS   Qp Quantity Physician   Qh Quantity Hospital   ♀ Female only   ♂ Male only   A Age   ♿ DMEPOS   A2-Z3 ASC Payment Indicator   A-Y ASC Status Indicator   Coding Clinic

D5916   Ocular prosthesis ⑧   B

Synonymous terminology: artificial eye, glass eye. A prosthesis, which artificially replaces an eye missing as a result of trauma, surgery or congenital absence. The prosthesis does not replace missing eyelids or adjacent skin, mucosa or muscle. Ocular prostheses require semiannual or annual cleaning and polishing. Also, occasional revisions to re-adapt the prosthesis to the tissue bed may be necessary. Glass eyes are rarely made and cannot be re-adapted.

Cross Reference V2623, V2629

D5919   Facial prosthesis ⑧   B

Synonymous terminology: prosthetic dressing. A removable prosthesis, which artificially replaces a portion of the face, lost due to surgery, trauma or congenital absence. Flexion of natural tissues may preclude adaptation and movement of the prosthesis to match the adjacent skin. Salivary leakage, when communicating with the oral cavity, adversely affects retention.

Cross Reference 21088

D5922   Nasal septal prosthesis ⑧   B

Synonymous terminology: septal plug, septal button. Removable prosthesis to occlude (obturate) a hole within the nasal septal wall. Adverse chemical degradation in this moist environment may require frequent replacement. Silicone prostheses are occasionally subject to fungal invasion.

Cross Reference 30220

D5923   Ocular prosthesis, interim ⑧   B

Synonymous terminology: eye shell, shell, ocular conformer, conformer. A temporary replacement generally made of clear acrylic resin for an eye lost due to surgery or trauma. No attempt is made to re-establish aesthetics. Fabrication of an interim ocular prosthesis generally implies subsequent fabrication of an aesthetic ocular prosthesis.

Cross Reference 92330

D5924   Cranial prosthesis ⑧   B

Synonymous terminology: skull plate, cranioplasty prosthesis, cranial implant. A biocompatible, permanently implanted replacement of a portion of the skull bones; an artificial replacement for a portion of the skull bone.

Cross Reference 62143

D5925   Facial augmentation implant prosthesis ⑧   B

Synonymous terminology: facial implant. An implantable biocompatible material generally onlayed upon an existing bony area beneath the skin tissue to fill in or collectively raise portions of the overlaying facial skin tissues to create acceptable contours. Although some forms of pre-made surgical implants are commercially available, the facial augmentation is usually custom made for surgical implantation for each individual patient due to the irregular or extensive nature of the facial deficit.

Cross Reference 21208

D5926   Nasal prosthesis, replacement ⑧   B

Synonymous terminology: replacement nose. An artificial nose produced from a previously made mold. A replacement prosthesis does not require fabrication of a new mold. Generally, several prostheses can be made from the same mold assuming no changes occur in the tissue bed due to surgery or age related topographical variations.

Cross Reference 21087

D5927   Auricular prosthesis, replacement ⑧   B

Synonymous terminology: replacement ear. An artificial ear produced from a previously made mold. A replacement prosthesis does not require fabrication of a new mold. Generally, several prostheses can be made from the same mold assuming no changes occur in the tissue bed due to surgery or age related topographical variations.

Cross Reference 21086

▶ **New**   ↻ **Revised**   ✔ **Reinstated**   ~~deleted~~ **Deleted**   ⊘ **Not covered or valid by Medicare**   ✪ **Special coverage instructions**   ✳ **Carrier discretion**   ⑧ **Bill Part B MAC**   ⑧ **Bill DME MAC**

D5928   Orbital prosthesis, replacement ⓑ   **B**

A replacement for a previously made orbital prosthesis. A replacement prosthesis does not require fabrication of a new mold. Generally, several prostheses can be made from the same mold assuming no changes occur in the tissue bed due to surgery or age related topographical variations.

Cross Reference 67550

D5929   Facial prosthesis, replacement ⓑ   **B**

A replacement facial prosthesis made from the original mold. A replacement prosthesis does not require fabrication of a new mold. Generally, several prostheses can be made from the same mold assuming no changes occur in the tissue bed due to further surgery or age related topographical variations.

Cross Reference 21088

D5931   Obturator prosthesis, surgical ⓑ   **B**

Synonymous terminology: obturator, surgical stayplate, immediate temporary obturator. A temporary prosthesis inserted during or immediately following surgical or traumatic loss of a portion or all of one or both maxillary bones and contiguous alveolar structures (e.g., gingival tissue, teeth). Frequent revisions of surgical obturators are necessary during the ensuing healing phase (approximately six months). Some dentists prefer to replace many or all teeth removed by the surgical procedure in the surgical obturator, while others do not replace any teeth. Further surgical revisions may require fabrication of another surgical obturator (e.g., an initially planned small defect may be revised and greatly enlarged after the final pathology report indicates margins are not free of tumor).

Cross Reference 21079

D5932   Obturator prosthesis, definitive ⓑ   **B**

Synonymous terminology: obturator. A prosthesis, which artificially replaces part or all of the maxilla and associated teeth, lost due to surgery, trauma or congenital defects. A definitive obturator is made when it is deemed that further tissue changes or recurrence of tumor are unlikely and a more permanent prosthetic rehabilitation can be achieved; it is intended for long-term use.

Cross Reference 21080

D5933   Obturator prosthesis, modification ⓑ   **B**

Synonymous terminology: adjustment, denture adjustment, temporary or office reline. Revision or alteration of an existing obturator (surgical, interim, or definitive); possible modifications include relief of the denture base due to tissue compression, augmentation of the seal or peripheral areas to affect adequate sealing or separation between the nasal and oral cavities.

Cross Reference 21080

D5934   Mandibular resection prosthesis with guide flange ⓑ   **B**

Synonymous terminology: resection device, resection appliance. A prosthesis which guides the remaining portion of the mandible, left after a partial resection, into a more normal relationship with the maxilla. This allows for some tooth-to-tooth or an improved tooth contact. It may also artificially replace missing teeth and thereby increase masticatory efficiency.

Cross Reference 21081

D5935   Mandibular resection prosthesis without guide flange ⓑ   **B**

A prosthesis which helps guide the partially resected mandible to a more normal relation with the maxilla allowing for increased tooth contact. It does not have a flange or ramp, however, to assist in directional closure. It may replace missing teeth and thereby increase masticatory efficiency. Dentists who treat mandibulectomy patients may prefer to replace some, all or none of the teeth in the defect area. Frequently, the defect's margins preclude even partial replacement. Use of a guide (a mandibular resection prosthesis with a guide flange) may not be possible due to anatomical limitations or poor patient tolerance. Ramps, extended occlusal arrangements and irregular occlusal positioning relative to the denture foundation frequently preclude stability of the prostheses, and thus some prostheses are poorly tolerated under such adverse circumstances.

Cross Reference 21081

D5936 Obturator/prosthesis, interim ⓑ   B

Synonymous terminology: immediate postoperative obturator. A prosthesis which is made following completion of the initial healing after a surgical resection of a portion or all of one or both the maxillae; frequently many or all teeth in the defect area are replaced by this prosthesis. This prosthesis replaces the surgical obturator, which is usually inserted at, or immediately following the resection.

Generally, an interim obturator is made to facilitate closure of the resultant defect after initial healing has been completed. Unlike the surgical obturator, which usually is made prior to surgery and frequently revised in the operating room during surgery, the interim obturator is made when the defect margins are clearly defined and further surgical revisions are not planned. It is a provisional prosthesis, which may replace some or all lost teeth, and other lost bone and soft tissue structures. Also, it frequently must be revised (termed an obturator prosthesis modification) during subsequent dental procedures (e.g., restorations, gingival surgery) as well as to compensate for further tissue shrinkage before a definitive obturator prosthesis is made.

Cross Reference 21079

D5937 Trismus appliance (not for tm treatment) ⓑ   B

Synonymous terminology: occlusal device for mandibular trismus, dynamic bite opener. A prosthesis, which assists the patient in increasing their oral aperture width in order to eat as well as maintain oral hygiene. Several versions and designs are possible, all intending to ease the severe lack of oral opening experienced by many patients immediately following extensive intraoral surgical procedures.

D5951 Feeding aid ⓑ   B

Synonymous terminology: feeding prosthesis. A prosthesis, which maintains the right and left maxillary segments of an infant cleft palate patient in their proper orientation until surgery is performed to repair the cleft. It closes the oral-nasal cavity defect, thus enhancing sucking and swallowing. Used on an interim basis, this prosthesis achieves separation of the oral and nasal cavities in infants born with wide clefts necessitating delayed closure. It is eliminated if surgical closure can be affected or, alternatively, with eruption of the deciduous dentition a pediatric speech aid may be made to facilitate closure of the defect.

D5952 Speech aid prosthesis, pediatric ⓑ Ⓐ B

Synonymous terminology: nasopharyngeal obturator, speech appliance, obturator, cleft palate appliance, prosthetic speech aid, speech bulb. A temporary or interim prosthesis used to close a defect in the hard and/ or soft palate. It may replace tissue lost due to developmental or surgical alterations. It is necessary for the production of intelligible speech. Normal lateral growth of the palatal bones necessitates occasional replacement of this prosthesis. Intermittent revisions of the obturator section can assist in maintenance of palatalpharyngeal closure (termed a speech aid prosthesis modification). Frequently, such prostheses are not fabricated before the deciduous dentition is fully erupted since clasp retention is often essential.

Cross Reference 21084

D5953 Speech aid prosthesis, adult ⒼＡ B

Synonymous terminology: prosthetic speech appliance, speech aid, speech bulb. A definitive prosthesis, which can improve speech in adult cleft palate patients either by obturating (sealing off) a palatal cleft or fistula, or occasionally by assisting an incompetent soft palate. Both mechanisms are necessary to achieve velopharyngeal competency. Generally, this prosthesis is fabricated when no further growth is anticipated and the objective is to achieve long-term use. Hence, more precise materials and techniques are utilized. Occasionally such procedures are accomplished in conjunction with precision attachments in crown work undertaken on some or all maxillary teeth to achieve improved aesthetics.

Cross Reference 21084

D5954 Palatal augmentation prosthesis Ⓑ B

Synonymous terminology: superimposed prosthesis, maxillary glossectomy prosthesis, maxillary speech prosthesis, palatal drop prosthesis. A removable prosthesis which alters the hard and/or soft palate's topographical form adjacent to the tongue.

Cross Reference 21082

D5955 Palatal lift prosthesis, definitive Ⓑ B

A prosthesis which elevates the soft palate superiorly and aids in restoration of soft palate functions which may be lost due to an acquired, congenital or developmental defect. A definitive palatal lift is usually made for patients whose experience with an interim palatal lift has been successful, especially if surgical alterations are deemed unwarranted.

Cross Reference 21083

D5958 Palatal lift prosthesis, interim Ⓑ B

Synonymous terminology: diagnostic palatal lift. A prosthesis which elevates and assists in restoring soft palate function which may be lost due to clefting, surgery, trauma or unknown paralysis. It is intended for interim use to determine its usefulness in achieving palatalpharyngeal competency or enhance swallowing reflexes. This prosthesis is intended for interim use as a diagnostic aid to assess the level of possible improvement in speech intelligibility. Some clinicians believe use of a palatal lift on an interim basis may stimulate an otherwise flaccid soft palate to increase functional activity, subsequently lessening its need.

Cross Reference 21083

D5959 Palatal lift prosthesis, modification Ⓑ B

Synonymous terminology: revision of lift, adjustment. Alterations in the adaptation, contour, form or function of an existing palatal lift necessitated due to tissue impingement, lack of function, poor clasp adaptation or the like.

Cross Reference 21083

D5960 Speech aid prosthesis, modification Ⓑ B

Synonymous terminology: adjustment, repair, revision. Any revision of a pediatric or adult speech aid not necessitating its replacement. Frequently, revisions of the obturating section of any speech aid is required to facilitate enhanced speech intelligibility. Such revisions or repairs do not require complete remaking of the prosthesis, thus extending its longevity.

Cross Reference 21084

D5982 Surgical stent Ⓑ B

Synonymous terminology: periodontal stent, skin graft stent, columellar stent. Stents are utilized to apply pressure to soft tissues to facilitate healing and prevent cicatrization or collapse. A surgical stent may be required in surgical and post-surgical revisions to achieve close approximation of tissues. Usually such materials as temporary or interim soft denture liners, gutta percha, or dental modeling impression compound may be used.

Cross Reference 21085

D5983   Radiation carrier ⑧   S

Synonymous terminology: radiotherapy prosthesis, carrier prosthesis, radiation applicator, radium carrier, intracavity carrier, intracavity applicator. A device used to administer radiation to confined areas by means of capsules, beads or needles of radiation emitting materials such as radium or cesium. Its function is to hold the radiation source securely in the same location during the entire period of treatment. Radiation oncologists occasionally request these devices to achieve close approximation and controlled application of radiation to a tumor deemed amiable to eradication.

D5984   Radiation shield ⑧   S

Synonymous terminology: radiation stent, tongue protector, lead shield. An intraoral prosthesis designed to shield adjacent tissues from radiation during orthovoltage treatment of malignant lesions of the head and neck region.

D5985   Radiation cone locator ⑧   S

Synonymous terminology: docking device, cone locator. A prosthesis utilized to direct and reduplicate the path of radiation to an oral tumor during a split course of irradiation.

D5986   Fluoride gel carrier ⑧   B

Synonymous terminology: fluoride applicator. A prosthesis, which covers the teeth in either dental arch and is used to apply topical fluoride in close proximity to tooth enamel and dentin for several minutes daily.

D5987   Commissure splint ⑧   S

Synonymous terminology: lip splint. A device placed between the lips, which assists in achieving increased opening between the lips. Use of such devices enhances opening where surgical, chemical or electrical alterations of the lips has resulted in severe restriction or contractures.

D5988   Surgical splint ⑧   B

Synonymous terminology: Gunning splint, modified Gunning splint, labiolingual splint, fenestrated splint, Kingsley splint, cast metal splint. Splints are designed to utilize existing teeth and/or alveolar processes as points of anchorage to assist in stabilization and immobilization of broken bones during healing. They are used to re-establish, as much as possible, normal occlusal relationships during the process of immobilization. Frequently, existing prostheses (e.g., a patient's complete dentures) can be modified to serve as surgical splints. Frequently, surgical splints have arch bars added to facilitate intermaxillary fixation. Rubber elastics may be used to assist in this process. Circummandibular eyelet hooks can be utilized for enhanced stabilization with wiring to adjacent bone.

D5991   Vesicobullous disease medicament carrier ⑧   B

A custom fabricated carrier that covers the teeth and alveolar mucosa, or alveolar mucosa alone, and is used to deliver prescription medicaments for treatment of immunologically mediated vesiculobullous disease.

D5992   Adjust maxillofacial prosthetic appliance, by report ⑧   B

D5993   Maintenance and cleaning of a maxillofacial prosthesis (extra or intra-oral) other than required adjustments, by report ⑧   B

D5995   Periodontal medicament carrier with peripheral seal – laboratory processed – maxillary

A custom fabricated, laboratory processed carrier for the maxillary arch that covers the teeth and alveolar mucosa. Used as a vehicle to deliver prescribed medicaments for sustained contact with the gingiva, alveolar mucosa, and into the periodontal sulcus or pocket.

▶ New	↻ Revised	✔ Reinstated	~~deleted~~ Deleted	⊘ Not covered or valid by Medicare
✷ Special coverage instructions		✳ Carrier discretion	⑧ Bill Part B MAC	⑧ Bill DME MAC

D5996 Periodontal medicament carrier with peripheral seal – laboratory processed – mandibular

A custom fabricated, laboratory processed carrier for the mandibular arch that covers the teeth and alveolar mucosa. Used as a vehicle to deliver prescribed medicaments for sustained contact with the gingiva, alveolar mucosa, and into the periodontal sulcus or pocket.

D5999 Unspecified maxillofacial prosthesis, by report Ⓑ   **B**

Used for procedure that is not adequately described by a code. Describe procedure.

Implant Services (D6010-D6199)

D6010-D6199: FPD = fixed partial denture

Surgical Services

D6010 Surgical placement of implant body: endosteal implant Ⓑ   **B**

Cross Reference 21248

D6011 Surgical access to an implant body (second stage implant surgery) Ⓑ   **B**

This procedure, also known as second stage implant surgery, involves removal of tissue that covers the implant body so that a fixture of any type can be placed, or an existing fixture be replaced with another. Examples of fixtures include but are not limited to healing caps, abutments shaped to help contour the gingival margins or the final restorative prosthesis.

D6012 Surgical placement of interim implant body for transitional prosthesis: endosteal implant Ⓑ   **B**

D6013 Surgical placement of mini implant Ⓑ   **B**

D6040 Surgical placement: eposteal implant Ⓑ   **B**

An eposteal (subperiosteal) framework of a biocompatible material designed and fabricated to fit on the surface of the bone of the mandible or maxilla with permucosal extensions which provide support and attachment of a prosthesis. This may be a complete arch or unilateral appliance. Eposteal implants rest upon the bone and under the periosteum.

Cross Reference 21245

D6050 Surgical placement: transosteal implant Ⓑ   **B**

A transosteal (transosseous) biocompatible device with threaded posts penetrating both the superior and inferior cortical bone plates of the mandibular symphysis and exiting through the permucosa providing support and attachment for a dental prosthesis. Transosteal implants are placed completely through the bone and into the oral cavity from extraoral or intraoral.

Cross Reference 21244

Implant Supported Prosthetics

D6051 Interim abutment placement implant Ⓑ   **B**

A healing cap is not an interim abutment.

D6055 Connecting bar — implant supported or abutment supported Ⓑ   **B**

Utilized to stabilize and anchor a prosthesis.

D6056 Prefabricated abutment - includes modification and placement Ⓑ   **B**

Modification of a prefabricated abutment may be necessary.

D6057 Custom fabricated abutment - includes placement Ⓑ   **B**

Created by a laboratory process, specific for an individual application.

D6058 Abutment supported porcelain/ceramic crown Ⓑ   **B**

A single crown restoration that is retained, supported and stabilized by an abutment on an implant.

D6059 Abutment supported porcelain fused to metal crown (high noble metal) Ⓑ   **B**

A single metal-ceramic crown restoration that is retained, supported and stabilized by an abutment on an implant.

D6060 Abutment supported porcelain fused to metal crown (predominantly base metal) Ⓑ   **B**

A single metal-ceramic crown restoration that is retained, supported and stabilized by an abutment on an implant.

🐾 MIPS	𝗤𝗽 Quantity Physician	𝗤𝗵 Quantity Hospital	♀ Female only
♂ Male only Ⓐ Age ⅛ DMEPOS	A2-Z3 ASC Payment Indicator	A-Y ASC Status Indicator	Coding Clinic

DENTAL PROCEDURES   D5996 – D6060

191

D6061 Abutment supported porcelain fused to metal crown (noble metal) ⑬   **B**

A single metal-ceramic crown restoration that is retained, supported and stabilized by an abutment on an implant.

D6062 Abutment supported cast metal crown (high noble metal) ⑬   **B**

A single cast metal crown restoration that is retained, supported and stabilized by an abutment on an implant.

D6063 Abutment supported cast metal crown (predominantly base metal) ⑬   **B**

A single cast metal crown restoration that is retained, supported and stabilized by an abutment on an implant.

D6064 Abutment supported cast metal crown (noble metal) ⑬   **B**

A single cast metal crown restoration that is retained, supported and stabilized by an abutment on an implant.

D6065 Implant supported porcelain/ceramic crown ⑬   **B**

A single crown restoration that is retained, supported and stabilized by an implant.

D6066 Implant supported crown - porcelain fused to high noble alloys ⑬   **B**

A single metal-ceramic crown restoration that is retained, supported and stabilized by an implant.

D6067 Implant supported crown - high noble alloys ⑬   **B**

A single cast metal or milled crown restoration that is retained, supported and stabilized by an implant.

D6068 Abutment supported retainer for porcelain/ceramic FPD ⑬   **B**

A ceramic retainer for a fixed partial denture that gains retention, support and stability from an abutment on an implant.

D6069 Abutment supported retainer for porcelain fused to metal FPD (high noble metal) ⑬   **B**

A metal-ceramic retainer for a fixed partial denture that gains retention, support and stability from an abutment on an implant.

D6070 Abutment supported retainer for porcelain fused to metal FPD (predominantly base metal) ⑬   **B**

A metal-ceramic retainer for a fixed partial denture that gains retention, support and stability from an abutment on an implant.

D6071 Abutment supported retainer for porcelain fused to metal FPD (noble metal) ⑬   **B**

A metal-ceramic retainer for a fixed partial denture that gains retention, support and stability from an abutment on an implant.

D6072 Abutment supported retainer for cast metal FPD (high noble metal) ⑬   **B**

A cast metal retainer for a fixed partial denture that gains retention, support and stability from an abutment on an implant.

D6073 Abutment supported retainer for cast metal FPD (predominantly base metal) ⑬   **B**

A cast metal retainer for a fixed partial denture that gains retention, support and stability from an abutment on an implant.

D6074 Abutment supported retainer for cast metal FPD (noble metal) ⑬   **B**

A cast metal retainer for a fixed partial denture that gains retention, support and stability from an abutment on an implant.

D6075 Implant supported retainer for ceramic FPD ⑬   **B**

A ceramic retainer for a fixed partial denture that gains retention, support and stability from an implant.

D6076 Implant supported retainer for FPD - porcelain fused to high noble alloys ⑬   **B**

A metal-ceramic retainer for a fixed partial denture that gains retention, support and stability from an implant.

D6077 Implant supported retainer for metal FPD - high noble alloys ⑬   **B**

A cast metal retainer for a fixed partial denture that gains retention, support and stability from an implant.

▶ **New**   ⤺ **Revised**   ✓ **Reinstated**   ~~deleted~~ **Deleted**   ⊘ **Not covered or valid by Medicare**

⊛ **Special coverage instructions**   ✳ **Carrier discretion**   ⑬ **Bill Part B MAC**   Ⓖ **Bill DME MAC**

Other Implant Services

D6080 Implant maintenance procedures when prostheses are removed and reinserted, including cleansing of prostheses and abutments Ⓑ   B

This procedure includes active debriding of the implant(s) and examination of all aspects of the implant system(s), including the occlusion and stability of the superstructure. The patient is also instructed in thorough daily cleansing of the implant(s). This is not a per implant code, and is indicated for implant supported fixed prostheses.

D6081 Scaling and debridement in the presence of inflammation or mucositis of a single implant, including cleaning of the implant surfaces, without flap entry and closure Ⓑ   B

This procedure is not performed in conjunction with D1110, D4910, or D4346.

D6082 Implant supported crown - porcelain fused to predominantly base alloys   B

D6083 Implant supported crown - porcelain fused to noble alloys   B

D6084 Implant supported crown - porcelain fused to titanium and titanium alloys   B

D6085 Interim implant crown Ⓑ   B

Placed when a period of healing is necessary prior to fabrication and placement of definitive prosthetic.

D6086 Implant supported crown - predominantly base alloys   B

D6087 Implant supported crown - noble alloys   B

D6088 Implant supported crown - titanium and titanium alloys   B

▶ **D6089** Accessing and retorquing loose implant screw - per screw   B

D6090 Repair implant supported prosthesis by report Ⓑ   B

This procedure involves the repair or replacement of any part of the implant supported prosthesis.

Cross Reference 21299

D6091 Replacement of replaceable part of semi-precision or precision attachment of implant/abutment supported prosthesis, per attachment Ⓑ   B

D6092 Re-cement or re-bond implant/abutment supported crown Ⓑ   B

D6093 Re-cement or re-bond implant/abutment supported fixed partial denture Ⓑ   B

D6094 Abutment supported crown - titanium and titanium alloys Ⓑ   B

A single crown restoration that is retained, supported and stabilized by an abutment on an implant. May be cast or milled.

D6095 Repair implant abutment, by report Ⓑ   B

This procedure involves the repair or replacement of any part of the implant abutment.

Cross Reference 21299

D6096 Remove broken implant retaining screw Ⓑ   B

D6097 Abutment supported crown - porcelain fused to titanium and titanium alloys   B

A single metal-ceramic crown restoration that is retained, supported, and stabilized by an abutment on an implant.

D6098 Implant supported retainer - porcelain fused to predominantly base alloys   B

A metal-ceramic retainer for a fixed partial denture that gains retention, support, and stability from an implant.

D6099 Implant supported retainer for FPD - porcelain fused to noble alloys   B

A metal-ceramic retainer for a fixed partial denture that gains retention, support, and stability from an implant.

Surgical Services

D6100 Surgical removal, of implant body Ⓑ   B

Cross Reference 21299

D6101 Debridement of a peri-implant defect or defects surrounding a single implant, and surface cleaning of exposed implant surfaces, including flap entry and closure Ⓑ   B

D6102 Debridement and osseous contouring of a peri-implant defect or defects surrounding a single implant and includes surface cleaning of the exposed implant surfaces and flap entry and closure Ⓑ   B

D6103 Bone graft for repair of peri-implant defect - does not include flap entry and closure ⓑ B

Placement of a barrier membrane or biologic materials to aid in osseous regeneration, are reported separately.

D6104 Bone graft at time of implant placement ⓑ B

Placement of a barrier membrane, or biologic materials to aid in osseous regeneration are reported separately.

D6105 Removal of implant body not requiring bone removal or flap elevation ⓑ B

D6106 Guided tissue regeneration - resorbable barrier, per implant ⓑ B

This procedure does not include flap entry and closure, or, when indicated, wound debridement, osseous contouring, bone replacement grafts, and placement of biologic materials to aid in osseous regeneration. This procedure is used for peri-implant defects and during implant placement.

D6107 Guided tissue regeneration - non-resorbable barrier, per implant ⓑ B

This procedure does not include flap entry and closure, or, when indicated, wound debridement, osseous contouring, bone replacement grafts, and placement of biologic materials to aid in osseous regeneration. This procedure is used for peri-implant defects and during implant placement.

Implant Supported Prosthetics

D6110 Implant /abutment supported removable denture for edentulous arch - maxillary ⓑ B

D6111 Implant /abutment supported removable denture for edentulous arch - mandibular ⓑ B

D6112 Implant/abutment supported removable denture for partially edentulous arch - maxillary ⓑ B

D6113 Implant/abutment supported removable denture for partially edentulous arch - mandibular ⓑ B

D6114 Implant/abutment supported fixed denture for edentulous arch - maxillary ⓑ B

D6115 Implant/abutment supported fixed denture for edentulous arch - mandibular ⓑ B

D6116 Implant/abutment supported fixed denture for partially edentulous arch - maxillary ⓑ B

D6117 Implant/abutment supported fixed denture for partially edentulous arch - mandibular ⓑ B

D6118 Implant/abutment supported interim fixed denture for edentulous arch mandibular ⓑ B

Used when a period of healing is necessary prior to fabrication and placement of a permanent prosthetic.

D6119 Implant/abutment supported interim fixed denture for edentulous arch maxillary ⓑ B

Used when a period of healing is necessary prior to fabrication and placement of a permanent prosthetic.

D6120 Implant supported retainer - porcelain fused to titanium and titanium alloys B

A metal-ceramic retainer for a fixed partial denture that gains retention, support, and stability from an implant.

D6121 Implant supported retainer for metal FPD - predominantly base alloys B

A metal-ceramic retainer for a fixed partial denture that gains retention, support, and stability from an implant.

D6122 Implant supported retainer for metal FPD - noble alloys B

A metal retainer for a fixed partial denture that gains retention, support, and stability from an implant.

D6123 Implant supported retainer for metal FPD - titanium and titanum alloys B

A metal retainer for a fixed partial denture that gains retention, support, and stability from an implant.

D6190 Radiographic/surgical implant index, by report ⓑ B

An appliance, designed to relate osteotomy or fixture position to existing anatomic structures, to be utilized during radiographic exposure for treatment planning and/or during osteotomy creation for fixture installation.

D6191 Semi-precision abutment – placement B

This procedure is the initial placement, or replacement, of a semi-precision abutment on the implant body.

▶ **New**   ⟳ **Revised**   ✔ **Reinstated**   ~~deleted~~ **Deleted**   ⊘ **Not covered or valid by Medicare**
☼ **Special coverage instructions**   ✳ **Carrier discretion**   ⓑ **Bill Part B MAC**   ⓑ **Bill DME MAC**

D6192 Semi-precision attachment – placement B

This procedure involves the luting of the initial, or replacement, semi-precision attachment to the removable prosthesis.

D6194 Abutment supported retainer crown for FPD – titanium and titanium alloys ⓑ B

A retainer for a fixed partial denture that gains retention, support and stability from an abutment on an implant. May be cast or milled.

D6195 Abutment supported retainer - porcelain fused to titanium and titanium alloys B

A metal retainer for a fixed partial denture that gains retention, support, and stability from an implant.

D6197 Replacement of restorative material used to close an access opening of a screw-retained implant supported prosthesis, per implant B

D6198 Remove interim implant component B

Removal of implant component (e.g., interim abutment; provisional implant crown) originally placed for a specific clinical purpose and period of time determined by the dentist.

None

D6199 Unspecified implant procedure, by report ⓑ B

Use for procedure that is not adequately described by a code. Describe procedure.

Cross Reference 21299

Prosthodontics, fixed (D6205-D6999)
Fixed Partial Denture Pontics

D6205 Pontic - indirect resin based composite ⓑ B

Not to be used as a temporary or provisional prosthesis.

D6210 Pontic - cast high noble metal ⓑ B

D6211 Pontic - cast predominantly base metal ⓑ B

D6212 Pontic - cast noble metal ⓑ B

D6214 Pontic - titanium and titanium alloys ⓑ B

D6240 Pontic - porcelain fused to high noble metal ⓑ B

D6241 Pontic - porcelain fused to predominantly base metal ⓑ B

D6242 Pontic - porcelain fused to noble metal ⓑ B

IOM: 100-02, 15, 150

D6243 Pontic - porcelain fused to titanium and titanium alloys B

D6245 Pontic - porcelain/ceramic ⓑ B

D6250 Pontic - resin with high noble metal ⓑ B

D6251 Pontic - resin with predominantly base metal ⓑ B

D6252 Pontic - resin with noble metal ⓑ B

D6253 Interim pontic - further treatment or completion of diagnosis necessary prior to final impression ⓑ B

Not to be used as a temporary pontic for routine prosthetic restoration.

Fixed Partial Denture Retainers – Inlays/Onlays

D6545 Retainer - cast metal for resin bonded fixed prosthesis ⓑ B

D6548 Retainer - porcelain/ceramic for resin bonded fixed prosthesis ⓑ B

D6549 Retainer - for resin bonded fixed prosthesis ⓑ B

D6600 Retainer inlay - porcelain/ceramic, two surfaces ⓑ B

D6601 Retainer inlay - porcelain/ceramic, three or more surfaces ⓑ B

D6602 Retainer inlay - cast high noble metal, two surfaces ⓑ B

D6603 Retainer inlay - cast high noble metal, three or more surfaces ⓑ B

D6604 Retainer inlay - cast predominantly base metal, two surfaces ⓑ B

D6605 Retainer inlay - cast predominantly base metal, three or more surfaces ⓑ B

D6606 Retainer inlay - cast noble metal, two surfaces ⓑ B

D6607 Retainer inlay - cast noble metal, three or more surfaces ⓑ B

D6608 Retainer onlay - porcelain/ceramic, two surfaces ⓑ B

D6609 Retainer onlay - porcelain/ceramic, three or more surfaces ⓑ B

D6610 Retainer onlay - cast high noble metal, two surfaces ⓑ B

D6611 Retainer onlay - cast high noble metal, three or more surfaces ⓑ B

D6612 Retainer onlay - cast predominantly base metal, two surfaces ⓑ B

D6613 Retainer onlay - cast predominantly base metal, three or more surfaces ⓑ B

🐾 MIPS Qp Quantity Physician Qh Quantity Hospital ♀ Female only ♂ Male only A Age ♿ DMEPOS A2-Z3 ASC Payment Indicator A-Y ASC Status Indicator Coding Clinic

D6614 Retainer onlay - cast noble metal, two surfaces Ⓑ　　　B

D6615 Retainer onlay - cast noble metal, three or more surfaces Ⓑ　　　B

D6624 Retainer inlay - titanium Ⓑ　　　B

D6634 Retainer onlay - titanium Ⓑ　　　B

Fixed Partial Denture Retainers – Crowns

D6710 Retainer crown - indirect resin based composite Ⓑ　　　B

Not to be used as a temporary or provisional prosthesis.

D6720 Retainer crown - resin with high noble metal Ⓑ　　　B

D6721 Retainer crown - resin with predominantly base metal Ⓑ　　　B

D6722 Retainer crown - resin with noble metal Ⓑ　　　B

D6740 Retainer crown - porcelain/ceramic Ⓑ　　　B

D6750 Retainer crown - porcelain fused to high noble metal Ⓑ　　　B

D6751 Retainer crown - porcelain fused to predominantly base metal Ⓑ　　　B

D6752 Retainer crown - porcelain fused to noble metal Ⓑ　　　B

D6753 Retainer crown - porcelain fused to titanium and titanium alloys　　　B

D6780 Retainer crown - 3/4 cast high noble metal Ⓑ　　　B

D6781 Retainer crown - 3/4 cast predominantly based metal Ⓑ　　　B

D6782 Retainer crown - 3/4 cast noble metal Ⓑ　　　B

D6783 Retainer crown - 3/4 porcelain/ceramic Ⓑ　　　B

D6784 Retainer crown 3/4 - titanium and titanium alloys　　　B

D6790 Retainer crown - full cast high noble metal Ⓑ　　　B

D6791 Retainer crown - full cast predominantly base metal Ⓑ　　　B

D6792 Retainer crown - full cast noble metal Ⓑ　　　B

D6793 Interim retainer crown - further treatment or completion of diagnosis necessary prior to final impression Ⓑ　B

Not to be used as a temporary retainer crown for routine prosthetic restoration.

D6794 Retainer crown - titanium and titanium alloys Ⓑ　　　B

Other Fixed Partial Denture Services

D6920 Connector bar Ⓑ　　　S

A device attached to fixed partial denture retainer or coping which serves to stabilize and anchor a removable overdenture prosthesis.

D6930 Re-cement or re-bond fixed partial denture Ⓑ　　　B

D6940 Stress breaker Ⓑ　　　B

A non-rigid connector.

D6950 Precision attachment Ⓑ　　　B

A pair of components constitutes one precision attachment that is separate from the prosthesis.

D6980 Bridge repair necessitated by restorative material failure Ⓑ　　　B

D6985 Pediatric partial denture, fixed Ⓑ Ⓐ　　　B

This prosthesis is used primarily for aesthetic purposes.

None

D6999 Unspecified fixed prosthodontic procedure, by report Ⓑ　　　B

Used for procedure that is not adequately described by a code. Describe procedure.

Oral and Maxillofacial Surgery (D7111-D7999)
Extractions (Includes Local Anesthesia, Suturing, If Needed, and Routine Postoperative Care)

D7111 Extraction, coronal remnants - primary tooth Ⓑ　　　S

Removal of soft tissue-retained coronal remnants.

D7140 Extraction, erupted tooth or exposed root (elevation and/or forceps removal) Ⓑ　　　S

Includes removal of tooth structure, minor smoothing of socket bone, and closure, as necessary.

D7210 Extraction, erupted tooth requiring removal of bone and/or sectioning of tooth, and including elevation of mucoperiosteal flap if indicated Ⓑ　S

Includes related cutting of gingiva and bone, removal of tooth structure, minor smoothing of socket bone and closure.

D7220 Removal of impacted tooth - soft tissue Ⓑ　　　S

Occlusal surface of tooth covered by soft tissue; requires mucoperiosteal flap elevation.

▶ New　↻ Revised　✔ Reinstated　deleted Deleted　⊘ Not covered or valid by Medicare　✵ Special coverage instructions　✳ Carrier discretion　Ⓑ Bill Part B MAC　Ⓖ Bill DME MAC

D7230 Removal of impacted tooth - partially bony Ⓑ S

Part of crown covered by bone; requires mucoperiosteal flap elevation and bone removal.

D7240 Removal of impacted tooth - completely bony Ⓑ S

Most or all of crown covered by bone; requires mucoperiosteal flap elevation and bone removal.

D7241 Removal of impacted tooth - completely bony, with unusual surgical complications Ⓑ S

Most or all of crown covered by bone; unusually difficult or complicated due to factors such as nerve dissection required, separate closure of maxillary sinus required or aberrant tooth position.

D7250 Removal of residual tooth roots (cutting procedure) Ⓑ S

Includes cutting of soft tissue and bone, removal of tooth structure, and closure.

D7251 Coronectomy — intentional partial tooth removal, impacted teeth only Ⓑ B

Intentional partial tooth removal is performed when a neurovascular complication is likely if the entire impacted tooth is removed.

Other Surgical Procedures

D7260 Oroantral fistula closure Ⓑ S

Excision of fistulous tract between maxillary sinus and oral cavity and closure by advancement flap.

D7261 Primary closure of a sinus perforation Ⓑ S

Subsequent to surgical removal of tooth, exposure of sinus requiring repair, or immediate closure of oroantral or oralnasal communication in absence of fistulous tract.

D7270 Tooth reimplantation and/or stabilization of accidentally evulsed or displaced tooth Ⓑ B

Includes splinting and/or stabilization.

D7272 Tooth transplantation (includes reimplantation from one site to another and splinting and/or stabilization) Ⓑ B

D7280 Exposure of an unerupted tooth Ⓑ B

An incision is made and the tissue is reflected and bone removed as necessary to expose the crown of an impacted tooth not intended to be extracted.

D7282 Mobilization of erupted or malpositioned tooth to aid eruption Ⓑ B

To move/luxate teeth to eliminate ankylosis; not in conjunction with an extraction.

D7283 Placement of device to facilitate eruption of impacted tooth Ⓑ B

Placement of an orthodontic bracket, band or other device on an unerupted tooth, after its exposure, to aid in its eruption. Report the surgical exposure separately using D7280.

▶ **D7284** Excisional biopsy of minor salivary glands

D7285 Incisional biopsy of oral tissue - hard (bone, tooth) Ⓑ B

For partial removal of specimen only. This procedure involves biopsy of osseous lesions and is not used for apicoectomy/periradicular surgery. This procedure does not entail an excision.

Cross Reference 20220, 20225, 20240, 20245

D7286 Incisional biopsy of oral tissue - soft Ⓑ B

For partial removal of an architecturally intact specimen only. This procedure is not used at the same time as codes for apicoectomy/periradicular curettage. This procedure does not entail an excision.

Cross Reference 40808

D7287 Exfoliative cytological sample collection Ⓑ B

For collection of non-transepithelial cytology sample via mild scraping of the oral mucosa.

D7288 Brush biopsy - transepithelial sample collection Ⓑ B

For collection of oral disaggregated transepithelial cells via rotational brushing of the oral mucosa.

D7290 Surgical repositioning of teeth Ⓑ B

Grafting procedure(s) is/are additional.

🐾 **MIPS**   🆀🅿 **Quantity Physician**   🆀🅷 **Quantity Hospital**   ♀ **Female only**

♂ **Male only**   🅰 **Age**   🦽 **DMEPOS**   A2-Z3 **ASC Payment Indicator**   A-Y **ASC Status Indicator**   Coding Clinic

D7291 Transseptal fiberotomy/supra-crestal fiberotomy, by report Ⓑ   S

The supraosseous connective tissue attachment is surgically severed around the involved teeth. Where there are adjacent teeth, the transseptal fiberotomy of a single tooth will involve a minimum of three teeth. Since the incisions are within the gingival sulcus and tissue and the root surface is not instrumented, this procedure heals by the reunion of connective tissue with the root surface on which viable periodontal tissue is present (reattachment).

D7292 Placement of temporary anchorage device [screw retained plate] requiring flap Ⓑ   B

D7293 Placement of temporary anchorage device requiring flap Ⓑ   B

D7294 Placement of temporary anchorage device without flap Ⓑ   B

D7295 Harvest of bone for use in autogenous grafting procedure Ⓑ   B

Reported in addition to those autogenous graft placement procedures that do not include harvesting of bone.

D7296 Corticotomy one to three teeth or tooth spaces, per quadrant Ⓑ   B

This procedure involves creating multiple cuts, perforations, or removal of cortical, alveolar or basal bone of the jaw for the purpose of facilitating orthodontic repositioning of the dentition. This procedure includes flap entry and closure. Graft material and membrane, if used, should be reported separately.

D7297 Corticotomy four or more teeth or tooth spaces, per quadrant Ⓑ   B

This procedure involves creating multiple cuts, perforations, or removal of cortical, alveolar or basal bone of the jaw for the purpose of facilitating orthodontic repositioning of the dentition. This procedure includes flap entry and closure. Graft material and membrane, if used, should be reported separately.

D7298 Removal of temporary anchorage device [screw retained plate], requiring flap Ⓑ   B

D7299 Removal of temporary anchorage device, requiring flap Ⓑ   B

D7300 Removal of temporary anchorage device without flap Ⓑ   B

Alveoloplasty – Preparation of Ridge

D7310 Alveoloplasty in conjunction with extractions - four or more teeth or tooth spaces, per quadrant Ⓑ   B

The alveoloplasty is distinct (separate procedure) from extractions. Usually in preparation for a prosthesis or other treatments such as radiation therapy and transplant surgery.

Cross Reference 41874

D7311 Alveoloplasty in conjunction with extractions - one to three teeth or tooth spaces, per quadrant Ⓑ   B

The alveoloplasty is distinct (separate procedure) from extractions. Usually in preparation for a prosthesis or other treatments such as radiation therapy and transplant surgery.

D7320 Alveoloplasty not in conjunction with extractions - four or more teeth or tooth spaces, per quadrant Ⓑ   B

No extractions performed in an edentulous area. See D7310 if teeth are being extracted concurrently with the alveoloplasty. Usually in preparation for a prosthesis or other treatments such as radiation therapy and transplant surgery.

Cross Reference 41870

D7321 Alveoloplasty not in conjunction with extractions - one to three teeth or tooth spaces, per quadrant Ⓑ   B

No extractions performed in an edentulous area. See D7311 if teeth are being extracted concurrently with the alveoloplasty. Usually in preparation for a prosthesis or other treatments such as radiation therapy and transplant surgery.

Vestibuloplasty

D7340 Vestibuloplasty - ridge extension (second epithelialization) Ⓑ   B

Cross Reference 40840, 40842, 40843, 40844

D7350 Vestibuloplasty - ridge extension (including soft tissue grafts, muscle reattachments, revision of soft tissue attachment, and management of hypertrophied and hyperplastic tissue) Ⓑ   B

Cross Reference 40845

▶ **New**   ⟲ **Revised**   ✔ **Reinstated**   ~~deleted~~ **Deleted**   ⊘ **Not covered or valid by Medicare**
⊗ **Special coverage instructions**   ✳ **Carrier discretion**   Ⓑ **Bill Part B MAC**   Ⓓ **Bill DME MAC**

Excision of Soft Tissue Lesions

D7410 Excision of benign lesion up to 1.25 cm ⑧   B

D7411 Excision of benign lesion greater than 1.25 cm ⑧   B

D7412 Excision of benign lesion, complicated ⑧   B

Requires extensive undermining with advancement or rotational flap closure.

D7413 Excision of malignant lesion up to 1.25 cm ⑧   B

D7414 Excision of malignant lesion greater than 1.25 cm ⑧   B

D7415 Excision of malignant lesion, complicated ⑧   B

Requires extensive undermining with advancement or rotational flap closure.

Excision of Intra-Osseous Lesions

D7440 Excision of malignant tumor - lesion diameter up to 1.25 cm ⑧   B

D7441 Excision of malignant tumor - lesion diameter greater than 1.25 cm ⑧   B

D7450 Removal of benign odontogenic cyst or tumor - lesion diameter up to 1.25 cm ⑧   B

D7451 Removal of benign odontogenic cyst or tumor - lesion diameter greater than 1.25 cm ⑧   B

D7460 Removal of benign nonodontogenic cyst or tumor - lesion diameter up to 1.25 cm ⑧   B

D7461 Removal of benign nonodontogenic cyst or tumor - lesion diameter greater than 1.25 cm ⑧   B

Excision of Soft Tissue Lesions

D7465 Destruction of lesion(s) by physical or chemical methods, by report ⑧   B

Examples include using cryo, laser or electro surgery.

Cross Reference 41850

Excision of Bone Tissue

D7471 Removal of lateral exostosis (maxilla or mandible) ⑧   B

Cross Reference 21031, 21032

D7472 Removal of torus palatinus ⑧   B

D7473 Removal of torus mandibularis ⑧   B

D7485 Reduction of osseous tuberosity ⑧   B

D7490 Radical resection of maxilla or mandible ⑧   B

Partial resection of maxilla or mandible; removal of lesion and defect with margin of normal appearing bone. Reconstruction and bone grafts should be reported separately.

Cross Reference 21095

Surgical Incision

D7509 Marsupialization of odontogenic cyst ⑧   B

Surgical decompression of a large cystic lesion by creating a long-term open pocket or pouch.

D7510 Incision and drainage of abscess - intraoral soft tissue ⑧   B

Involves incision through mucosa, including periodontal origins.

Cross Reference 41800

D7511 Incision and drainage of abscess - intraoral soft tissue - complicated (includes drainage of multiple fascial spaces) ⑧   B

Incision is made intraorally and dissection is extended into adjacent fascial space(s) to provide adequate drainage of abscess/cellulitis.

D7520 Incision and drainage of abscess - extraoral soft tissue ⑧   B

Involves incision through skin.

Cross Reference 41800

D7521 Incision and drainage of abscess - extraoral soft tissue - complicated (includes drainage of multiple fascial spaces) ⑧   B

Incision is made extraorally and dissection is extended into adjacent fascial space(s) to provide adequate drainage of abscess/cellulitis.

D7530 Removal of foreign body from mucosa, skin, or subcutaneous alveolar tissue ⑧   B

Cross Reference 41805, 41828

D7540 Removal of reaction-producing foreign bodies, musculoskeletal system ⑧   B

May include, but is not limited to, removal of splinters, pieces of wire, etc., from muscle and/or bone.

Cross Reference 20520, 41800, 41806

🐾 MIPS   **Qp** Quantity Physician   **Qh** Quantity Hospital   ♀ Female only

♂ **Male only**   **A** Age   **&** DMEPOS   **A2-Z3** ASC Payment Indicator   **A-Y** ASC Status Indicator   Coding Clinic

DENTAL PROCEDURES   D7410 – D7540

D7550 Partial ostectomy/sequestrectomy for removal of non-vital bone Ⓑ   B

Removal of loose or sloughed-off dead bone caused by infection or reduced blood supply.

Cross Reference 20999

D7560 Maxillary sinusotomy for removal of tooth fragment or foreign body Ⓑ   B

Cross Reference 31020

Treatment of Closed Fractures

D7610 Maxilla - open reduction (teeth immobilized, if present) Ⓑ   B

Teeth may be wired, banded or splinted together to prevent movement. Incision required for interosseous fixation.

D7620 Maxilla - closed reduction (teeth immobilized if present) Ⓑ   B

No incision required to reduce fracture. See D7610 if interosseous fixation is applied.

D7630 Mandible - open reduction (teeth immobilized, if present) Ⓑ   B

Teeth may be wired, banded or splinted together to prevent movement. Incision required to reduce fracture.

D7640 Mandible - closed reduction (teeth immobilized if present) Ⓑ   B

No incision required to reduce fracture. See D7630 if interosseous fixation is applied.

D7650 Malar and/or zygomatic arch - open reduction Ⓑ   B

D7660 Malar and/or zygomatic arch - closed reduction Ⓑ   B

D7670 Alveolus - closed reduction, may include stabilization of teeth Ⓑ   B

Teeth may be wired, banded or splinted together to prevent movement.

D7671 Alveolus - open reduction, may include stabilization of teeth Ⓑ   B

Teeth may be wired, banded or splinted together to prevent movement.

D7680 Facial bones - complicated reduction with fixation and multiple surgical approaches Ⓑ   B

Facial bones include upper and lower jaw, cheek, and bones around eyes, nose, and ears.

Treatment of Open Fractures

D7710 Maxilla - open reduction Ⓑ   B

Incision required to reduce fracture.

Cross Reference 21346

D7720 Maxilla - closed reduction Ⓑ   B

Cross Reference 21345

D7730 Mandible - open reduction Ⓑ   B

Incision required to reduce fracture.

Cross Reference 21461, 21462

D7740 Mandible - closed reduction Ⓑ   B

Cross Reference 21455

D7750 Malar and/or zygomatic arch - open reduction Ⓑ   B

Incision required to reduce fracture.

Cross Reference 21360, 21365

D7760 Malar and/or zygomatic arch - closed reduction Ⓑ   B

Cross Reference 21355

D7770 Alveolus - open reduction stabilization of teeth Ⓑ   B

Fractured bone(s) are exposed to mouth or outside the face. Incision required to reduce fracture.

Cross Reference 21422

D7771 Alveolus, closed reduction stabilization of teeth Ⓑ   B

Fractured bone(s) are exposed to mouth or outside the face.

D7780 Facial bones - complicated reduction with fixation and multiple approaches Ⓑ   B

Incision required to reduce fracture. Facial bones include upper and lower jaw, cheek, and bones around eyes, nose, and ears.

Cross Reference 21433, 21435

Reduction of Dislocation and Management of Other Temporomandibular Joint Dysfunction

D7810 Open reduction of dislocation Ⓑ   B

Access to TMJ via surgical opening.

Cross Reference 21490

D7820 Closed reduction of dislocation Ⓑ   B

Joint manipulated into place; no surgical exposure.

Cross Reference 21480

▶ **New**   ⟳ **Revised**   ✔ **Reinstated**   ~~deleted~~ **Deleted**   ⊘ **Not covered or valid by Medicare**
⟳ **Special coverage instructions**   ✳ **Carrier discretion**   Ⓑ **Bill Part B MAC**   Ⓖ **Bill DME MAC**

D7830 Manipulation under anesthesia ⓑ   B

Usually done under general anesthesia or intravenous sedation.

Cross Reference 00190

D7840 Condylectomy ⓑ   B

Removal of all or portion of the mandibular condyle (separate procedure).

Cross Reference 21050

D7850 Surgical discectomy, with/without implant ⓑ   B

Excision of the intra-articular disc of a joint.

Cross Reference 21060

D7852 Disc repair ⓑ   B

Repositioning and/or sculpting of disc; repair of perforated posterior attachment.

Cross Reference 21299

D7854 Synovectomy ⓑ   B

Excision of a portion or all of the synovial membrane of a joint.

Cross Reference 21299

D7856 Myotomy ⓑ   B

Cutting of muscle for therapeutic purposes (separate procedure).

Cross Reference 21299

D7858 Joint reconstruction ⓑ   B

Reconstruction of osseous components including or excluding soft tissues of the joint with autogenous, homologous, or alloplastic materials.

Cross Reference 21242, 21243

D7860 Arthrotomy ⓑ   B

Cutting into joint (separate procedure).

D7865 Arthroplasty ⓑ   B

Reduction of osseous components of the joint to create a pseudoarthrosis or eliminate an irregular remodeling pattern (osteophytes).

Cross Reference 21240

D7870 Arthrocentesis ⓑ   B

Withdrawal of fluid from a joint space by aspiration.

Cross Reference 21060

D7871 Non-arthroscopic lysis and lavage ⓑ   B

Inflow and outflow catheters are placed into the joint space. The joint is lavaged and manipulated as indicated in an effort to release minor adhesions and synovial vacuum phenomenon as well as to remove inflammation products from the joint space.

D7872 Arthroscopy - diagnosis, with or without biopsy ⓑ   B

Cross Reference 29800

D7873 Arthroscopy: lavage and lysis of adhesions ⓑ   B

Removal of adhesions using the arthroscope and lavage of the joint cavities.

Cross Reference 29804

D7874 Arthroscopy: disc repositioning and stabilization ⓑ   B

Repositioning and stabilization of disc using arthroscopic techniques.

Cross Reference 29804

D7875 Arthroscopy: synovectomy ⓑ   B

Removal of inflamed and hyperplastic synovium (partial/complete) via an arthroscopic technique.

Cross Reference 29804

D7876 Arthroscopy: discectomy ⓑ   B

Removal of disc and remodeled posterior attachment via the arthroscope.

Cross Reference 29804

D7877 Arthroscopy: debridement ⓑ   B

Removal of pathologic hard and/or soft tissue using the arthroscope.

Cross Reference 29804

D7880 Occlusal orthotic device, by report ⓑ   B

Presently includes splints provided for treatment of temporomandibular joint dysfunction.

Cross Reference 21499

D7881 Occlusal orthotic device adjustment ⓑ   B

D7899 Unspecified TMD therapy, by report ⓑ   B

Used for procedure that is not adequately described by a code. Describe procedure.

Cross Reference 21499

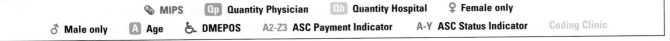

Repair of Traumatic Wounds

D7910 Suture of recent small wounds up to 5 cm Ⓑ   B

Cross Reference 12011, 12013

Complicated Suturing (Reconstruction Requiring Delicate Handling of Tissue and Wide Undermining for Meticulous Closure)

D7911 Complicated suture - up to 5 cm Ⓑ   B

Cross Reference 12051, 12052

D7912 Complicated suture - greater than 5 cm Ⓑ   B

Cross Reference 13132

Other Repair Procedures

D7920 Skin graft (identify defect covered, location, and type of graft) Ⓑ   B

D7921 Collection and application of autologous blood concentrate product Ⓑ   B

D7922 Placement of intra-socket biological dressing to aid in hemostasis or clot stabilization, per site   B

This procedure can be performed at time and/or after extraction to aid in hemostasis. The socket is packed with a hemostatic agent to aid in hemostasis and or clot stabilization.

▶ **D7939** Indexing for osteotomy using dynamic robotic assisted or dynamic navigation

A guide is stabilized to the teeth and/or the bone to allow for virtual guidance of osteotomy.

D7940 Osteoplasty - for orthognathic deformities Ⓑ   S

Reconstruction of jaws for correction of congenital, developmental or acquired traumatic or surgical deformity.

D7941 Osteotomy - mandibular rami Ⓑ   B

Cross Reference 21193, 21195, 21196

D7943 Osteotomy - mandibular rami with bone graft; includes obtaining the graft Ⓑ   B

Cross Reference 21194

D7944 Osteotomy - segmented or subapical Ⓑ   B

Report by range of tooth numbers within segment.

Cross Reference 21198, 21206

D7945 Osteotomy - body of mandible Ⓑ   B

Sectioning of lower jaw. This includes exposure, bone cut, fixation, routine wound closure and normal post-operative follow-up care.

Cross Reference 21193, 21194, 21195, 21196

D7946 LeFort I (maxilla - total) Ⓑ   B

Sectioning of the upper jaw. This includes exposure, bone cuts, downfracture, repositioning, fixation, routine wound closure and normal post-operative follow-up care.

Cross Reference 21147

D7947 LeFort I (maxilla - segmented) Ⓑ   B

When reporting a surgically assisted palatal expansion without downfracture, this code would entail a reduced service and should be "by report."

Cross Reference 21145, 21146

D7948 LeFort II or LeFort III (osteoplasty of facial bones for midface hypoplasia or retrusion) - without bone graft Ⓑ   B

Sectioning of upper jaw. This includes exposure, bone cuts, downfracture, segmentation of maxilla, repositioning, fixation, routine wound closure and normal post-operative follow-up care.

Cross Reference 21150

D7949 LeFort II or LeFort III - with bone graft Ⓑ   B

Includes obtaining autografts.

D7950 Osseous, osteoperiosteal, or cartilage graft of the mandible or maxilla - autogenous or nonautogenous, by report Ⓑ   B

This procedure is for ridge augmentation or reconstruction to increase height, width and/or volume of residual alveolar ridge. It includes obtaining graft material. Placement of a barrier membrane, if used, should be reported separately.

Cross Reference 21247

D7951 Sinus augmentation with bone or bone substitutes Ⓑ   B

The augmentation of the sinus cavity to increase alveolar height for reconstruction of edentulous portions of the maxilla. This procedure is performed via a lateral open approach. This includes obtaining the bone or bone substitutes. Placement of a barrier membrane if used should be reported separately.

▶ **New**   ⮌ **Revised**   ✔ **Reinstated**   ~~deleted~~ **Deleted**   ⊘ **Not covered or valid by Medicare**
✛ **Special coverage instructions**   ✳ **Carrier discretion**   Ⓑ **Bill Part B MAC**   Ⓑ **Bill DME MAC**

D7952 Sinus augmentation via a vertical approach ⒷB

The augmentation of the sinus to increase alveolar height by vertical access through the ridge crest by raising the floor of the sinus and grafting as necessary. This includes obtaining the bone or bone substitutes.

D7953 Bone replacement graft for ridge preservation - per site ⒷB

Graft is placed in an extraction or implant removal site at the time of the extraction or removal to preserve ridge integrity (e.g., clinically indicated in preparation for implant reconstruction or where alveolar contour is critical to planned prosthetic reconstruction). Does not include obtaining graft material. Membrane, if used should be reported separately.

D7955 Repair of maxillofacial soft and/or hard tissue defect ⒷB

Reconstruction of surgical, traumatic, or congenital defects of the facial bones, including the mandible, may utilize graft materials in conjunction with soft tissue procedures to repair and restore the facial bones to form and function. This does not include obtaining the graft and these procedures may require multiple surgical approaches. This procedure does not include edentulous maxilla and mandibular reconstruction for prosthetic considerations.

Cross Reference 21299

D7956 Guided tissue regeneration, edentulous area - resorbable barrier, per site ⒷB

This procedure does not include flap entry and closure, or, when indicated, wound debridement, osseous contouring, bone replacement grafts, and placement of biologic materials to aid in osseous regeneration. This procedure may be used for ridge augmentation, sinus lift procedures, and after tooth extraction.

D7957 Guided tissue regeneration, edentulous area - non-resorbable barrier, per site ⒷB

This procedure does not include flap entry and closure, or, when indicated, wound debridement, osseous contouring, bone replacement grafts, and placement of biologic materials to aid in osseous regeneration. This procedure may be used for ridge augmentation, sinus lift procedures, and after tooth extraction.

D7961 Buccal / labial frenectomy (frenulectomy)

D7962 Lingual frenectomy (frenulectomy)

D7963 Frenuloplasty ⒷB

Excision of frenum with accompanying excision or repositioning of aberrant muscle and z-plasty or other local flap closure.

D7970 Excision of hyperplastic tissue - per arch ⒷB

D7971 Excision of pericoronal gingival ⒷB

Removal of inflammatory or hypertrophied tissues surrounding partially erupted/impacted teeth.

Cross Reference 41821

D7972 Surgical reduction of fibrous tuberosity ⒷB

D7979 Non surgical sialolithotomy ⒷB

A sialolith is removed from the gland or ductal portion of the gland without surgical incision into the gland or the duct of the gland; for example via manual manipulation, ductal dilation, or any other non-surgical method.

D7980 Surgical sialolithotomy ⒷB

Procedure by which a stone within a salivary gland or its duct is removed, either intraorally or extraorally.

Cross Reference 42330, 42335, 42340

D7981 Excision of salivary gland, by report ⒷB

Cross Reference 42408

D7982 Sialodochoplasty ⒷB

Procedure for the repair of a defect and/or restoration of a portion of a salivary gland duct.

Cross Reference 42500

D7983 Closure of salivary fistula ⒷB

Closure of an opening between a salivary duct and/or gland and the cutaneous surface, or an opening into the oral cavity through other than the normal anatomic pathway.

Cross Reference 42600

D7990 Emergency tracheotomy ⒷB

Formation of a tracheal opening usually below the cricoid cartilage to allow for respiratory exchange.

Cross Reference 21070

🐾 MIPS	Ⓠᴾ Quantity Physician	Ⓠʰ Quantity Hospital	♀ Female only
♂ Male only	Ⓐ Age	♿ DMEPOS	A2-Z3 ASC Payment Indicator	A-Y ASC Status Indicator	Coding Clinic

D7991 Coronoidectomy Ⓑ B

Removal of the coronoid process of the mandible.

Cross Reference 21070

D7993 Surgical placement of craniofacial implant – extra oral

Surgical placement of a craniofacial implant to aid in retention of an auricular, nasal, or orbital prosthesis.

D7994 Surgical placement: zygomatic implant

An implant placed in the zygomatic bone and exiting though the maxillary mucosal tissue providing support and attachment of a maxillary dental prosthesis.

D7995 Synthetic graft - mandible or facial bones, by report Ⓑ B

Includes allogenic material.

Cross Reference 21299

D7996 Implant-mandible for augmentation purposes (excluding alveolar ridge), by report Ⓑ B

Cross Reference 21299

D7997 Appliance removal (not by dentist who placed appliance), includes removal of archbar Ⓑ B

D7998 Intraoral placement of a fixation device not in conjunction with a fracture Ⓑ B

The placement of intermaxillary fixation appliance for documented medically accepted treatments not in association with fractures.

None

D7999 Unspecified oral surgery procedure, by report Ⓑ B

Used for procedure that is not adequately described by a code. Describe procedure.

Cross Reference 21299

Orthodontics (D8010-D8999)
Limited Orthodontic Treatment

D8010 Limited orthodontic treatment of the primary dentition Ⓑ B

D8020 Limited orthodontic treatment of the transitional dentition Ⓑ B

D8030 Limited orthodontic treatment of the adolescent dentition Ⓑ Ⓐ B

D8040 Limited orthodontic treatment of the adult dentition Ⓑ Ⓐ B

Comprehensive Orthodontic Treatment

D8070 Comprehensive orthodontic treatment of the transitional dentition Ⓑ B

D8080 Comprehensive orthodontic treatment of the adolescent dentition Ⓑ Ⓐ B

D8090 Comprehensive orthodontic treatment of the adult dentition Ⓑ Ⓐ B

Minor Treatment to Control Harmful Habits

D8210 Removable appliance therapy Ⓑ B

Removable indicates patient can remove; includes appliances for thumb sucking and tongue thrusting.

D8220 Fixed appliance therapy Ⓑ B

Fixed indicates patient cannot remove appliance; includes appliances for thumb sucking and tongue thrusting.

Other Orthodontic Services

D8660 Pre-orthodontic treatment examination to monitor growth and development Ⓑ B

Periodic observation of patient dentition, at intervals established by the dentist, to determine when orthodontic treatment should begin. Diagnostic procedures are documented separately.

D8670 Periodic orthodontic treatment visit Ⓑ B

D8680 Orthodontic retention (removal of appliances, construction and placement of retainer(s)) Ⓑ B

D8681 Removable orthodontic retainer adjustment Ⓑ B

D8695 Removal of fixed orthodontic appliances for reasons other than completion of treatment Ⓑ B

D8696 Repair of orthodontic appliance - maxillary B

Does not include bracket and standard fixed orthodontic appliances. It does include functional appliances and palatal expanders.

D8697 Repair of orthodontic appliance - mandibular B

Does not include bracket and standard fixed orthodontic appliances. It does include functional appliances and palatal expanders.

▶ New   ↻ Revised   ✔ Reinstated   ~~deleted~~ Deleted   ⊘ Not covered or valid by Medicare
Ⓢ Special coverage instructions   ✳ Carrier discretion   Ⓑ Bill Part B MAC   Ⓑ Bill DME MAC

D8698 Re-cement or re-bond fixed retainer - maxillary   B

D8699 Re-cement or re-bond fixed retainer - mandibular   B

D8701 Repair of fixed retainer, includes reattachment - maxillary   B

D8702 Repair of fixed retainer, includes reattachment - mandibular   B

D8703 Replacement of lost or broken retainer - maxillary   B

D8704 Replacement of lost or broken retainer - mandibular   B

None

D8999 Unspecified orthodontic procedure, by report ⑧   B

Used for procedure that is not adequately described by a code. Describe procedure.

Adjunctive General Services (D9110-D9999)
Unclassified Treatment

D9110 Palliative treatment of dental pain - per visit ⑧   N

Treatment that relieves pain but is not curative; services provided do not have distinct procedure codes.

D9120 Fixed partial denture sectioning ⑧   B

Separation of one or more connections between abutments and/or pontics when some portion of a fixed prosthesis is to remain intact and serviceable following sectioning and extraction or other treatment. Includes all recontouring and polishing of retained portions.

D9130 Temporomandibular joint dysfunction - non-invasive physical therapies ⑧   B

Anesthesia

D9210 Local anesthesia not in conjunction with operative or surgical procedures ⑧   B

Cross Reference 90784

D9211 Regional block anesthesia ⑧   B

Cross Reference 01995

D9212 Trigeminal division block anesthesia ⑧   B

Cross Reference 64400

D9215 Local anesthesia in conjunction with operative or surgical procedures ⑧   B

Cross Reference 90784

D9219 Evaluation for moderate sedation or general anesthesia ⑧ Ⓐ   B

D9222 Deep sedation/general anesthesia first 15 minutes ⑧   B

Anesthesia time begins when the doctor administering the anesthetic agent initiates the appropriate anesthesia and non-invasive monitoring protocol and remains in continuous attendance of the patient. Anesthesia services are considered completed when the patient may be safely left under the observation of trained personnel and the doctor may safely leave the room to attend to other patients or duties.

The level of anesthesia is determined by the anesthesia provider's documentation of the anesthetic effects upon the central nervous system and not dependent upon the route of administration.

D9223 Deep sedation/general anesthesia - each subsequent 15 minute increment ⑧   B

D9230 Inhalation of nitrous oxide/analgesia, anxiolysis ⑧   N

D9239 Intravenous moderate (conscious) sedation/analgesia - first 15 minutes ⑧   B

Anesthesia time begins when the doctor administering the anesthetic agent initiates the appropriate anesthesia and non-invasive monitoring protocol and remains in continuous attendance of the patient. Anesthesia services are considered completed when the patient may be safely left under the observation of trained personnel and the doctor may safely leave the room to attend to other patients or duties.

The level of anesthesia is determined by the anesthesia provider's documentation of the anesthetic effects upon the central nervous system and not dependent upon the route of administration.

D9243 Intravenous moderate (conscious) sedation/analgesia - each subsequent 15 minute increment ⑧   B

D9248   Non-intravenous conscious sedation Ⓑ N

This includes non-IV minimal and moderate sedation. A medically controlled state of depressed consciousness while maintaining the patient's airway, protective reflexes and the ability to respond to stimulation or verbal commands. It includes non-intravenous administration of sedative and/or analgesic agent(s) and appropriate monitoring.

The level of anesthesia is determined by the anesthesia provider's documentation of the anesthetic's effects upon the central nervous system and not dependent upon the route of administration.

Professional Consultation

D9310   Consultation - diagnostic service provided by dentist or physician other than requesting dentist or physician Ⓑ   B

A patient encounter with a practitioner whose opinion or advice regarding evaluation and/or management of a specific problem; may be requested by another practitioner or appropriate source. The consultation includes an oral evaluation. The consulted practitioner may initiate diagnostic and/or therapeutic services.

D9311   Consultation with a medical health care professional Ⓑ   B

Treating dentist consults with a medical health care professional concerning medical issues that may affect patient's planned dental treatment.

Professional Visits

D9410   House/extended care facility call Ⓑ   B

Includes visits to nursing homes, long-term care facilities, hospice sites, institutions, etc. Report in addition to reporting appropriate code numbers for actual services performed.

D9420   Hospital or ambulatory surgical center call Ⓑ   B

Care provided outside the dentist's office to a patient who is in a hospital or ambulatory surgical center. Services delivered to the patient on the date of service are documented separately using the applicable procedure codes.

D9430   Office visit for observation (during regularly scheduled hours) - no other services performed Ⓑ   B

D9440   Office visit-after regularly scheduled hours Ⓑ   B

Cross Reference 99050

D9450   Case presentation, subsequent to detailed and extensive treatment planning Ⓑ   B

Established patient. Not performed on same day as evaluation.

Drugs

D9610   Therapeutic parenteral drug, single administration Ⓑ   B

Includes single administration of antibiotics, steroids, anti-inflammatory drugs, or other therapeutic medications. This code should not be used to report administration of sedative, anesthetic or reversal agents.

D9612   Therapeutic parenteral drugs, two or more administrations, different medications Ⓑ   B

Includes multiple administrations of antibiotics, steroids, anti-inflammatory drugs or other therapeutic medications. This code should not be used to report administration of sedatives, anesthetic or reversal agents. This code should be reported when two or more different medications are necessary and should not be reported in addition to code D9610 on the same date.

D9613   Infiltration of sustained release therapeutic drug, per quadrant   B

Infiltration of a sustained release pharmacologic agent for long acting surgical site pain control. Not for local anesthesia purposes.

D9630   Drugs or medicaments dispensed in the office for home use Ⓑ   B

Includes, but is not limited to oral antibiotics, oral analgesics, and topical fluoride; does not include writing prescriptions.

Miscellaneous Services

D9910   Application of desensitizing medicament Ⓑ   B

Includes in-office treatment for root sensitivity. Typically reported on a "per visit" basis for application of topical fluoride. This code is not to be used for bases, liners or adhesives used under restorations.

▶ New   ↻ Revised   ✔ Reinstated   ~~deleted~~ Deleted   ⊘ Not covered or valid by Medicare

❋ Special coverage instructions   ✳ Carrier discretion   Ⓑ Bill Part B MAC   Ⓑ Bill DME MAC

D9911 Application of desensitizing resin for cervical and/or root surface, per tooth ⒷB

Typically reported on a "per tooth" basis for application of adhesive resins. This code is not to be used for bases, liners, or adhesives used under restorations.

D9912 Pre-visit patient screening

Capture and documentation of a patient's health status prior to or on the scheduled date of service to evaluate risk of infectious disease transmission if the patient is to be treated within the dental practice.

D9920 Behavior management, by report ⒷB

May be reported in addition to treatment provided. Should be reported in 15-minute increments.

D9930 Treatment of complications (postsurgical) - unusual circumstances, by report ⒷS

For example, treatment of a dry socket following extraction or removal of bony sequestrum.

D9932 Cleaning and inspection of removable complete denture, maxillary ⒷB

This procedure does not include any adjustments.

D9933 Cleaning and inspection of removable complete denture, mandibular ⒷB

This procedure does not include any adjustments.

D9934 Cleaning and inspection of removable partial denture, maxillary ⒷB

This procedure does not include any adjustments.

D9935 Cleaning and inspection of removable partial denture, mandibular ⒷB

This procedure does not include any adjustments.

▶ **D9938** Fabrication of a custom removable clear plastic temporary aesthetic appliance B

▶ **D9939** Placement of a custom removable clear plastic temporary aesthetic appliance B

D9941 Fabrication of athletic mouthguard ⒷB

Cross Reference 21089

D9942 Repair and/or reline of occlusal guard ⒷB

D9943 Occlusal guard adjustment ⒷB

D9944 Occlusal guard - hard appliance, full arch B

D9945 Occlusal guard - soft appliance, full arch B

D9946 Occlusal guard - hard appliance, partial arch ⒷB

D9947 Custom sleep apnea appliance fabrication and placement B

D9948 Adjustment of custom sleep apnea appliance B

D9949 Repair of custom sleep apnea appliance B

D9950 Occlusion analysis - mounted case ⒷS

Includes, but is not limited to, facebow, interocclusal records tracings, and diagnostic wax-up; for diagnostic casts, see D0470.

D9951 Occlusal adjustment - limited ⒷS

May also be known as equilibration; reshaping the occlusal surfaces of teeth to create harmonious contact relationships between the maxillary and mandibular teeth. Presently includes discing/odontoplasty/enamoplasty. Typically reported on a "per visit" basis. This should not be reported when the procedure only involves bite adjustment in the routine post-delivery care for a direct/indirect restoration or fixed/removable prosthodontics.

D9952 Occlusal adjustment - complete ⒷS

Occlusal adjustment may require several appointments of varying length, and sedation may be necessary to attain adequate relaxation of the musculature. Study casts mounted on an articulating instrument may be utilized for analysis of occlusal disharmony. It is designed to achieve functional relationships and masticatory efficiency in conjunction with restorative treatment, orthodontics, orthognathic surgery, or jaw trauma when indicated. Occlusal adjustment enhances the healing potential of tissues affected by the lesions of occlusal trauma.

D9953 Reline custom sleep apnea appliance (indirect) ⒷB

Resurface dentition side of appliance with new soft or hard base material as required to restore original form and function.

▶ **D9954** Fabrication and delivery of oral appliance therapy (OAT) morning repositioning device

Device for use immediately after removing a mandibular advancement device to aid in relieving muscle/jaw pain and occlusal changes.

🔊 MIPS	Ⓠᵖ Quantity Physician	Ⓠʰ Quantity Hospital	♀ Female only
♂ Male only Ⓐ Age ♿ DMEPOS A2-Z3 ASC Payment Indicator		A-Y ASC Status Indicator Coding Clinic	

▶ **D9955** Oral appliance therapy (OAT) titration visit

Post-delivery visit for titration of a mandibular advancement device and to subsequently evaluate the patient's response to treatment, integrity of the device, and management of side effects

▶ **D9956** Administration of home sleep apnea test

Sleep apnea test, for patients who are at risk for sleep related breathing disorders and appropriate candidates, as allowed by applicable laws. Also, to help the dentist in defining the optimal position of the mandible.

▶ **D9957** Screening for sleep related breathing disorders

Screening activities, performed alone or in conjunction with another evaluation, to identify signs and symptoms of sleep-related breathing disorders.

D9961 Duplicate/copy of patient's records ⑬ B

D9970 Enamel microabrasion ⑬ B

The removal of discolored surface enamel defects resulting from altered mineralization or decalcification of the superficial enamel layer. Submit per treatment visit.

D9971 Odontoplasty - per tooth ⑬ B

Removal/reshaping of enamel surfaces or projections

D9972 External bleaching - per arch - performed in office ⑬ B

D9973 External bleaching - per tooth ⑬ B

D9974 Internal bleaching - per tooth ⑬ B

D9975 External bleaching for home application, per arch; includes materials and fabrication of custom trays ⑬ B

Non-Clinical Procedures

D9985 Sales tax ⑬ B

D9986 Missed appointment ⑬ B

D9987 Cancelled appointment ⑬ B

D9990 Certified translation or sign-language services - per visit ⑬ B

D9991 Dental case management - addressing appointment compliance barriers ⑬ B

Individualized efforts to assist a patient to maintain scheduled appointments by solving transportation challenges or other barriers.

D9992 Dental case management - care coordination ⑬ B

Assisting in a patient's decisions regarding the coordination of oral health care services across multiple providers, provider types, specialty areas of treatment, health care settings, health care organizations and payment systems. This is the additional time and resources expended to provide experience or expertise beyond that possessed by the patient.

D9993 Dental case management - motivational interviewing ⑬ B

Patient-centered, personalized counseling using methods such as Motivational Interviewing (MI) to identify and modify behaviors interfering with positive oral health outcomes. This is a separate service from traditional nutritional or tobacco counseling.

D9994 Dental case management - patient education to improve oral health literacy ⑬ B

Individual, customized communication of information to assist the patient in making appropriate health decisions designed to improve oral health literacy, explained in a manner acknowledging economic circumstances and different cultural beliefs, values, attitudes, traditions and language preferences, and adopting information and services to these differences, which requires the expenditure of time and resources beyond that of an oral evaluation or case presentation.

D9995 Teledentistry synchronous; real-time encounter ⑬ B

Reported in addition to other procedures (e.g., diagnostic) delivered to the patient on the date of service.

D9996 Teledentistry asynchronous; information stored and forwarded to dentist for subsequent review ⑬ B

Reported in addition to other procedures (e.g., diagnostic) delivered to the patient on the date of service.

▶ **New** ↻ **Revised** ✔ **Reinstated** ~~deleted~~ **Deleted** ⊘ **Not covered or valid by Medicare**
✲ **Special coverage instructions** ✳ **Carrier discretion** ⑬ **Bill Part B MAC** ⑬ **Bill DME MAC**

DURABLE MEDICAL EQUIPMENT (E0100-E8002)

Canes

⊘ **E0100** Cane, includes canes of all materials, adjustable or fixed, with tip ⑧ Qp Qh ⅋   Y

IOM: 100-02, 15, 110.1; 100-03, 4, 280.1; 100-03, 4, 280.2

⊘ **E0105** Cane, quad or three prong, includes canes of all materials, adjustable or fixed, with tips ⑧ Qp Qh ♿   Y

IOM: 100-02, 15, 110.1; 100-03, 4, 280.1; 100-03, 4, 280.2

Coding Clinic: 2016, Q3, P3

Crutches

⊘ **E0110** Crutches, forearm, includes crutches of various materials, adjustable or fixed, pair, complete with tips and handgrips ⑧ Qp Qh ⅋   Y

Crutches are covered when prescribed for a patient who is normally ambulatory but suffers from a condition that impairs ambulation. Provides minimal to moderate weight support while ambulating.

IOM: 100-02, 15, 110.1; 100-03, 4, 280.1

⊘ **E0111** Crutch forearm, includes crutches of various materials, adjustable or fixed, each, with tips and handgrips ⑧ Qp Qh ⅋   Y

IOM: 100-02, 15, 110.1; 100-03, 4, 280.1

⊘ **E0112** Crutches, underarm, wood, adjustable or fixed, pair, with pads, tips, and handgrips ⑧ Qp Qh ⅋   Y

IOM: 100-02, 15, 110.1; 100-03, 4, 280.1

⊘ **E0113** Crutch underarm, wood, adjustable or fixed, each, with pad, tip, and handgrip ⑧ Qp Qh ⅋   Y

IOM: 100-02, 15, 110.1; 100-03, 4, 280.1

⊘ **E0114** Crutches, underarm, other than wood, adjustable or fixed, pair, with pads, tips and handgrips ⑧ Qp Qh ♿   Y

IOM: 100-02, 15, 110.1; 100-03, 4, 280.1

⊘ **E0116** Crutch, underarm, other than wood, adjustable or fixed, with pad, tip, handgrip, with or without shock absorber, each ⑧ Qp Qh ♿   Y

IOM: 100-02, 15, 110.1; 100-03, 4, 280.1

⊘ **E0117** Crutch, underarm, articulating, spring assisted, each ⑧ Qp Qh ⅋   Y

IOM: 100-02, 15, 110.1

✳ **E0118** Crutch substitute, lower leg platform, with or without wheels, each ⑧ Qp Qh   E1

Walkers

⊘ **E0130** Walker, rigid (pickup), adjustable or fixed height ⑧ Qp Qh ⅋   Y

Standard walker criteria for payment: Individual has a mobility limitation that significantly impairs ability to participate in mobility-related activities of daily living that cannot be adequately or safely addressed by a cane. The patient is able to use the walker safely; the functional mobility deficit can be resolved with use of a standard walker.

IOM: 100-02, 15, 110.1; 100-03, 4, 280.1

⊘ **E0135** Walker, folding (pickup), adjustable or fixed height ⑧ Qp Qh ⅋   Y

IOM: 100-02, 15, 110.1; 100-03, 4, 280.1

⊘ **E0140** Walker, with trunk support, adjustable or fixed height, any type ⑧ Qp Qh ⅋   Y

IOM: 100-02, 15, 110.1; 100-03, 4, 280.1

⊘ **E0141** Walker, rigid, wheeled, adjustable or fixed height ⑧ Qp Qh ⅋   Y

IOM: 100-02, 15, 110.1; 100-03, 4, 280.1

⊘ **E0143** Walker, folding, wheeled, adjustable or fixed height ⑧ Qp Qh ⅋   Y

IOM: 100-02, 15, 110.1; 100-03, 4, 280.1

⊘ **E0144** Walker, enclosed, four sided framed, rigid or folding, wheeled, with posterior seat ⑧ Qp Qh ♿   Y

IOM: 100-02, 15, 110.1; 100-03, 4, 280.1

⊘ **E0147** Walker, heavy duty, multiple braking system, variable wheel resistance ⑧ Qp Qh ⅋   Y

Heavy-duty walker is labeled as capable of supporting more than 300 pounds

IOM: 100-02, 15, 110.1; 100-03, 4, 280.1

Figure 11 Walkers.

* **E0148** Walker, heavy duty, without wheels, rigid or folding, any type, each ⑤ Qp Qh ♿   Y

Heavy-duty walker is labeled as capable of supporting more than 300 pounds

* **E0149** Walker, heavy duty, wheeled, rigid or folding, any type ⑤ Qp Qh ♿   Y

Heavy-duty walker is labeled as capable of supporting more than 300 pounds

* **E0153** Platform attachment, forearm crutch, each ⑤ Qp Qh ♿   Y

* **E0154** Platform attachment, walker, each ⑤ Qp Qh ♿   Y

* **E0155** Wheel attachment, rigid pick-up walker, per pair ⑤ Qp Qh ♿   Y

Attachments

* **E0156** Seat attachment, walker ⑤ Qp Qh ♿ Y

* **E0157** Crutch attachment, walker, each ⑤ Qp Qh ♿   Y

* **E0158** Leg extensions for walker, per set of four (4) ⑤ Qp Qh ♿   Y

Leg extensions are considered medically necessary DME for patients 6 feet tall or more.

* **E0159** Brake attachment for wheeled walker, replacement, each ⑤ Qp Qh ♿   Y

Sitz Bath/Equipment

⊘ **E0160** Sitz type bath or equipment, portable, used with or without commode ⑤ Qp Qh ♿   Y

IOM: 100-03, 4, 280.1

⊘ **E0161** Sitz type bath or equipment, portable, used with or without commode, with faucet attachment/s ⑤ Qp Qh ♿   Y

IOM: 100-03, 4, 280.1

⊘ **E0162** Sitz bath chair ⑤ Qp Qh ♿   Y

IOM: 100-03, 4, 280.1

Commodes

⊘ **E0163** Commode chair, mobile or stationary, with fixed arms ⑤ Qp Qh ♿   Y

IOM: 100-02, 15, 110.1; 100-03, 4, 280.1

⊘ **E0165** Commode chair, mobile or stationary, with detachable arms ⑤ Qp Qh ♿   Y

IOM: 100-02, 15, 110.1; 100-03, 4, 280.1

⊘ **E0167** Pail or pan for use with commode chair, replacement only ⑤ Qp Qh ♿ Y

IOM: 100-03, 4, 280.1

* **E0168** Commode chair, extra wide and/or heavy duty, stationary or mobile, with or without arms, any type, each ⑤ Qp Qh ♿   Y

Extra-wide or heavy duty commode chair is labeled as capable of supporting more than 300 pounds

* **E0170** Commode chair with integrated seat lift mechanism, electric, any type ⑤ Qp Qh ♿   Y

* **E0171** Commode chair with integrated seat lift mechanism, non-electric, any type ⑤ Qp Qh ♿   Y

⊘ **E0172** Seat lift mechanism placed over or on top of toilet, any type ⑤ Qp Qh   E1

Medicare Statute 1861 SSA

* **E0175** Foot rest, for use with commode chair, each ⑤ Qp Qh ♿   Y

Decubitus Care Equipment

⊘ **E0181** Powered pressure reducing mattress overlay/pad, alternating, with pump, includes heavy duty ⑤ Qp Qh ♿   Y

Requires the provider to determine medical necessity compliance. To demonstrate the requirements in the medical policy were met, attach KX.

IOM: 100-03, 4, 280.1; 100-08, 5, 5.2.3

⊘ **E0182** Pump for alternating pressure pad, for replacement only ⑤ Qp Qh ♿   Y

IOM: 100-03, 4, 280.1; 100-08, 5, 5.2.3

* **E0183** Powered pressure reducing underlay/pad, alternating, with pump, includes heavy duty ⑤ Qp Qh ♿   Y

⊘ **E0184** Dry pressure mattress ⑤ Qp Qh ♿ Y

IOM: 100-03, 4, 280.1; 100-08, 5, 5.2.3

⊘ **E0185** Gel or gel-like pressure pad for mattress, standard mattress length and width ⑤ Qp Qh ♿   Y

IOM: 100-03, 4, 280.1; 100-08, 5, 5.2.3

⊘ **E0186** Air pressure mattress ⑤ Qp Qh ♿ Y

IOM: 100-03, 4, 280.1

⊘ **E0187** Water pressure mattress ⑤ Qp Qh ♿ Y

IOM: 100-03, 4, 280.1

⊘ **E0188** Synthetic sheepskin pad ⑤ Qp Qh ♿ Y

IOM: 100-03, 4, 280.1; 100-08, 5, 5.2.3

▶ New   ↻ Revised   ✔ Reinstated   ~~deleted~~ Deleted   ⊘ Not covered or valid by Medicare

⊘ Special coverage instructions   * Carrier discretion   ⑧ Bill Part B MAC   ⑤ Bill DME MAC

E0189 Lambswool sheepskin pad, any size ⊚ Qp Qh ♿   Y

IOM: 100-03, 4, 280.1; 100-08, 5, 5.2.3

E0190 Positioning cushion/pillow/wedge, any shape or size, includes all components and accessories ⊚ Qp Qh   E1

IOM: 100-02, 15, 110.1

* E0191 Heel or elbow protector, each ⊚ Qp Qh ♿   Y

* E0193 Powered air flotation bed (low air loss therapy) ⊚ Qp Qh ♿   Y

E0194 Air fluidized bed ⓑ Qp Qh ♿   Y

IOM: 100-03, 4, 280.1

E0196 Gel pressure mattress ⓑ Qp Qh ♿   Y

IOM: 100-03, 4, 280.1

E0197 Air pressure pad for mattress, standard mattress length and width ⓑ Qp Qh ♿   Y

IOM: 100-03, 4, 280.1

E0198 Water pressure pad for mattress, standard mattress length and width ⓑ Qp Qh ♿   Y

IOM: 100-03, 4, 280.1

E0199 Dry pressure pad for mattress, standard mattress length and width ⓑ Qp Qh ♿   Y

IOM: 100-03, 4, 280.1

Heat/Cold Application

E0200 Heat lamp, without stand (table model), includes bulb, or infrared element ⓑ Qp Qh ♿   Y

Covered when medical review determines patient's medical condition is one for which application of heat by heat lamp is therapeutically effective

IOM: 100-02, 15, 110.1; 100-03, 4, 280.1

* E0202 Phototherapy (bilirubin) light with photometer ⓑ Qp Qh ♿   Y

⊘ E0203 Therapeutic lightbox, minimum 10,000 lux, table top model ⓑ Qp Qh   E1

IOM: 100-03, 4, 280.1

E0205 Heat lamp, with stand, includes bulb, or infrared element ⓑ Qp Qh ♿   Y

IOM: 100-02, 15, 110.1; 100-03, 4, 280.1

E0210 Electric heat pad, standard ⓑ Qp Qh ♿   Y

Flexible device containing electric resistive elements producing heat; has fabric cover to prevent burns; with or without timing devices for automatic shut-off

IOM: 100-03, 4, 280.1

E0215 Electric heat pad, moist ⓑ Qp Qh ♿ Y

Flexible device containing electric resistive elements producing heat. Must have component that will absorb and retain liquid (water).

IOM: 100-03, 4, 280.1

E0217 Water circulating heat pad with pump ⓑ Qp Qh ♿   Y

Consists of flexible pad containing series of channels through which water is circulated by means of electrical pumping mechanism and heated in external reservoir

IOM: 100-03, 4, 280.1

E0218 Fluid circulating cold pad with pump, any type ⓑ Qp Qh   Y

IOM: 100-03, 4, 280.1

* E0221 Infrared heating pad system ⓑ Qp Qh   Y

E0225 Hydrocollator unit, includes pads ⓑ Qp Qh ♿   Y

IOM: 100-02, 15, 230; 100-03, 4, 280.1

⊘ E0231 Non-contact wound warming device (temperature control unit, AC adapter and power cord) for use with warming card and wound cover ⓑ Qp Qh   E1

IOM: 100-02, 16, 20

⊘ E0232 Warming card for use with the non-contact wound warming device and non-contact wound warming wound cover ⓑ Qp Qh   E1

IOM: 100-02, 16, 20

E0235 Paraffin bath unit, portable, (see medical supply code A4265 for paraffin) ⓑ Qp Qh ♿   Y

Ordered by physician and patient's condition expected to be relieved by long-term use of modality

IOM: 100-02, 15, 230; 100-03, 4, 280.1

E0236 Pump for water circulating pad ⓑ Qp Qh ♿   Y

IOM: 100-03, 4, 280.1

E0239 Hydrocollator unit, portable ⓑ Qp Qh ♿   Y

IOM: 100-02, 15, 230; 100-03, 4, 280.1

🐾 MIPS   Qp Quantity Physician   Qh Quantity Hospital   ♀ Female only

♂ Male only   A Age   ♿ DMEPOS   A2-Z3 ASC Payment Indicator   A-Y ASC Status Indicator   Coding Clinic

Bath and Toilet Aids

⊘ **E0240** Bath/shower chair, with or without wheels, any size ⑧ Qp Qh E1
IOM: 100-03, 4, 280.1

⊘ **E0241** Bath tub wall rail, each ⑧ Qp Qh E1
IOM: 100-02, 15, 110.1; 100-03, 4, 280.1

⊘ **E0242** Bath tub rail, floor base ⑧ Qp Qh E1
IOM: 100-02, 15, 110.1; 100-03, 4, 280.1

⊘ **E0243** Toilet rail, each ⑧ Qp Qh E1
IOM: 100-02, 15, 110.1; 100-03, 4, 280.1

⊘ **E0244** Raised toilet seat ⑧ Qp Qh E1
IOM: 100-03, 4, 280.1

⊘ **E0245** Tub stool or bench ⑧ Qp Qh E1
IOM: 100-03, 4, 280.1

✳ **E0246** Transfer tub rail attachment ⑧ Qp Qh E1

⊘ **E0247** Transfer bench for tub or toilet with or without commode opening ⑧ Qp Qh E1
IOM: 100-03, 4, 280.1

⊘ **E0248** Transfer bench, heavy duty, for tub or toilet with or without commode opening ⑧ Qp Qh E1
Heavy duty transfer bench is labeled as capable of supporting more than 300 pounds
IOM: 100-03, 4, 280.1

Pad for Heating Unit

⊘ **E0249** Pad for water circulating heat unit, for replacement only ⑧ Qp Qh & Y
Describes durable replacement pad used with water circulating heat pump system
IOM: 100-03, 4, 280.1

Hospital Beds and Accessories

⊘ **E0250** Hospital bed, fixed height, with any type side rails, with mattress ⑧ Qp Qh & Y
IOM: 100-02, 15, 110.1; 100-03, 4, 280.7

⊘ **E0251** Hospital bed, fixed height, with any type side rails, without mattress ⑧ Qp Qh & Y
IOM: 100-02, 15, 110.1; 100-03, 4, 280.7

⊘ **E0255** Hospital bed, variable height, hi-lo, with any type side rails, with mattress ⑧ Qp Qh & Y
IOM: 100-02, 15, 110.1; 100-03, 4, 280.7

⊘ **E0256** Hospital bed, variable height, hi-lo, with any type side rails, without mattress ⑧ Qp Qh & Y
IOM: 100-02, 15, 110.1; 100-03, 4, 280.7

⊘ **E0260** Hospital bed, semi-electric (head and foot adjustment), with any type side rails, with mattress ⑧ Qp Qh & Y
IOM: 100-02, 15, 110.1; 100-03, 4, 280.7

⊘ **E0261** Hospital bed, semi-electric (head and foot adjustment), with any type side rails, without mattress ⑧ Qp Qh & Y
IOM: 100-02, 15, 110.1; 100-03, 4, 280.7

⊘ **E0265** Hospital bed, total electric (head, foot and height adjustments), with any type side rails, with mattress ⑧ Qp Qh & Y
IOM: 100-02, 15, 110.1; 100-03, 4, 280.7

⊘ **E0266** Hospital bed, total electric (head, foot and height adjustments), with any type side rails, without mattress ⑧ Qp Qh & Y
IOM: 100-02, 15, 110.1; 100-03, 4, 280.7

⊘ **E0270** Hospital bed, institutional type includes: oscillating, circulating and Stryker frame, with mattress ⑧ Qp Qh E1
IOM: 100-03, 4, 280.1

⊘ **E0271** Mattress, innerspring ⑧ Qp Qh & Y
IOM: 100-03, 4, 280.1; 100-03, 4, 280.7

⊘ **E0272** Mattress, foam rubber ⑧ Qp Qh & Y
IOM: 100-03, 4, 280.1; 100-03, 4, 280.7

⊘ **E0273** Bed board ⑧ Qp Qh E1
IOM: 100-03, 4, 280.1

⊘ **E0274** Over-bed table ⑧ Qp Qh E1
IOM: 100-03, 4, 280.1

⊘ **E0275** Bed pan, standard, metal or plastic ⑧ Qp Qh & Y
IOM: 100-03, 4, 280.1

⊘ **E0276** Bed pan, fracture, metal or plastic ⑧ Qp Qh & Y
IOM: 100-03, 4, 280.1

⊘ **E0277** Powered pressure-reducing air mattress ⑧ Qp Qh & Y
IOM: 100-03, 4, 280.1

✳ **E0280** Bed cradle, any type ⑧ Qp Qh & Y

E0290 Hospital bed, fixed height, without side rails, with mattress Ⓑ Qp Qh ♿ Y
IOM: 100-02, 15, 110.1; 100-03, 4, 280.7

E0291 Hospital bed, fixed height, without side rails, without mattress Ⓑ Qp Qh ♿ Y
IOM: 100-02, 15, 110.1; 100-03, 4, 280.7

E0292 Hospital bed, variable height, hi-lo, without side rails, with mattress Ⓑ Qp Qh ♿ Y
IOM: 100-02, 15, 110.1; 100-03, 4, 280.7

E0293 Hospital bed, variable height, hi-lo, without side rails, without mattress Ⓑ Qp Qh ♿ Y
IOM: 100-02, 15, 110.1; 100-03, 4, 280.7

E0294 Hospital bed, semi-electric (head and foot adjustment), without side rails, with mattress Ⓑ Qp Qh ♿ Y
IOM: 100-02, 15, 110.1; 100-03, 4, 280.7

E0295 Hospital bed, semi-electric (head and foot adjustment), without side rails, without mattress Ⓑ Qp Qh ♿ Y
IOM: 100-02, 15, 110.1; 100-03, 4, 280.7

E0296 Hospital bed, total electric (head, foot and height adjustments), without side rails, with mattress Ⓑ Qp Qh ♿ Y
IOM: 100-02, 15, 110.1; 100-03, 4, 280.7

E0297 Hospital bed, total electric (head, foot and height adjustments), without side rails, without mattress Ⓑ Qp Qh ♿ Y
IOM: 100-02, 15, 110.1; 100-03, 4, 280.7

E0300 Pediatric crib, hospital grade, fully enclosed, with or without top enclosure Ⓑ Qp Qh A ♿ Y

E0301 Hospital bed, heavy duty, extra wide, with weight capacity greater than 350 pounds, but less than or equal to 600 pounds, with any type side rails, without mattress Ⓑ Qp Qh ♿ Y
IOM: 100-03, 4, 280.7

E0302 Hospital bed, extra heavy duty, extra wide, with weight capacity greater than 600 pounds, with any type side rails, without mattress Ⓑ Qp Qh ♿ Y
IOM: 100-03, 4, 280.7

E0303 Hospital bed, heavy duty, extra wide, with weight capacity greater than 350 pounds, but less than or equal to 600 pounds, with any type side rails, with mattress Ⓑ Qp Qh ♿ Y
IOM: 100-03, 4, 280.7

E0304 Hospital bed, extra heavy duty, extra wide, with weight capacity greater than 600 pounds, with any type side rails, with mattress Ⓑ Qp Qh ♿ Y
IOM: 100-03, 4, 280.7

E0305 Bed side rails, half length Ⓑ Qp Qh ♿ Y
IOM: 100-03, 4, 280.7

E0310 Bed side rails, full length Ⓑ Qp Qh ♿ Y
IOM: 100-03, 4, 280.7

E0315 Bed accessory: board, table, or support device, any type Ⓑ Qp Qh E1
IOM: 100-03, 4, 280.1

E0316 Safety enclosure frame/canopy for use with hospital bed, any type Ⓑ Qp Qh ♿ Y

E0325 Urinal; male, jug-type, any material Ⓑ Qp Qh ♂ ♿ Y
IOM: 100-03, 4, 280.1

E0326 Urinal; female, jug-type, any material Ⓑ Qp Qh ♀ ♿ Y
IOM: 100-03, 4, 280.1

E0328 Hospital bed, pediatric, manual, 360 degree side enclosures, top of headboard, footboard and side rails up to 24 inches above the spring, includes mattress Ⓑ Qp Qh A Y

E0329 Hospital bed, pediatric, electric or semi-electric, 360 degree side enclosures, top of headboard, footboard and side rails up to 24 inches above the spring, includes mattress Ⓑ Qp Qh A Y

E0350 Control unit for electronic bowel irrigation/evacuation system Ⓑ Qp Qh E1

Pulsed Irrigation Enhanced Evacuation (PIEE) is pulsed irrigation of severely impacted fecal material and may be necessary for patients who have not responded to traditional bowel program.

E0352 Disposable pack (water reservoir bag, speculum, valving mechanism and collection bag/box) for use with the electronic bowel irrigation/evacuation system Ⓑ Qp Qh E1

Therapy kit includes 1 B-Valve circuit, 2 containment bags, 1 lubricating jelly, 1 bed pad, 1 tray liner-waste disposable bag, and 2 hose clamps

E0370 Air pressure elevator for heel Ⓑ Qp Qh E1

* **E0371** Non powered advanced pressure reducing overlay for mattress, standard mattress length and width Ⓑ Qp Qh ♿   Y

  Patient has at least one large Stage III or Stage IV pressure sore (greater than 2 × 2 cm.) on trunk, with only two turning surfaces on which to lie

* **E0372** Powered air overlay for mattress, standard mattress length and width Ⓑ Qp Qh ♿   Y

* **E0373** Non powered advanced pressure reducing mattress Ⓑ Qp Qh ♿   Y

Oxygen and Related Respiratory Equipment

○ **E0424** Stationary compressed gaseous oxygen system, rental; includes container, contents, regulator, flowmeter, humidifier, nebulizer, cannula or mask, and tubing Ⓑ Qp Qh ♿   Y

  IOM: 100-03, 4, 280.1; 100-04, 20, 30.6

○ **E0425** Stationary compressed gas system, purchase; includes regulator, flowmeter, humidifier, nebulizer, cannula or mask, and tubing Ⓑ Qp Qh   E1

  IOM: 100-03, 4, 280.1; 100-04, 20, 30.6

○ **E0430** Portable gaseous oxygen system, purchase; includes regulator, flowmeter, humidifier, cannula or mask, and tubing Ⓑ Qp Qh   E1

  IOM: 100-03, 4, 280.1; 100-04, 20, 30.6

○ **E0431** Portable gaseous oxygen system, rental; includes portable container, regulator, flowmeter, humidifier, cannula or mask, and tubing Ⓑ Qp Qh ♿   Y

  IOM: 100-03, 4, 280.1; 100-04, 20, 30.6

* **E0433** Portable liquid oxygen system, rental; home liquefier used to fill portable liquid oxygen containers, includes portable containers, regulator, flowmeter, humidifier, cannula or mask and tubing, with or without supply reservoir and contents gauge Ⓑ Qh ♿   Y

○ **E0434** Portable liquid oxygen system, rental; includes portable container, supply reservoir, humidifier, flowmeter, refill adaptor, contents gauge, cannula or mask, and tubing Ⓑ Qp Qh ♿   Y

  Fee schedule payments for stationary oxygen system rentals are all-inclusive and represent monthly allowance for beneficiary. Non-Medicare payers may rent device to beneficiaries, or arrange for purchase of device.

  IOM: 100-03, 4, 280.1; 100-04, 20, 30.6

○ **E0435** Portable liquid oxygen system, purchase; includes portable container, supply reservoir, flowmeter, humidifier, contents gauge, cannula or mask, tubing and refill adaptor Ⓑ Qp Qh   E1

  IOM: 100-03, 4, 280.1; 100-04, 20, 30.6

○ **E0439** Stationary liquid oxygen system, rental; includes container, contents, regulator, flowmeter, humidifier, nebulizer, cannula or mask, and tubing Ⓑ Qp Qh ♿   Y

  This allowance includes payment for equipment, contents, and accessories furnished during rental month

  IOM: 100-03, 4, 280.1; 100-04, 20, 30.6

○ **E0440** Stationary liquid oxygen system, purchase; includes use of reservoir, contents indicator, regulator, flowmeter, humidifier, nebulizer, cannula or mask, and tubing Ⓑ Qp Qh   E1

  IOM: 100-03, 4, 280.1; 100-04, 20, 30.6

○ **E0441** Stationary oxygen contents, gaseous, 1 month's supply = 1 unit Ⓑ Qp Qh ♿ Y

  IOM: 100-03, 4, 280.1; 100-04, 20, 30.6

○ **E0442** Stationary oxygen contents, liquid, 1 month's supply = 1 unit Ⓑ Qp Qh ♿ Y

  IOM: 100-03, 4, 280.1; 100-04, 20, 30.6

○ **E0443** Portable oxygen contents, gaseous, 1 month's supply = 1 unit Ⓑ Qp Qh ♿ Y

  IOM: 100-03, 4, 280.1; 100-04, 20, 30.6

○ **E0444** Portable oxygen contents, liquid, 1 month's supply = 1 unit Ⓑ Qp Qh ♿ Y

  IOM: 100-03, 4, 280.1; 100-04, 20, 30.6

Figure 12 Oximeter device.

▶ New   ↻ Revised   ✔ Reinstated   ~~deleted~~ Deleted   ⊘ Not covered or valid by Medicare

○ Special coverage instructions   * Carrier discretion   Ⓟ Bill Part B MAC   Ⓑ Bill DME MAC

✳ **E0445** Oximeter device for measuring blood oxygen levels non-invasively ⓑ Qp Qh　N

✳ **E0446** Topical oxygen delivery system, not otherwise specified, includes all supplies and accessories ⓑ Qp Qh　A

⊚ **E0447** Portable oxygen contents, liquid, 1 month's supply = 1 unit, prescribed amount at rest or nighttime exceeds 4 liters per minute (lpm) ⟨ᵭ⟩　Y

⊚ **E0455** Oxygen tent, excluding croup or pediatric tents ⓑ Qp Qh　Y

IOM: 100-03, 4, 280.1; 100-04, 20, 30.6

⊘ **E0457** Chest shell (cuirass) ⓑ Qp Qh　E1

⊘ **E0459** Chest wrap ⓑ Qp Qh　E1

✳ **E0462** Rocking bed with or without side rails ⓑ Qp Qh ⟨ᵭ⟩　Y

⊚ **E0465** Home ventilator, any type, used with invasive interface (e.g., tracheostomy tube) ⓑ Qp Qh ⟨ᵭ⟩　Y

IOM: 100-03, 4, 280.1

⊚ **E0466** Home ventilator, any type, used with non-invasive interface (e.g., mask, chest shell) ⓑ Qp Qh ⟨ᵭ⟩　Y

IOM: 100-03, 4, 280.1

⊚ **E0467** Home ventilator, multi-function respiratory device, also performs any or all of the additional functions of oxygen concentration, drug nebulization, aspiration, and cough stimulation, includes all accessories, components and supplies for all functions ⟨ᵭ⟩　Y

⊚ **E0470** Respiratory assist device, bi-level pressure capability, without backup rate feature, used with noninvasive interface, e.g., nasal or facial mask (intermittent assist device with continuous positive airway pressure device) ⓑ Qp Qh ⟨ᵭ⟩　Y

IOM: 100-03, 4, 240.2

⊚ **E0471** Respiratory assist device, bi-level pressure capability, with back-up rate feature, used with noninvasive interface, e.g., nasal or facial mask (intermittent assist device with continuous positive airway pressure device) ⓑ Qp Qh ⟨ᵭ⟩　Y

IOM: 100-03, 4, 240.2

⊚ **E0472** Respiratory assist device, bi-level pressure capability, with backup rate feature, used with invasive interface, e.g., tracheostomy tube (intermittent assist device with continuous positive airway pressure device) ⓑ Qp Qh ⟨ᵭ⟩　Y

IOM: 100-03, 4, 240.2

⊚ **E0480** Percussor, electric or pneumatic, home model ⓑ Qp Qh ⟨ᵭ⟩　Y

IOM: 100-03, 4, 240.2

⊘ **E0481** Intrapulmonary percussive ventilation system and related accessories ⓑ Qp Qh　E1

IOM: 100-03, 4, 240.2

✳ **E0482** Cough stimulating device, alternating positive and negative airway pressure ⓑ Qp Qh ⟨ᵭ⟩　Y

✳ **E0483** High frequency chest wall oscillation system, with full anterior and/or posterior thoracic region receiving simultaneous external oscillation, includes all accessories and supplies, each ⓑ Qp Qh ⟨ᵭ⟩　Y

✳ **E0484** Oscillatory positive expiratory pressure device, non-electric, any type, each ⓑ Qp Qh　Y

✳ **E0485** Oral device/appliance used to reduce upper airway collapsibility, adjustable or non-adjustable, prefabricated, includes fitting and adjustment ⓑ Qp Qh ⟨ᵭ⟩　Y

✳ **E0486** Oral device/appliance used to reduce upper airway collapsibility, adjustable or non-adjustable, custom fabricated, includes fitting and adjustment ⓑ Qp Qh ⟨ᵭ⟩　Y

⊚ **E0487** Spirometer, electronic, includes all accessories ⓑ Qp Qh　N

▶ **E0490** Power source and control electronics unit for oral device/appliance for neuromuscular electrical stimulation of the tongue muscle, controlled by hardware remote

▶ **E0491** Oral device/appliance for neuromuscular electrical stimulation of the tongue muscle, used in conjunction with the power source and control electronics unit, controlled by hardware remote, 90-day supply

IPPB Machines

⊚ **E0500** IPPB machine, all types, with built-in nebulization; manual or automatic valves; internal or external power source ⓑ Qp Qh ⟨ᵭ⟩　Y

IOM: 100-03, 4, 240.2

Humidifiers/Nebulizers/Compressors for Use with Oxygen IPPB Equipment

⊚ **E0550** Humidifier, durable for extensive supplemental humidification during IPPB treatments or oxygen delivery ⓑ Qp Qh ⟨ᵭ⟩　Y

IOM: 100-03, 4, 240.2

🖉 MIPS　Qp Quantity Physician　Qh Quantity Hospital　♀ Female only
♂ Male only　A Age　⟨ᵭ⟩ DMEPOS　A2-Z3 ASC Payment Indicator　A-Y ASC Status Indicator　Coding Clinic

Figure 13 Nebulizer

Suction Pump/CPAP

⊚ **E0600** Respiratory suction pump, home model, portable or stationary, electric Ⓑ Qp Qh ♿ Y

IOM: 100-03, 4, 240.2

⊚ **E0601** Continuous positive airway pressure (CPAP) device Ⓑ Qp Qh ♿ Y

IOM: 100-03, 4, 240.4

Breast Pump

✳ **E0602** Breast pump, manual, any type Ⓑ Qp Qh ♀ ♿ Y

Bill either manual breast pump or breast pump kit

✳ **E0603** Breast pump, electric (AC and/or DC), any type Ⓑ Qp Qh ♀ N

✳ **E0604** Breast pump, hospital grade, electric (AC and/or DC), any type Ⓑ Qp Qh ♀ A

Other Breathing Aids

⊚ **E0605** Vaporizer, room type Ⓑ Qp Qh ♿ Y

IOM: 100-03, 4, 240.2

⊚ **E0606** Postural drainage board Ⓑ Qp Qh ♿ Y

IOM: 100-03, 4, 240.2

Monitoring Equipment

⊚ **E0607** Home blood glucose monitor Ⓑ Qp Qh ♿ Y

Document recipient or caregiver is competent to monitor equipment and that device is designed for home rather than clinical use

IOM: 100-03, 4, 280.1; 100-03, 1, 40.2

⊚ **E0610** Pacemaker monitor, self-contained, (checks battery depletion, includes audible and visible check systems) Ⓑ Qp Qh ♿ Y

IOM: 100-03, 1, 20.8

⊚ **E0555** Humidifier, durable, glass or autoclavable plastic bottle type, for use with regulator or flowmeter Ⓑ Qp Qh Y

IOM: 100-03, 4, 280.1; 100-04, 20, 30.6

⊚ **E0560** Humidifier, durable for supplemental humidification during IPPB treatment or oxygen delivery Ⓑ Qp Qh ♿ Y

IOM: 100-03, 4, 280.1

✳ **E0561** Humidifier, non-heated, used with positive airway pressure device Ⓑ Qp Qh ♿ Y

✳ **E0562** Humidifier, heated, used with positive airway pressure device Ⓑ Qp Qh ♿ Y

✳ **E0565** Compressor, air power source for equipment which is not self-contained or cylinder driven Qp Qh ♿ Y

E0570 Nebulizer, with compressor Ⓑ Qp Qh ♿ Y

IOM: 100-03, 4, 240.2; 100-03, 4, 280.1

✳ **E0572** Aerosol compressor, adjustable pressure, light duty for intermittent use Ⓑ Qp Qh ♿ Y

✳ **E0574** Ultrasonic/electronic aerosol generator with small volume nebulizer Ⓑ Qp Qh ♿ Y

⊚ **E0575** Nebulizer, ultrasonic, large volume Ⓑ Qp Qh ♿ Y

IOM: 100-03, 4, 240.2

⊚ **E0580** Nebulizer, durable, glass or autoclavable plastic, bottle type, for use with regulator or flowmeter Ⓑ Qp Qh ♿ Y

IOM: 100-03, 4, 240.2; 100-03, 4, 280.1

⊚ **E0585** Nebulizer, with compressor and heater Ⓑ Qp Qh ♿ Y

IOM: 100-03, 4, 240.2; 100-03, 4, 280.1

Figure 14 Glucose monitor.

▶ **New**   ↻ **Revised**   ✔ **Reinstated**   ~~deleted~~ **Deleted**   ⊘ **Not covered or valid by Medicare**
⊚ **Special coverage instructions**   ✳ **Carrier discretion**   Ⓑ **Bill Part B MAC**   ⒹⓂ **Bill DME MAC**

⊙ **E0615** Pacemaker monitor, self-contained, checks battery depletion and other pacemaker components, includes digital/visible check systems ⑧ Qp Qh ⅙   Y

IOM: 100-03, 1, 20.8

✳ **E0616** Implantable cardiac event recorder with memory, activator and programmer ⊚ Qp Qh   N

Assign when two 30-day pre-symptom external loop recordings fail to establish a definitive diagnosis

✳ **E0617** External defibrillator with integrated electrocardiogram analysis ⑧ Qp Qh ⅙   Y

✳ **E0618** Apnea monitor, without recording feature ⑧ Qp Qh ⅙   Y

✳ **E0619** Apnea monitor, with recording feature ⑧ Qp Qh ⅙   Y

✳ **E0620** Skin piercing device for collection of capillary blood, laser, each ⑧ Qp Qh ⅙   Y

Patient Lifts

⊙ **E0621** Sling or seat, patient lift, canvas or nylon ⑧ Qp Qh ⅙   Y

IOM: 100-03, 4, 240.2, 280.4

⊘ **E0625** Patient lift, bathroom or toilet, not otherwise classified ⑧ Qp Qh   E1

IOM: 100-03, 4, 240.2

⊙ **E0627** Seat lift mechanism, electric, any type ⑧ Qp Qh ⅙   Y

IOM: 100-03, 4, 280.4; 100-04, 4, 20

⊙ **E0629** Seat lift mechanism, non-electric, any type ⑧ Qp Qh ⅙   Y

IOM: 100-04, 4, 20

⊙ **E0630** Patient lift, hydraulic or mechanical, includes any seat, sling, strap(s) or pad(s) ⑧ Qp Qh ⅙   Y

IOM: 100-03, 4, 240.2

⊙ **E0635** Patient lift, electric, with seat or sling ⑧ Qp Qh ⅙   Y

IOM: 100-03, 4, 240.2

✳ **E0636** Multipositional patient support system, with integrated lift, patient accessible controls ⑧ Qp Qh ⅙   Y

⊘ **E0637** Combination sit to stand frame/table system, any size including pediatric, with seat lift feature, with or without wheels ⑧ Qp Qh   E1

IOM: 100-03, 4, 240.2

⊘ **E0638** Standing frame/table system, one position (e.g., upright, supine or prone stander), any size including pediatric, with or without wheels ⑧ Qp Qh   E1

IOM: 100-03, 4, 240.2

✳ **E0639** Patient lift, moveable from room to room with disassembly and reassembly, includes all components/accessories ⑧ Qp Qh ⅙   E1

✳ **E0640** Patient lift, fixed system, includes all components/accessories ⑧ Qp Qh ⅙   E1

⊘ **E0641** Standing frame/table system, multi-position (e.g., three-way stander), any size including pediatric, with or without wheels ⑧ Qp Qh   E1

IOM: 100-03, 4, 240.2

⊘ **E0642** Standing frame/table system, mobile (dynamic stander), any size including pediatric ⑧ Qp Qh   E1

IOM: 100-03, 4, 240.2

Pneumatic Compressor and Appliances

⊙ **E0650** Pneumatic compressor, non-segmental home model ⑧ Qp Qh ⅙   Y

Lymphedema pumps are classified as segmented or nonsegmented, depending on whether distinct segments of devices can be inflated sequentially.

IOM: 100-03, 4, 280.6

⊙ **E0651** Pneumatic compressor, segmental home model without calibrated gradient pressure ⑧ Qp Qh ⅙   Y

IOM: 100-03, 4, 280.6

⊙ **E0652** Pneumatic compressor, segmental home model with calibrated gradient pressure ⑧ Qp Qh ⅙   Y

IOM: 100-03, 4, 280.6

⊙ **E0655** Non-segmental pneumatic appliance for use with pneumatic compressor, half arm ⑧ Qp Qh ⅙   Y

IOM: 100-03, 4, 280.6

⊙ **E0656** Segmental pneumatic appliance for use with pneumatic compressor, trunk ⑧ Qp Qh ⅙   Y

⊙ **E0657** Segmental pneumatic appliance for use with pneumatic compressor, chest ⑧ Qp Qh ⅙   Y

⊙ **E0660** Non-segmental pneumatic appliance for use with pneumatic compressor, full leg ⑧ Qp Qh ⅙   Y

IOM: 100-03, 4, 280.6

🝩 MIPS	Qp Quantity Physician	Qh Quantity Hospital	♀ Female only
♂ Male only Ⓐ Age ⅙ DMEPOS	A2-Z3 ASC Payment Indicator	A-Y ASC Status Indicator	Coding Clinic

⊛ **E0665** Non-segmental pneumatic appliance for use with pneumatic compressor, full arm ⑧ Qp Qh ♿   Y

IOM: 100-03, 4, 280.6

⊛ **E0666** Non-segmental pneumatic appliance for use with pneumatic compressor, half leg ⑧ Qp Qh ♿   Y

IOM: 100-03, 4, 280.6

⊛ **E0667** Segmental pneumatic appliance for use with pneumatic compressor, full leg ⑧ Qp Qh ♿   Y

IOM: 100-03, 4, 280.6

⊛ **E0668** Segmental pneumatic appliance for use with pneumatic compressor, full arm ⑧ Qp Qh ♿   Y

IOM: 100-03, 4, 280.6

⊛ **E0669** Segmental pneumatic appliance for use with pneumatic compressor, half leg ⑧ Qp Qh ♿   Y

IOM: 100-03, 4, 280.6

⊛ **E0670** Segmental pneumatic appliance for use with pneumatic compressor, integrated, 2 full legs and trunk ⑧ Qp Qh ♿   Y

IOM: 100-03, 4, 280.6

⊛ **E0671** Segmental gradient pressure pneumatic appliance, full leg ⑧ Qp Qh ♿   Y

IOM: 100-03, 4, 280.6

⊛ **E0672** Segmental gradient pressure pneumatic appliance, full arm ⑧ Qp Qh ♿   Y

IOM: 100-03, 4, 280.6

⊛ **E0673** Segmental gradient pressure pneumatic appliance, half leg ⑧ Qp Qh ♿   Y

IOM: 100-03, 4, 280.6

✳ **E0675** Pneumatic compression device, high pressure, rapid inflation/deflation cycle, for arterial insufficiency (unilateral or bilateral system) ⑧ Qp Qh ♿   Y

✳ **E0676** Intermittent limb compression device (includes all accessories), not otherwise specified ⑧ Qp Qh   Y

▶ **E0677** Non-pneumatic sequential compression garment, trunk   Y

Ultraviolet Light Therapy Systems

✳ **E0691** Ultraviolet light therapy system, includes bulbs/lamps, timer and eye protection; treatment area 2 square feet or less ⑧ Qp Qh ♿   Y

✳ **E0692** Ultraviolet light therapy system panel, includes bulbs/lamps, timer and eye protection, 4 foot panel ⑧ Qp Qh ♿ Y

✳ **E0693** Ultraviolet light therapy system panel, includes bulbs/lamps, timer and eye protection, 6 foot panel ⑧ Qp Qh ♿ Y

✳ **E0694** Ultraviolet multidirectional light therapy system in 6 foot cabinet, includes bulbs/lamps, timer and eye protection ⑧ Qp Qh ♿   Y

Safety Equipment

✳ **E0700** Safety equipment, device or accessory, any type ⑧ Qp Qh   E1

⊛ **E0705** Transfer device, any type, each ⑧ Qp Qh ♿   B

Restraints

✳ **E0710** Restraints, any type (body, chest, wrist or ankle) ⑧ Qp Qh   E1

▶ **E0711** Upper extremity medical tubing/lines enclosure or covering device, restricts elbow range of motion

Transcutaneous and/or Neuromuscular Electrical Nerve Stimulators (TENS)

⊛ **E0720** Transcutaneous electrical nerve stimulation (TENS) device, two lead, localized stimulation ⑧ Qp Qh ♿   Y

A Certificate of Medical Necessity (CMN) is not needed for a TENS rental, but is needed for purchase.

IOM: 100-03, 2, 160.2; 100-03, 4, 280.1

⊛ **E0730** Transcutaneous electrical nerve stimulation (TENS) device, four or more leads, for multiple nerve stimulation ⑧ Qp Qh ♿   Y

IOM: 100-03, 2, 160.2; 100-03, 4, 280.1

⊛ **E0731** Form-fitting conductive garment for delivery of TENS or NMES (with conductive fibers separated from the patient's skin by layers of fabric) ⑧ Qp Qh ♿   Y

IOM: 100-03, 2, 160.13

⊛ **E0740** Non-implanted pelvic floor electrical stimulator, complete system ⑧ Qp Qh ♿   Y

IOM: 100-03, 4, 230.8

✳ **E0744** Neuromuscular stimulator for scoliosis ⑧ Qp Qh ♿   Y

▶ New   ⟳ Revised   ✔ Reinstated   ~~deleted~~ Deleted   ⊘ Not covered or valid by Medicare

⊛ Special coverage instructions   ✳ Carrier discretion   ⑧ Bill Part B MAC   Ⓑ Bill DME MAC

⊛ **E0745** Neuromuscular stimulator, electronic shock unit Ⓑ Qp Qh ♿   Y

IOM: 100-03, 2, 160.12

⊛ **E0746** Electromyography (EMG), biofeedback device Ⓑ Qp Qh   N

IOM: 100-03, 1, 30.1

⊛ **E0747** Osteogenesis stimulator, electrical, non-invasive, other than spinal applications Ⓑ Qp Qh ♿   Y

Devices are composed of two basic parts: Coils that wrap around cast and pulse generator that produces electric current

⊛ **E0748** Osteogenesis stimulator, electrical, non-invasive, spinal applications Ⓑ Qp Qh ♿   Y

Device should be applied within 30 days as adjunct to spinal fusion surgery

⊛ **E0749** Osteogenesis stimulator, electrical, surgically implanted Ⓑ Qp Qh ♿   N

✳ **E0755** Electronic salivary reflex stimulator (intra-oral/non-invasive) Ⓑ Qp Qh   E1

✳ **E0760** Osteogenesis stimulator, low intensity ultrasound, non-invasive Ⓑ Qp Qh ♿   Y

Ultrasonic osteogenesis stimulator may not be used concurrently with other noninvasive stimulators

⊛ **E0761** Non-thermal pulsed high frequency radiowaves, high peak power electromagnetic energy treatment device Ⓑ Qp Qh   E1

✳ **E0762** Transcutaneous electrical joint stimulation device system, includes all accessories Ⓑ Qp Qh ♿   B

⊛ **E0764** Functional neuromuscular stimulator, transcutaneous stimulation of sequential muscle groups of ambulation with computer control, used for walking by spinal cord injured, entire system, after completion of training program Ⓑ Qp Qh ♿   Y

IOM: 100-03, 2, 160.12

✳ **E0765** FDA approved nerve stimulator, with replaceable batteries, for treatment of nausea and vomiting Ⓑ Qp Qh ♿   Y

✳ **E0766** Electrical stimulation device used for cancer treatment, includes all accessories, any type Ⓑ Qp Qh   Y

⊛ **E0769** Electrical stimulation or electromagnetic wound treatment device, not otherwise classified Ⓑ Qp Qh   B

IOM: 100-04, 32, 11.1

⊛ **E0770** Functional electrical stimulator, transcutaneous stimulation of nerve and/or muscle groups, any type, complete system, not otherwise specified Ⓑ Qp Qh   Y

Infusion Supplies

✳ **E0776** IV pole Ⓑ Qp Qh ♿   Y

PEN: On Fee Schedule

✳ **E0779** Ambulatory infusion pump, mechanical, reusable, for infusion 8 hours or greater Ⓑ Qp Qh ♿   Y

Requires prior authorization and copy of invoice

This is a capped rental infusion pump modifier. The correct monthly modifier (KH, KI, KJ) is used to indicate which month the rental is for (i.e., KH, month 1; KI, months 2 and 3; KJ, months 4 through 13).

✳ **E0780** Ambulatory infusion pump, mechanical, reusable, for infusion less than 8 hours Ⓑ Qp Qh ♿   Y

Requires prior authorization and copy of invoice

⊛ **E0781** Ambulatory infusion pump, single or multiple channels, electric or battery operated with administrative equipment, worn by patient Ⓑ Qp Qh ♿   Y

IOM: 100-03, 1, 50.3

⊛ **E0782** Infusion pump, implantable, non-programmable (includes all components, e.g., pump, cathether, connectors, etc.) Ⓑ Qp Qh ♿   N

IOM: 100-03, 1, 50.3

⊛ **E0783** Infusion pump system, implantable, programmable (includes all components, e.g., pump, catheter, connectors, etc.) Ⓑ Qp Qh ♿   N

IOM: 100-03, 1, 50.3

⊛ **E0784** External ambulatory infusion pump, insulin Ⓑ Qp Qh ♿   Y

IOM: 100-03, 4, 280.14

⊛ **E0785** Implantable intraspinal (epidural/intrathecal) catheter used with implantable infusion pump, replacement Ⓑ Qp Qh ♿   N

IOM: 100-03, 1, 50.3

⊛ **E0786** Implantable programmable infusion pump, replacement (excludes implantable intraspinal catheter) Ⓑ Qp Qh ♿   N

IOM: 100-03, 1, 50.3

---

* **E0787** External ambulatory infusion pump, insulin, dosage rate adjustment using therapeutic continuous glucose sensing ⊕   Y

✿ **E0791** Parenteral infusion pump, stationary, single or multi-channel ⊕ Qp Qh ♿ Y

IOM: 100-02, 15, 120; 100-03, 3, 180.2; 100-04, 20, 100.2.2

Traction Equipment and Orthopedic Devices

✿ **E0830** Ambulatory traction device, all types, each ⊕ Qp Qh   N

IOM: 100-03, 4, 280.1

✿ **E0840** Traction frame, attached to headboard, cervical traction ⊕ Qp Qh ♿ Y

IOM: 100-03, 4, 280.1

* **E0849** Traction equipment, cervical, free-standing stand/frame, pneumatic, applying traction force to other than mandible ⊕ Qp Qh ♿ Y

✿ **E0850** Traction stand, free standing, cervical traction ⊕ Qp Qh ♿ Y

IOM: 100-03, 4, 280.1

* **E0855** Cervical traction equipment not requiring additional stand or frame ⊕ Qp Qh ♿ Y

* **E0856** Cervical traction device, with inflatable air bladder(s) ⊕ Qp Qh ♿ Y

✿ **E0860** Traction equipment, overdoor, cervical ⊕ Qp Qh ♿ Y

IOM: 100-03, 4, 280.1

✿ **E0870** Traction frame, attached to footboard, extremity traction, (e.g., Buck's) ⊕ Qp Qh ♿ Y

IOM: 100-03, 4, 280.1

✿ **E0880** Traction stand, free standing, extremity traction ⊕ Qp Qh ♿ Y

IOM: 100-03, 4, 280.1

✿ **E0890** Traction frame, attached to footboard, pelvic traction ⊕ Qp Qh ♿ Y

IOM: 100-03, 4, 280.1

✿ **E0900** Traction stand, free standing, pelvic traction (e.g., Buck's) ⊕ Qp Qh ♿ Y

IOM: 100-03, 4, 280.1

✿ **E0910** Trapeze bars, A/K/A patient helper, attached to bed, with grab bar ⊕ Qp Qh ♿ Y

IOM: 100-03, 4, 280.1

✿ **E0911** Trapeze bar, heavy duty, for patient weight capacity greater than 250 pounds, attached to bed, with grab bar ⊕ Qp Qh ♿ Y

IOM: 100-03, 4, 280.1

✿ **E0912** Trapeze bar, heavy duty, for patient weight capacity greater than 250 pounds, free standing, complete with grab bar ⊕ Qp Qh ♿ Y

IOM: 100-03, 4, 280.1

✿ **E0920** Fracture frame, attached to bed, includes weights ⊕ Qp Qh ♿ Y

IOM: 100-03, 4, 280.1

✿ **E0930** Fracture frame, free standing, includes weights ⊕ Qp Qh ♿ Y

IOM: 100-03, 4, 280.1

✿ **E0935** Continuous passive motion exercise device for use on knee only ⊕ Qp Qh ♿ Y

To qualify for coverage, use of device must commence within two days following surgery

IOM: 100-03, 4, 280.1

⊘ **E0936** Continuous passive motion exercise device for use other than knee ⊕ Qp Qh E1

✿ **E0940** Trapeze bar, free standing, complete with grab bar ⊕ Qp Qh ♿ Y

IOM: 100-03, 4, 280.1

✿ **E0941** Gravity assisted traction device, any type ⊕ Qp Qh ♿ Y

IOM: 100-03, 4, 280.1

* **E0942** Cervical head harness/halter ⊕ Qp Qh ♿ Y

* **E0944** Pelvic belt/harness/boot ⊕ Qp Qh ♿ Y

* **E0945** Extremity belt/harness ⊕ Qp Qh ♿ Y

✿ **E0946** Fracture, frame, dual with cross bars, attached to bed (e.g., Balken, 4 poster) ⊕ Qp Qh ♿ Y

IOM: 100-03, 4, 280.1

✿ **E0947** Fracture frame, attachments for complex pelvic traction ⊕ Qp Qh ♿ Y

IOM: 100-03, 4, 280.1

✿ **E0948** Fracture frame, attachments for complex cervical traction ⊕ Qp Qh ♿ Y

IOM: 100-03, 4, 280.1

▶ New   ↻ Revised   ✔ Reinstated   deleted Deleted   ⊘ Not covered or valid by Medicare
✿ Special coverage instructions   * Carrier discretion   ⓑ Bill Part B MAC   ⊕ Bill DME MAC

Wheelchair Accessories

E0950 Wheelchair accessory, tray, each Ⓑ Qp Qh ♿   Y

IOM: 100-03, 4, 280.1

E0951 Heel loop/holder, any type, with or without ankle strap, each Ⓑ Qp Qh ♿   Y

E0952 Toe loop/holder, any type, each Ⓑ Qp Qh ♿   Y

IOM: 100-03, 4, 280.1

E0953 Wheelchair accessory, lateral thigh or knee support, any type, including fixed mounting hardware, each ♿   Y

E0954 Wheelchair accessory, foot box, any type, includes attachment and mounting hardware, each foot ♿   Y

E0955 Wheelchair accessory, headrest, cushioned, any type, including fixed mounting hardware, each Ⓑ Qp Qh ♿   Y

E0956 Wheelchair accessory, lateral trunk or hip support, any type, including fixed mounting hardware, each Ⓑ Qp Qh ♿   Y

E0957 Wheelchair accessory, medial thigh support, any type, including fixed mounting hardware, each Ⓑ Qp Qh ♿   Y

E0958 Manual wheelchair accessory, one-arm drive attachment, each Ⓑ Qp Qh ♿   Y

IOM: 100-03, 4, 280.1

E0959 Manual wheelchair accessory, adapter for amputee, each Ⓑ Qp Qh ♿   B

IOM: 100-03, 4, 280.1

E0960 Wheelchair accessory, shoulder harness/straps or chest strap, including any type mounting hardware Ⓑ Qp Qh ♿   Y

E0961 Manual wheelchair accessory, wheel lock brake extension (handle), each Ⓑ Qp Qh ♿   B

IOM: 100-03, 4, 280.1

E0966 Manual wheelchair accessory, headrest extension, each Ⓑ Qp Qh ♿   B

IOM: 100-03, 4, 280.1

E0967 Manual wheelchair accessory, hand rim with projections, any type, replacement only, each Ⓑ Qp Qh ♿   Y

IOM: 100-03, 4, 280.1

E0968 Commode seat, wheelchair Ⓑ Qp Qh ♿   Y

IOM: 100-03, 4, 280.1

E0969 Narrowing device, wheelchair Ⓑ ♿   Y

IOM: 100-03, 4, 280.1

E0970 No. 2 footplates, except for elevating leg rest Ⓑ Qp Qh   E1

IOM: 100-03, 4, 280.1

Cross Reference K0037, K0042

E0971 Manual wheelchair accessory, anti-tipping device, each Ⓑ Qp Qh ♿   B

IOM: 100-03, 4, 280.1

Cross Reference K0021

E0973 Wheelchair accessory, adjustable height, detachable armrest, complete assembly, each Ⓑ Qp Qh ♿   B

IOM: 100-03, 4, 280.1

E0974 Manual wheelchair accessory, anti-rollback device, each Ⓑ Qp Qh ♿   B

IOM: 100-03, 4, 280.1

E0978 Wheelchair accessory, positioning belt/safety belt/pelvic strap, each Ⓑ Qp Qh ♿   B

E0980 Safety vest, wheelchair Ⓑ ♿   Y

E0981 Wheelchair accessory, seat upholstery, replacement only, each Ⓑ Qp Qh ♿   Y

E0982 Wheelchair accessory, back upholstery, replacement only, each Ⓑ Qp Qh ♿   Y

E0983 Manual wheelchair accessory, power add-on to convert manual wheelchair to motorized wheelchair, joystick control Ⓑ Qp Qh ♿   Y

E0984 Manual wheelchair accessory, power add-on to convert manual wheelchair to motorized wheelchair, tiller control Ⓑ Qp Qh ♿   Y

E0985 Wheelchair accessory, seat lift mechanism Ⓑ Qp Qh ♿   Y

E0986 Manual wheelchair accessory, push-rim activated power assist system Ⓑ Qp Qh ♿   Y

E0988 Manual wheelchair accessory, lever-activated, wheel drive, pair Ⓑ Qp Qh ♿   Y

E0990 Wheelchair accessory, elevating leg rest, complete assembly, each Ⓑ Qp Qh ♿   B

IOM: 100-03, 4, 280.1

E0992 Manual wheelchair accessory, solid seat insert Ⓑ Qp Qh ♿   B

E0994 Arm rest, each Ⓑ Qp Qh ♿   Y

IOM: 100-03, 4, 280.1

MIPS   Qp Quantity Physician   Qh Quantity Hospital   ♀ Female only   ♂ Male only   A Age   ♿ DMEPOS   A2-Z3 ASC Payment Indicator   A-Y ASC Status Indicator   Coding Clinic

DURABLE MEDICAL EQUIPMENT   E0950 – E0994

221

* **E0995** Wheelchair accessory, calf rest/pad, replacement only, each ⑧ Qp Qh ⑤   B

IOM: 100-03, 4, 280.1

* **E1002** Wheelchair accessory, power seating system, tilt only ⑧ Qp Qh ⑤   Y

* **E1003** Wheelchair accessory, power seating system, recline only, without shear reduction ⑧ Qp Qh ⑤   Y

* **E1004** Wheelchair accessory, power seating system, recline only, with mechanical shear reduction ⑧ Qp Qh ⑤   Y

* **E1005** Wheelchair accessory, power seating system, recline only, with power shear reduction ⑧ Qp Qh ⑤   Y

* **E1006** Wheelchair accessory, power seating system, combination tilt and recline, without shear reduction ⑧ Qp Qh ⑤   Y

* **E1007** Wheelchair accessory, power seating system, combination tilt and recline, with mechanical shear reduction ⑧ Qp Qh ⑤   Y

* **E1008** Wheelchair accessory, power seating system, combination tilt and recline, with power shear reduction ⑧ Qp Qh ⑤   Y

* **E1009** Wheelchair accessory, addition to power seating system, mechanically linked leg elevation system, including pushrod and leg rest, each ⑧ Qp Qh ⑤   Y

* **E1010** Wheelchair accessory, addition to power seating system, power leg elevation system, including leg rest, pair ⑧ Qp Qh ⑤   Y

⊘ **E1011** Modification to pediatric size wheelchair, width adjustment package (not to be dispensed with initial chair) ⑧ Qp Qh A ⑤   Y

IOM: 100-03, 4, 280.1

* **E1012** Wheelchair accessory, addition to power seating system, center mount power elevating leg rest/platform, complete system, any type, each Qp Qh ⑤   Y

⊘ **E1014** Reclining back, addition to pediatric size wheelchair ⑧ Qp Qh A ⑤   Y

IOM: 100-03, 4, 280.1

⊘ **E1015** Shock absorber for manual wheelchair, each ⑧ Qp Qh ⑤   Y

IOM: 100-03, 4, 280.1

⊘ **E1016** Shock absorber for power wheelchair, each ⑧ Qp Qh ⑤   Y

IOM: 100-03, 4, 280.1

⊘ **E1017** Heavy duty shock absorber for heavy duty or extra heavy duty manual wheelchair, each ⑧ Qp Qh ⑤   Y

IOM: 100-03, 4, 280.1

⊘ **E1018** Heavy duty shock absorber for heavy duty or extra heavy duty power wheelchair, each ⑧ Qp Qh ⑤   Y

IOM: 100-03, 4, 280.1

⊘ **E1020** Residual limb support system for wheelchair, any type ⑧ Qp Qh ⑤   Y

IOM: 100-03, 3, 280.3

* **E1028** Wheelchair accessory, manual swing-away, retractable or removable mounting hardware for joystick, other control interface or positioning accessory ⑧ Qp Qh   Y

* **E1029** Wheelchair accessory, ventilator tray, fixed ⑧ Qp Qh ⑤   Y

* **E1030** Wheelchair accessory, ventilator tray, gimbaled ⑧ Qp Qh ⑤   Y

Rollabout Chair, Transfer System, Transport Chair

⊘ **E1031** Rollabout chair, any and all types with casters 5" or greater ⑧ Qp Qh ⑤   Y

IOM: 100-⊠03, 4, 280.1

⊘ **E1035** Multi-positional patient transfer system, with integrated seat, operated by care giver, patient weight capacity up to and including 300 lbs ⑧ Qp Qh ⑤   Y

IOM: 100-02, 15, 110

* **E1036** Multi-positional patient transfer system, extra-wide, with integrated seat, operated by caregiver, patient weight capacity greater than 300 lbs ⑧ Qh ⑤   Y

⊘ **E1037** Transport chair, pediatric size ⑧ Qp Qh A ⑤   Y

IOM: 100-03, 4, 280.1

⊘ **E1038** Transport chair, adult size, patient weight capacity up to and including 300 pounds ⑧ Qp Qh A ⑤   Y

IOM: 100-03, 4, 280.1

* **E1039** Transport chair, adult size, heavy duty, patient weight capacity greater than 300 pounds ⑧ Qp Qh A ⑤   Y

▶ New   ↻ Revised   ✔ Reinstated   ~~deleted~~ Deleted   ⊘ Not covered or valid by Medicare

⊘ Special coverage instructions   * Carrier discretion   ⑧ Bill Part B MAC   ⑧ Bill DME MAC

Wheelchair: Fully Reclining

⚙ **E1050** Fully-reclining wheelchair, fixed full length arms, swing away detachable elevating leg rests Ⓑ **Qp** **Qh** ♿   Y

IOM: 100-03, 4, 280.1

⚙ **E1060** Fully-reclining wheelchair, detachable arms, desk or full length, swing away detachable elevating legrests Ⓑ **Qp** **Qh** ♿   Y

IOM: 100-03, 4, 280.1

⚙ **E1070** Fully-reclining wheelchair, detachable arms (desk or full length), swing away detachable footrests Ⓑ **Qp** **Qh** ♿   Y

IOM: 100-03, 4, 280.1

Wheelchair: Hemi

⚙ **E1083** Hemi-wheelchair, fixed full length arms, swing away detachable elevating leg rest Ⓑ **Qp** **Qh** ♿   Y

IOM: 100-03, 4, 280.1

⚙ **E1084** Hemi-wheelchair, detachable arms desk or full length arms, swing away detachable elevating leg rests Ⓑ **Qp** **Qh** ♿   Y

IOM: 100-03, 4, 280.1

⊘ **E1085** Hemi-wheelchair, fixed full length arms, swing away detachable foot rests Ⓑ **Qp** **Qh**   E1

IOM: 100-03, 4, 280.1

Cross Reference K0002

⊘ **E1086** Hemi-wheelchair, detachable arms desk or full length, swing away detachable footrests Ⓑ **Qp** **Qh**   E1

IOM: 100-03, 4, 280.1

Cross Reference K0002

Wheelchair: High-strength Lightweight

⚙ **E1087** High strength lightweight wheelchair, fixed full length arms, swing away detachable elevating leg rests Ⓑ **Qp** **Qh** ♿   Y

IOM: 100-03, 4, 280.1

⚙ **E1088** High strength lightweight wheelchair, detachable arms desk or full length, swing away detachable elevating leg rests Ⓑ **Qp** **Qh** ♿   Y

IOM: 100-03, 4, 280.1

⊘ **E1089** High strength lightweight wheelchair, fixed length arms, swing away detachable footrest Ⓑ **Qp** **Qh**   E1

IOM: 100-03, 4, 280.1

Cross Reference K0004

⊘ **E1090** High strength lightweight wheelchair, detachable arms desk or full length, swing away detachable foot rests Ⓑ **Qp** **Qh**   E1

IOM: 100-03, 4, 280.1

Cross Reference K0004

Wheelchair: Wide Heavy Duty

⚙ **E1092** Wide heavy duty wheelchair, detachable arms (desk or full length), swing away detachable elevating leg rests Ⓑ **Qp** **Qh** ♿   Y

IOM: 100-03, 4, 280.1

⚙ **E1093** Wide heavy duty wheelchair, detachable arms (desk or full length arms), swing away detachable foot rests Ⓑ **Qp** **Qh** ♿   Y

IOM: 100-03, 4, 280.1

Wheelchair: Semi-reclining

⚙ **E1100** Semi-reclining wheelchair, fixed full length arms, swing away detachable elevating leg rests Ⓑ **Qp** **Qh** ♿   Y

IOM: 100-03, 4, 280.1

⚙ **E1110** Semi-reclining wheelchair, detachable arms (desk or full length), elevating leg rest Ⓑ **Qp** **Qh** ♿   Y

IOM: 100-03, 4, 280.1

Wheelchair: Standard

⊘ **E1130** Standard wheelchair, fixed full length arms, fixed or swing away detachable footrests Ⓑ **Qp** **Qh**   E1

IOM: 100-03, 4, 280.1

Cross Reference K0001

⊘ **E1140** Wheelchair, detachable arms, desk or full length, swing away detachable footrests Ⓑ **Qp** **Qh**   E1

IOM: 100-03, 4, 280.1

Cross Reference K0001

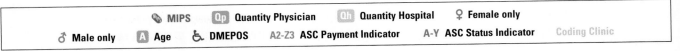

🖐 MIPS   **Qp** Quantity Physician   **Qh** Quantity Hospital   ♀ Female only

♂ Male only   **A** Age   ♿ DMEPOS   A2-Z3 ASC Payment Indicator   A-Y ASC Status Indicator   Coding Clinic

⊛ **E1150** Wheelchair, detachable arms, desk or full length, swing away detachable elevating legrests ⑧ Qp Qh ♿ Y

IOM: 100-03, 4, 280.1

⊛ **E1160** Wheelchair, fixed full length arms, swing away detachable elevating legrests ⑧ Qp Qh ♿ Y

IOM: 100-03, 4, 280.1

✳ **E1161** Manual adult size wheelchair, includes tilt in space ⑧ Qp Qh A ♿ Y

Wheelchair: Amputee

⊛ **E1170** Amputee wheelchair, fixed full length arms, swing away detachable elevating legrests ⑧ Qp Qh ♿ Y

IOM: 100-03, 4, 280.1

⊛ **E1171** Amputee wheelchair, fixed full length arms, without footrests or legrest ⑧ Qp Qh ♿ Y

IOM: 100-03, 4, 280.1

⊛ **E1172** Amputee wheelchair, detachable arms (desk or full length) without footrests or legrest ⑧ Qp Qh ♿ Y

IOM: 100-03, 4, 280.1

⊛ **E1180** Amputee wheelchair, detachable arms (desk or full length) swing away detachable footrests ⑧ Qp Qh ♿ Y

IOM: 100-03, 4, 280.1

⊛ **E1190** Amputee wheelchair, detachable arms (desk or full length), swing away detachable elevating legrests ⑧ Qp Qh ♿ Y

IOM: 100-03, 4, 280.1

⊛ **E1195** Heavy duty wheelchair, fixed full length arms, swing away detachable elevating legrests ⑧ Qp Qh ♿ Y

IOM: 100-03, 4, 280.1

⊛ **E1200** Amputee wheelchair, fixed full length arms, swing away detachable footrest ⑧ Qp Qh ♿ Y

IOM: 100-03, 4, 280.1

Wheelchair: Other and Accessories

⊛ **E1220** Wheelchair; specially sized or constructed (indicate brand name, model number, if any) and justification ⑧ Qp Qh Y

IOM: 100-03, 4, 280.3

⊛ **E1221** Wheelchair with fixed arm, footrests ⑧ Qp Qh ♿ Y

IOM: 100-03, 4, 280.3

⊛ **E1222** Wheelchair with fixed arm, elevating legrests ⑧ Qp Qh ♿ Y

IOM: 100-03, 4, 280.3

⊛ **E1223** Wheelchair with detachable arms, footrests ⑧ Qp Qh ♿ Y

IOM: 100-03, 4, 280.3

⊛ **E1224** Wheelchair with detachable arms, elevating legrests ⑧ Qp Qh ♿ Y

IOM: 100-03, 4, 280.3

⊛ **E1225** Wheelchair accessory, manual semi-reclining back, (recline greater than 15 degrees, but less than 80 degrees), each ⑧ Qp Qh ♿ Y

IOM: 100-03, 4, 280.3

⊛ **E1226** Wheelchair accessory, manual fully reclining back, (recline greater than 80 degrees), each ⑧ Qp Qh ♿ B

IOM: 100-03, 4, 280.1

⊛ **E1227** Special height arms for wheelchair ⑧ ♿ Y

IOM: 100-03, 4, 280.3

⊛ **E1228** Special back height for wheelchair ⑧ Qp Qh ♿ Y

IOM: 100-03, 4, 280.3

Wheelchair: Pediatric

✳ **E1229** Wheelchair, pediatric size, not otherwise specified ⑧ Qp Qh A Y

⊛ **E1230** Power operated vehicle (three or four wheel non-highway), specify brand name and model number ⑧ Qp Qh ♿ Y

Patient is unable to operate manual wheelchair; patient capable of safely operating controls for scooter; patient can transfer safely in and out of scooter

IOM: 100-08, 5, 5.2.3

⊛ **E1231** Wheelchair, pediatric size, tilt-in-space, rigid, adjustable, with seating system ⑧ Qp Qh A ♿ Y

IOM: 100-03, 4, 280.1

⊛ **E1232** Wheelchair, pediatric size, tilt-in-space, folding, adjustable, with seating system ⑧ Qp Qh A ♿ Y

IOM: 100-03, 4, 280.1

⊛ **E1233** Wheelchair, pediatric size, tilt-in-space, rigid, adjustable, without seating system ⑧ Qp Qh A ♿ Y

IOM: 100-03, 4, 280.1

▶ New   ↻ Revised   ✔ Reinstated   ~~deleted~~ Deleted   ⊘ Not covered or valid by Medicare
⊛ Special coverage instructions   ✳ Carrier discretion   ⑧ Bill Part B MAC   ⑧ Bill DME MAC

⊚ **E1234** Wheelchair, pediatric size, tilt-in-space, folding, adjustable, without seating system Ⓑ Qp Qh A &   Y

IOM: 100-03, 4, 280.1

⊚ **E1235** Wheelchair, pediatric size, rigid, adjustable, with seating system Ⓑ Qp Qh A &   Y

IOM: 100-03, 4, 280.1

⊚ **E1236** Wheelchair, pediatric size, folding, adjustable, with seating system Ⓑ Qp Qh A &   Y

IOM: 100-03, 4, 280.1

⊚ **E1237** Wheelchair, pediatric size, rigid, adjustable, without seating system Ⓑ Qp Qh A &   Y

IOM: 100-03, 4, 280.1

⊚ **E1238** Wheelchair, pediatric size, folding, adjustable, without seating system Ⓑ Qp Qh A &   Y

IOM: 100-03, 4, 280.1

✳ **E1239** Power wheelchair, pediatric size, not otherwise specified Ⓑ Qh A   Y

Wheelchair: Lightweight

⊚ **E1240** Lightweight wheelchair, detachable arms (desk or full length), swing-away detachable elevating leg rests Ⓑ Qp Qh &   Y

IOM: 100-03, 4, 280.1

⊘ **E1250** Lightweight wheelchair, fixed full length arms, swing away detachable footrest Ⓑ Qp Qh   E1

IOM: 100-03, 4, 280.1

Cross Reference K0003

⊘ **E1260** Lightweight wheelchair, detachable arms (desk or full length), swing-away detachable footrest Ⓑ Qp Qh   E1

IOM: 100-03, 4, 280.1

Cross Reference K0003

⊚ **E1270** Lightweight wheelchair, fixed full length arms, swing away detachable elevating legrests Ⓑ Qp Qh &   Y

IOM: 100-03, 4, 280.1

Wheelchair: Heavy Duty

⊚ **E1280** Heavy duty wheelchair, detachable arms (desk or full length), elevating legrests Ⓑ Qp Qh &   Y

IOM: 100-03, 4, 280.1

⊘ **E1285** Heavy duty wheelchair, fixed full length arms, swing away detachable footrest Ⓑ Qp Qh   E1

IOM: 100-03, 4, 280.1

Cross Reference K0006

⊘ **E1290** Heavy duty wheelchair, detachable arms (desk or full length), swing-away detachable footrest Ⓑ Qp Qh   E1

IOM: 100-03, 4, 280.1

Cross Reference K0006

⊚ **E1295** Heavy duty wheelchair, fixed full length arms, elevating legrest Ⓑ Qp Qh & Y

IOM: 100-03, 4, 280.1

⊚ **E1296** Special wheelchair seat height from floor Ⓑ &   Y

IOM: 100-03, 4, 280.3

⊚ **E1297** Special wheelchair seat depth, by upholstery Ⓑ &   Y

IOM: 100-03, 4, 280.3

⊚ **E1298** Special wheelchair seat depth and/or width, by construction Ⓑ &   Y

IOM: 100-03, 4, 280.3

Whirlpool Equipment

⊘ **E1300** Whirlpool, portable (overtub type) Ⓑ Qp Qh   E1

IOM: 100-03, 4, 280.1

⊚ **E1310** Whirlpool, non-portable (built-in type) Ⓑ Qp Qh &   Y

IOM: 100-03, 4, 280.1

Additional Oxygen Related Equipment

✳ **E1352** Oxygen accessory, flow regulator capable of positive inspiratory pressure Ⓑ Qp Qh   Y

⊚ **E1353** Regulator Ⓑ Qp Qh &   Y

IOM: 100-03, 4, 240.2

✳ **E1354** Oxygen accessory, wheeled cart for portable cylinder or portable concentrator, any type, replacement only, each Ⓑ Qp Qh   Y

⊚ **E1355** Stand/rack Ⓑ Qp Qh &   Y

IOM: 100-03, 4, 240.2

✳ **E1356** Oxygen accessory, battery pack/cartridge for portable concentrator, any type, replacement only, each Ⓑ Qp Qh   Y

⠿ MIPS   Qp Quantity Physician   Qh Quantity Hospital   ♀ Female only
♂ Male only   A Age   & DMEPOS   A2-Z3 ASC Payment Indicator   A-Y ASC Status Indicator   Coding Clinic

DURABLE MEDICAL EQUIPMENT   E1234 – E1356

225

✳ **E1357** Oxygen accessory, battery charger for portable concentrator, any type, replacement only, each Ⓖ **Qp** **Qh** Y

❂ **E1358** Oxygen accessory, DC power adapter for portable concentrator, any type, replacement only, each Ⓖ **Qp** **Qh** Y

❂ **E1372** Immersion external heater for nebulizer Ⓖ **Qp** **Qh** ♿ Y
IOM: 100-03, 4, 240.2

❂ **E1390** Oxygen concentrator, single delivery port, capable of delivering 85 percent or greater oxygen concentration at the prescribed flow rate Ⓑ **Qp** **Qh** ♿ Y
IOM: 100-03, 4, 240.2

❂ **E1391** Oxygen concentrator, dual delivery port, capable of delivering 85 percent or greater oxygen concentration at the prescribed flow rate, each Ⓑ **Qp** **Qh** ♿ Y
IOM: 100-03, 4, 240.2

❂ **E1392** Portable oxygen concentrator, rental Ⓑ **Qp** **Qh** ♿ Y
IOM: 100-03, 4, 240.2

✳ **E1399** Durable medical equipment, miscellaneous Ⓑ Ⓖ Y
Example: Therapeutic exercise putty; rubber exercise tubing; anti-vibration gloves
On DMEPOS fee schedule as a payable replacement for miscellaneous implanted or non-implanted items

❂ **E1405** Oxygen and water vapor enriching system with heated delivery Ⓑ **Qp** **Qh** ♿ Y
IOM: 100-03, 4, 240.2

❂ **E1406** Oxygen and water vapor enriching system without heated delivery Ⓖ **Qp** **Qh** ♿ Y
IOM: 100-03, 4, 240.2

Artificial Kidney Machines and Accessories

❂ **E1500** Centrifuge, for dialysis Ⓖ **Qp** **Qh** A

❂ **E1510** Kidney, dialysate delivery system, kidney machine, pump recirculating, air removal system, flowrate meter, power off, heater and temperature control with alarm, I.V. poles, pressure gauge, concentrate container Ⓖ **Qp** **Qh** A

❂ **E1520** Heparin infusion pump for hemodialysis Ⓑ **Qp** **Qh** A

❂ **E1530** Air bubble detector for hemodialysis, each, replacement Ⓑ **Qp** **Qh** A

❂ **E1540** Pressure alarm for hemodialysis, each, replacement Ⓑ **Qp** **Qh** A

❂ **E1550** Bath conductivity meter for hemodialysis, each Ⓖ **Qp** **Qh** A

❂ **E1560** Blood leak detector for hemodialysis, each, replacement Ⓑ **Qp** **Qh** A

❂ **E1570** Adjustable chair, for ESRD patients Ⓖ **Qp** **Qh** A

❂ **E1575** Transducer protectors/fluid barriers for hemodialysis, any size, per 10 Ⓑ **Qp** **Qh** A

❂ **E1580** Unipuncture control system for hemodialysis Ⓖ **Qp** **Qh** A

❂ **E1590** Hemodialysis machine Ⓑ **Qp** **Qh** A

❂ **E1592** Automatic intermittent peritoneal dialysis system Ⓑ **Qp** **Qh** A

❂ **E1594** Cycler dialysis machine for peritoneal dialysis Ⓖ **Qp** **Qh** A

❂ **E1600** Delivery and/or installation charges for hemodialysis equipment Ⓖ **Qp** **Qh** A

❂ **E1610** Reverse osmosis water purification system, for hemodialysis Ⓖ **Qp** **Qh** A
IOM: 100-03, 4, 230.7

❂ **E1615** Deionizer water purification system, for hemodialysis Ⓖ **Qp** **Qh** A
IOM: 100-03, 4, 230.7

❂ **E1620** Blood pump for hemodialysis replacement Ⓖ **Qp** **Qh** A

❂ **E1625** Water softening system, for hemodialysis Ⓑ **Qp** **Qh** A
IOM: 100-03, 4, 230.7

❂ **E1629** Tablo hemodialysis system for the billable dialysis service A

✳ **E1630** Reciprocating peritoneal dialysis system Ⓑ **Qp** **Qh** A

❂ **E1632** Wearable artificial kidney, each Ⓖ **Qp** **Qh** A

❂ **E1634** Peritoneal dialysis clamps, each Ⓖ **Qp** **Qh** B
IOM: 100-04, 8, 60.4.2; 100-04, 8, 90.1; 100-04, 18, 80; 100-04, 18, 90

❂ **E1635** Compact (portable) travel hemodialyzer system Ⓖ **Qp** **Qh** A

❂ **E1636** Sorbent cartridges, for hemodialysis, per 10 Ⓑ **Qp** **Qh** A

❂ **E1637** Hemostats, each Ⓖ **Qp** **Qh** A

❂ **E1639** Scale, each Ⓖ **Qp** **Qh** A

❂ **E1699** Dialysis equipment, not otherwise specified Ⓖ A

▶ **New** ↻ **Revised** ✔ **Reinstated** ~~deleted~~ **Deleted** ⊘ **Not covered or valid by Medicare**
❂ **Special coverage instructions** ✳ **Carrier discretion** Ⓑ **Bill Part B MAC** Ⓖ **Bill DME MAC**

Jaw Motion Rehabilitation System

✳ **E1700** Jaw motion rehabilitation system Ⓑ Qp Qh 👤   Y

    Must be prescribed by physician

✳ **E1701** Replacement cushions for jaw motion rehabilitation system, pkg. of 6 Ⓑ Qp Qh 👤   Y

✳ **E1702** Replacement measuring scales for jaw motion rehabilitation system, pkg. of 200 Ⓑ Qp Qh 👤   Y

Other Orthopedic Devices

✳ **E1800** Dynamic adjustable elbow extension/flexion device, includes soft interface material Ⓑ Qp Qh 👤   Y

✳ **E1801** Static progressive stretch elbow device, extension and/or flexion, with or without range of motion adjustment, includes all components and accessories Ⓑ Qp Qh 👤   Y

✳ **E1802** Dynamic adjustable forearm pronation/supination device, includes soft interface material Ⓑ Qp Qh 👤   Y

✳ **E1805** Dynamic adjustable wrist extension/flexion device, includes soft interface material Ⓑ Qp Qh 👤   Y

✳ **E1806** Static progressive stretch wrist device, flexion and/or extension, with or without range of motion adjustment, includes all components and accessories Ⓑ Qp Qh 👤   Y

✳ **E1810** Dynamic adjustable knee extension/flexion device, includes soft interface material Ⓑ Qp Qh 👤   Y

✳ **E1811** Static progressive stretch knee device, extension and/or flexion, with or without range of motion adjustment, includes all components and accessories Ⓑ Qp Qh 👤   Y

✳ **E1812** Dynamic knee, extension/flexion device with active resistance control Ⓑ Qp Qh 👤   Y

✳ **E1815** Dynamic adjustable ankle extension/flexion device, includes soft interface material Ⓑ Qp Qh 👤   Y

✳ **E1816** Static progressive stretch ankle device, flexion and/or extension, with or without range of motion adjustment, includes all components and accessories Ⓑ Qp Qh 👤   Y

✳ **E1818** Static progressive stretch forearm pronation/supination device with or without range of motion adjustment, includes all components and accessories Ⓑ Qp Qh 👤   Y

✳ **E1820** Replacement soft interface material, dynamic adjustable extension/flexion device Ⓑ Qp Qh 👤   Y

✳ **E1821** Replacement soft interface material/cuffs for bi-directional static progressive stretch device Ⓑ Qp Qh 👤   Y

✳ **E1825** Dynamic adjustable finger extension/flexion device, includes soft interface material Ⓑ Qp Qh 👤   Y

✳ **E1830** Dynamic adjustable toe extension/flexion device, includes soft interface material Ⓑ Qp Qh 👤   Y

✳ **E1831** Static progressive stretch toe device, extension and/or flexion, with or without range of motion adjustment, includes all components and accessories Ⓑ Qp Qh 👤   Y

✳ **E1840** Dynamic adjustable shoulder flexion/abduction/rotation device, includes soft interface material Ⓑ Qp Qh 👤   Y

✳ **E1841** Static progressive stretch shoulder device, with or without range of motion adjustment, includes all components and accessories Ⓑ Qp Qh 👤   Y

Miscellaneous

✳ **E1902** Communication board, non-electronic augmentative or alternative communication device Ⓑ Qp Qh   Y

▶ **E1905** Virtual reality cognitive behavioral therapy device (cbt), including pre-programmed therapy software   Y

✳ **E2000** Gastric suction pump, home model, portable or stationary, electric Ⓑ Qp Qh 👤   Y

◉ **E2100** Blood glucose monitor with integrated voice synthesizer Ⓑ Qp Qh 👤   Y

    IOM: 100-03, 4, 230.16

◉ **E2101** Blood glucose monitor with integrated lancing/blood sample Ⓑ Qp Qh 👤   Y

    IOM: 100-03, 4, 230.16

✳ **E2102** Adjunctive, non-implanted continuous glucose monitor or receiver 👤   Y

✳ **E2103** Non-adjunctive, non-implanted continuous glucose monitor or receiver 👤   Y

✳ **E2120** Pulse generator system for tympanic treatment of inner ear endolymphatic fluid Ⓑ Qp Qh 👤   Y

🔊 **MIPS**   Qp **Quantity Physician**   Qh **Quantity Hospital**   ♀ **Female only**

♂ **Male only**   A **Age**   👤 **DMEPOS**   A2-Z3 **ASC Payment Indicator**   A-Y **ASC Status Indicator**   Coding Clinic

Wheelchair Assessories: Manual and Power

* **E2201** Manual wheelchair accessory, nonstandard seat frame, width greater than or equal to 20 inches and less than 24 inches ⑧ Qp Qh ♿ Y

* **E2202** Manual wheelchair accessory, nonstandard seat frame width, 24-27 inches ⑧ Qp Qh ♿ Y

* **E2203** Manual wheelchair accessory, nonstandard seat frame depth, 20 to less than 22 inches ⑧ Qp Qh ♿ Y

* **E2204** Manual wheelchair accessory, nonstandard seat frame depth, 22 to 25 inches ⑧ Qp Qh ♿ Y

* **E2205** Manual wheelchair accessory, handrim without projections (includes ergonomic or contoured), any type, replacement only, each ⑧ Qp Qh ♿ Y

* **E2206** Manual wheelchair accessory, wheel lock assembly, complete, replacement only, each ⑧ Qp Qh ♿ Y

* **E2207** Wheelchair accessory, crutch and cane holder, each ⑧ Qp Qh ♿ Y

* **E2208** Wheelchair accessory, cylinder tank carrier, each ⑧ Qp Qh ♿ Y

* **E2209** Accessory arm trough, with or without hand support, each ⑧ Qp Qh ♿ Y

* **E2210** Wheelchair accessory, bearings, any type, replacement only, each ⑧ Qp Qh ♿ Y

* **E2211** Manual wheelchair accessory, pneumatic propulsion tire, any size, each ⑧ Qp Qh ♿ Y

* **E2212** Manual wheelchair accessory, tube for pneumatic propulsion tire, any size, each ⑧ Qp Qh ♿ Y

* **E2213** Manual wheelchair accessory, insert for pneumatic propulsion tire (removable), any type, any size, each ⑧ Qp Qh ♿ Y

* **E2214** Manual wheelchair accessory, pneumatic caster tire, any size, each ⑧ Qp Qh ♿ Y

* **E2215** Manual wheelchair accessory, tube for pneumatic caster tire, any size, each ⑧ Qp Qh ♿ Y

* **E2216** Manual wheelchair accessory, foam filled propulsion tire, any size, each ⑧ Qp Qh ♿ Y

* **E2217** Manual wheelchair accessory, foam filled caster tire, any size, each ⑧ Qp Qh ♿ Y

* **E2218** Manual wheelchair accessory, foam propulsion tire, any size, each ⑧ Qp Qh ♿ Y

* **E2219** Manual wheelchair accessory, foam caster tire, any size, each ⑧ Qp Qh ♿ Y

* **E2220** Manual wheelchair accessory, solid (rubber/plastic) propulsion tire, any size, replacement only, each ⑧ Qp Qh ♿ Y

* **E2221** Manual wheelchair accessory, solid (rubber/plastic) caster tire (removable), any size, replacement only, each ⑧ Qp Qh ♿ Y

* **E2222** Manual wheelchair accessory, solid (rubber/plastic) caster tire with integrated wheel, any size, replacement only, each ⑧ Qp Qh ♿ Y

* **E2224** Manual wheelchair accessory, propulsion wheel excludes tire, any size, replacement only, each ⑧ Qp Qh ♿ Y

* **E2225** Manual wheelchair accessory, caster wheel excludes tire, any size, replacement only, each ⑧ Qp Qh ♿ Y

* **E2226** Manual wheelchair accessory, caster fork, any size, replacement only, each ⑧ Qp Qh ♿ Y

* **E2227** Manual wheelchair accessory, gear reduction drive wheel, each ⑧ Qp Qh ♿ Y

* **E2228** Manual wheelchair accessory, wheel braking system and lock, complete, each ⑧ Qp Qh ♿ Y

* **E2230** Manual wheelchair accessory, manual standing system ⑧ Qp Qh Y

* **E2231** Manual wheelchair accessory, solid seat support base (replaces sling seat), includes any type mounting hardware ⑧ Qp Qh ♿ Y

* **E2291** Back, planar, for pediatric size wheelchair including fixed attaching hardware ⑧ Qp Qh A Y

* **E2292** Seat, planar, for pediatric size wheelchair including fixed attaching hardware ⑧ Qp Qh A Y

* **E2293** Back, contoured, for pediatric size wheelchair including fixed attaching hardware ⑧ Qp Qh A Y

* **E2294** Seat, contoured, for pediatric size wheelchair including fixed attaching hardware ⑧ Qp Qh A Y

* **E2295** Manual wheelchair accessory, for pediatric size wheelchair, dynamic seating frame, allows coordinated movement of multiple positioning features ⑧ Qp Qh A Y

* **E2300** Wheelchair accessory, power seat elevation system, any type ⑧ Qp Qh Y

▶ New ↻ Revised ✔ Reinstated ~~deleted~~ Deleted ⊘ Not covered or valid by Medicare ⊕ Special coverage instructions ✳ Carrier discretion ⑧ Bill Part B MAC ⑥ Bill DME MAC

* **E2301** Wheelchair accessory, power standing system, any type Ⓑ Qp Qh   Y

* **E2310** Power wheelchair accessory, electronic connection between wheelchair controller and one power seating system motor, including all related electronics, indicator feature, mechanical function selection switch, and fixed mounting hardware Ⓑ Qp Qh &   Y

* **E2311** Power wheelchair accessory, electronic connection between wheelchair controller and two or more power seating system motors, including all related electronics, indicator feature, mechanical function selection switch, and fixed mounting hardware Ⓑ Qp Qh &   Y

* **E2312** Power wheelchair accessory, hand or chin control interface, mini-proportional remote joystick, proportional, including fixed mounting hardware Ⓑ Qp Qh &   Y

* **E2313** Power wheelchair accessory, harness for upgrade to expandable controller, including all fasteners, connectors and mounting hardware, each Ⓑ Qp Qh &   Y

* **E2321** Power wheelchair accessory, hand control interface, remote joystick, nonproportional, including all related electronics, mechanical stop switch, and fixed mounting hardware Ⓑ Qp Qh &   Y

* **E2322** Power wheelchair accessory, hand control interface, multiple mechanical switches, nonproportional, including all related electronics, mechanical stop switch, and fixed mounting hardware Ⓑ Qp Qh &   Y

* **E2323** Power wheelchair accessory, specialty joystick handle for hand control interface, prefabricated Ⓑ Qp Qh &   Y

* **E2324** Power wheelchair accessory, chin cup for chin control interface Ⓑ Qp Qh &   Y

* **E2325** Power wheelchair accessory, sip and puff interface, nonproportional, including all related electronics, mechanical stop switch, and manual swingaway mounting hardware Ⓑ Qp Qh &   Y

* **E2326** Power wheelchair accessory, breath tube kit for sip and puff interface Ⓑ Qp Qh &   Y

* **E2327** Power wheelchair accessory, head control interface, mechanical, proportional, including all related electronics, mechanical direction change switch, and fixed mounting hardware Ⓑ Qp Qh &   Y

* **E2328** Power wheelchair accessory, head control or extremity control interface, electronic, proportional, including all related electronics and fixed mounting hardware Ⓑ Qp Qh &   Y

* **E2329** Power wheelchair accessory, head control interface, contact switch mechanism, nonproportional, including all related electronics, mechanical stop switch, mechanical direction change switch, head array, and fixed mounting hardware Ⓑ Qp Qh &   Y

* **E2330** Power wheelchair accessory, head control interface, proximity switch mechanism, nonproportional, including all related electronics, mechanical stop switch, mechanical direction change switch, head array, and fixed mounting hardware Ⓑ Qp Qh &   Y

* **E2331** Power wheelchair accessory, attendant control, proportional, including all related electronics and fixed mounting hardware Ⓑ Qp Qh   Y

* **E2340** Power wheelchair accessory, nonstandard seat frame width, 20-23 inches Qp Qh &   Y

* **E2341** Power wheelchair accessory, nonstandard seat frame width, 24-27 inches Ⓑ Qp Qh &   Y

* **E2342** Power wheelchair accessory, nonstandard seat frame depth, 20 or 21 inches Ⓑ Qp Qh &   Y

* **E2343** Power wheelchair accessory, nonstandard seat frame depth, 22-25 inches Ⓑ Qp Qh &   Y

* **E2351** Power wheelchair accessory, electronic interface to operate speech generating device using power wheelchair control interface Ⓑ Qp Qh &   Y

* **E2358** Power wheelchair accessory, Group 34 non-sealed lead acid battery, each Ⓑ Qp Qh   Y

* **E2359** Power wheelchair accessory, Group 34 sealed lead acid battery, each (e.g., gel cell, absorbed glassmat) Ⓑ Qp Qh &   Y

* **E2360** Power wheelchair accessory, 22 NF non-sealed lead acid battery, each Ⓑ &   Y

🅜 MIPS	Qp Quantity Physician	Qh Quantity Hospital	♀ Female only
♂ Male only	A Age	& DMEPOS	A2-Z3 ASC Payment Indicator	A-Y ASC Status Indicator	Coding Clinic

* **E2361** Power wheelchair accessory, 22NF sealed lead acid battory, each (e.g., gel cell, absorbed glassmat) ⑧ Qp Qh ♿ Y

* **E2362** Power wheelchair accessory, group 24 non-sealed lead acid battery, each ⑧ ♿ Y

* **E2363** Power wheelchair accessory, group 24 sealed lead acid battery, each (e.g., gel cell, absorbed glassmat) ⑧ Qp Qh ♿ Y

* **E2364** Power wheelchair accessory, U-1 non-sealed lead acid battery, each ⑧ ♿ Y

* **E2365** Power wheelchair accessory, U-1 sealed lead acid battery, each (e.g., gel cell, absorbed glassmat) ⑧ Qp Qh ♿ Y

* **E2366** Power wheelchair accessory, battery charger, single mode, for use with only one battery type, sealed or non-sealed, each ⑧ Qp Qh ♿ Y

* **E2367** Power wheelchair accessory, battery charger, dual mode, for use with either battery type, sealed or non-sealed, each ⑧ Qp Qh ♿ Y

* **E2368** Power wheelchair component, drive wheel motor, replacement only ⑧ Qp Qh ♿ Y

* **E2369** Power wheelchair component, drive wheel gear box, replacement only ⑧ Qp Qh ♿ Y

* **E2370** Power wheelchair component, integrated drive wheel motor and gear box combination, replacement only ⑧ Qp Qh ♿ Y

* **E2371** Power wheelchair accessory, group 27 sealed lead acid battery, (e.g., gel cell, absorbed glass mat), each ⑧ Qp Qh ♿ Y

* **E2372** Power wheelchair accessory, group 27 non-sealed lead acid battery, each ⑧ ♿ Y

* **E2373** Power wheelchair accessory, hand or chin control interface, compact remote joystick, proportional, including fixed mounting hardware ⑧ Qp Qh ♿ Y

⊛ **E2374** Power wheelchair accessory, hand or chin control interface, standard remote joystick (not including controller), proportional, including all related electronics and fixed mounting hardware, replacement only ⑧ Qp Qh ♿ Y

⊛ **E2375** Power wheelchair accessory, non-expandable controller, including all related electronics and mounting hardware, replacement only ⑧ Qp Qh ♿ Y

⊛ **E2376** Power wheelchair accessory, expandable controller, including all related electronics and mounting hardware, replacement only ⑧ Qp Qh ♿ Y

⊛ **E2377** Power wheelchair accessory, expandable controller, including all related electronics and mounting hardware, upgrade provided at initial issue ⑧ Qp Qh ♿ Y

* **E2378** Power wheelchair component, actuator, replacement only ⑧ Qp Qh ♿ Y

⊛ **E2381** Power wheelchair accessory, pneumatic drive wheel tire, any size, replacement only, each ⑧ Qp Qh ♿ Y

⊛ **E2382** Power wheelchair accessory, tube for pneumatic drive wheel tire, any size, replacement only, each ⑧ Qp Qh ♿ Y

⊛ **E2383** Power wheelchair accessory, insert for pneumatic drive wheel tire (removable), any type, any size, replacement only, each ⑧ Qp Qh ♿ Y

⊛ **E2384** Power wheelchair accessory, pneumatic caster tire, any size, replacement only, each ⑧ Qp Qh ♿ Y

⊛ **E2385** Power wheelchair accessory, tube for pneumatic caster tire, any size, replacement only, each ⑧ Qp Qh ♿ Y

⊛ **E2386** Power wheelchair accessory, foam filled drive wheel tire, any size, replacement only, each ⑧ Qp Qh ♿ Y

⊛ **E2387** Power wheelchair accessory, foam filled caster tire, any size, replacement only, each ⑧ Qp Qh ♿ Y

⊛ **E2388** Power wheelchair accessory, foam drive wheel tire, any size, replacement only, each ⑧ Qp Qh ♿ Y

⊛ **E2389** Power wheelchair accessory, foam caster tire, any size, replacement only, each ⑧ Qp Qh ♿ Y

⊛ **E2390** Power wheelchair accessory, solid (rubber/plastic) drive wheel tire, any size, replacement only, each ⑧ Qp Qh ♿ Y

⊛ **E2391** Power wheelchair accessory, solid (rubber/plastic) caster tire (removable), any size, replacement only, each ⑧ Qp Qh ♿ Y

⊛ **E2392** Power wheelchair accessory, solid (rubber/plastic) caster tire with integrated wheel, any size, replacement only, each ⑧ Qp Qh ♿ Y

▶ **New**   ↻ **Revised**   ✔ **Reinstated**   ~~deleted~~ **Deleted**   ⊘ **Not covered or valid by Medicare**
⊛ **Special coverage instructions**   * **Carrier discretion**   ⑧ **Bill Part B MAC**   ⑥ **Bill DME MAC**

⊘ **E2394** Power wheelchair accessory, drive wheel excludes tire, any size, replacement only, each Ⓑ Qp Qh ♿ Y

⊘ **E2395** Power wheelchair accessory, caster wheel excludes tire, any size, replacement only, each Ⓑ Qp Qh ♿ Y

⊘ **E2396** Power wheelchair accessory, caster fork, any size, replacement only, each Ⓑ Qp Qh ♿ Y

✳ **E2397** Power wheelchair accessory, lithium-based battery, each Ⓑ Qp Qh ♿ Y

✳ **E2398** Wheelchair accessory, dynamic positioning hardware for back Y

Negative Pressure

✳ **E2402** Negative pressure wound therapy electrical pump, stationary or portable Ⓑ Qp Qh ♿ Y

Document at least every 30 calendar days the quantitative wound characteristics, including wound surface area (length, width and depth).

Medicare coverage up to a maximum of 15 dressing kits (A6550) per wound per month unless documentation states that the wound size requires more than one dressing kit for each dressing change.

Speech Device

⊘ **E2500** Speech generating device, digitized speech, using pre-recorded messages, less than or equal to 8 minutes recording time Ⓑ Qp Qh ♿ Y

IOM: 100-03, 1, 50.1

⊘ **E2502** Speech generating device, digitized speech, using pre-recorded messages, greater than 8 minutes but less than or equal to 20 minutes recording time Ⓑ Qp Qh ♿ Y

IOM: 100-03, 1, 50.1

⊘ **E2504** Speech generating device, digitized speech, using pre-recorded messages, greater than 20 minutes but less than or equal to 40 minutes recording time Ⓑ Qp Qh ♿ Y

IOM: 100-03, 1, 50.1

⊘ **E2506** Speech generating device, digitized speech, using pre-recorded messages, greater than 40 minutes recording time Ⓑ Qp Qh ♿ Y

IOM: 100-03, 1, 50.1

⊘ **E2508** Speech generating device, synthesized speech, requiring message formulation by spelling and access by physical contact with the device Ⓑ Qp Qh ♿ Y

IOM: 100-03, 1, 50.1

⊘ **E2510** Speech generating device, synthesized speech, permitting multiple methods of message formulation and multiple methods of device access Ⓑ Qp Qh ♿ Y

IOM: 100-03, 1, 50.1

⊘ **E2511** Speech generating software program, for personal computer or personal digital assistant Ⓑ Qp Qh ♿ Y

IOM: 100-03, 1, 50.1

⊘ **E2512** Accessory for speech generating device, mounting system Ⓑ Qp Qh ♿ Y

IOM: 100-03, 1, 50.1

⊘ **E2599** Accessory for speech generating device, not otherwise classified Ⓑ Y

IOM: 100-03, 1, 50.1

Wheelchair: Cushion

✳ **E2601** General use wheelchair seat cushion, width less than 22 inches, any depth Ⓑ Qp Qh ♿ Y

✳ **E2602** General use wheelchair seat cushion, width 22 inches or greater, any depth Ⓑ Qp Qh ♿ Y

✳ **E2603** Skin protection wheelchair seat cushion, width less than 22 inches, any depth Ⓑ Qp Qh ♿ Y

✳ **E2604** Skin protection wheelchair seat cushion, width 22 inches or greater, any depth Ⓑ Qp Qh ♿ Y

✳ **E2605** Positioning wheelchair seat cushion, width less than 22 inches, any depth Ⓑ Qp Qh ♿ Y

✳ **E2606** Positioning wheelchair seat cushion, width 22 inches or greater, any depth Ⓑ Qp Qh ♿ Y

✳ **E2607** Skin protection and positioning wheelchair seat cushion, width less than 22 inches, any depth Ⓑ Qp Qh ♿ Y

✳ **E2608** Skin protection and positioning wheelchair seat cushion, width 22 inches or greater, any depth Ⓑ Qp Qh ♿ Y

✳ **E2609** Custom fabricated wheelchair seat cushion, any size Ⓑ Qp Qh Y

✳ **E2610** Wheelchair seat cushion, powered Ⓑ B

| 🅜 MIPS | Qp Quantity Physician | Qh Quantity Hospital | ♀ Female only |
| ♂ Male only | 🅐 Age | ♿ DMEPOS | A2-Z3 ASC Payment Indicator | A-Y ASC Status Indicator | Coding Clinic |

DURABLE MEDICAL EQUIPMENT E2394 – E2610

231

✳ **E2611** General use wheelchair back cushion, width less than 22 inches, any height, including any type mounting hardware Ⓑ Qp Qh ♿   Y

✳ **E2612** General use wheelchair back cushion, width 22 inches or greater, any height, including any type mounting hardware Ⓑ Qp Qh ♿   Y

✳ **E2613** Positioning wheelchair back cushion, posterior, width less than 22 inches, any height, including any type mounting hardware Ⓑ Qp Qh ♿   Y

✳ **E2614** Positioning wheelchair back cushion, posterior, width 22 inches or greater, any height, including any type mounting hardware Ⓑ Qp Qh ♿   Y

✳ **E2615** Positioning wheelchair back cushion, posterior-lateral, width less than 22 inches, any height, including any type mounting hardware Ⓑ Qp Qh ♿   Y

✳ **E2616** Positioning wheelchair back cushion, posterior-lateral, width 22 inches or greater, any height, including any type mounting hardware Ⓑ Qp Qh ♿   Y

✳ **E2617** Custom fabricated wheelchair back cushion, any size, including any type mounting hardware Ⓑ Qp Qh   Y

✳ **E2619** Replacement cover for wheelchair seat cushion or back cushion, each Ⓑ Qp Qh ♿   Y

✳ **E2620** Positioning wheelchair back cushion, planar back with lateral supports, width less than 22 inches, any height, including any type mounting hardware Ⓑ Qp Qh ♿   Y

✳ **E2621** Positioning wheelchair back cushion, planar back with lateral supports, width 22 inches or greater, any height, including any type mounting hardware Ⓑ Qp Qh ♿   Y

Wheelchair: Skin Protection

✳ **E2622** Skin protection wheelchair seat cushion, adjustable, width less than 22 inches, any depth Ⓑ Qp Qh ♿   Y

✳ **E2623** Skin protection wheelchair seat cushion, adjustable, width 22 inches or greater, any depth Ⓑ Qp Qh ♿   Y

✳ **E2624** Skin protection and positioning wheelchair seat cushion, adjustable, width less than 22 inches, any depth Ⓑ Qp Qh ♿   Y

✳ **E2625** Skin protection and positioning wheelchair seat cushion, adjustable, width 22 inches or greater, any depth Ⓑ Qp Qh ♿   Y

Wheelchair: Arm Support

✳ **E2626** Wheelchair accessory, shoulder elbow, mobile arm support attached to wheelchair, balanced, adjustable Ⓑ Qp Qh ♿   Y

✳ **E2627** Wheelchair accessory, shoulder elbow, mobile arm support attached to wheelchair, balanced, adjustable rancho type Ⓑ Qp Qh ♿   Y

✳ **E2628** Wheelchair accessory, shoulder elbow, mobile arm support attached to wheelchair, balanced, reclining Ⓑ Qp Qh ♿   Y

✳ **E2629** Wheelchair accessory, shoulder elbow, mobile arm support attached to wheelchair, balanced, friction arm support (friction dampening to proximal and distal joints) Ⓑ Qp Qh ♿   Y

✳ **E2630** Wheelchair accessory, shoulder elbow, mobile arm support, monosuspension arm and hand support, overhead elbow forearm hand sling support, yoke type suspension support Ⓑ Qp Qh ♿   Y

✳ **E2631** Wheelchair accessory, addition to mobile arm support, elevating proximal arm Ⓑ Qp Qh ♿   Y

✳ **E2632** Wheelchair accessory, addition to mobile arm support, offset or lateral rocker arm with elastic balance control Ⓑ Qp Qh ♿   Y

✳ **E2633** Wheelchair accessory, addition to mobile arm support, supinator Ⓑ Qp Qh ♿   Y

Pediatric Gait Trainer

⊘ **E8000** Gait trainer, pediatric size, posterior support, includes all accessories and components Ⓑ Ⓐ   E1

⊘ **E8001** Gait trainer, pediatric size, upright support, includes all accessories and components Ⓑ Ⓐ   E1

⊘ **E8002** Gait trainer, pediatric size, anterior support, includes all accessories and components Ⓑ Ⓐ   E1

▶ **New**   ⊃ **Revised**   ✔ **Reinstated**   ~~deleted~~ **Deleted**   ⊘ **Not covered or valid by Medicare**
✳ **Special coverage instructions**   ✳ **Carrier discretion**   Ⓑ **Bill Part B MAC**   Ⓖ **Bill DME MAC**

TEMPORARY PROCEDURES/ PROFESSIONAL SERVICES (G0000-G9999)

NOTE: Series "G", "K", and "Q" in the Level II coding are reserved for CMS assignment. "G", "K", and "Q" codes are temporary national codes for items or services requiring uniform national coding between one year's update and the next. Sometimes "temporary" codes remain for more than one update. If "G", "K", and "Q" codes are not converted to permanent codes in Level I or Level II series in the following update, they will remain active until converted in following years or until CMS notifies contractors to delete them. All active "G", "K", and "Q" codes at the time of update will be included on the update file for contractors. In addition, deleted codes are retained on the file for informational purposes, with a deleted indicator, for four years.

Vaccine Administration

❋ **G0008** Administration of influenza virus vaccine ⑧ `Qp` `Qh`   S

Coinsurance and deductible do not apply. If provided, report significant, separately identifiable E/M for medically necessary services (Z23).

Coding Clinic: 2016, Q4, P3

❋ **G0009** Administration of pneumococcal vaccine ⑧ `Qp` `Qh`   S

Reported once in a lifetime based on risk; Medicare covers cost of vaccine and administration (Z23)

Copayment, coinsurance, and deductible waived. (https://www.cms.gov/MLNProducts/downloads/MPS_QuickReferenceChart_1.pdf)

Coding Clinic: 2016, Q4, P3

❋ **G0010** Administration of hepatitis B vaccine ⑧ `Qp` `Qh`   S

Report for other than OPPs. Coinsurance and deductible apply; Medicare covers both cost of vaccine and administration (Z23)

Copayment/coinsurance and deductible are waived. (https://www.cms.gov/MLNProducts/downloads/MPS_QuickReferenceChart_1.pdf)

Coding Clinic: 2016, Q4, P3

Semen Analysis

❋ **G0027** Semen analysis; presence and/or motility of sperm excluding Huhner ⑧ `Qp` `Qh` ♂   Q4

Laboratory Certification: Hematology

❋ **G0029** Tobacco screening not performed or tobacco cessation intervention not provided during the measurement period or in the six months prior to the measurement period   M

❋ **G0030** Patient screened for tobacco use and received tobacco cessation intervention during the measurement period or in the six months prior to the measurement period (counseling, pharmacotherapy, or both), if identified as a tobacco user   M

❋ **G0031** Palliative care services given to patient any time during the measurement period   M

❋ **G0032** Two or more antipsychotic prescriptions ordered for patients who had a diagnosis of schizophrenia, schizoaffective disorder, or bipolar disorder on or between January 1 of the year prior to the measurement period and the index prescription start date (ipsd) for antipsychotics   M

❋ **G0033** Two or more benzodiazepine prescriptions ordered for patients who had a diagnosis of seizure disorders, rapid eye movement sleep behavior disorder, benzodiazepine withdrawal, ethanol withdrawal, or severe generalized anxiety disorder on or between January 1 of the year prior to the measurement period and the ipsd for benzodiazepines   M

❋ **G0034** Patients receiving palliative care during the measurement period   M

❋ **G0035** Patient has any emergency department encounter during the performance period with place of service indicator 23   M

❋ **G0036** Patient or care partner decline assessment   M

❋ **G0037** On date of encounter, patient is not able to participate in assessment or screening, including non-verbal patients, delirious, severely aphasic, severely developmentally delayed, severe visual or hearing impairment and for those patients, no knowledgeable informant available   M

❋ **G0038** Clinician determines patient does not require referral   M

🐦 **MIPS**	`Qp` **Quantity Physician**	`Qh` **Quantity Hospital**	♀ **Female only**
♂ **Male only** `A` **Age** ♿ **DMEPOS** **A2-Z3 ASC Payment Indicator** **A-Y ASC Status Indicator** *Coding Clinic*			

* **G0039** Patient not referred, reason not otherwise specified M

* **G0040** Patient already receiving physical/ occupational/speech/recreational therapy during the measurement period M

* **G0041** Patient and/or care partner decline referral M

* **G0042** Referral to physical, occupational, speech, or recreational therapy M

* **G0043** Patients with mechanical prosthetic heart valve M

* **G0044** Patients with moderate or severe mitral stenosis M

* **G0045** Clinical follow-up and mrs score assessed at 90 days following endovascular stroke intervention M

* **G0046** Clinical follow-up and mrs score not assessed at 90 days following endovascular stroke intervention M

* **G0047** Pediatric patient with minor blunt head trauma and pecarn prediction criteria are not assessed M

* **G0048** Patients who receive palliative care services any time during the intake period through the end of the measurement year M

* **G0049** With maintenance hemodialysis (in-center and home hd) for the complete reporting month M

* **G0050** Patients with a catheter that have limited life expectancy M

* **G0051** Patients under hospice care in the current reporting month M

* **G0052** Patients on peritoneal dialysis for any portion of the reporting month M

* **G0053** Advancing rheumatology patient care mips value pathways M

* **G0054** Coordinating stroke care to promote prevention and cultivate positive outcomes mips value pathways M

* **G0055** Advancing care for heart disease mips value pathways M

* **G0056** Optimizing chronic disease management mips value pathways M

* **G0057** Proposed adopting best practices and promoting patient safety within emergency medicine mips value pathways M

* **G0058** Improving care for lower extremity joint repair mips value pathways M

* **G0059** Patient safety and support of positive experiences with anesthesia mips value pathways M

* **G0060** Allergy/immunology mips specialty set M

* **G0061** Anesthesiology mips specialty set M

* **G0062** Audiology mips specialty set M

* **G0063** Cardiology mips specialty set M

* **G0064** Certified nurse midwife mips specialty set M

* **G0065** Chiropractic medicine mips specialty set M

* **G0066** Clinical social work mips specialty set M

* **G0067** Dentistry mips specialty set M

Administration, Payment and Care Management Services

* **G0068** Professional services for the administration of anti-infective, pain management, chelation, pulmonary hypertension, or other intravenous infusion drug or biological (excluding chemotherapy or other highly complex drug or biological) inotropic for each infusion drug administration calendar day in the individual's home, each 15 minutes ⑧ A

* **G0069** Professional services for the administration of subcutaneous immunotherapy or other subcutaneous infusion drug or biological for each infusion drug administration calendar day in the individual's home, each 15 minutes ⑧ A

* **G0070** Professional services for the administration of intravenous chemotherapy or other intravenous highly complex drug or biological infusion for each infusion drug administration calendar day in the individual's home, each 15 minutes ⑧ A

* **G0071** Payment for communication technology-based services for 5 minutes or more of a virtual (non-face-to-face) communication between an rural health clinic (RHC) or federally qualified health center (FQHC) practitioner and RHC or FQHC patient, or 5 minutes or more of remote evaluation of recorded video and/or images by an RHC or FQHC practitioner, occurring in lieu of an office visit; RHC or FQHC only ⑧ A

* **G0076** Brief (20 minutes) care management home visit for a new patient. For use only in a Medicare-approved CMMI model. (Services must be furnished within a beneficiary's home, domiciliary, rest home, assisted living and/or nursing facility.) ⑧ B

* **G0077** Limited (30 minutes) care management home visit for a new patient. For use only in a Medicare-approved CMMI model. (Services must be furnished within a beneficiary's home, domiciliary, rest home, assisted living and/or nursing facility.) ⑧ B

▶ **New**   ↻ **Revised**   ✔ **Reinstated**   ~~deleted~~ **Deleted**   ⊘ **Not covered or valid by Medicare**

⊛ **Special coverage instructions**   ✳ **Carrier discretion**   ⑧ **Bill Part B MAC**   ⑧ **Bill DME MAC**

* **G0078** Moderate (45 minutes) care management home visit for a new patient. For use only in a Medicare-approved CMMI model. (Services must be furnished within a beneficiary's home, domiciliary, rest home, assisted living and/or nursing facility.) ⓑ B

* **G0079** Comprehensive (60 minutes) care management home visit for a new patient. For use only in a Medicare-approved CMMI model. (Services must be furnished within a beneficiary's home, domiciliary, rest home, assisted living and/or nursing facility.) ⓑ B

* **G0080** Extensive (75 minutes) care management home visit for a new patient. For use only in a Medicare-approved CMMI model. (Services must be furnished within a beneficiary's home, domiciliary, rest home, assisted living and/or nursing facility.) ⓑ B

* **G0081** Brief (20 minutes) care management home visit for an existing patient. For use only in a Medicare-approved CMMI model. (Services must be furnished within a beneficiary's home, domiciliary, rest home, assisted living and/or nursing facility.) ⓑ B

* **G0082** Limited (30 minutes) care management home visit for an existing patient. For use only in a Medicare-approved CMMI model. (Services must be furnished within a beneficiary's home, domiciliary, rest home, assisted living and/or nursing facility.) ⓑ B

* **G0083** Moderate (45 minutes) care management home visit for an existing patient. For use only in a Medicare-approved CMMI model. (Services must be furnished within a beneficiary's home, domiciliary, rest home, assisted living and/or nursing facility.) ⓑ B

* **G0084** Comprehensive (60 minutes) care management home visit for an existing patient. For use only in a Medicare-approved CMMI model. (Services must be furnished within a beneficiary's home, domiciliary, rest home, assisted living and/or nursing facility.) ⓑ B

* **G0085** Extensive (75 minutes) care management home visit for an existing patient. For use only in a Medicare-approved CMMI model. (Services must be furnished within a beneficiary's home, domiciliary, rest home, assisted living and/or nursing facility.) ⓑ B

* **G0086** Limited (30 minutes) care management home care plan oversight. For use only in a Medicare-approved CMMI model. (Services must be furnished within a beneficiary's home, domiciliary, rest home, assisted living and/or nursing facility.) ⓑ B

* **G0087** Comprehensive (60 minutes) care management home care plan oversight. For use only in a Medicare-approved CMMI model. (Services must be furnished within a beneficiary's home, domiciliary, rest home, assisted living and/or nursing facility.) ⓑ B

* **G0088** Professional services, initial visit, for the administration of anti-infective, pain management, chelation, pulmonary hypertension, inotropic, or other intravenous infusion drug or biological (excluding chemotherapy or other highly complex drug or biological) for each infusion drug administration calendar day in the individual's home, each 15 minutes A

* **G0089** Professional services, initial visit, for the administration of subcutaneous immunotherapy or other subcutaneous infusion drug or biological for each infusion drug administration calendar day in the individual's home, each 15 minutes A

* **G0090** Professional services, initial visit, for the administration of intravenous chemotherapy or other highly complex infusion drug or biological for each infusion drug administration calendar day in the individual's home, each 15 minutes A

Screening Services

⊙ **G0101** Cervical or vaginal cancer screening; pelvic and clinical breast examination ⓑ Qp Qh S

Covered once every two years and annually if high risk for cervical/vaginal cancer, or if childbearing age patient has had an abnormal Pap smear in preceding three years. High risk diagnosis, Z77.9

Coding Clinic: 2002, Q4, P8

⊙ **G0102** Prostate cancer screening; digital rectal examination ⓑ Qp Qh N

Covered annually by Medicare (Z12.5). Not separately payable with an E/M code (99201-99499).

IOM: 100-02, 6, 10; 100-04, 4, 240; 100-04, 18, 50.1

⊙ **G0103** Prostate cancer screening; prostate specific antigen test (PSA) ⓑ Qp Qh A

Covered annually by Medicare (Z12.5)

IOM: 100-02, 6, 10; 100-04, 4, 240; 100-04, 18, 50

Laboratory Certification: Routine chemistry

⊛ MIPS Qp Quantity Physician Qh Quantity Hospital ♀ Female only
♂ Male only A Age ⅃ DMEPOS A2-Z3 ASC Payment Indicator A-Y ASC Status Indicator Coding Clinic

G0104 Colorectal cancer screening; flexible sigmoidoscopy ⑧ **Qp** **Qh**   T

Covered once every 48 months for beneficiaries age 50+

Co-insurance waived under Section 4104.

Coding Clinic: 2011, Q2, P4

G0105 Colorectal cancer screening; colonoscopy on individual at high risk ⑧ **Qp** **Qh**   T

Screening colonoscopy covered once every 24 months for high risk for developing colorectal cancer. May use modifier 53 if appropriate (physician fee schedule).

Co-insurance waived under Section 4104.

Coding Clinic: 2023, Q3, P12; 2018, Q2, P4; 2011, Q2, P4

G0106 Colorectal cancer screening; alternative to G0104, screening sigmoidoscopy, barium enema ⑧ **Qp** **Qh**   S

Barium enema (not high risk) (alternative to G0104). Covered once every 4 years for beneficiaries age 50+. Use modifier 26 for professional component only.

Coding Clinic: 2011, Q2, P4

Diabetes Management Training Services

* G0108 Diabetes outpatient self-management training services, individual, per 30 minutes ⑧ **Qp** **Qh**   A

Report for beneficiaries diagnosed with diabetes.

Effective January 2011, DSMT will be included in the list of reimbursable Medicare telehealth services.

* G0109 Diabetes outpatient self-management training services, group session (2 or more) per 30 minutes ⑧ **Qp** **Qh**   A

Report for beneficiaries diagnosed with diabetes.

Effective January 2011, DSMT will be included in the list of reimbursable Medicare telehealth services.

Screening Services

* G0117 Glaucoma screening for high risk patients furnished by an optometrist or ophthalmologist ⑧ **Qp** **Qh**   S

Covered once per year (full 11 months between screenings). Bundled with all other ophthalmic services provided on same day. Diagnosis code Z13.5.

* G0118 Glaucoma screening for high risk patient furnished under the direct supervision of an optometrist or ophthalmologist ⑧ **Qp** **Qh**   S

Covered once per year (full 11 months between screenings). Diagnosis code Z13.5.

G0120 Colorectal cancer screening; alternative to G0105, screening colonoscopy, barium enema. ⑧ **Qp** **Qh**   S

Barium enema for patients with a high risk of developing colorectal. Covered once every 2 years. Used as an alternative to G0105. Use modifier 26 for professional component only.

G0121 Colorectal cancer screening; colonoscopy on individual not meeting criteria for high risk ⑧ **Qp** **Qh**   T

Screening colonoscopy for patients that are not high risk. Covered once every 10 years, but not within 48 months of a G0104. For non-Medicare patients report 45378.

Co-insurance waived under Section 4104.

Coding Clinic: 2023, Q3, P12; 2018, Q2, P4

⊘ G0122 Colorectal cancer screening; barium enema ⑧   E1

Medicare: this service is denied as noncovered, because it fails to meet the requirements of the benefit. The beneficiary is liable for payment.

G0123 Screening cytopathology, cervical or vaginal (any reporting system), collected in preservative fluid, automated thin layer preparation, screening by cytotechnologist under physician supervision ⑧ **Qp** **Qh** ♀   A

Use G0123 or G0143 or G0144 or G0145 or G0147 or G0148 or P3000 for Pap smears NOT requiring physician interpretation (technical component).

IOM: 100-03, 3, 190.2; 100-04, 18, 30

Laboratory Certification: Cytology

G0124 Screening cytopathology, cervical or vaginal (any reporting system), collected in preservative fluid, automated thin layer preparation, requiring interpretation by physician ⑧ **Qp** **Qh** ♀   B

Report professional component for Pap smears requiring physician interpretation.

IOM: 100-03, 3, 190.2; 100-04, 18, 30

Laboratory Certification: Cytology

▶ New   ↺ Revised   ✔ Reinstated   ~~deleted~~ Deleted   ⊘ Not covered or valid by Medicare
◎ Special coverage instructions   * Carrier discretion   ⑧ Bill Part B MAC   ⑨ Bill DME MAC

Miscellaneous Services, Diagnostic and Therapeutic

⊘ **G0127** Trimming of dystrophic nails, any number Ⓑ [Qp] [Qh]   Q1

Must be used with a modifier (Q7, Q8, or Q9) to show that the foot care service is needed because the beneficiary has a systemic disease. Limit 1 unit of service.

IOM: 100-02, 15, 290

⊘ **G0128** Direct (face-to-face with patient) skilled nursing services of a registered nurse provided in a comprehensive outpatient rehabilitation facility, each 10 minutes beyond the first 5 minutes Ⓑ [Qp] [Qh]   B

A separate nursing service that is clearly identifiable in the Plan of Treatment and not part of other services. Documentation must support this service. Examples include: Insertion of a urinary catheter, intramuscular injections, bowel disimpaction, nursing assessment, and education. Restricted coverage by Medicare.

Medicare Statute 1833(a)

✳ **G0129** Occupational therapy services requiring the skills of a qualified occupational therapist, furnished as a component of a partial hospitalization treatment program, per session (45 minutes or more) Ⓑ [Qh]   P

⊘ **G0130** Single energy x-ray absorptiometry (SEXA) bone density study, one or more sites; appendicular skeleton (peripheral) (e.g., radius, wrist, heel) Ⓑ [Qp] [Qh]   Z3 S

Covered every 24 months (more frequently if medically necessary). Use modifier 26 for professional component only.

Preventive service; no deductible

IOM: 100-03, 2, 150.3; 100-04, 13, 140.1

✳ **G0141** Screening cytopathology smears, cervical or vaginal, performed by automated system, with manual rescreening, requiring interpretation by physician Ⓑ [Qp] [Qh] ♀   B

Co-insurance, copay, and deductible waived

Report professional component for Pap smears requiring physician interpretation. Refer to diagnosis of Z92.89, Z12.4, Z12.72, or Z12.89 to report appropriate risk level.

Laboratory Certification: Cytology

✳ **G0143** Screening cytopathology, cervical or vaginal (any reporting system), collected in preservative fluid, automated thin layer preparation, with manual screening and rescreening by cytotechnologist under physician supervision Ⓑ [Qp] [Qh] ♀   A

Co-insurance, copay, and deductible waived

Laboratory Certification: Cytology

✳ **G0144** Screening cytopathology, cervical or vaginal (any reporting system), collected in preservative fluid, automated thin layer preparation, with screening by automated system, under physician supervision Ⓑ [Qp] [Qh] ♀   A

Co-insurance, copay, and deductible waived

Laboratory Certification: Cytology

✳ **G0145** Screening cytopathology, cervical or vaginal (any reporting system), collected in preservative fluid, automated thin layer preparation, with screening by automated system and manual rescreening under physician supervision Ⓑ [Qp] [Qh] ♀   A

Co-insurance, copay, and deductible waived

Laboratory Certification: Cytology

✳ **G0147** Screening cytopathology smears, cervical or vaginal; performed by automated system under physician supervision Ⓑ [Qp] [Qh] ♀   A

Co-insurance, copay, and deductible waived

Laboratory Certification: Cytology

✳ **G0148** Screening cytopathology smears, cervical or vaginal; performed by automated system with manual rescreening Ⓑ [Qp] [Qh] ♀   A

Co-insurance, copay, and deductible waived

Laboratory Certification: Cytology

✳ **G0151** Services performed by a qualified physical therapist in the home health or hospice setting, each 15 minutes Ⓑ   B

✳ **G0152** Services performed by a qualified occupational therapist in the home health or hospice setting, each 15 minutes Ⓑ   B

✳ **G0153** Services performed by a qualified speech-language pathologist in the home health or hospice setting, each 15 minutes Ⓑ   B

✳ **G0155** Services of clinical social worker in home health or hospice settings, each 15 minutes Ⓑ   B

✳ **G0156** Services of home health/health aide in home health or hospice settings, each 15 minutes Ⓑ   B

🐾 **MIPS**   [Qp] **Quantity Physician**   [Qh] **Quantity Hospital**   ♀ **Female only**

♂ **Male only**   Ⓐ **Age**   ☪ **DMEPOS**   A2-Z3 **ASC Payment Indicator**   A-Y **ASC Status Indicator**   Coding Clinic

* **G0157** Services performed by a qualified physical therapist assistant in the home health or hospice setting, each 15 minutes Ⓑ   B

* **G0158** Services performed by a qualified occupational therapist assistant in the home health or hospice setting, each 15 minutes Ⓑ   B

* **G0159** Services performed by a qualified physical therapist, in the home health setting, in the establishment or delivery of a safe and effective physical therapy maintenance program, each 15 minutes Ⓑ   B

* **G0160** Services performed by a qualified occupational therapist, in the home health setting, in the establishment or delivery of a safe and effective occupational therapy maintenance program, each 15 minutes Ⓑ   B

* **G0161** Services performed by a qualified speech-language pathologist, in the home health setting, in the establishment or delivery of a safe and effective speech-language pathology maintenance program, each 15 minutes Ⓑ   B

* **G0162** Skilled services by a registered nurse (RN) for management and evaluation of the plan of care; each 15 minutes (the patient's underlying condition or complication requires an RN to ensure that essential non-skilled care achieves its purpose in the home health or hospice setting) Ⓑ   B

  Transmittal No. 824 (CR7182)

○ **G0166** External counterpulsation, per treatment session Ⓑ Qp Qh   Q1

  IOM: 100-03, 1, 20.20

* **G0168** Wound closure utilizing tissue adhesive(s) only Ⓑ Qp Qh   B

  Report for wound closure with only tissue adhesive. If a practitioner utilizes tissue adhesive in addition to staples or sutures to close a wound, HCPCS code G0168 is not separately reportable, but is included in the tissue repair.

  The only closure material used for a simple repair, coverage based on payer.

  Coding Clinic: 2005, Q1, P5; 2001, Q4, P12; Q3, P13

Figure 15 Tissue adhesive.

* **G0175** Scheduled interdisciplinary team conference (minimum of three exclusive of patient care nursing staff) with patient present Ⓑ Qp Qh   V

○ **G0176** Activity therapy, such as music, dance, art or play therapies not for recreation, related to the care and treatment of patient's disabling mental health problems, per session (45 minutes or more) ⊚ Qh   P

  Paid in partial hospitalization

○ **G0177** Training and educational services related to the care and treatment of patient's disabling mental health problems per session (45 minutes or more) ⊚ Qp Qh   N

  Paid in partial hospitalization

* **G0179** Physician recertification for Medicare-covered home health services under a home health plan of care (patient not present), including contacts with home health agency and review of reports of patient status required by physicians to affirm the initial implementation of the plan of care that meets patient's needs, per recertification period Ⓑ Qp Qh   M

  The recertification code is used after a patient has received services for at least 60 days (or one certification period) when the physician signs the certification after the initial certification period.

* **G0180** Physician certification for Medicare-covered home health services under a home health plan of care (patient not present), including contacts with home health agency and review of reports of patient status required by physicians to affirm the initial implementation of the plan of care that meets patient's needs, per certification period Ⓑ Qp Qh   M

  This code can be billed only when the patient has not received Medicare covered home health services for at least 60 days.

* **G0181** Physician supervision of a patient receiving Medicare-covered services provided by a participating home health agency (patient not present) requiring complex and multidisciplinary care modalities involving regular physician development and/or revision of care plans, review of subsequent reports of patient status, review of laboratory and other studies, communication (including telephone calls) with other health care professionals involved in the patient's care, integration of new information into the medical treatment plan and/or adjustment of medical therapy, within a calendar month, 30 minutes or more Ⓑ Qp Qh   M

  Coding Clinic: 2015, Q2, P10

▶ New   ↻ Revised   ✔ Reinstated   deleted Deleted   ⊘ Not covered or valid by Medicare
○ Special coverage instructions   * Carrier discretion   Ⓑ Bill Part B MAC   Ⓑ Bill DME MAC

Figure 16 PET scan.

* **G0182** Physician supervision of a patient under a Medicare-approved hospice (patient not present) requiring complex and multidisciplinary care modalities involving regular physician development and/or revision of care plans, review of subsequent reports of patient status, review of laboratory and other studies, communication (including telephone calls) with other health care professionals involved in the patient's care, integration of new information into the medical treatment plan and/or adjustment of medical therapy, within a calendar month, 30 minutes or more ⑧ Qp Qh **M**

Coding Clinic: 2015, Q2, P10

* **G0186** Destruction of localized lesion of choroid (for example, choroidal neovascularization); photocoagulation, feeder vessel technique (one or more sessions) ⑧ Qp Qh **T**

⊘ **G0219** PET imaging whole body; melanoma for non-covered indications ⑧ **E1**

Example: Assessing regional lymph nodes in melanoma.

IOM: 100-03, 4, 220.6

Coding Clinic: 2007, Q1, P6

⊘ **G0235** PET imaging, any site, not otherwise specified ⑧ Qp Qh **E1**

Example: Prostate cancer diagnosis and initial staging.

IOM: 100-03, 4, 220.6

Coding Clinic: 2007, Q1, P6

* **G0237** Therapeutic procedures to increase strength or endurance of respiratory muscles, face to face, one on one, each 15 minutes (includes monitoring) ⑧ Qp Qh **S**

* **G0238** Therapeutic procedures to improve respiratory function, other than described by G0237, one on one, face to face, per 15 minutes (includes monitoring) ⑧ Qp Qh **S**

* **G0239** Therapeutic procedures to improve respiratory function or increase strength or endurance of respiratory muscles, two or more individuals (includes monitoring) ⑧ Qp Qh **S**

⊛ **G0245** Initial physician evaluation and management of a diabetic patient with diabetic sensory neuropathy resulting in a loss of protective sensation (LOPS) which must include (1) the diagnosis of LOPS, (2) a patient history, (3) a physical examination that consist of at least the following elements: (A) visual inspection of the forefoot, hindfoot and toe web spaces, (B) evaluation of a protective sensation, (C) evaluation of foot structure and biomechanics, (D) evaluation of vascular status and skin integrity, and (E) evaluation and recommendation of footwear, and (4) patient education ⑧ Qp Qh **V**

IOM: 100-03, 1, 70.2.1

⊛ **G0246** Follow-up physician evaluation and management of a diabetic patient with diabetic sensory neuropathy resulting in a loss of protective sensation (LOPS) to include at least the following: (1) a patient history, (2) a physical examination that includes: (A) visual inspection of the forefoot, hindfoot and toe web spaces, (B) evaluation of protective sensation, (C) evaluation of foot structure and biomechanics, (D) evaluation of vascular status and skin integrity, and (E) evaluation and recommendation of footwear, and (3) patient education ⑧ Qp Qh **V**

IOM: 100-03, 1, 70.2.1; 100-02, 15, 290

⊛ **G0247** Routine foot care by a physician of a diabetic patient with diabetic sensory neuropathy resulting in a loss of protective sensation (LOPS) to include, the local care of superficial wounds (i.e., superficial to muscle and fascia) and at least the following if present: (1) local care of superficial wounds, (2) debridement of corns and calluses, and (3) trimming and debridement of nails ⑧ Qp Qh **Q1**

IOM: 100-03, 1, 70.2.1

⊛ **G0248** Demonstration, prior to initiation, of home INR monitoring for patient with either mechanical heart valve(s), chronic atrial fibrillation, or venous thromboembolism who meets Medicare coverage criteria, under the direction of a physician; includes: face-to-face demonstration of use and care of the INR monitor, obtaining at least one blood sample, provision of instructions for reporting home INR test results, and documentation of patient's ability to perform testing and report results ⑨ Qp Qh **V**

⬢ MIPS Qp **Quantity Physician** Qh **Quantity Hospital** ♀ **Female only**

♂ **Male only** A **Age** & **DMEPOS** A2-Z3 **ASC Payment Indicator** A-Y **ASC Status Indicator** *Coding Clinic*

⊚ **G0249** Provision of test materials and equipment for home INR monitoring of patient with either mechanical heart valve(s), chronic atrial fibrillation, or venous thromboembolism who meets Medicare coverage criteria; includes provision of materials for use in the home and reporting of test results to physician; testing not occurring more frequently than once a week; testing materials, billing units of service include 4 tests ⑧ **Qp** **Qh**   V

⊚ **G0250** Physician review, interpretation, and patient management of home INR testing for patient with either mechanical heart valve(s), chronic atrial fibrillation, or venous thromboembolism who meets Medicare coverage criteria; testing not occurring more frequently than once a week; billing units of service include 4 tests ⑧ **Qp** **Qh**   M

⊘ **G0252** PET imaging, full and partial-ring PET scanners only, for initial diagnosis of breast cancer and/or surgical planning for breast cancer (e.g., initial staging of axillary lymph nodes) ⑧   E1

IOM: 100-03, 4, 220.6

Coding Clinic: 2007, Q1, P6

⊘ **G0255** Current perception threshold/sensory nerve conduction test (SNCT), per limb, any nerve ⑧   E1

IOM: 100-03, 2, 160.23

⊚ **G0257** Unscheduled or emergency dialysis treatment for an ESRD patient in a hospital outpatient department that is not certified as an ESRD facility ⑧ **Qp** **Qh**   S

Coding Clinic: 2003, Q1, P9

⊚ **G0259** Injection procedure for sacroiliac joint; arthrography ⑨ **Qp** **Qh**   N

Replaces 27096 for reporting injections for Medicare beneficiaries

Used by Part A only (facility), not priced by Part B Medicare.

⊚ **G0260** Injection procedure for sacroiliac joint; provision of anesthetic, steroid and/or other therapeutic agent, with or without arthrography ⑨ **Qp** **Qh**   T

ASCs report when a therapeutic sacroiliac joint injection is administered in ASC

✻ **G0268** Removal of impacted cerumen (one or both ears) by physician on same date of service as audiologic function testing ⑧ **Qp** **Qh**   N

Report only when a physician, not an audiologist, performs the procedure.

Use with DX H61.2- when performed by physician.

Coding Clinic: 2016, Q2, P2-3; 2003, Q1, P12

⊚ **G0269** Placement of occlusive device into either a venous or arterial access site, post surgical or interventional procedure (e.g., angioseal plug, vascular plug) ⑨ **Qh**   N

Report for replacement of vasoseal. Hospitals may report the closure device as a supply with C1760. Bundled status on Physician Fee Schedule.

Coding Clinic: 2011, Q3, P4; 2010, Q4, P6

✻ **G0270** Medical nutrition therapy; reassessment and subsequent intervention(s) following second referral in same year for change in diagnosis, medical condition or treatment regimen (including additional hours needed for renal disease), individual, face to face with the patient, each 15 minutes ⑨ **Qp** **Qh**   A

Requires physician referral for beneficiaries with diabetes or renal disease. Services must be provided by dietitian/nutritionist. Co-insurance and deductible waived.

✻ **G0271** Medical nutrition therapy, reassessment and subsequent intervention(s) following second referral in same year for change in diagnosis, medical condition, or treatment regimen (including additional hours needed for renal disease), group (2 or more individuals), each 30 minutes ⑧ **Qp** **Qh**   A

Requires physician referral for beneficiaries with diabetes or renal disease. Services must be provided by dietitian/nutritionist. Co-insurance and deductible waived.

⊚ **G0276** Blinded procedure for lumbar stenosis, percutaneous image-guided lumbar decompression (PILD) or placebo-control, performed in an approved coverage with evidence development (CED) clinical trial ⑧ **Qp** **Qh**   J1

⊚ **G0277** Hyperbaric oxygen under pressure, full body chamber, per 30 minute interval ⑧ **Qp** **Qh**   S

IOM: 100-03, 1, 20.29

Coding Clinic: 2015, Q3, P7

✻ **G0278** Iliac and/or femoral artery angiography, non-selective, bilateral or ipsilateral to catheter insertion, performed at the same time as cardiac catheterization and/or coronary angiography, includes positioning or placement of the catheter in the distal aorta or ipsilateral femoral or iliac artery, injection of dye, production of permanent images, and radiologic supervision and interpretation (list separately in addition to primary procedure) ⑧ **Qp** **Qh**   N

Medicare specific code not reported for iliac injection used as a guiding shot for a closure device

Coding Clinic: 2011, Q3, P4; 2006, Q4, P7

▶ **New**   ⤶ **Revised**   ✔ **Reinstated**   ~~deleted~~ **Deleted**   ⊘ **Not covered or valid by Medicare**
⊚ **Special coverage instructions**   ✻ **Carrier discretion**   ⑧ **Bill Part B MAC**   ⑨ **Bill DME MAC**

* **G0279** Diagnostic digital breast tomosynthesis, unilateral or bilateral (list separately in addition to 77065 or 77066) Ⓑ   **A**

* **G0281** Electrical stimulation, (unattended), to one or more areas, for chronic stage III and stage IV pressure ulcers, arterial ulcers, diabetic ulcers, and venous stasis ulcers not demonstrating measurable signs of healing after 30 days of conventional care, as part of a therapy plan of care Ⓑ Qp Qh   **A**

  Reported by encounter/areas and not by site. Therapists report G0281 and G0283 rather than 97014.

⊘ **G0282** Electrical stimulation, (unattended), to one or more areas, for wound care other than described in G0281 Ⓑ   **E1**

  IOM: 100-03, 4, 270.1

* **G0283** Electrical stimulation, (unattended), to one or more areas for indication(s) other than wound care, as part of a therapy plan of care Ⓑ Qp Qh   **A**

  Reported by encounter/areas and not by site. Therapists report G0281 and G0283 rather than 97014.

* **G0288** Reconstruction, computed tomographic angiography of aorta for surgical planning for vascular surgery Ⓑ Qp Qh   **N**

* **G0289** Arthroscopy, knee, surgical, for removal of loose body, foreign body, debridement/shaving of articular cartilage (chondroplasty) at the time of other surgical knee arthroscopy in a different compartment of the same knee Ⓑ Qp Qh   **N**

  Add-on code reported with knee arthroscopy code for major procedure performed-reported once per extra compartment

  "The code may be reported twice (or with a unit of two) if the physician performs these procedures in two compartments, in addition to the compartment where the main procedure was performed." (http://www.ama-assn.org/resources/doc/cpt/orthopaedics.pdf)

⊚ **G0293** Noncovered surgical procedure(s) using conscious sedation, regional, general or spinal anesthesia in a Medicare qualifying clinical trial, per day Ⓑ Qp Qh   **Q1**

⊚ **G0294** Noncovered procedure(s) using either no anesthesia or local anesthesia only, in a Medicare qualifying clinical trial, per day Ⓑ Qp Qh   **Q1**

⊘ **G0295** Electromagnetic therapy, to one or more areas, for wound care other than described in G0329 or for other uses Ⓑ **E1**

  IOM: 100-03, 4, 270.1

* **G0296** Counseling visit to discuss need for lung cancer screening (LDCT) using low dose CT scan (service is for eligibility determination and shared decision making) Ⓑ Qp Qh   **S**

* **G0299** Direct skilled nursing services of a registered nurse (RN) in the home health or hospice setting, each 15 minutes Ⓑ   **B**

* **G0300** Direct skilled nursing services of a licensed practical nurse (LPN) in the home health or hospice setting, each 15 minutes Ⓑ   **B**

* **G0302** Pre-operative pulmonary surgery services for preparation for LVRS, complete course of services, to include a minimum of 16 days of services Ⓑ Qp Qh   **S**

* **G0303** Pre-operative pulmonary surgery services for preparation for LVRS, 10 to 15 days of services Ⓑ Qp Qh   **S**

* **G0304** Pre-operative pulmonary surgery services for preparation for LVRS, 1 to 9 days of services Ⓑ Qp Qh   **S**

* **G0305** Post-discharge pulmonary surgery services after LVRS, minimum of 6 days of services Ⓑ Qp Qh   **S**

* **G0306** Complete CBC, automated (HgB, HCT, RBC, WBC, without platelet count) and automated WBC differential count Ⓑ Qp Qh   **Q4**

  Laboratory Certification: Hematology

* **G0307** Complete CBC, automated (HgB, HCT, RBC, WBC; without platelet count) Ⓑ Qp Qh   **Q4**

  Laboratory Certification: Hematology

   G0310 Immunization counseling by a physician or other qualified health care professional when the vaccine(s) is not administered on the same date of service, 5 to 15 mins time (this code is used for Medicaid billing purposes)   **E1**

   G0311 Immunization counseling by a physician or other qualified health care professional when the vaccine(s) is not administered on the same date of service, 16-30 mins time (this code is used for Medicaid billing purposes)   **E1**

   G0312 Immunization counseling by a physician or other qualify ED health care professional when the vaccine(s) is not administered on the same date of service for ages under 21, 5 to 15 mins time (this code is used for Medicaid billing purposes)   **E1**

G0313 Immunization counseling by a physician or other qualified health care professional when the vaccine(s) is not administered on the same date of service for ages under 21, 16-30 mins time (this code is used for Medicaid billing purposes)   E1

G0314 Immunization counseling by a physician or other qualified health care professional for covid-19, ages under 21, 16-30 mins time (this code is used for the medicaid early and periodic screening, diagnostic, and treatment benefit [EPSDT])   E1

G0315 Immunization counseling by a physician or other qualified health care professional for covid-19, ages under 21, 5-15 mins time (this code is used for the medicaid early and periodic screening, diagnostic, and treatment benefit [EPSDT])   E1

G0316 Prolonged hospital inpatient or observation care evaluation and management service(s) beyond the total time for the primary service (when the primary service has been selected using time on the date of the primary service); each additional 15 minutes by the physician or qualified healthcare professional, with or without direct patient contact (list separately in addition to CPT codes 99223, 99233, and 99236 for hospital inpatient or observation care evaluation and management services). (do not report G0316 on the same date of service as other prolonged services for evaluation and management 99358, 99359, 99418, 99415, 99416). (do not report G0316 for any time unit less than 15 minutes)   N

G0317 Prolonged nursing facility evaluation and management service(s) beyond the total time for the primary service (when the primary service has been selected using time on the date of the primary service); each additional 15 minutes by the physician or qualified healthcare professional, with or without direct patient contact (list separately in addition to CPT codes 99306, 99310 for nursing facility evaluation and management services). (do not report G0317 on the same date of service as other prolonged services for evaluation and management 99358, 99359, 99418). (do not report G0317 for any time unit less than 15 minutes)   B

G0318 Prolonged home or residence evaluation and management service(s) beyond the total time for the primary service (when the primary service has been selected using time on the date of the primary service); each additional 15 minutes by the physician or qualified healthcare professional, with or without direct patient contact (list separately in addition to CPT codes 99345, 99350 for home or residence evaluation and management services). (do not report G0318 on the same date of service as other prolonged services for evaluation and management 99358, 99359, 99417). (do not report G0318 for any time unit less than 15 minutes)   B

G0320 Home health services furnished using synchronous telemedicine rendered via a real-time two-way audio and video telecommunications system   A

G0321 Home health services furnished using synchronous telemedicine rendered via telephone or other real-time interactive audio-only telecommunications system   A

G0322 The collection of physiologic data digitally stored and/or transmitted by the patient to the home health agency (i.e., remote patient monitoring)   A

G0323 Care management services for behavioral health conditions, at least 20 minutes of clinical psychologist or clinical social worker time, per calendar month. (these services include the following required elements: initial assessment or follow-up monitoring, including the use of applicable validated rating scales; behavioral health care planning in relation to behavioral/psychiatric health problems, including revision for patients who are not progressing or whose status changes; facilitating and coordinating treatment such as psychotherapy, coordination with and/or referral to physicians and practitioners who are authorized by Medicare to prescribe medications and furnish e/m services, counseling and/or psychiatric consultation; and continuity of care with a designated member of the care team)   S

✱ **G0327** Colorectal cancer screening; blood-based biomarker   A

▶ **New**   ↻ **Revised**   ✔ **Reinstated**   ~~deleted~~ **Deleted**   ⊘ **Not covered or valid by Medicare**

⊛ **Special coverage instructions**   ✱ **Carrier discretion**   Ⓑ **Bill Part B MAC**   Ⓓ **Bill DME MAC**

US machine

Electromagnetic device

Figure 17 Electromagnetic device.

⊛ **G0328** Colorectal cancer screening; fecal occult blood test, immunoassay, 1-3 simultaneous ⑧ **Qp** **Qh**   A

Co-insurance and deductible waived

Reported for Medicare patients 501; one FOBT per year, with either G0107 (guaiac-based) or G0328 (immunoassay-based)

Laboratory Certification: Routine chemistry, Hematology

Coding Clinic: 2023, Q3, P12; 2012, Q2, P9

✳ **G0329** Electromagnetic therapy, to one or more areas for chronic stage III and stage IV pressure ulcers, arterial ulcers, and diabetic ulcers and venous stasis ulcers not demonstrating measurable signs of healing after 30 days of conventional care as part of a therapy plan of care ⑧ **Qp** **Qh**   A

G0330 Facility services for dental rehabilitation procedure(s) performed on a patient who requires monitored anesthesia (e.g., general, intravenous sedation (monitored anesthesia care) and use of an operating room   S

⊛ **G0333** Pharmacy dispensing fee for inhalation drug(s); initial 30-day supply as a beneficiary ⑧ **Qp** **Qh**   M

Medicare will reimburse an initial dispensing fee to a pharmacy for initial 30-day period of inhalation drugs furnished through DME.

✳ **G0337** Hospice evaluation and counseling services, pre-election ⑧ **Qp** **Qh**   B

✳ **G0339** Image-guided robotic linear accelerator-based stereotactic radiosurgery, complete course of therapy in one session or first session of fractionated treatment ⑧ **Qp** **Qh**   B

✳ **G0340** Image-guided robotic linear accelerator-based stereotactic radiosurgery, delivery including collimator changes and custom plugging, fractionated treatment, all lesions, per session, second through fifth sessions, maximum five sessions per course of treatment ⑧ **Qp** **Qh**   B

⊛ **G0341** Percutaneous islet cell transplant, includes portal vein catheterization and infusion ⑧ **Qp** **Qh**   C

IOM: 100-03, 4, 260.3; 100-04, 32, 70

⊛ **G0342** Laparoscopy for islet cell transplant, includes portal vein catheterization and infusion ⑧ **Qp** **Qh**   C

IOM: 100-03, 4, 260.3

⊛ **G0343** Laparotomy for islet cell transplant, includes portal vein catheterization and infusion ⑧ **Qp** **Qh**   C

IOM: 100-03, 4, 260.3

⊛ **G0372** Physician service required to establish and document the need for a power mobility device ⑧ **Qp** **Qh**   M

Providers should bill the E/M code and G0372 on the same claim.

Hospital Services: Observation and Emergency Department

⊛ **G0378** Hospital observation service, per hour ⑧ **Qh**   N

Report all related services in addition to G0378. Report units of hours spent in observation (rounded to the nearest hour). Hospitals report the ED or clinic visit with a CPT code or, if applicable, G0379 (direct admit to observation) and G0378 (hospital observation services, per hour).

Coding Clinic: 2007, Q1, P10; 2006, Q3, P7-8

⊛ **G0379** Direct admission of patient for hospital observation care ⑧ **Qp** **Qh**   J2

Report all related services in addition to G0379. Report units of hours spent in observation (rounded to the nearest hour). Hospitals report the ED or clinic visit with a CPT code or, if applicable, G0379 (direct admit to observation) and G0378 (hospital observation services, per hour).

Coding Clinic: 2007, Q1, P7

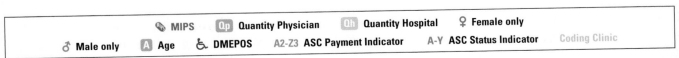

🏷 MIPS   **Qp** Quantity Physician   **Qh** Quantity Hospital   ♀ Female only

♂ Male only   **A** Age   ♿ DMEPOS   A2-Z3 ASC Payment Indicator   A-Y ASC Status Indicator   Coding Clinic

* **G0380** Level 1 hospital emergency department visit provided in a type B emergency department; (the ED must meet at least one of the following requirements: (1) it is licensed by the state in which it is located under applicable state law as an emergency room or emergency department; (2) it is held out to the public (by name, posted signs, advertising, or other means) as a place that provides care for emergency medical conditions on an urgent basis without requiring a previously scheduled appointment; or (3) during the calendar year immediately preceding the calendar year in which a determination under 42 CFR 489.24 is being made, based on a representative sample of patient visits that occurred during that calendar year, it provides at least one-third of all of its outpatient visits for the treatment of emergency medical conditions on an urgent basis without requiring a previously scheduled appointment) ⑧ 〔Oh〕 **J2**

Coding Clinic: 2009, Q1, P4; 2007, Q2, P1

* **G0381** Level 2 hospital emergency department visit provided in a type B emergency department; (the ED must meet at least one of the following requirements: (1) it is licensed by the state in which it is located under applicable state law as an emergency room or emergency department; (2) it is held out to the public (by name, posted signs, advertising, or other means) as a place that provides care for emergency medical conditions on an urgent basis without requiring a previously scheduled appointment; or (3) during the calendar year immediately preceding the calendar year in which a determination under 42 CFR 489.24 is being made, based on a representative sample of patient visits that occurred during that calendar year, it provides at least one-third of all of its outpatient visits for the treatment of emergency medical conditions on an urgent basis without requiring a previously scheduled appointment) ⑧ 〔Oh〕 **J2**

Coding Clinic: 2009, Q1, P4; 2007, Q2, P1

* **G0382** Level 3 hospital emergency department visit provided in a type B emergency department; (the ED must meet at least one of the following requirements: (1) it is licensed by the state in which it is located under applicable state law as an emergency room or emergency department; (2) it is held out to the public (by name, posted signs, advertising, or other means) as a place that provides care for emergency medical conditions on an urgent basis without requiring a previously scheduled appointment; or (3) during the calendar year immediately preceding the calendar year in which a determination under 42 CFR 489.24 is being made, based on a representative sample of patient visits that occurred during that calendar year, it provides at least one-third of all of its outpatient visits for the treatment of emergency medical conditions on an urgent basis without requiring a previously scheduled appointment) ⑧ 〔Oh〕 **J2**

Coding Clinic: 2009, Q1, P4; 2007, Q2, P1

* **G0383** Level 4 hospital emergency department visit provided in a type B emergency department; (the ED must meet at least one of the following requirements: (1) it is licensed by the state in which it is located under applicable state law as an emergency room or emergency department; (2) it is held out to the public (by name, posted signs, advertising, or other means) as a place that provides care for emergency medical conditions on an urgent basis without requiring a previously scheduled appointment; or (3) during the calendar year immediately preceding the calendar year in which a determination under 42 CFR 489.24 is being made, based on a representative sample of patient visits that occurred during that calendar year, it provides at least one-third of all of its outpatient visits for the treatment of emergency medical conditions on an urgent basis without requiring a previously scheduled appointment) ⑧ 〔Oh〕 **J2**

Coding Clinic: 2009, Q1, P4; 2007, Q2, P1

TEMPORARY PROCEDURES/PROFESSIONAL SERVICES

G0380 – G0383

▶ **New**   ⟳ **Revised**   ✔ **Reinstated**   ~~deleted~~ **Deleted**   ⊘ **Not covered or valid by Medicare**
⊛ **Special coverage instructions**   * **Carrier discretion**   ⑧ **Bill Part B MAC**   ⑨ **Bill DME MAC**

✳ **G0384** Level 5 hospital emergency department visit provided in a type B emergency department; (the ED must meet at least one of the following requirements: (1) it is licensed by the state in which it is located under applicable state law as an emergency room or emergency department; (2) it is held out to the public (by name, posted signs, advertising, or other means) as a place that provides care for emergency medical conditions on an urgent basis without requiring a previously scheduled appointment; or (3) during the calendar year immediately preceding the calendar year in which a determination under 42 CFR 489.24 is being made, based on a representative sample of patient visits that occurred during that calendar year, it provides at least one-third of all of its outpatient visits for the treatment of emergency medical conditions on an urgent basis without requiring a previously scheduled appointment) ⑧ 𝗤𝗵 **J2**

Coding Clinic: 2009, Q1, P4; 2007, Q2, P1

Trauma Response Team

◎ **G0390** Trauma response team associated with hospital critical care service ⑧ 𝗤𝗵 **S**

Coding Clinic: 2007, Q2, P5

Alcohol Substance Abuse Assessment and Intervention

🔖 ✳ **G0396** Alcohol and/or substance (other than tobacco) misuse structured assessment (e.g., audit) and brief intervention 15 to 30 minutes ⑧ 𝗤𝗽 𝗤𝗵 **S**

Bill instead of 99408 and 99409

🔖 ✳ **G0397** Alcohol and/or substance (other than tobacco) misuse structured assessment (e.g., audit) and intervention, greater than 30 minutes ⑧ 𝗤𝗽 𝗤𝗵 **S**

Bill instead of 99408 and 99409

Home Sleep Study Test

✳ **G0398** Home sleep study test (HST) with type II portable monitor, unattended; minimum of 7 channels: EEG, EOG, EMG, ECG/heart rate, airflow, respiratory effort and oxygen saturation ⑧ 𝗤𝗽 𝗤𝗵 **S**

✳ **G0399** Home sleep test (HST) with type III portable monitor, unattended; minimum of 4 channels: 2 respiratory movement/airflow, 1 ECG/heart rate and 1 oxygen saturation ⑧ 𝗤𝗽 𝗤𝗵 **S**

✳ **G0400** Home sleep test (HST) with type IV portable monitor, unattended; minimum of 3 channels ⑧ 𝗤𝗽 𝗤𝗵 **S**

Initial Examination for Medicare Enrollment

🔖 ✳ **G0402** Initial preventive physical examination; face-to-face visit, services limited to new beneficiary during the first 12 months of Medicare enrollment ⑧ 𝗤𝗽 𝗤𝗵 **V**

Depending on circumstances, 99201-99215 may be assigned with modifier 25 to report an E/M service as a significant, separately identifiable service in addition to the Initial Preventive Physical Examination (IPPE), G0402.

Copayment and coinsurance waived, deductible waived.

Coding Clinic: 2009, Q4, P8

Electrocardiogram

✳ **G0403** Electrocardiogram, routine ECG with 12 leads; performed as a screening for the initial preventive physical examination with interpretation and report ⑧ 𝗤𝗽 𝗤𝗵 **M**

Optional service may be ordered or performed at discretion of physician. Once in a lifetime screening, stemming from a referral from Initial Preventive Physical Examination (IPPE). Both deductible and co-payment apply.

✳ **G0404** Electrocardiogram, routine ECG with 12 leads; tracing only, without interpretation and report, performed as a screening for the initial preventive physical examination ⑧ 𝗤𝗽 𝗤𝗵 **S**

✳ **G0405** Electrocardiogram, routine ECG with 12 leads; interpretation and report only, performed as a screening for the initial preventive physical examination ⑧ 𝗤𝗽 𝗤𝗵 **B**

🔖 MIPS	𝗤𝗽 Quantity Physician	𝗤𝗵 Quantity Hospital	♀ Female only
♂ Male only · A Age · ⅊ DMEPOS	A2-Z3 ASC Payment Indicator	A-Y ASC Status Indicator	Coding Clinic

Follow-up Telehealth Consultation

✻ **G0406** Follow-up inpatient consultation, limited, physicians typically spend 15 minutes communicating with the patient via telehealth ⑧ **Qp** **Qh**   B

These telehealth modifers are required when billing for telehealth services with codes G0406-G0408 and G0425-G0427:

- GT, via interactive audio and video telecommunications system
- GQ, via asynchronous telecommunications system

✻ **G0407** Follow-up inpatient consultation, intermediate, physicians typically spend 25 minutes communicating with the patient via telehealth ⑧ **Qp** **Qh**   B

✻ **G0408** Follow-up inpatient consultation, complex, physicians typically spend 35 minutes communicating with the patient via telehealth ⑧ **Qp** **Qh**   B

Psychological Services

✻ **G0409** Social work and psychological services, directly relating to and/or furthering the patient's rehabilitation goals, each 15 minutes, face-to-face; individual (services provided by a CORF-qualified social worker or psychologist in a CORF) ⑧   B

✻ **G0410** Group psychotherapy other than of a multiple-family group, in a partial hospitalization setting, approximately 45 to 50 minutes ⑧ **Qp** **Qh**   P

Coding Clinic: 2009, Q4, P9, 10

✻ **G0411** Interactive group psychotherapy, in a partial hospitalization setting, approximately 45 to 50 minutes ⑧ **Qp** **Qh**   P

Coding Clinic: 2009, Q4, P9, 10

Fracture Treatment

✻ **G0412** Open treatment of iliac spine(s), tuberosity avulsion, or iliac wing fracture(s), unilateral or bilateral for pelvic bone fracture patterns which do not disrupt the pelvic ring, includes internal fixation, when performed ⑧ **Qp** **Qh**   C

✻ **G0413** Percutaneous skeletal fixation of posterior pelvic bone fracture and/or dislocation, for fracture patterns which disrupt the pelvic ring, unilateral or bilateral, (includes ilium, sacroiliac joint and/or sacrum) ⑧ **Qp** **Qh**   J1

✻ **G0414** Open treatment of anterior pelvic bone fracture and/or dislocation for fracture patterns which disrupt the pelvic ring, unilateral or bilateral, includes internal fixation when performed (includes pubic symphysis and/or superior/inferior rami) ⑧ **Qp** **Qh**   C

✻ **G0415** Open treatment of posterior pelvic bone fracture and/or dislocation, for fracture patterns which disrupt the pelvic ring, unilateral or bilateral, includes internal fixation, when performed (includes ilium, sacroiliac joint and/or sacrum) ⑧ **Qp** **Qh**   C

Surgical Pathology: Prostate Biopsy

✻ **G0416** Surgical pathology, gross and microscopic examinations for prostate needle biopsy, any method ⑧ **Qp** **Qh** ♂   Q2

This testing requires a facility to have either a CLIA certificate of registration (certificate type code 9), a CLIA certificate of compliance (certificate type code 1), or a CLIA certificate of accreditation (certificate type code 3). A facility without a valid, current, CLIA certificate, with a current CLIA certificate of waiver (certificate type code 2) or with a current CLIA certificate for provider-performed microscopy procedures (certificate type code 4), must not be permitted to be paid for these tests. This code has a TC, 26 (physician), or global component.

Laboratory Certification: Histopathology

Coding Clinic: 2013, Q2, P6

Educational Services

✳ **G0420** Face-to-face educational services related to the care of chronic kidney disease; individual, per session, per one hour Ⓑ Qp Qh   A

CKD is kidney damage of 3 months or longer, regardless of the cause of kidney damage. Sessions billed in increments of one hour (if session is less than one hour, it must last at least 31 minutes to be billable. Sessions less than one hour and longer than 31 minutes are billable as one session. No more than 6 sessions of KDE services in a beneficiary's lifetime.

✳ **G0421** Face-to-face educational services related to the care of chronic kidney disease; group, per session, per one hour Ⓑ Qp Qh   A

Group setting: 2 to 20, report codes G0420 and G0421 with diagnosis code N18.4.

Cardiac and Pulmonary Rehabilitation

✳ **G0422** Intensive cardiac rehabilitation; with or without continuous ECG monitoring with exercise, per session Ⓑ Qp Qh   S

Includes the same service as 93798 but at a greater frequency; may be reported with as many as six hourly sessions on a single date of service. Includes medical nutrition services to reduce cardiac disease risk factors.

✳ **G0423** Intensive cardiac rehabilitation; with or without continuous ECG monitoring; without exercise, per session Ⓑ Qp Qh   S

Includes the same service as 93797 but at a greater frequency; may be reported with as many as six hourly sessions on a single date of service. Includes medical nutrition services to reduce cardiac disease risk factors.

Initial Telehealth Consultation

✳ **G0425** Telehealth consultation, emergency department or initial inpatient, typically 30 minutes communicating with the patient via telehealth Ⓑ Qp Qh   B

Problem Focused: Problem focused history and examination, with straightforward medical decision-making complexity. Typically 30 minutes communicating with patient via telehealth.

✳ **G0426** Initial inpatient telehealth consultation, emergency department or initial inpatient, typically 50 minutes communicating with the patient via telehealth Ⓑ Qp Qh   B

Detailed: Detailed history and examination, with moderate medical decision-making complexity. Typically 50 minutes communicating with patient via telehealth.

✳ **G0427** Initial inpatient telehealth consultation, emergency department or initial inpatient, typically 70 minutes or more communicating with the patient via telehealth Ⓑ Qp Qh   B

Comprehensive: Comprehensive history and examination, with high medical decision-making complexity. Typically 70 minutes or more communicating with patient via telehealth.

Fillers

⊘ **G0428** Collagen meniscus implant procedure for filling meniscal defects (e.g., cmi, collagen scaffold, menaflex) Ⓑ   E1

✳ **G0429** Dermal filler injection(s) for the treatment of facial lipodystrophy syndrome (LDS) (e.g., as a result of highly active antiretroviral therapy) Ⓑ Qp Qh   T

Designated for dermal fillers Sculptra and Radiesse (Medicare). (https://www.cms.gov/ContractorLearningResources/downloads/JA6953.pdf)

Coding Clinic: 2010, Q3, P8

🔖 MIPS   Qp Quantity Physician   Qh Quantity Hospital   ♀ Female only

♂ Male only   A Age   ⅙ DMEPOS   A2-Z3 ASC Payment Indicator   A-Y ASC Status Indicator   Coding Clinic

Laboratory Screening

✻ **G0432** Infectious agent antibody detection by enzyme immunoassay (EIA) technique, HIV-1 and/or HIV-2, screening ⑧ Qp Qh   A

Laboratory Certification: Virology, General immunology

Coding Clinic: 2010, Q2, P10

✻ **G0433** Infectious agent antibody detection by enzyme-linked immunosorbent assay (ELISA) technique, HIV-1 and/or HIV-2, screening ⑨ Qp Qh   A

Laboratory Certification: Virology, General immunology

Coding Clinic: 2010, Q2, P10

✻ **G0435** Infectious agent antibody detection by rapid antibody test, HIV-1 and/or HIV-2, screening ⑧ Qp Qh   A

Coding Clinic: 2010, Q2, P10

Counselling, Wellness, and Screening Services

✻ **G0438** Annual wellness visit; includes a personalized prevention plan of service (pps), initial visit ⑧ Qp Qh   A

✻ **G0439** Annual wellness visit, includes a personalized prevention plan of service (pps), subsequent visit ⑨ Qp Qh   A

✻ **G0442** Annual alcohol misuse screening, 5 to 15 minutes ⑧ Qp Qh   S

Coding Clinic: 2012, Q1, P7

✻ **G0443** Brief face-to-face behavioral counseling for alcohol misuse, 15 minutes ⑧ Qp Qh   S

Coding Clinic: 2012, Q1, P7

✻ **G0444** Annual depression screening, 5 to 15 minutes ⑧ Qp Qh   S

✻ **G0445** High intensity behavioral counseling to prevent sexually transmitted infection; face-to-face, individual, includes: education, skills training and guidance on how to change sexual behavior; performed semi-annually, 30 minutes ⑧ Qp Qh   S

✻ **G0446** Annual, face-to-face intensive behavioral therapy for cardiovascular disease, individual, 15 minutes ⑧ Qp Qh   S

Coding Clinic: 2012, Q2, P8

✻ **G0447** Face-to-face behavioral counseling for obesity, 15 minutes ⑧ Qp Qh   S

Coding Clinic: 2012, Q1, P8

✻ **G0448** Insertion or replacement of a permanent pacing cardioverter-defibrillator system with transvenous lead(s), single or dual chamber with insertion of pacing electrode, cardiac venous system, for left ventricular pacing ⑧ Qp Qh   B

✻ **G0451** Development testing, with interpretation and report, per standardized instrument form ⑧ Qp Qh   Q3

Miscellaneous Services

✻ **G0452** Molecular pathology procedure; physician interpretation and report ⑧ Qp Qh   B

✻ **G0453** Continuous intraoperative neurophysiology monitoring, from outside the operating room (remote or nearby), per patient (attention directed exclusively to one patient), each 15 minutes (list in addition to primary procedure) ⑧ Qp Qh   N

✻ **G0454** Physician documentation of face-to-face visit for durable medical equipment determination performed by nurse practitioner, physician assistant or clinical nurse specialist ⑧ Qp Qh   B

✻ **G0455** Preparation with instillation of fecal microbiota by any method, including assessment of donor specimen ⑧ Qp Qh   Q1

Coding Clinic: 2013, Q3, P8

✻ **G0458** Low dose rate (LDR) prostate brachytherapy services, composite rate ⑧ Qp Qh   B

✻ **G0459** Inpatient telehealth pharmacologic management, including prescription, use, and review of medication with no more than minimal medical psychotherapy ⑧ Qp Qh   B

⟲ ✻ **G0460** Autologous platelet rich plasma or other blood-derived product for non-diabetic chronic wounds/ulcers, including phlebotomy, centrifugation or mixing, and all other preparatory procedures, administration and dressings, per treatment ⑨ Qp Qh   T

▶ New   ⟲ Revised   ✔ Reinstated   ~~deleted~~ Deleted   ⊘ Not covered or valid by Medicare
⊙ Special coverage instructions   ✻ Carrier discretion   ⑧ Bill Part B MAC   ⑨ Bill DME MAC

* **G0463** Hospital outpatient clinic visit for assessment and management of a patient ⓑ Qp Qh   J2

* **G0464** Colorectal cancer screening; stool-based DNA and fecal occult hemoglobin (e.g., KRAS, NDRG4 and BMP3) ⓑ

  Cross Reference 81528

  Laboratory Certification: General immunology, Routine chemistry, Clinical cytogenetics

↻ * **G0465** Autologous platelet rich plasma (prp) or other blood-derived product for diabetic chronic wounds/ulcers, using an FDA-cleared device for this indication, (includes administration, dressings, phlebotomy, centrifugation or mixing, and all other preparatory procedures, per treatment)   T

Federally Qualified Health Center Visits

* **G0466** Federally qualified health center (FQHC) visit, new patient; a medically-necessary, face-to-face encounter (one-on-one) between a new patient and a FQHC practitioner during which time one or more FQHC services are rendered and includes a typical bundle of Medicare-covered services that would be furnished per diem to a patient receiving a FQHC visit ⓑ Qp Qh   A

* **G0467** Federally qualified health center (FQHC) visit, established patient; a medically-necessary, face-to-face encounter (one-on-one) between an established patient and a FQHC practitioner during which time one or more FQHC services are rendered and includes a typical bundle of Medicare-covered services that would be furnished per diem to a patient receiving a FQHC visit ⓑ Qp Qh   A

* **G0468** Federally qualified health center (FQHC) visit, IPPE or AWV; a FQHC visit that includes an initial preventive physical examination (IPPE) or annual wellness visit (AWV) and includes a typical bundle of Medicare-covered services that would be furnished per diem to a patient receiving an IPPE or AWV ⓑ * Qp Qh   A

* **G0469** Federally qualified health center (FQHC) visit, mental health, new patient; a medically-necessary, face-to-face mental health encounter (one-on-one) between a new patient and a FQHC practitioner during which time one or more FQHC services are rendered and includes a typical bundle of Medicare-covered services that would be furnished per diem to a patient receiving a mental health visit ⓑ Qp Qh   A

* **G0470** Federally qualified health center (FQHC) visit, mental health, established patient; a medically-necessary, face-to-face mental health encounter (one-on-one) between an established patient and a FQHC practitioner during which time one or more FQHC services are rendered and includes a typical bundle of Medicare-covered services that would be furnished per diem to a patient receiving a mental health visit ⓑ Qp Qh   A

Other Miscellaneous Services

* **G0471** Collection of venous blood by venipuncture or urine sample by catheterization from an individual in a skilled nursing facility (SNF) or by a laboratory on behalf of a home health agency (HHA) ⓑ Qp Qh   A

⊙ **G0472** Hepatitis C antibody screening, for individual at high risk and other covered indication(s) ⓑ Qp Qh   A

  Medicare Statute 1861SSA

  Laboratory Certification: General immunology

* **G0473** Face-to-face behavioral counseling for obesity, group (2-10), 30 minutes ⓑ Qp Qh   S

* **G0475** HIV antigen/antibody, combination assay, screening ⓑ Qp Qh   A

  Laboratory Certification: Virology, General immunology

* **G0476** Infectious agent detection by nucleic acid (DNA or RNA); human papillomavirus (HPV), high-risk types (e.g., 16, 18, 31, 33, 35, 39, 45, 51, 52, 56, 58, 59, 68) for cervical cancer screening, must be performed in addition to pap test ⓑ Qp Qh   A

  Laboratory Certification: Virology

🅜 MIPS	Qp **Quantity Physician**	Qh **Quantity Hospital**	♀ **Female only**
♂ **Male only**	A **Age**	⅙ **DMEPOS**	A2-Z3 **ASC Payment Indicator**	A-Y **ASC Status Indicator**	Coding Clinic

Drug Tests

* **G0480** Drug test(s), definitive, utilizing drug identification methods able to identify individual drugs and distinguish between structural isomers (but not necessarily stereoisomers), including, but not limited to GC/MS (any type, single or tandem) and LC/MS (any type, single or tandem and excluding immunoassays (e.g., IA, EIA, ELISA, EMIT, FPIA) and enzymatic methods (e.g., alcohol dehydrogenase)); qualitative or quantitative, all sources(s), includes specimen validity testing, per day, 1-7 drug class(es), including metabolite(s) if performed ⑧ **Qp** **Qh** Q4

Coding Clinic: 2018, Q1, P5

* **G0481** Drug test(s), definitive, utilizing drug identification methods able to identify individual drugs and distinguish between structural isomers (but not necessarily stereoisomers), including, but not limited to GC/MS (any type, single or tandem) and LC/MS (any type, single or tandem and excluding immunoassays (e.g., IA, EIA, ELISA, EMIT, FPIA) and enzymatic methods (e.g., alcohol dehydrogenase)); qualitative or quantitative, all sources(s), includes specimen validity testing, per day, 8-14 drug class(es), including metabolite(s) if performed ⑧ **Qp** **Qh** Q4

Coding Clinic: 2018, Q1, P5

* **G0482** Drug test(s), definitive, utilizing drug identification methods able to identify individual drugs and distinguish between structural isomers (but not necessarily stereoisomers), including, but not limited to GC/MS (any type, single or tandem) and LC/MS (any type, single or tandem and excluding immunoassays (e.g., IA, EIA, ELISA, EMIT, FPIA) and enzymatic methods (e.g., alcohol dehydrogenase)); qualitative or quantitative, all sources(s), includes specimen validity testing, per day, 15-21 drug class(es), including metabolite(s) if performed ⑨ **Qp** **Qh** Q4

Coding Clinic: 2018, Q1, P5

* **G0483** Drug test(s), definitive, utilizing drug identification methods able to identify individual drugs and distinguish between structural isomers (but not necessarily stereoisomers), including, but not limited to GC/MS (any type, single or tandem) and LC/MS (any type, single or tandem and excluding immunoassays (e.g., IA, EIA, ELISA, EMIT, FPIA) and enzymatic methods (e.g., alcohol dehydrogenase); qualitative or quantitative, all sources(s), includes specimen validity testing, per day, 22 or more drug class(es), including metabolite(s) if performed ⑨ **Qp** **Qh** Q4

Coding Clinic: 2018, Q1, P5

Home Health Nursing Visit: Area of Shortage

* **G0490** Face-to-face home health nursing visit by a rural health clinic (RHC) or federally qualified health center (FQHC) in an area with a shortage of home health agencies (services limited to RN or LPN only) ⑧ A

Dialysis Procedure

* **G0491** Dialysis procedure at a Medicare certified ESRD facility for acute kidney injury without ESRD ⑨ **Qp** **Qh** B

* **G0492** Dialysis procedure with single evaluation by a physician or other qualified health care professional for acute kidney injury without ESRD ⑨ **Qp** **Qh** B

Home Health or Hospice: Skilled Services

* **G0493** Skilled services of a registered nurse (RN) for the observation and assessment of the patient's condition, each 15 minutes (the change in the patient's condition requires skilled nursing personnel to identify and evaluate the patient's need for possible modification of treatment in the home health or hospice setting) ⑧ B

▶ New ⟲ Revised ✓ Reinstated ~~deleted~~ Deleted ⊘ Not covered or valid by Medicare
⊛ Special coverage instructions ✳ Carrier discretion ⑧ Bill Part B MAC ⑨ Bill DME MAC

✳ **G0494** Skilled services of a licensed practical nurse (LPN) for the observation and assessment of the patient's condition, each 15 minutes (the change in the patient's condition requires skilled nursing personnel to identify and evaluate the patient's need for possible modification of treatment in the home health or hospice setting) Ⓑ   **B**

✳ **G0495** Skilled services of a registered nurse (RN), in the training and/or education of a patient or family member, in the home health or hospice setting, each 15 minutes Ⓑ   **B**

✳ **G0496** Skilled services of a licensed practical nurse (LPN), in the training and/or education of a patient or family member, in the home health or hospice setting, each 15 minutes Ⓑ   **B**

Chemotherapy Administration

✳ **G0498** Chemotherapy administration, intravenous infusion technique; initiation of infusion in the office/clinic setting using office/clinic pump/supplies, with continuation of the infusion in the community setting (e.g., home, domiciliary, rest home or assisted living) using a portable pump provided by the office/clinic, includes follow up office/clinic visit at the conclusion of the infusion Ⓥ **Qp** **Qh**   **S**

Hepatitis B Screening

✳ **G0499** Hepatitis B screening in non-pregnant, high risk individual includes hepatitis B surface antigen (HBsAG), antibodies to HBsAG (anti-HBs) and antibodies to hepatitis B core antigen (anti-hbc), and is followed by a neutralizing confirmatory test, when performed, only for an initially reactive HBsAG result Ⓑ **Qp** **Qh**   **A**

Laboratory Certification: Virology

Moderate Sedation Services

✳ **G0500** Moderate sedation services provided by the same physician or other qualified health care professional performing a gastrointestinal endoscopic service that sedation supports, requiring the presence of an independent trained observer to assist in the monitoring of the patient's level of consciousness and physiological status; initial 15 minutes of intra-service time; patient age 5 years or older (additional time may be reported with 99153, as appropriate) Ⓥ **Qp** **Qh**   **N**

Resource-Intensive Service

✳ **G0501** Resource-intensive services for patients for whom the use of specialized mobility-assistive technology (such as adjustable height chairs or tables, patient lift, and adjustable padded leg supports) is medically necessary and used during the provision of an office/outpatient, evaluation and management visit (list separately in addition to primary service) Ⓑ   **N**

Psychiatric Care Management

✳ **G0506** Comprehensive assessment of and care planning for patients requiring chronic care management services (list separately in addition to primary monthly care management service) Ⓥ **Qp** **Qh**   **N**

Critical Care Telehealth Consultation

✳ **G0508** Telehealth consultation, critical care, initial, physicians typically spend 60 minutes communicating with the patient and providers via telehealth Ⓑ **Qp** **Qh**   **B**

✳ **G0509** Telehealth consultation, critical care, subsequent, physicians typically spend 50 minutes communicating with the patient and providers via telehealth Ⓥ **Qp** **Qh**   **B**

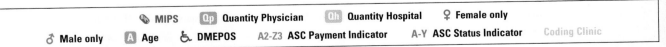

🐾 MIPS   **Qp** Quantity Physician   **Qh** Quantity Hospital   ♀ Female only

♂ Male only   **A** Age   ♿ DMEPOS   A2-Z3 **ASC Payment Indicator**   A-Y **ASC Status Indicator**   Coding Clinic

Rural Health Clinic: Management and Care

⊙ **G0511**   Rural health clinic or federally qualified health center (RHC or FQHC) only, general care management, 20 minutes or more of clinical staff time for chronic care management services or behavioral health integration services directed by an RHC or FQHC practitioner (physician, NP, PA, or CNM), per calendar month   A

⊙ **G0512**   Rural health clinic or federally qualified health center (RHC/FQHC) only, psychiatric collaborative care model (psychiatric CoCM), 60 minutes or more of clinical staff time for psychiatric CoCM services directed by an RHC or FQHC practitioner (physician, NP, PA, or CNM) and including services furnished by a behavioral health care manager and consultation with a psychiatric consultant, per calendar month   A

Prolonged Preventive Services

✳ **G0513**   Prolonged preventive service(s) (beyond the typical service time of the primary procedure), in the office or other outpatient setting requiring direct patient contact beyond the usual service; first 30 minutes (list separately in addition to code for preventive service)   N

✳ **G0514**   Prolonged preventive service(s) (beyond the typical service time of the primary procedure), in the office or other outpatient setting requiring direct patient contact beyond the usual service; each additional 30 minutes (list separately in addition to code G0513 for additional 30 minutes of preventive service)   N

Non-biodegradable Drug Delivery Implants: Removal and Insertion

✳ **G0516**   Insertion of non-biodegradable drug delivery implants, 4 or more (services for subdermal rod implant)   Q1

✳ **G0517**   Removal of non-biodegradable drug delivery implants, 4 or more (services for subdermal implants)   Q1

✳ **G0518**   Removal with reinsertion, non-biodegradable drug delivery implants, 4 or more (services for subdermal implants)   Q1

Drug Test

✳ **G0659**   Drug test(s), definitive, utilizing drug identification methods able to identify individual drugs and distinguish between structural isomers (but not necessarily stereoisomers), including but not limited to GC/MS (any type, single or tandem) and LC/MS (any type, single or tandem), excluding immunoassays (e.g., IA, EIA, ELISA, EMIT, FPIA) and enzymatic methods (e.g., alcohol dehydrogenase), performed without method or drug-specific calibration, without matrix-matched quality control material, or without use of stable isotope or other universally recognized internal standard(s) for each drug, drug metabolite or drug class per specimen; qualitative or quantitative, all sources, includes specimen validity testing, per day, any number of drug classes   Q4

Quality Care Measures: Cataract Surgery

MIPS ✳ **G0913**   Improvement in visual function achieved within 90 days following cataract surgery Ⓑ   M

MIPS ✳ **G0914**   Patient care survey was not completed by patient Ⓑ   M

MIPS ✳ **G0915**   Improvement in visual function not achieved within 90 days following cataract surgery Ⓑ   M

MIPS ✳ **G0916**   Satisfaction with care achieved within 90 days following cataract surgery Ⓑ   M

MIPS ✳ **G0917**   Patient care survey was not completed by patient Ⓑ   M

MIPS ✳ **G0918**   Satisfaction with care not achieved within 90 days following cataract surgery Ⓑ   M

Clinical Decision Support Mechanism

✳ **G1001**   Clinical decision support mechanism eviCore, as defined by the Medicare Appropriate Use Criteria Program   E1

✳ **G1002**   Clinical decision support mechanism MedCurrent, as defined by the Medicare Appropriate Use Criteria Program   E1

✳ **G1003**   Clinical decision support mechanism Medicalis, as defined by the Medicare Appropriate Use Criteria Program   E1

✳ **G1004** Clinical decision support mechanism National Decision Support Company, as defined by the Medicare Appropriate Use Criteria Program E1

✳ **G1007** Clinical decision support mechanism AIM Specialty Health, as defined by the Medicare Appropriate Use Criteria Program E1

✳ **G1008** Clinical decision support mechanism Cranberry Peak, as defined by the Medicare Appropriate Use Criteria Program E1

✳ **G1009** Clinical decision support mechanism Sage Health Management Solutions, as defined by the Medicare Appropriate Use Criteria Program E1

✳ **G1010** Clinical decision support mechanism Stanson, as defined by the Medicare Appropriate Use Criteria Program E1

✳ **G1011** Clinical decision support mechanism, qualified tool not otherwise specified, as defined by the Medicare Appropriate Use Criteria Program E1

✳ **G1012** Clinical decision support mechanism AgileMD, as defined by the Medicare appropriate use criteria program E1

✳ **G1013** Clinical decision support mechanism EvidenceCare ImagingCare, as defined by the Medicare appropriate use criteria program E1

✳ **G1014** Clinical decision support mechanism InveniQA semantic answers in medicine, as defined by the Medicare appropriate use criteria program E1

✳ **G1015** Clinical decision support mechanism Reliant Medical Group, as defined by the Medicare appropriate use criteria program E1

✳ **G1016** Clinical decision support mechanism Speed of Care, as defined by the Medicare appropriate use criteria program E1

✳ **G1017** Clinical decision support mechanism HealthHelp, as defined by the Medicare appropriate use criteria program E1

✳ **G1018** Clinical decision support mechanism Infinx, as defined by the Medicare appropriate use criteria program E1

✳ **G1019** Clinical decision support mechanism LogicNets, as defined by the Medicare appropriate use criteria program E1

✳ **G1020** Clinical decision support mechanism Curbside Clinical Augmented Workflow, as defined by the Medicare appropriate use criteria program E1

✳ **G1021** Clinical decision support mechanism E*HealthLine clinical decision support mechanism, as defined by the Medicare appropriate use criteria program E1

✳ **G1022** Clinical decision support mechanism Intermountain clinical decision support mechanism, as defined by the Medicare appropriate use criteria program E1

✳ **G1023** Clinical decision support mechanism Persivia clinical decision support, as defined by the Medicare appropriate use criteria program E1

✳ **G1024** Clinical decision support mechanism radrite, as defined by the medicare appropriate use criteria program E1

✳ **G1025** Patient-months where there are more than one medicare capitated payment (mcp) provider listed for the month M

✳ **G1026** The number of adult patient-months in the denominator who were on maintenance hemodialysis using a catheter continuously for three months or longer under the care of the same practitioner or group partner as of the last hemodialysis session of the reporting month M

✳ **G1027** The number of adult patient-months in the denominator who were on maintenance hemodialysis under the care of the same practitioner or group partner as of the last hemodialysis session of the reporting month using a catheter continuously for less than three months M

✳ **G1028** Take-home supply of nasal naloxone; 2-pack of 8mg per 0.1 ml nasal spray (provision of the services by a medicare-enrolled opioid treatment program); list separately in addition to code for primary procedure A

Therapy, Evaluation and Assessment

✳ **G2000** Blinded administration of convulsive therapy procedure, either electroconvulsive therapy (ECT, current covered gold standard) or magnetic seizure therapy (MST, non-covered experimental therapy), performed in an approved IDE-based clinical trial, per treatment session S

* **G2010** Remote evaluation of recorded video and/or images submitted by an established patient (e.g., store and forward), including interpretation with follow-up with the patient within 24 business hours, not originating from a related E/M service provided within the previous 7 days nor leading to an E/M service or procedure within the next 24 hours or soonest available appointment **M**

* **G2011** Alcohol and/or substance (other than tobacco) misuse structured assessment (e.g., audit, dast), and brief intervention, 5-14 minutes **S**

* **G2012** Brief communication technology-based service, e.g., virtual check-in, by a physician or other qualified health care professional who can report evaluation and management services, provided to an established patient, not originating from a related E/M service provided within the previous 7 days nor leading to an E/M service or procedure within the next 24 hours or soonest available appointment; 5-10 minutes of medical discussion **M**

* **G2020** Services for high intensity clinical services associated with the initial engagement and outreach of beneficiaries assigned to the sip component of the pcf model (do not bill with chronic care management codes) **A**

* **G2021** Health care practitioners rendering treatment in place (TIP) **E1**

* **G2022** A model participant (ambulance supplier/provider), the beneficiary refuses services covered under the model (transport to an alternate destination/treatment in place) **E1**

G2023 ~~Specimen collection for severe acute respiratory syndrome coronavirus 2 (SARS CoV 2) (coronavirus disease [COVID 19]), any specimen source~~ **B**

G2024 ~~Specimen collection for severe acute respiratory syndrome coronavirus 2 (SARS CoV 2) (coronavirus disease [COVID 19]) from an individual in a SNF or by a laboratory on behalf of a HHA, any specimen source~~ **B**

* **G2025** Payment for a telehealth distant site service furnished by a rural health clinic (RHC) or federally qualified health center (FQHC) only **A**

* **G2061** Qualified nonphysician healthcare professional online assessment and management service, for an established patient, for up to seven days, cumulative time during the 7 days; 5-10 minutes **M**

* **G2062** Qualified nonphysician healthcare professional online assessment and management service, for an established patient, for up to seven days, cumulative time during the 7 days; 11-20 minutes **M**

* **G2063** Qualified nonphysician qualified healthcare professional assessment and management service, for an established patient, for up to seven days, cumulative time during the 7 days; 21 or more minutes **M**

* **G2066** Interrogation device evaluation(s), (remote) up to 30 days; implantable cardiovascular physiologic monitor system, implantable loop recorder system, or subcutaneous cardiac rhythm monitor system, remote data acquisition(s), receipt of transmissions and technician review, technical support and distribution of results **Q1**

* **G2067** Medication assisted treatment, methadone; weekly bundle including dispensing and/or administration, substance use counseling, individual and group therapy, and toxicology testing, if performed (provision of the services by a Medicare-enrolled opioid treatment program) **E1**

* **G2068** Medication assisted treatment, buprenorphine (oral); weekly bundle including dispensing and/or administration, substance use counseling, individual and group therapy, and toxicology testing if performed (provision of the services by a Medicare-enrolled opioid treatment program) **E1**

* **G2069** Medication assisted treatment, buprenorphine (injectable); weekly bundle including dispensing and/or administration, substance use counseling, individual and group therapy, and toxicology testing if performed (provision of the services by a Medicare-enrolled opioid treatment program) **E1**

▶ New   ↻ Revised   ✔ Reinstated   ~~deleted~~ Deleted   ⊘ Not covered or valid by Medicare
⊙ Special coverage instructions   ✳ Carrier discretion   Ⓑ Bill Part B MAC   Ⓓ Bill DME MAC

G2010 – G2069   TEMPORARY PROCEDURES/PROFESSIONAL SERVICES

254

✳ **G2070** Medication assisted treatment, buprenorphine (implant insertion); weekly bundle including dispensing and/or administration, substance use counseling, individual and group therapy, and toxicology testing if performed (provision of the services by a Medicare-enrolled opioid treatment program)   E1

✳ **G2071** Medication assisted treatment, buprenorphine (implant removal); weekly bundle including dispensing and/or administration, substance use counseling, individual and group therapy, and toxicology testing if performed (provision of the services by a Medicare-enrolled opioid treatment program)   E1

✳ **G2072** Medication assisted treatment, buprenorphine (implant insertion and removal); weekly bundle including dispensing and/or administration, substance use counseling, individual and group therapy, and toxicology testing if performed (provision of the services by a Medicare-enrolled opioid treatment program)   E1

✳ **G2073** Medication assisted treatment, naltrexone; weekly bundle including dispensing and/or administration, substance use counseling, individual and group therapy, and toxicology testing if performed (provision of the services by a Medicare-enrolled opioid treatment program)   E1

✳ **G2074** Medication assisted treatment, weekly bundle not including the drug, including substance use counseling, individual and group therapy, and toxicology testing if performed (provision of the services by a Medicare-enrolled opioid treatment program)   E1

✳ **G2075** Medication assisted treatment, medication not otherwise specified; weekly bundle including dispensing and/or administration, substance use counseling, individual and group therapy, and toxicology testing, if performed (provision of the services by a Medicare-enrolled opioid treatment program)   E1

✳ **G2076** Intake activities, including initial medical examination that is a complete, fully documented physical evaluation and initial assessment by a program physician or a primary care physician, or an authorized healthcare professional under the supervision of a program physician qualified personnel that includes preparation of a treatment plan that includes the patient's short-term goals and the tasks the patient must perform to complete the short-term goals; the patient's requirements for education, vocational rehabilitation, and employment; and the medical, psycho-social, economic, legal, or other supportive services that a patient needs, conducted by qualified personnel (provision of the services by a Medicare-enrolled opioid treatment program); list separately in addition to code for primary procedure   E1

✳ **G2077** Periodic assessment; assessing periodically by qualified personnel to determine the most appropriate combination of services and treatment (provision of the services by a Medicare-enrolled opioid treatment program); list separately in addition to code for primary procedure   E1

✳ **G2078** Take-home supply of methadone; up to 7 additional day supply (provision of the services by a Medicare-enrolled opioid treatment program); list separately in addition to code for primary procedure   E1

✳ **G2079** Take-home supply of buprenorphine (oral); up to 7 additional day supply (provision of the services by a Medicare-enrolled opioid treatment program); list separately in addition to code for primary procedure   E1

✳ **G2080** Each additional 30 minutes of counseling in a week of medication assisted treatment, (provision of the services by a Medicare-enrolled opioid treatment program); list separately in addition to code for primary procedure   E1

✳ **G2081** Patients age 66 and older in institutional special needs plans (SNP) or residing in long-term care with a POS code 32, 33, 34, 54 or 56 for more than 90 consecutive days during the measurement period   M

---

* **G2082**   Office or other outpatient visit for the evaluation and management of an established patient that requires the supervision of a physician or other qualified health care professional and provision of up to 56 mg of esketamine nasal self-administration, includes 2 hours post-administration observation   S

* **G2083**   Office or other outpatient visit for the evaluation and management of an established patient that requires the supervision of a physician or other qualified health care professional and provision of greater than 56 mg esketamine nasal self-administration, includes 2 hours post-administration observation   S

* **G2086**   Office-based treatment for opioid use disorder, including development of the treatment plan, care coordination, individual therapy and group therapy and counseling; at least 70 minutes in the first calendar month   S

* **G2087**   Office-based treatment for opioid use disorder, including care coordination, individual therapy and group therapy and counseling; at least 60 minutes in a subsequent calendar month   S

* **G2088**   Office-based treatment for opioid use disorder, including care coordination, individual therapy and group therapy and counseling; each additional 30 minutes beyond the first 120 minutes (list separately in addition to code for primary procedure)   N

* **G2090**   Patients 66 years of age and older with at least one claim/encounter for frailty during the measurement period and a dispensed medication for dementia during the measurement period or the year prior to the measurement period   N1 M

* **G2091**   Patients 66 years of age and older with at least one claim/encounter for frailty during the measurement period and either one acute inpatient encounter with a diagnosis of advanced illness or two outpatient, observation, ED or nonacute inpatient encounters on different dates of service with an advanced illness diagnosis during the measurement period or the year prior to the measurement period   N1 M

* **G2092**   Angiotensin converting enzyme (ACE) inhibitor or angiotensin receptor blocker (ARB) or angiotensin receptor-neprilysin inhibitor (AMI) therapy prescribed or currently being taken   N1 M

* **G2093**   Documentation of medical reason(s) for not prescribing ACE inhibitor or ARB or AMI therapy (e.g., hypotensive patients who are at immediate risk of cardiogenic shock, hospitalized patients who have experienced marked azotemia, allergy, intolerance, other medical reasons)   N1 M

* **G2094**   Documentation of patient reason(s) for not prescribing ACE inhibitor or ARB or AMI therapy (e.g., patient declined, other patient reasons)   N1 M

* **G2096**   Angiotensin converting enzyme (ACE) inhibitor or angiotensin receptor blocker (ARB) or angiotensin receptor-neprilysin inhibitor (AMI) therapy was not prescribed, reason not given   N1 M

* **G2097**   Episodes where the patient had a competing diagnosis on or within three days after the episode date (e.g., intestinal infection, pertussis, bacterial infection, Lyme disease, otitis media, acute sinusitis, acute pharyngitis, acute tonsillitis, chronic sinusitis, infection of the pharynx/larynx/tonsils/adenoids, prostatitis, cellulitis, mastoiditis, or bone infections, acute lymphadenitis, impetigo, skin staph infections, pneumonia/gonococcal infections, venereal disease (syphilis, chlamydia, inflammatory diseases [female reproductive organs]), infections of the kidney, cystitis or UTI   N1 M

* **G2098**   Patients 66 years of age and older with at least one claim/encounter for frailty during the measurement period and a dispensed medication for dementia during the measurement period or the year prior to the measurement period   N1 M

* **G2099**   Patients 66 years of age and older with at least one claim/encounter for frailty during the measurement period and either one acute inpatient encounter with a diagnosis of advanced illness or two outpatient, observation, ED or nonacute inpatient encounters on different dates of service with an advanced illness diagnosis during the measurement period or the year prior to the measurement period   N1 M

▶ **New**   ↻ **Revised**   ✓ **Reinstated**   ~~deleted~~ **Deleted**   ⊘ **Not covered or valid by Medicare**

✪ **Special coverage instructions**   * **Carrier discretion**   Ⓑ **Bill Part B MAC**   Ⓓ **Bill DME MAC**

✳ **G2100** Patients 66 years of age and older with at least one claim/encounter for frailty during the measurement period and a dispensed medication for dementia during the measurement period or the year prior to the measurement period **N1 M**

✳ **G2101** Patients 66 years of age and older with at least one claim/encounter for frailty during the measurement period and either one acute inpatient encounter with a diagnosis of advanced illness or two outpatient, observation, ED or nonacute inpatient encounters on different dates of service with an advanced illness diagnosis during the measurement period or the year prior to the measurement period **N1 M**

✳ **G2105** Patients age 66 or older in institutional special needs plans (SNP) or residing in long-term care with POS code 32, 33, 34, 54 or 56 for more than 90 days consecutive during the measurement period **N1 M**

✳ **G2106** Patients 66 years of age and older with at least one claim/encounter for frailty during the measurement period and a dispensed medication for dementia during the measurement period or the year prior to the measurement period **N1 M**

✳ **G2107** Patients 66 years of age and older with at least one claim/encounter for frailty during the measurement period and either one acute inpatient encounter with a diagnosis of advanced illness or two outpatient, observation, ED or nonacute inpatient encounters on different dates of service with an advanced illness diagnosis during the measurement period or the year prior to the measurement period **N1 M**

✳ **G2108** Patients age 66 or older in institutional special needs plans (SNP) or residing in long-term care with POS code 32, 33, 34, 54 or 56 for more than 90 days consecutive during the measurement period **N1 M**

✳ **G2109** Patients 66 years of age and older with at least one claim/encounter for frailty during the measurement period and a dispensed medication for dementia during the measurement period or the year prior to the measurement period **N1 M**

✳ **G2110** Patients 66 years of age and older with at least one claim/encounter for frailty during the measurement period and either one acute inpatient encounter with a diagnosis of advanced illness or two outpatient, observation, ED or nonacute inpatient encounters on different dates of service with an advanced illness diagnosis during the measurement period or the year prior to the measurement period **N1 M**

✳ **G2112** Patient receiving <=5 mg daily prednisone (or equivalent), or RA activity is worsening, or glucocorticoid use is for less than 6 months **N1 M**

✳ **G2113** Patient receiving >5 mg daily prednisone (or equivalent) for longer than 6 months, and improvement or no change in disease activity **N1 M**

✳ **G2115** Patients 66-80 years of age with at least one claim/encounter for frailty during the measurement period and a dispensed medication for dementia during the measurement period or the year prior to the measurement period **N1 M**

✳ **G2116** Patients 66-80 years of age with at least one claim/encounter for frailty during the measurement period and either one acute inpatient encounter with a diagnosis of advanced illness or two outpatient, observation, ED or nonacute inpatient encounters on different dates of service with an advanced illness diagnosis during the measurement period or the year prior to the measurement period **N1 M**

✳ **G2118** Patients 81 years of age and older with at least one claim/encounter for frailty during the measurement period **N1 M**

✳ **G2121** Depression, anxiety, apathy, and psychosis assessed **N1 M**

✳ **G2122** Depression, anxiety, apathy, and psychosis not assessed **N1 M**

✳ **G2125** Patients 81 years of age and older with at least one claim/encounter for frailty during the six months prior to the measurement period through December 31 of the measurement period **N1 M**

🐾 **MIPS**   　**Qp** **Quantity Physician**   　**Qh** **Quantity Hospital**   　♀ **Female only**

♂ **Male only**   　**A** **Age**   　♿ **DMEPOS**   　**A2-Z3** **ASC Payment Indicator**   　**A-Y** **ASC Status Indicator**   　Coding Clinic

* **G2126** Patients 66-80 years of age with at least one claim/encounter for frailty during the measurement period and either one acute inpatient encounter with a diagnosis of advanced illness or two outpatient, observation, ED or nonacute inpatient encounters on different dates of service with an advanced illness diagnosis during the measurement period or the year prior to the measurement period   N1 M

* **G2127** Patients 66-80 years of age with at least one claim/encounter for frailty during the measurement period and a dispensed dementia medication   N1 M

* **G2128** Documentation of medical reason(s) for not on a daily aspirin or other antiplatelet (e.g. history of gastrointestinal bleed, intra-cranial bleed, blood disorders, idiopathic thrombocytopenic purpura [ITP], gastric bypass or documentation of active anticoagulant use during the measurement period)   N1 M

* **G2129** Procedure-related BP's not taken during an outpatient visit. Examples include same day surgery, ambulatory service center, G.I. lab, dialysis, infusion center, chemotherapy   N1 M

* **G2136** Back pain measured by the Visual Analog Scale (VAS) or numeric pain scale at three months (6 - 20 weeks) postoperatively was less than or equal to 3.0 or back pain measured by the Visual Analog Scale (VAS) or numeric pain scale within three months preoperatively and at three months (6 - 20 weeks) postoperatively demonstrated an improvement of 5.0 points or greater   N1 M

* **G2137** Back pain measured by the Visual Analog Scale (VAS) or numeric pain scale at three months (6 - 20 weeks) postoperatively was greater than 3.0 and back pain measured by the Visual Analog Scale (VAS) or numeric pain scale within three months preoperatively and at three months (6 - 20 weeks) postoperatively demonstrated a change of less than an improvement of 5.0 points   N1 M

* **G2138** Back pain as measured by the Visual Analog Scale (VAS) or numeric pain scale at one year (9 to 15 months) postoperatively was less than or equal to 3.0 or back pain measured by the Visual Analog Scale (VAS) or numeric pain scale within three months preoperatively and at one year (9 to 15 months) postoperatively demonstrated a change of 5.0 points or greater   N1 M

* **G2139** Back pain measured by the Visual Analog Scale (VAS) or numeric pain scale pain at one year (9 to 15 months) postoperatively was greater than 3.0 and back pain measured by the Visual Analog Scale (VAS) or numeric pain scale within three months preoperatively and at one year (9 to 15 months) postoperatively demonstrated a change of less than 5.0   N1 M

* **G2140** Leg pain measured by the Visual Analog Scale (VAS) or numeric pain scale at three months (6 - 20 weeks) postoperatively was less than or equal to 3.0 or leg pain measured by the Visual Analog Scale (VAS) or numeric pain scale within three months preoperatively and at three months (6 - 20 weeks) postoperatively demonstrated an improvement of 5.0 points or greater   N1 M

* **G2141** Leg pain measured by the Visual Analog Scale (VAS) or numeric pain scale at three months (6 - 20 weeks) postoperatively was greater than 3.0 and leg pain measured by the Visual Analog Scale (VAS) or numeric pain scale within three months preoperatively and at three months (6 - 20 weeks) postoperatively demonstrated less than an improvement of 5.0 points   N1 M

* **G2142** Functional status measured by the Oswestry Disability Index (ODI version 2.1a) at one year (9 to 15 months) postoperatively was less than or equal to 22 or functional status measured by the ODI version 2.1a within three months preoperatively and at one year (9 to 15 months) postoperatively demonstrated an improvement of 30 points or greater   N1 M

✳ **G2143** Functional status measured by the Oswestry Disability Index (ODI version 2.1a) at one year (9 to 15 months) postoperatively was greater than 22 and functional status measured by the ODI version 2.1a within three months preoperatively and at one year (9 to 15 months) postoperatively demonstrated an improvement of less than 30 points　**N1 M**

✳ **G2144** Functional status measured by the Oswestry Disability Index (ODI version 2.1a) at three months (6 - 20 weeks) postoperatively was less than or equal to 22 or functional status measured by the ODI version 2.1a within three months preoperatively and at three months (6 - 20 weeks) postoperatively demonstrated an improvement of 30 points or greater

✳ **G2145** Functional status measured by the Oswestry Disability Index (ODI version 2.1a) at three months (6 - 20 weeks) postoperatively was greater than 22 and functional status measured by the ODI version 2.1a within three months preoperatively and at three months (6 - 20 weeks) postoperatively demonstrated an improvement of less than 30 points　**N1 M**

✳ **G2146** Leg pain as measured by the Visual Analog Scale (VAS) or numeric pain scale at one year (9 to 15 months) postoperatively was less than or equal to 3.0 or leg pain measured by the Visual Analog Scale (VAS) or numeric pain scale within three months preoperatively and at one year (9 to 15 months) postoperatively demonstrated an improvement of 5.0 points or greater　**N1 M**

✳ **G2147** Leg pain measured by the Visual Analog Scale (VAS) or numeric pain scale at one year (9 to 15 months) postoperatively was greater than 3.0 and leg pain measured by the Visual Analog Scale (VAS) or numeric pain scale within three months preoperatively and at one year (9 to 15 months) postoperatively demonstrated less than an improvement of 5.0 points　**N1 M**

✳ **G2148** Multimodal pain management was used　**N1 M**

✳ **G2149** Documentation of medical reason(s) for not using multimodal pain management (e.g., allergy to multiple classes of analgesics, intubated patient, hepatic failure, patient reports no pain during PACU stay, other medical reason(s))　**N1 M**

✳ **G2150** Multimodal pain management was not used　**N1 M**

✳ **G2151** Documentation stating patient has a diagnosis of a degenerative neurological condition such as ALS, MS, Parkinson's diagnosed at any time before or during the episode of care　**N1 M**

✳ **G2152** Residual score for the neck impairment successfully calculated and the score was equal to zero (0) or greater than zero (> 0)　**N1 M**

✳ **G2167** Residual score for the neck impairment successfully calculated and the score was less than zero (< 0)　**N1 M**

✳ **G2168** Services performed by a physical therapist assistant in the home health setting in the delivery of a safe and effective physical therapy maintenance program, each 15 minutes　**B**

✳ **G2169** Services performed by an occupational therapist assistant in the home health setting in the delivery of a safe and effective occupational therapy maintenance program, each 15 minutes　**B**

✳ **G2172** All inclusive payment for services related to highly coordinated and integrated opioid use disorder (oud) treatment services furnished for the demonstration project　**A**

✳ **G2173** URI episodes where the patient had a comorbid condition during the 12 months prior to or on the episode date (e.g., tuberculosis, neutropenia, cystic fibrosis, chronic bronchitis, pulmonary edema, respiratory failure, rheumatoid lung disease)　**M**

🖉 MIPS　　**Qp** Quantity Physician　　**Qh** Quantity Hospital　　♀ Female only

♂ Male only　　**A** Age　　♿ DMEPOS　　A2-Z3 ASC Payment Indicator　　A-Y ASC Status Indicator　　Coding Clinic

* **G2174** URI episodes when the patient had an active prescription of antibiotics in the 30 days prior to the episode date or is still active the same day of the encounter **M**

* **G2175** Episodes where the patient had a comorbid condition during the 12 months prior to or on the episode date (e.g., tuberculosis, neutropenia, cystic fibrosis, chronic bronchitis, pulmonary edema, respiratory failure, rheumatoid lung disease) **M**

* **G2176** Outpatient, ED, or observation visits that result in an inpatient admission **M**

* **G2177** Acute bronchitis/bronchiolitis episodes when the patient had a new or refill prescription of antibiotics (table 1) in the 30 days prior to the episode date

* **G2178** Clinician documented that patient was not an eligible candidate for lower extremity neurological exam measure, for example patient bilateral amputee; patient has condition that would not allow them to accurately respond to a neurological exam (dementia, Alzheimer's, etc.); patient has previously documented diabetic peripheral neuropathy with loss of protective sensation **M**

* **G2179** Clinician documented that patient had medical reason for not performing lower extremity neurological exam **M**

* **G2180** Clinician documented that patient was not an eligible candidate for evaluation of footwear as patient is bilateral lower extremity amputee **M**

* **G2181** BMI not documented due to medical reason or patient refusal of height or weight measurement **M**

* **G2182** Patient receiving first-time biologic and/or immune response modifier therapy **M**

* **G2183** Documentation patient unable to communicate and informant not available **M**

* **G2184** Patient does not have a caregiver **M**

* **G2185** Documentation caregiver is trained and certified in dementia care **M**

* **G2186** Patient /caregiver dyad has been referred to appropriate resources and connection to those resources is confirmed **M**

* **G2187** Patients with clinical indications for imaging of the head: Head trauma **M**

* **G2188** Patients with clinical indications for imaging of the head: New or change in headache above 50 years of age **M**

* **G2189** Patients with clinical indications for imaging of the head: Abnormal neurologic exam **M**

* **G2190** Patients with clinical indications for imaging of the head: Headache radiating to the neck **M**

* **G2191** Patients with clinical indications for imaging of the head: Positional headaches **M**

* **G2192** Patients with clinical indications for imaging of the head: Temporal headaches in patients over 55 years of age **M**

* **G2193** Patients with clinical indications for imaging of the head: New onset headache in pre-school children or younger (<6 years of age) **M**

* **G2194** Patients with clinical indications for imaging of the head: New onset headache in pediatric patients with disabilities for which headache is a concern as inferred from behavior **M**

* **G2195** Patients with clinical indications for imaging of the head: Occipital headache in children **M**

* **G2196** Patient identified as an unhealthy alcohol user when screened for unhealthy alcohol use using a systematic screening method **M**

* **G2197** Patient screened for unhealthy alcohol use using a systematic screening method and not identified as an unhealthy alcohol user **M**

* **G2199** Patient not screened for unhealthy alcohol use using a systematic screening method **M**

* **G2200** Patient identified as an unhealthy alcohol user received brief counseling **M**

* **G2202** Patient did not receive brief counseling if identified as an unhealthy alcohol user **M**

* **G2204** Patients between 45 and 85 years of age who received a screening colonoscopy during the performance period **M**

▶ **New**   ↻ **Revised**   ✔ **Reinstated**   ~~deleted~~ **Deleted**   ⊘ **Not covered or valid by Medicare**
⊛ **Special coverage instructions**   * **Carrier discretion**   Ⓑ **Bill Part B MAC**   Ⓓ **Bill DME MAC**

* **G2205** Patients with pregnancy during adjuvant treatment course **M**

* **G2206** Patient received adjuvant treatment course including both chemotherapy and her 2-targeted therapy **M**

* **G2207** Reason for not administering adjuvant treatment course including both chemotherapy and her2-targeted therapy (e.g., poor performance status (ECOG 3-4; Karnofsky < 50), cardiac contraindications, insufficient renal function, insufficient hepatic function, other active or secondary cancer diagnoses, other medical contraindications, patients who died during initial treatment course or transferred during or after initial treatment course) **M**

* **G2208** Patient did not receive adjuvant treatment course including both chemotherapy and her 2-targeted therapy **M**

* **G2209** Patient refused to participate **M**

* **G2210** Residual score for the neck impairment not measured because the patient did not complete the neck fs prom at initial evaluation and/or near discharge, reason not given **M**

* **G2211** Visit complexity inherent to evaluation and management associated with medical care services that serve as the continuing focal point for all needed health care services and/or with medical care services that are part of ongoing care related to a patient's single, serious condition or a complex condition. (Add-on code, list separately in addition to office/outpatient evaluation and management visit, new or established) **N**

* **G2212** Prolonged office or other outpatient evaluation and management service(s) beyond the maximum required time of the primary procedure which has been selected using total time on the date of the primary service; each additional 15 minutes by the physician or qualified healthcare professional, with or without direct patient contact (list separately in addition to CPT codes 99205, 99215, 99483 for office or other outpatient evaluation and management services) (do not report G2212 on the same date of service as 99358, 99359, 99415, 99416). (Do not report G2212 for any time unit less than 15 minutes) **N**

* **G2213** Initiation of medication for the treatment of opioid use disorder in the emergency department setting, including assessment, referral to ongoing care, and arranging access to supportive services (list separately in addition to code for primary procedure) **N**

* **G2214** Initial or subsequent psychiatric collaborative care management, first 30 minutes in a month of behavioral health care manager activities, in consultation with a psychiatric consultant, and directed by the treating physician or other qualified health care professional **S**

* **G2215** Take-home supply of nasal naloxone; 2-pack of 4mg per 0.1 ml nasal spray (provision of the services by a Medicare-enrolled opioid treatment program); list separately in addition to code for primary procedure **A**

* **G2216** Take-home supply of injectable naloxone (provision of the services by a Medicare-enrolled opioid treatment program); list separately in addition to code for primary procedure **A**

* **G2250** Remote assessment of recorded video and/or images submitted by an established patient (e.g., store and forward), including interpretation with follow-up with the patient within 24 business hours, not originating from a related service provided within the previous 7 days nor leading to a service or procedure within the next 24 hours or soonest available appointment **A**

* **G2251** Brief communication technology-based service, e.g., virtual check-in, by a qualified health care professional who cannot report Evaluation and Management services, provided to an established patient, not originating from a related service provided within the previous 7 days nor leading to a service or procedure within the next 24 hours or soonest available appointment; 5-10 minutes of clinical discussion **A**

* **G2252** Brief communication technology-based service, e.g., virtual check-in, by a physician or other qualified health care professional who can report Evaluation and Management services, provided to an established patient, not originating from a related e/m service provided within the previous 7 days nor leading to an e/m service or procedure within the next 24 hours or soonest available appointment; 11-20 minutes of medical discussion **A**

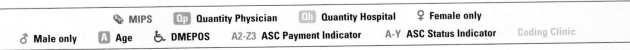

Pain Management

G3002   Chronic pain management and treatment, monthly bundle including, diagnosis; assessment and monitoring; administration of a validated pain rating scale or tool; the development, implementation, revision, and/or maintenance of a person-centered care plan that includes strengths, goals, clinical needs, and desired outcomes; overall treatment management; facilitation and coordination of any necessary behavioral health treatment; medication management; pain and health literacy counseling; any necessary chronic pain related crisis care; and ongoing communication and care coordination between relevant practitioners furnishing care, e.g. physical therapy and occupational therapy, complementary and integrative approaches, and community-based care, as appropriate. Required initial face-to-face visit at least 30 minutes provided by a physician or other qualified health professional; first 30 minutes personally provided by physician or other qualified health care professional, per calendar month. (When using G3002, 30 minutes must be met or exceeded.)   M

G3003   Each additional 15 minutes of chronic pain management and treatment by a physician or other qualified health care professional, per calendar month. (List separately in addition to code for G3002. When using G3003, 15 minutes must be met or exceeded.)   M

Specialty Set

✳ G4000	Dermatology mips specialty set	M
✳ G4001	Diagnostic radiology mips specialty set	M
✳ G4002	Electrophysiology cardiac specialist mips specialty set	M
✳ G4003	Emergency medicine mips specialty set	M
✳ G4004	Endocrinology mips specialty set	M
✳ G4005	Family medicine mips specialty set	M
✳ G4006	Gastro-enterology mips specialty set	M
✳ G4007	General surgery mips specialty set	M
✳ G4008	Geriatrics mips specialty set	M
✳ G4009	Hospitalists mips specialty set	M
✳ G4010	Infectious disease mips specialty set	M
✳ G4011	Internal medicine mips specialty set	M
✳ G4012	Interventional radiology mips specialty set	M
✳ G4013	Mental/behavioral and psychiatry mips specialty set	M
✳ G4014	Nephrology mips specialty set	M
✳ G4015	Neurology mips specialty set	M
✳ G4016	Neurosurgical mips specialty set	M
✳ G4017	Nutrition/dietician mips specialty set	M
✳ G4018	Obstetrics/gynecology mips specialty set	M
✳ G4019	Oncology/hematology mips specialty set	M
✳ G4020	Ophthalmology/optometry mips specialty set	M
✳ G4021	Orthopedic surgery mips specialty set	M
✳ G4022	Otolaryngology mips specialty set	M
✳ G4023	Pathology mips specialty set	M
✳ G4024	Pediatrics mips specialty set	M
✳ G4025	Physical medicine mips specialty set	M
✳ G4026	Physical therapy/occupational therapy mips specialty set	M
✳ G4027	Plastic surgery mips specialty set	M
✳ G4028	Podiatry mips specialty set	M
✳ G4029	Preventive medicine mips specialty set	M
✳ G4030	Pulmonology mips specialty set	M
✳ G4031	Radiation oncology mips specialty set	M
✳ G4032	Rheumatology mips specialty set	M
✳ G4033	Skilled nursing facility mips specialty set	M
✳ G4034	Speech language pathology mips specialty set	M
✳ G4035	Thoracic surgery mips specialty set	M
✳ G4036	Urgent care mips specialty set	M
✳ G4037	Urology mips specialty set	M
✳ G4038	Vascular surgery mips specialty set	M

Guidance

G6001   Ultrasonic guidance for placement of radiation therapy fields Ⓑ Qp Qh   B

✳ G6002   Stereoscopic x-ray guidance for localization of target volume for the delivery of radiation therapy Ⓑ Qp Qh   B

Radiation Treatment

✳ G6003   Radiation treatment delivery, single treatment area, single port or parallel opposed ports, simple blocks or no blocks: up to 5 mev Ⓑ Qp Qh   B

▶ New   ↷ Revised   ✔ Reinstated   deleted Deleted   ⊘ Not covered or valid by Medicare
◉ Special coverage instructions   ✳ Carrier discretion   Ⓑ Bill Part B MAC   Ⓑ Bill DME MAC

* **G6004** Radiation treatment delivery, single treatment area, single port or parallel opposed ports, simple blocks or no blocks: 6-10 mev Ⓑ Ⓠᵖ Ⓠₕ   B

* **G6005** Radiation treatment delivery, single treatment area, single port or parallel opposed ports, simple blocks or no blocks: 11-19 mev Ⓑ Ⓠᵖ Ⓠₕ   B

* **G6006** Radiation treatment delivery, single treatment area, single port or parallel opposed ports, simple blocks or no blocks: 20 mev or greater Ⓑ Ⓠᵖ Ⓠₕ   B

* **G6007** Radiation treatment delivery, 2 separate treatment areas, 3 or more ports on a single treatment area, use of multiple blocks: up to 5 mev Ⓑ Ⓠᵖ Ⓠₕ   B

* **G6008** Radiation treatment delivery, 2 separate treatment areas, 3 or more ports on a single treatment area, use of multiple blocks: 6-10 mev Ⓑ Ⓠᵖ Ⓠₕ   B

* **G6009** Radiation treatment delivery, 2 separate treatment areas, 3 or more ports on a single treatment area, use of multiple blocks: 11-19 mev Ⓑ Ⓠᵖ Ⓠₕ   B

* **G6010** Radiation treatment delivery, 2 separate treatment areas, 3 or more ports on a single treatment area, use of multiple blocks: 20 mev or greater Ⓑ Ⓠᵖ Ⓠₕ   B

* **G6011** Radiation treatment delivery, 3 or more separate treatment areas, custom blocking, tangential ports, wedges, rotational beam, compensators, electron beam; up to 5 mev Ⓑ Ⓠᵖ Ⓠₕ   B

* **G6012** Radiation treatment delivery, 3 or more separate treatment areas, custom blocking, tangential ports, wedges, rotational beam, compensators, electron beam; 6-10 mev Ⓑ Ⓠᵖ Ⓠₕ   B

* **G6013** Radiation treatment delivery, 3 or more separate treatment areas, custom blocking, tangential ports, wedges, rotational beam, compensators, electron beam; 11-19 mev Ⓑ Ⓠᵖ Ⓠₕ   B

* **G6014** Radiation treatment delivery, 3 or more separate treatment areas, custom blocking, tangential ports, wedges, rotational beam, compensators, electron beam; 20 mev or greater Ⓑ Ⓠᵖ Ⓠₕ   B

* **G6015** Intensity modulated treatment delivery, single or multiple fields/arcs, via narrow spatially and temporally modulated beams, binary, dynamic MLC, per treatment session Ⓑ Ⓠᵖ Ⓠₕ   B

* **G6016** Compensator-based beam modulation treatment delivery of inverse planned treatment using 3 or more high resolution (milled or cast) compensator, convergent beam modulated fields, per treatment session Ⓑ Ⓠᵖ Ⓠₕ   B

* **G6017** Intra-fraction localization and tracking of target or patient motion during delivery of radiation therapy (e.g., 3D positional tracking, gating, 3D surface tracking), each fraction of treatment Ⓑ Ⓠᵖ Ⓠₕ   B

Quality Measures

* **G8395** Left ventricular ejection fraction (LVEF) >=40% or documentation as normal or mildly depressed left ventricular systolic function Ⓑ   M

* **G8396** Left ventricular ejection fraction (LVEF) not performed or documented Ⓑ   M

🅜 * **G8397** Dilated macular or fundus exam performed, including documentation of the presence or absence of macular edema and level of severity of retinopathy Ⓑ   M

🅜 * **G8399** Patient with documented results of a central dual-energy x-ray absorptiometry (DXA) ever being performed Ⓑ   M

🅜 * **G8400** Patient with central dual-energy x-ray absorptiometry (DXA) results not documented Ⓑ   M

🅜 * **G8404** Lower extremity neurological exam performed and documented Ⓑ   M

🅜 * **G8405** Lower extremity neurological exam not performed Ⓑ   M

🅜 * **G8410** Footwear evaluation performed and documented Ⓑ   M

🅜 * **G8415** Footwear evaluation was not performed Ⓑ   M

🅜 * **G8416** Clinician documented that patient was not an eligible candidate for footwear evaluation measure Ⓑ   M

🅜 * **G8417** BMI is documented above normal parameters and a follow-up plan is documented Ⓑ   M

🅜 * **G8418** BMI is documented below normal parameters and a follow-up plan is documented Ⓑ   M

🅜 * **G8419** BMI is documented outside normal parameters, no follow-up plan documented, no reason given Ⓑ   M

🅜 * **G8420** BMI is documented within normal parameters and no follow-up plan is required Ⓑ   M

🅜 * **G8421** BMI not documented and no reason is given Ⓑ   M

🅜 * **G8427** Eligible clinician attests to documenting in the medical record they obtained, updated, or reviewed the patient's current medications Ⓑ   M

🅜 MIPS   Ⓠᵖ Quantity Physician   Ⓠₕ Quantity Hospital   ♀ Female only

♂ Male only   Ⓐ Age   ♿ DMEPOS   A2-Z3 ASC Payment Indicator   A-Y ASC Status Indicator   Coding Clinic

* **G8428** Current list of medications not documented as obtained, updated, or reviewed by the eligible clinician, reason not given ⑧ M

* **G8430** Documentation of a medical reason(s) for not documenting, updating, or reviewing the patient's current medications list (e.g., patient is in an urgent or emergent medical situation) ⑧ M

* **G8431** Screening for depression is documented as being positive and a follow-up plan is documented ⑧ M

* **G8432** Depression screening not documented, reason not given ⑧ M

* **G8433** Screening for depression not completed, documented patient or medical reason ⑧ M

* **G8450** Beta-blocker therapy prescribed ⑧ M

* **G8451** Beta-blocker therapy for LVEF <40% not prescribed for reasons documented by the clinician (e.g., low blood pressure, fluid overload, asthma, patients recently treated with an intravenous positive inotropic agent, allergy, intolerance, other medical reasons, patient declined, other patient reasons ⑧ M

* **G8452** Beta-blocker therapy not prescribed ⑧ M

* **G8465** High or very high risk of recurrence of prostate cancer ⑧ ♂ M

* **G8473** Angiotensin converting enzyme (ACE) inhibitor or angiotensin receptor blocker (ARB) therapy prescribed ⑧ M

* **G8474** Angiotensin converting enzyme (ACE) inhibitor or angiotensin receptor blocker (ARB) therapy not prescribed for reasons documented by the clinician (e.g., allergy, intolerance, pregnancy, renal failure due to ACE inhibitor, diseases of the aortic or mitral valve, other medical reasons) or (e.g., patient declined, other patient reasons) or (e.g., lack of drug availability, other reasons attributable to the health care system) ⑧ M

* **G8475** Angiotensin converting enzyme (ACE) inhibitor or angiotensin receptor blocker (ARB) therapy not prescribed, reason not given ⑧ M

* **G8476** Most recent blood pressure has a systolic measurement of <140 mmHg and a diastolic measurement of <90 mmHg ⑧ M

* **G8477** Most recent blood pressure has a systolic measurement of >=140 mmHg and/or a diastolic measurement of >=90 mmHg ⑧ M

* **G8478** Blood pressure measurement not performed or documented, reason not given ⑧ M

* **G8482** Influenza immunization administered or previously received ⑧ M

* **G8483** Influenza immunization was not administered for reasons documented by clinician (e.g., patient allergy or other medical reasons, patient declined or other patient reasons, vaccine not available or other system reasons) ⑧ M

* **G8484** Influenza immunization was not administered, reason not given ⑧ M

* **G8506** Patient receiving angiotensin converting enzyme (ACE) inhibitor or angiotensin receptor blocker (ARB) therapy ⑧ M

* **G8510** Screening for depression is documented as negative, a follow-up plan is not required ⑧ M

* **G8511** Screening for depression documented as positive, follow up plan not documented, reason not given ⑧ M

* **G8535** Elder maltreatment screen not documented; documentation that patient is not eligible for the elder maltreatment screen at the time of the encounter ⑧ Ⓐ M

* **G8536** No documentation of an elder maltreatment screen, reason not given ⑧ Ⓐ M

* **G8539** Functional outcome assessment documented as positive using a standardized tool and a care plan based on identified deficiencies is documented within two days of the functional outcome assessment ⑧ M

* **G8540** Functional outcome assessment not documented as being performed, documentation the patient is not eligible for a functional outcome assessment using a standardized tool at the time of the encounter ⑧ M

* **G8541** Functional outcome assessment using a standardized tool not documented, reason not given ⑧ M

* **G8542** Functional outcome assessment using a standardized tool is documented; no functional deficiencies identified, care plan not required ⑧ M

* **G8543** Documentation of a positive functional outcome assessment using a standardized tool; care plan not documented within two days of assessment, reason not given ⑧ M

* **G8559** Patient referred to a physician (preferably a physician with training in disorders of the ear) for an otologic evaluation ⑧ M

* **G8560** Patient has a history of active drainage from the ear within the previous 90 days ⑧ M

▶ New   ↻ Revised   ✔ Reinstated   ~~deleted~~ Deleted   ⊘ Not covered or valid by Medicare
✿ Special coverage instructions   ✱ Carrier discretion   Ⓑ Bill Part B MAC   Ⓓ Bill DME MAC

* **G8561** Patient is not eligible for the referral for otologic evaluation for patients with a history of active drainage measure Ⓑ M

* **G8562** Patient does not have a history of active drainage from the ear within the previous 90 days Ⓑ M

* **G8563** Patient not referred to a physician (preferably a physician with training in disorders of the ear) for an otologic evaluation, reason not given Ⓑ M

* **G8564** Patient was referred to a physician (preferably a physician with training in disorders of the ear) for an otologic evaluation, reason not specified Ⓑ M

* **G8565** Verification and documentation of sudden or rapidly progressive hearing loss Ⓑ M

* **G8566** Patient is not eligible for the "referral for otologic evaluation for sudden or rapidly progressive hearing loss" measure Ⓑ M

* **G8567** Patient does not have verification and documentation of sudden or rapidly progressive hearing loss Ⓑ M

* **G8568** Patient was not referred to a physician (preferably a physician with training in disorders of the ear) for an otologic evaluation, reason not given Ⓑ M

* **G8569** Prolonged postoperative intubation (>24 hrs) required Ⓑ M

* **G8570** Prolonged postoperative intubation (>24 hrs) not required Ⓑ M

* **G8575** Developed postoperative renal failure or required dialysis Ⓑ M

* **G8576** No postoperative renal failure/dialysis not required Ⓑ M

* **G8577** Re-exploration required due to mediastinal bleeding with or without tamponade, graft occlusion, valve disfunction, or other cardiac reason Ⓑ M

* **G8578** Re-exploration not required due to mediastinal bleeding with or without tamponade, graft occlusion, valve dysfunction, or other cardiac reason Ⓑ M

* **G8598** Aspirin or another antiplatelet therapy used Ⓑ M

* **G8599** Aspirin or another antiplatelet therapy not used, reason not given Ⓑ M

* **G8600** IV thrombolytic therapy initiated within 4.5 hours (<= 270 minutes) of time last known well Ⓑ M

* **G8601** IV thrombolytic therapy not initiated within 4.5 hours (= 270 minutes) of time last known well for reasons documented by clinician (e.g. patient enrolled in clinical trial for stroke, patient admitted for elective carotid intervention, patient received tenecteplase [tnk]) Ⓑ M

* **G8602** IV thrombolytic therapy not initiated within 4.5 hours (= 270 minutes) of time last known well, reason not given Ⓑ M

* **G8633** Pharmacologic therapy (other than minerals/vitamins) for osteoporosis prescribed Ⓑ M

* **G8635** Pharmacologic therapy for osteoporosis was not prescribed, reason not given Ⓑ M

* **G8647** Residual score for the knee impairment successfully calculated and the score was equal to zero (0) or greater than zero (>0) Ⓑ M

* **G8648** Residual score for the knee impairment successfully calculated and the score was less than zero (<0) Ⓑ M

* **G8650** Residual scores for the knee impairment not measured because the patient did not complete the LEPT prom at initial evaluation and/or near discharge, reason not given Ⓑ M

* **G8651** Residual score for the hip impairment successfully calculated and the score was equal to zero (0) or greater than zero (>0) Ⓑ M

* **G8652** Residual score for the hip impairment successfully calculated and the score was less than zero (<0) Ⓑ M

* **G8654** Residual scores for the hip impairment not measured because the patient did not complete LEPT prom at initial evaluation and/or follow up status survey near discharge, reason not given Ⓑ M

* **G8655** Residual score for the foot or ankle impairment successfully calculated and the score was equal to zero (0) or greater than zero (>0) Ⓑ M

* **G8656** Residual score for the foot or ankle impairment successfully calculated and the score was less than zero (<0) Ⓑ M

* **G8658** Residual scores for the lower leg, foot or ankle impairment not measured because the patient did not complete LEPT prom at initial evaluation and/or follow up status survey near discharge, reason not given Ⓑ M

* **G8659** Residual score for the low back impairment successfully calculated and the score was equal to zero (0) or greater than zero (>0) Ⓑ M

* **G8660** Residual score for the low back impairment successfully calculated and the score was less than zero (<0) Ⓑ M

🔖 MIPS   Ⓠp Quantity Physician   Ⓠh Quantity Hospital   ♀ Female only

♂ Male only   Ⓐ Age   ♿ DMEPOS   A2-Z3 ASC Payment Indicator   A-Y ASC Status Indicator   Coding Clinic

* **G8661** Risk-adjusted functional status change residual scores for the low back impairment not measured because the patient did not complete FOTO'S status survey near discharge, patient not appropriate Ⓑ M

* **G8662** Residual scores for the low back impairment not measured because the patient did not complete the low back FS prom at initial evaluation and/or near discharge, reason not given Ⓑ M

* **G8663** Residual score for the shoulder impairment successfully calculated and the score was equal to zero (0) or greater than zero (>0) Ⓑ M

* **G8664** Residual score for the shoulder impairment successfully calculated and the score was less than zero (<0) Ⓑ M

* **G8666** Residual scores for the shoulder impairment not measured because the patient did not complete the shoulder FS prom at initial evaluation and/or near discharge, reason not given Ⓑ M

* **G8667** Residual score for the elbow, wrist or hand impairment successfully calculated and the score was equal to zero (0) or greater than zero (>0) Ⓑ M

* **G8668** Residual score for the elbow, wrist or hand impairment successfully calculated and the score was less than zero (<0) Ⓑ M

* **G8670** Residual scores for the elbow, wrist or hand impairment not measured because the patient did not complete the the elbow/wrist/hand FS prom at initial evaluation near discharge, reason not given Ⓑ M

* **G8694** Left ventriucular ejection fraction (LVEF) <=40% or documentation of moderate or severe LVSD Ⓑ M

* **G8708** Patient not prescribed antibiotic Ⓑ M

* **G8709** URI episodes when the patient had competing diagnoses on or three days after the episode date (e.g., intestinal infection, pertussis, bacterial infection, Lyme disease, otitis media, acute sinusitis, acute pharyngitis, acute tonsillitis, chronic sinusitis, infection of the pharynx/larynx/tonsils/adenoids, prostatitis, cellulitis, mastoiditis, or bone infections, acute lymphadenitis, impetigo, skin staph infections, pneumonia/gonococcal infections, venereal disease [syphilis, chlamydia, inflammatory diseases (female reproductive organs)], infections of the kidney, cystitis or UTI, and acne) Ⓑ M

* **G8710** Patient prescribed antibiotic Ⓑ M

* **G8711** Prescribed antibiotic on or within 3 days after the episode date Ⓑ M

* **G8712** Antibiotic not prescribed or dispensed Ⓑ M

* **G8721** PT category (primary tumor), PN category (regional lymph nodes), and histologic grade were documented in pathology report Ⓑ M

* **G8722** Documentation of medical reason(s) for not including the PT category, the PN category or the histologic grade in the pathology report (e.g., re-excision without residual tumor; non-carcinomasanal canal) Ⓑ M

* **G8723** Specimen site is other than anatomic location of primary tumor Ⓑ M

* **G8724** PT category, PN category and histologic grade were not documented in the pathology report, reason not given Ⓑ M

* **G8733** Elder maltreatment screen documented as positive and a follow-up plan is documented Ⓑ Ⓐ M

* **G8734** Elder maltreatment screen documented as negative, follow-up is not required Ⓑ Ⓐ M

* **G8735** Elder maltreatment screen documented as positive, follow-up plan not documented, reason not given Ⓑ Ⓐ M

* **G8749** Absence of signs of melanoma (tenderness, jaundice, localized neurologic signs such as weakness, or any other sign suggesting systemic spread) or absence of symptoms of melanoma (cough, dyspnea, pain, paresthesia, or any other symptom suggesting the possibility of systemic spread of melanoma) Ⓑ M

* **G8752** Most recent systolic blood pressure <140 mmhg Ⓑ M

* **G8753** Most recent systolic blood pressure >=140 mmhg Ⓑ M

* **G8754** Most recent diastolic blood pressure <90 mmhg Ⓑ M

* **G8755** Most recent diastolic blood pressure >=90 mmhg Ⓑ M

* **G8756** No documentation of blood pressure measurement, reason not given Ⓑ M

* **G8783** Normal blood pressure reading documented, follow-up not required Ⓑ M

* **G8785** Blood pressure reading not documented, reason not given Ⓑ M

* **G8797** Specimen site other than anatomic location of esophagus Ⓑ M

▶ **New** ⟳ **Revised** ✔ **Reinstated** ~~deleted~~ **Deleted** ⊘ **Not covered or valid by Medicare**
Ⓢ **Special coverage instructions** * **Carrier discretion** Ⓑ **Bill Part B MAC** Ⓑ **Bill DME MAC**

* **G8798** Specimen site other than anatomic location of prostate Ⓑ M

* **G8806** Performance of trans-abdominal or trans-vaginal ultrasound and pregnancy location documented Ⓑ M

* **G8807** Trans-abdominal or trans-vaginal ultrasound not performed for reasons documented by clinician (e.g., patient has visited the ED multiple times within 72 hours, patient has a documented intrauterine pregnancy [IUP]) Ⓑ M

* **G8808** Trans-abdominal or trans-vaginal ultrasound not performed, reason not given Ⓑ M

* **G8815** Documented reason in the medical records for why the statin therapy was not prescribed (i.e., lower extremity bypass was for a patient with non-artherosclerotic disease) Ⓑ M

* **G8816** Statin medication prescribed at discharge Ⓑ M

* **G8817** Statin therapy not prescribed at discharge, reason not given Ⓑ M

* **G8818** Patient discharge to home no later than post-operative day #7 Ⓑ M

* **G8825** Patient not discharged to home by post-operative day #7 Ⓑ M

* **G8826** Patient discharged to home no later than post-operative day #2 following EVAR Ⓑ M

* **G8833** Patient not discharged to home by post-operative day #2 following EVAR Ⓑ M

* **G8834** Patient discharged to home no later than post-operative day #2 following CEA Ⓑ M

* **G8838** Patient not discharged to home by post-operative day #2 following CEA Ⓑ M

* **G8839** Sleep apnea symptoms assessed, including presence or absence of snoring and daytime sleepiness Ⓑ M

* **G8840** Documentation of reason(s) for not documenting an assessment of sleep symptoms (e.g., patient didn't have initial daytime sleepiness, patient visited between initial testing and initiation of therapy) Ⓑ M

* **G8841** Sleep apnea symptoms not assessed, reason not given Ⓑ M

* **G8842** Apnea Hypopnea Index (AHI) or Respiratory Disturbance Index (RDI), or Respiratory Event Index (REI) documented or measured within 2 months of initial evaluation for suspected obstructive sleep apnea Ⓑ M

* **G8843** Documentation of reason(s) for not measuring an Apnea Hypopnea Index (AHI) or a Respiratory Disturbance Index (RDI), or a Respiratory Event Index (REI) within 2 months of initial evaluation for suspected obstructive sleep apnea (e.g., medical, neurological, or psychiatric disease that prohibits successful completion of a sleep study, patients for whom a sleep study would present a bigger risk than benefit or would pose an undue burden, dementia, patients who decline AHI/RDI/REI measurement, patients who had a financial reason for not completing testing, test was ordered but not completed, patients decline because their insurance [payer] does not cover the expense) Ⓑ M

* **G8844** Apnea Hypopnea Index (AHI) or Respiratory Disturbance Index (RDI), or Respiratory Event Index (REI) not documented or measured within 2 months of initial evaluation for suspected obstructive sleep apnea, reason not given Ⓑ M

* **G8845** Positive airway pressure therapy prescribed Ⓑ M

* **G8846** Moderate or severe obstructive sleep apnea (Apnea Hypopnea Index (AHI) or Respiratory Disturbance Index (RDI) of 15 or greater) Ⓑ M

* **G8849** Documentation of reason(s) for not prescribing positive airway pressure therapy (e.g., patient unable to tolerate, alternative therapies use, patient declined, financial, insurance coverage) Ⓑ M

* **G8850** Positive airway pressure therapy not prescribed, reason not given Ⓑ M

* **G8851** Objective measurement of adherence to positive airway pressure therapy, documented Ⓑ M

* **G8852** Positive airway pressure therapy was prescribed Ⓑ M

* **G8854** Documentation of reason(s) for not objectively measuring adherence to positive airway pressure therapy (e.g., patient didn't bring data from continuous positive airway pressure [CPAP], therapy not yet initiated, not available on machine) Ⓑ M

* **G8855** Objective measurement of adherence to positive airway pressure therapy not performed, reason not given Ⓑ M

* **G8856** Referral to a physician for an otologic evaluation performed Ⓑ M

✳ **G8857** Patient is not eligible for the referral for otologic evaluation measure (e.g., patients who are already under the care of a physician for acute or chronic dizziness) Ⓑ M

✳ **G8858** Referral to a physician for an otologic evaluation not performed, reason not given Ⓑ M

✳ **G8863** Patients not assessed for risk of bone loss, reason not given Ⓑ M

✳ **G8864** Pneumococcal vaccine administered or previously received Ⓑ M

✳ **G8865** Documentation of medical reason(s) for not administering or previously receiving pneumococcal vaccine (e.g., patient allergic reaction, potential adverse drug reaction) Ⓑ M

✳ **G8866** Documentation of patient reason(s) for not administering or previously receiving pneumococcal vaccine (e.g., patient refusal) Ⓑ M

✳ **G8867** Pneumococcal vaccine not administered or previously received, reason not given Ⓑ M

✳ **G8869** Patient has documented immunity to hepatitis B and initiating anti-TNF therapy Ⓑ M

✳ **G8875** Clinician diagnosed breast cancer preoperatively by a minimally invasive biopsy method Ⓑ M

✳ **G8876** Documentation of reason(s) for not performing minimally invasive biopsy to diagnose breast cancer preoperatively (e.g., lesion too close to skin, implant, chest wall, etc., lesion could not be adequately visualized for needle biopsy, patient condition prevents needle biopsy [weight, breast thickness, etc.], duct excision without imaging abnormality, prophylactic mastectomy, reduction mammoplasty, excisional biopsy performed by another physician) Ⓑ M

✳ **G8877** Clinician did not attempt to achieve the diagnosis of breast cancer preoperatively by a minimally invasive biopsy method, reason not given Ⓑ M

✳ **G8878** Sentinel lymph node biopsy procedure performed Ⓑ M

✳ **G8880** Documentation of reason(s) sentinel lymph node biopsy not performed (e.g., reasons could include but not limited to: non-invasive cancer, incidental discovery of breast cancer on prophylactic mastectomy, incidental discovery of breast cancer on reduction mammoplasty, pre-operative biopsy proven lymph node (LN) metastases, inflammatory carcinoma, stage 3 locally advanced cancer, recurrent invasive breast cancer, clinically node positive after neoadjuvant systemic therapy, patient refusal after informed consent; patient with significant age, comorbidities, or limited life expectancy and favorable tumor; adjuvant systemic therapy unlikely to change) Ⓑ M

✳ **G8881** Stage of breast cancer is greater than T1N0M0 or T2N0M0 Ⓑ M

✳ **G8882** Sentinel lymph node biopsy procedure not performed, reason not given Ⓑ M

✳ **G8883** Biopsy results reviewed, communicated, tracked and documented Ⓑ M

✳ **G8884** Clinician documented reason that patient's biopsy results were not reviewed Ⓑ M

✳ **G8885** Biopsy results not reviewed, communicated, tracked or documented Ⓑ M

✳ **G8907** Patient documented not to have experienced any of the following events: a burn prior to discharge; a fall within the facility; wrong site/side/patient/ procedure/implant event; or a hospital transfer or hospital admission upon discharge from the facility Ⓑ M

✳ **G8908** Patient documented to have received a burn prior to discharge Ⓑ M

✳ **G8909** Patient documented not to have received a burn prior to discharge Ⓑ M

✳ **G8910** Patient documented to have experienced a fall within ASC Ⓑ M

✳ **G8911** Patient documented not to have experienced a fall within ambulatory surgical center Ⓑ M

✳ **G8912** Patient documented to have experienced a wrong site, wrong side, wrong patient, wrong procedure or wrong implant event Ⓑ M

✳ **G8913** Patient documented not to have experienced a wrong site, wrong side, wrong patient, wrong procedure or wrong implant event Ⓑ M

▶ **New**   ↻ **Revised**   ✔ **Reinstated**   ~~deleted~~ **Deleted**   ⊘ **Not covered or valid by Medicare**
⊛ **Special coverage instructions**   ✳ **Carrier discretion**   Ⓑ **Bill Part B MAC**   Ⓖ **Bill DME MAC**

* **G8914** Patient documented to have experienced a hospital transfer or hospital admission upon discharge from ASC ⓑ   M

* **G8915** Patient documented not to have experienced a hospital transfer or hospital admission upon discharge from ASC ⓑ   M

* **G8916** Patient with preoperative order for IV antibiotic surgical site infection (SSI) prophylaxis, antibiotic initiated on time ⓑ   M

* **G8917** Patient with preoperative order for IV antibiotic surgical site infection (SSI) prophylaxis, antibiotic not initiated on time ⓑ   M

* **G8918** Patient without preoperative order for IV antibiotic surgical site infection(SSI) prophylaxis ⓑ   M

* **G8923** Left ventricular ejection fraction (LVEF) <=40% or documentation of moderately or severely depressed left ventricular systolic function ⓑ   M

* **G8924** Spirometry test results demonstrate FEV1/FVC <70%, FEV 1 <60% predicted and patient has COPD symptoms (e.g., dyspnea, cough/sputum, wheezing) ⓑ   M

* **G8934** Left ventricular ejection fraction (LVEF) <=40% or documentation of moderately or severely depressed left ventricular systolic function ⓑ   M

* **G8935** Clinician prescribed angiotensin converting enzyme (ACE) inhibitor or angiotensin receptor blocker (ARB) therapy ⓑ   M

* **G8937** Clinician did not prescribe angiotensin converting enzyme (ACE) inhibitor or angiotensin receptor blocker (ARB) therapy, reason not given ⓑ   M

* **G8939** Pain assessment documented as positive, follow-up plan not documented, documentation the patient is not eligible at the time of the encounter at the time of the encounter ⓑ   M

* **G8941** Elder maltreatment screen documented as positive, follow-up plan not documented, documentation the patient is not eligible for follow-up plan at the time of the encounter ⓑ Ⓐ   M

* **G8942** Functional outcomes assessment using a standardized tool is documented within the previous 30 days and care plan, based on identified deficiencies is documented within two days of the functional outcome assessment ⓑ   M

* **G8944** AJCC melanoma cancer stage 0 through IIC melanoma ⓑ   M

* **G8946** Minimally invasive biopsy method attempted but not diagnostic of breast cancer (e.g., high risk lesion of breast such as atypical ductal hyperplasia, lobular neoplasia, atypical lobular hyperplasia, lobular carcinoma in situ, atypical columnar hyperplasia, flat epithelial atypia, radial scar, complex sclerosing lesion, papillary lesion, or any lesion with spindle cells) ⓑ   M

* **G8950** Elevated or hypertensive blood pressure reading documented, and the indicated follow-up documented ⓑ   M

* **G8952** Elevated or hypertensive blood pressure reading documented, indicated follow-up not documented, reason not given ⓑ   M

* **G8955** Most recent assessment of adequacy of volume management documented ⓑ M

* **G8956** Patient receiving maintenance hemodialysis in an outpatient dialysis facility ⓑ   M

* **G8958** Assessment of adequacy of volume management not documented, reason not given ⓑ   M

* **G8961** Cardiac stress imaging test primarily performed on low-risk surgery patient for preoperative evaluation within 30 days preceding this surgery ⓑ   M

* **G8962** Cardiac stress imaging test performed on patient for any reason including those who did not have low risk surgery or test that was performed more than 30 days preceding low risk surgery ⓑ   M

* **G8963** Cardiac stress imaging performed primarily for monitoring of asymptomatic patient who had PCI within 2 years ⓑ   M

* **G8964** Cardiac stress imaging test performed primarily for any other reason than monitoring of asymptomatic patient who had PCI within 2 years (e.g., symptomatic patient, patient greater than 2 years since PCI, initial evaluation, etc.) ⓑ   M

* **G8965** Cardiac stress imaging test primarily performed on low CHD risk patient for initial detection and risk assessment ⓑ   M

* **G8966** Cardiac stress imaging test performed on symptomatic or higher than low CHD risk patient or for any reason other than initial detection and risk assessment ⓑ   M

---

* **G8967**   FDA-approved oral anticoagulant is prescribed Ⓑ   M

* **G8968**   Documentation of medical reason(s) for not prescribing an FDA-approved anticoagulant (e.g., present or planned atrial appendage occlusion or ligation Ⓑ   M

* **G8969**   Documentation of patient reason(s) for not prescribing an oral anticoagulant that is FDA approved for the prevention of thromboembolism (e.g., patient choice of having atrial appendage device placed) Ⓑ   M

* **G8970**   No risk factors or one moderate risk factor for thromboembolism Ⓑ   M

Coordinated Care

G9001   Coordinated care fee, initial rate Ⓑ   B

G9002   Coordinated care fee, maintenance rate Ⓑ   B

G9003   Coordinated care fee, risk adjusted high, initial Ⓑ   B

G9004   Coordinated care fee, risk adjusted low, initial Ⓑ   B

G9005   Coordinated care fee, risk adjusted maintenance Ⓑ   B

G9006   Coordinated care fee, home monitoring Ⓑ   B

G9007   Coordinated care fee, scheduled team conference Ⓑ   B

G9008   Coordinated care fee, physician coordinated care oversight services Ⓑ B   B

G9009   Coordinated care fee, risk adjusted maintenance, level 3 Ⓑ   B

G9010   Coordinated care fee, risk adjusted maintenance, level 4 Ⓑ   B

G9011   Coordinated care fee, risk adjusted maintenance, level 5 Ⓑ   B

G9012   Other specified case management services not elsewhere classified Ⓑ   B

Demonstration Project

⊘ **G9013**   ESRD demo basic bundle Level I Ⓑ   E1

⊘ **G9014**   ESRD demo expanded bundle including venous access and related services Ⓑ   E1

⊘ **G9016**   Smoking cessation counseling, individual, in the absence of or in addition to any other evaluation and management service, per session (6-10 minutes) [demo project code only] Ⓑ   E1

⊘ **G9050**   Oncology; primary focus of visit; work-up, evaluation, or staging at the time of cancer diagnosis or recurrence (for use in a Medicare-approved demonstration project) Ⓑ   E1

⊘ **G9051**   Oncology; primary focus of visit; treatment decision-making after disease is staged or restaged, discussion of treatment options, supervising/coordinating active cancer directed therapy or managing consequences of cancer directed therapy (for use in a Medicare-approved demonstration project) Ⓑ   E1

⊘ **G9052**   Oncology; primary focus of visit; surveillance for disease recurrence for patient who has completed definitive cancer-directed therapy and currently lacks evidence of recurrent disease; cancer directed therapy might be considered in the future (for use in a Medicare-approved demonstration project) Ⓑ   E1

⊘ **G9053**   Oncology; primary focus of visit; expectant management of patient with evidence of cancer for whom no cancer directed therapy is being administered or arranged at present; cancer directed therapy might be considered in the future (for use in a Medicare-approved demonstration project) Ⓑ   E1

⊘ **G9054**   Oncology; primary focus of visit; supervising, coordinating or managing care of patient with terminal cancer or for whom other medical illness prevents further cancer treatment; includes symptom management, end-of-life care planning, management of palliative therapies (for use in a Medicare-approved demonstration project) Ⓑ   E1

⊘ **G9055**   Oncology; primary focus of visit; other, unspecified service not otherwise listed (for use in a Medicare-approved demonstration project) Ⓑ   E1

⊘ **G9056**   Oncology; practice guidelines; management adheres to guidelines (for use in a Medicare-approved demonstration project) Ⓑ   E1

▶ New   ↻ Revised   ✔ Reinstated   ~~deleted~~ Deleted   ⊘ Not covered or valid by Medicare

⊛ Special coverage instructions   * Carrier discretion   Ⓟ Bill Part B MAC   Ⓓ Bill DME MAC

⊘ **G9057** Oncology; practice guidelines; management differs from guidelines as a result of patient enrollment in an institutional review board approved clinical trial (for use in a Medicare-approved demonstration project) Ⓑ E1

⊘ **G9058** Oncology; practice guidelines; management differs from guidelines because the treating physician disagrees with guideline recommendations (for use in a Medicare-approved demonstration project) Ⓑ E1

⊘ **G9059** Oncology; practice guidelines; management differs from guidelines because the patient, after being offered treatment consistent with guidelines, has opted for alternative treatment or management, including no treatment (for use in a Medicare-approved demonstration project) Ⓑ E1

⊘ **G9060** Oncology; practice guidelines; management differs from guidelines for reason(s) associated with patient comorbid illness or performance status not factored into guidelines (for use in a Medicare-approved demonstration project) Ⓑ E1

⊘ **G9061** Oncology; practice guidelines; patient's condition not addressed by available guidelines (for use in a Medicare-approved demonstration project) Ⓑ E1

⊘ **G9062** Oncology; practice guidelines; management differs from guidelines for other reason(s) not listed (for use in a Medicare-approved demonstration project) Ⓑ E1

✳ **G9063** Oncology; disease status; limited to non-small cell lung cancer; extent of disease initially established as stage I (prior to neo-adjuvant therapy, if any) with no evidence of disease progression, recurrence, or metastases (for use in a Medicare-approved demonstration project) Ⓑ M

✳ **G9064** Oncology; disease status; limited to non-small cell lung cancer; extent of disease initially established as stage II (prior to neo-adjuvant therapy, if any) with no evidence of disease progression, recurrence, or metastases (for use in a Medicare-approved demonstration project) Ⓑ M

✳ **G9065** Oncology; disease status; limited to non-small cell lung cancer; extent of disease initially established as stage IIIA (prior to neo-adjuvant therapy, if any) with no evidence of disease progression, recurrence, or metastases (for use in a Medicare-approved demonstration project) Ⓑ M

✳ **G9066** Oncology; disease status; limited to non-small cell lung cancer; stage IIIB-IV at diagnosis, metastatic, locally recurrent, or progressive (for use in a Medicare-approved demonstration project) Ⓑ M

✳ **G9067** Oncology; disease status; limited to non-small cell lung cancer; extent of disease unknown, staging in progress, or not listed (for use in a Medicare-approved demonstration project) Ⓑ M

✳ **G9068** Oncology; disease status; limited to small cell and combined small cell/non-small cell; extent of disease initially established as limited with no evidence of disease progression, recurrence, or metastases (for use in a Medicare-approved demonstration project) Ⓑ M

✳ **G9069** Oncology; disease status; small cell lung cancer, limited to small cell and combined small cell/non-small cell; extensive stage at diagnosis, metastatic, locally recurrent, or progressive (for use in a Medicare-approved demonstration project) Ⓑ M

✳ **G9070** Oncology; disease status; small cell lung cancer, limited to small cell and combined small cell/non-small cell; extent of disease unknown, staging in progress, or not listed (for use in a Medicare-approved demonstration project) Ⓑ M

✳ **G9071** Oncology; disease status; invasive female breast cancer (does not include ductal carcinoma in situ); adenocarcinoma as predominant cell type; stage I or stage IIA-IIB; or T3, N1, M0; and ER and/or PR positive; with no evidence of disease progression, recurrence, or metastases (for use in a Medicare-approved demonstration project) Ⓑ ♀ M

✳ **G9072** Oncology; disease status; invasive female breast cancer (does not include ductal carcinoma in situ); adenocarcinoma as predominant cell type; stage I, or stage IIA-IIB; or T3, N1, M0; and ER and PR negative; with no evidence of disease progression, recurrence, or metastases (for use in a Medicare-approved demonstration project) Ⓑ ♀ M

🏷 MIPS   Qp Quantity Physician   Qh Quantity Hospital   ♀ Female only

♂ Male only   Ⓐ Age   ♿ DMEPOS   A2-Z3 ASC Payment Indicator   A-Y ASC Status Indicator   Coding Clinic

✳ **G9073**   Oncology; disease status; invasive female breast cancer (does not include ductal carcinoma in situ); adenocarcinoma as predominant cell type; stage IIIA-IIIB; and not T3, N1, M0; and ER and/or PR positive; with no evidence of disease progression, recurrence, or metastases (for use in a Medicare-approved demonstration project) ⑧ ♀   M

✳ **G9074**   Oncology; disease status; invasive female breast cancer (does not include ductal carcinoma in situ); adenocarcinoma as predominant cell type; stage IIIA-IIIB; and not T3, N1, M0; and ER and PR negative; with no evidence of disease progression, recurrence, or metastases (for use in a Medicare-approved demonstration project) ⑧ ♀   M

✳ **G9075**   Oncology; disease status; invasive female breast cancer (does not include ductal carcinoma in situ); adenocarcinoma as predominant cell type; M1 at diagnosis, metastatic, locally recurrent, or progressive (for use in a Medicare-approved demonstration project) ⑧ ♀   M

✳ **G9077**   Oncology; disease status; prostate cancer, limited to adenocarcinoma as predominant cell type; T1-T2c and Gleason 2-7 and PSA < or equal to 20 at diagnosis with no evidence of disease progression, recurrence, or metastases (for use in a Medicare-approved demonstration project) ⑧ ♂   M

✳ **G9078**   Oncology; disease status; prostate cancer, limited to adenocarcinoma as predominant cell type; T2 or T3a Gleason 8-10 or PSA >20 at diagnosis with no evidence of disease progression, recurrence, or metastases (for use in a Medicare-approved demonstration project) ⑧ ♂   M

✳ **G9079**   Oncology; disease status; prostate cancer, limited to adenocarcinoma as predominant cell type; T3b-T4, any N; any T, N1 at diagnosis with no evidence of disease progression, recurrence, or metastases (for use in a Medicare-approved demonstration project) ⑧ ♂M

✳ **G9080**   Oncology; disease status; prostate cancer, limited to adenocarcinoma; after initial treatment with rising PSA or failure of PSA decline (for use in a Medicare-approved demonstration project) ⑧ ♂   M

✳ **G9083**   Oncology; disease status; prostate cancer, limited to adenocarcinoma; extent of disease unknown, staging in progress, or not listed (for use in a Medicare-approved demonstration project) ⑧ ♂   M

✳ **G9084**   Oncology; disease status; colon cancer, limited to invasive cancer, adenocarcinoma as predominant cell type; extent of disease initially established as T1-3, N0, M0 with no evidence of disease progression, recurrence, or metastases (for use in a Medicare-approved demonstration project) ⑧   M

✳ **G9085**   Oncology; disease status; colon cancer, limited to invasive cancer, adenocarcinoma as predominant cell type; extent of disease initially established as T4, N0, M0 with no evidence of disease progression, recurrence, or metastases (for use in a Medicare-approved demonstration project) ⑧   M

✳ **G9086**   Oncology; disease status; colon cancer, limited to invasive cancer, adenocarcinoma as predominant cell type; extent of disease initially established as T1-4, N1-2, M0 with no evidence of disease progression, recurrence, or metastases (for use in a Medicare-approved demonstration project) ⑧   M

✳ **G9087**   Oncology; disease status; colon cancer, limited to invasive cancer, adenocarcinoma as predominant cell type; M1 at diagnosis, metastatic, locally recurrent, or progressive with current clinical, radiologic, or biochemical evidence of disease (for use in a Medicare-approved demonstration project) ⑧   M

✳ **G9088**   Oncology; disease status; colon cancer, limited to invasive cancer, adenocarcinoma as predominant cell type; M1 at diagnosis, metastatic, locally recurrent, or progressive without current clinical, radiologic, or biochemical evidence of disease (for use in a Medicare-approved demonstration project) ⑧   M

✳ **G9089**   Oncology; disease status; colon cancer, limited to invasive cancer, adenocarcinoma as predominant cell type; extent of disease unknown, staging in progress, or not listed (for use in a Medicare-approved demonstration project) ⑧   M

▶ **New**   ↻ **Revised**   ✔ **Reinstated**   ~~deleted~~ **Deleted**   ⊘ **Not covered or valid by Medicare**
✿ **Special coverage instructions**   ✳ **Carrier discretion**   ⑧ **Bill Part B MAC**   ⑧ **Bill DME MAC**

* **G9090** Oncology; disease status; rectal cancer, limited to invasive cancer, adenocarcinoma as predominant cell type; extent of disease initially established as T1-2, N0, M0 (prior to neo-adjuvant therapy, if any) with no evidence of disease progression, recurrence, or metastases (for use in a Medicare-approved demonstration project) Ⓑ   M

* **G9091** Oncology; disease status; rectal cancer, limited to invasive cancer, adenocarcinoma as predominant cell type; extent of disease initially established as T3, N0, M0 (prior to neo-adjuvant therapy, if any) with no evidence of disease progression, recurrence, or metastases (for use in a Medicare-approved demonstration project) Ⓑ   M

* **G9092** Oncology; disease status; rectal cancer, limited to invasive cancer, adenocarcinoma as predominant cell type; extent of disease initially established as T1-3, N1-2, M0 (prior to neo-adjuvant therapy, if any) with no evidence of disease progression, recurrence or metastases (for use in a Medicare-approved demonstration project) Ⓑ   M

* **G9093** Oncology; disease status; rectal cancer, limited to invasive cancer, adenocarcinoma as predominant cell type; extent of disease initially established as T4, any N, M0 (prior to neo-adjuvant therapy, if any) with no evidence of disease progression, recurrence, or metastases (for use in a Medicare-approved demonstration project) Ⓑ   M

* **G9094** Oncology; disease status; rectal cancer, limited to invasive cancer, adenocarcinoma as predominant cell type; M1 at diagnosis, metastatic, locally recurrent, or progressive (for use in a Medicare-approved demonstration project) Ⓑ   M

* **G9095** Oncology; disease status; rectal cancer, limited to invasive cancer, adenocarcinoma as predominant cell type; extent of disease unknown, staging in progress, or not listed (for use in a Medicare-approved demonstration project) Ⓑ   M

* **G9096** Oncology; disease status; esophageal cancer, limited to adenocarcinoma or squamous cell carcinoma as predominant cell type; extent of disease initially established as T1-T3, N0-N1 or NX (prior to neo-adjuvant therapy, if any) with no evidence of disease progression, recurrence, or metastases (for use in a Medicare-approved demonstration project) Ⓑ   M

* **G9097** Oncology; disease status; esophageal cancer, limited to adenocarcinoma or squamous cell carcinoma as predominant cell type; extent of disease initially established as T4, any N, M0 (prior to neo-adjuvant therapy, if any) with no evidence of disease progression, recurrence, or metastases (for use in a Medicare-approved demonstration project) Ⓑ   M

* **G9098** Oncology; disease status; esophageal cancer, limited to adenocarcinoma or squamous cell carcinoma as predominant cell type; M1 at diagnosis, metastatic, locally recurrent, or progressive (for use in a Medicare-approved demonstration project) Ⓑ   M

* **G9099** Oncology; disease status; esophageal cancer, limited to adenocarcinoma or squamous cell carcinoma as predominant cell type; extent of disease unknown, staging in progress, or not listed (for use in a Medicare-approved demonstration project) Ⓑ   M

* **G9100** Oncology; disease status; gastric cancer, limited to adenocarcinoma as predominant cell type; post R0 resection (with or without neoadjuvant therapy) with no evidence of disease recurrence, progression, or metastases (for use in a Medicare-approved demonstration project) Ⓑ   M

* **G9101** Oncology; disease status; gastric cancer, limited to adenocarcinoma as predominant cell type; post R1 or R2 resection (with or without neoadjuvant therapy) with no evidence of disease progression, or metastases (for use in a Medicare-approved demonstration project) Ⓑ   M

* **G9102** Oncology; disease status; gastric cancer, limited to adenocarcinoma as predominant cell type; clinical or pathologic M0, unresectable with no evidence of disease progression, or metastases (for use in a Medicare-approved demonstration project) Ⓑ   M

🐾 MIPS   Ⓠ Quantity Physician   Ⓠ Quantity Hospital   ♀ Female only
♂ Male only   Ⓐ Age   ♿ DMEPOS   A2-Z3 ASC Payment Indicator   A-Y ASC Status Indicator   Coding Clinic

✳ **G9103**   Oncology; disease status; gastric cancer, limited to adenocarcinoma as predominant cell type; clinical or pathologic M1 at diagnosis, metastatic, locally recurrent, or progressive (for use in a Medicare-approved demonstration project) Ⓑ   M

✳ **G9104**   Oncology; disease status; gastric cancer, limited to adenocarcinoma as predominant cell type; extent of disease unknown, staging in progress, or not listed (for use in a Medicare-approved demonstration project) Ⓑ   M

✳ **G9105**   Oncology; disease status; pancreatic cancer, limited to adenocarcinoma as predominant cell type; post R0 resection without evidence of disease progression, recurrence, or metastases (for use in a Medicare-approved demonstration project) Ⓑ   M

✳ **G9106**   Oncology; disease status; pancreatic cancer, limited to adenocarcinoma; post R1 or R2 resection with no evidence of disease progression or metastases (for use in a Medicare-approved demonstration project) Ⓑ   M

✳ **G9107**   Oncology; disease status; pancreatic cancer, limited to adenocarcinoma; unresectable at diagnosis, M1 at diagnosis, metastatic, locally recurrent, or progressive (for use in a Medicare-approved demonstration project) Ⓑ   M

✳ **G9108**   Oncology; disease status; pancreatic cancer, limited to adenocarcinoma; extent of disease unknown, staging in progress, or not listed (for use in a Medicare-approved demonstration project) Ⓑ   M

✳ **G9109**   Oncology; disease status; head and neck cancer, limited to cancers of oral cavity, pharynx and larynx with squamous cell as predominant cell type; extent of disease initially established as T1-T2 and N0, M0 (prior to neo-adjuvant therapy, if any) with no evidence of disease progression, recurrence, or metastases (for use in a Medicare-approved demonstration project) Ⓑ   M

✳ **G9110**   Oncology; disease status; head and neck cancer, limited to cancers of oral cavity, pharynx, and larynx with squamous cell as predominant cell type; extent of disease initially established as T3-4 and/ or N1-3, M0 (prior to neo-adjuvant therapy, if any) with no evidence of disease progression, recurrence, or metastases (for use in a Medicare-approved demonstration project) Ⓑ   M

✳ **G9111**   Oncology; disease status; head and neck cancer, limited to cancers of oral cavity, pharynx and larynx with squamous cell as predominant cell type; M1 at diagnosis, metastatic, locally recurrent, or progressive (for use in a Medicare-approved demonstration project) Ⓑ   M

✳ **G9112**   Oncology; disease status; head and neck cancer, limited to cancers of oral cavity, pharynx and larynx with squamous cell as predominant cell type; extent of disease unknown, staging in progress, or not listed (for use in a Medicare-approved demonstration project) Ⓑ   M

✳ **G9113**   Oncology; disease status; ovarian cancer, limited to epithelial cancer; pathologic stage IA-B (grade 1) without evidence of disease progression, recurrence, or metastases (for use in a Medicare-approved demonstration project) Ⓑ ♀   M

✳ **G9114**   Oncology; disease status; ovarian cancer, limited to epithelial cancer; pathologic stage IA-B (grade 2-3); or stage IC (all grades); or stage II; without evidence of disease progression, recurrence, or metastases (for use in a Medicare-approved demonstration project) Ⓑ ♀   M

✳ **G9115**   Oncology; disease status; ovarian cancer, limited to epithelial cancer; pathologic stage III-IV; without evidence of progression, recurrence, or metastases (for use in a Medicare-approved demonstration project) Ⓑ ♀   M

✳ **G9116**   Oncology; disease status; ovarian cancer, limited to epithelial cancer; evidence of disease progression, or recurrence and/or platinum resistance (for use in a Medicare-approved demonstration project) Ⓑ ♀   M

✳ **G9117**   Oncology; disease status; ovarian cancer, limited to epithelial cancer; extent of disease unknown, staging in progress, or not listed (for use in a Medicare-approved demonstration project) Ⓑ ♀   M

✳ **G9123**   Oncology; disease status; chronic myelogenous leukemia, limited to Philadelphia chromosome positive and/ or BCR-ABL positive; chronic phase not in hematologic, cytogenetic, or molecular remission (for use in a Medicare-approved demonstration project) Ⓑ   M

▶ **New**   ↻ **Revised**   ✔ **Reinstated**   ~~deleted~~ **Deleted**   ⊘ **Not covered or valid by Medicare**
Ⓢ **Special coverage instructions**   ✳ **Carrier discretion**   Ⓑ **Bill Part B MAC**   Ⓓ **Bill DME MAC**

* **G9124** Oncology; disease status; chronic myelogenous leukemia, limited to Philadelphia chromosome positive and/or BCR-ABL positive; accelerated phase not in hematologic cytogenetic, or molecular remission (for use in a Medicare-approved demonstration project) ⓑ M

* **G9125** Oncology; disease status; chronic myelogenous leukemia, limited to Philadelphia chromosome positive and/or BCR-ABL positive; blast phase not in hematologic, cytogenetic, or molecular remission (for use in a Medicare-approved demonstration project) ⓑ M

* **G9126** Oncology; disease status; chronic myelogenous leukemia, limited to Philadelphia chromosome positive and/or BCR-ABL positive; in hematologic, cytogenetic, or molecular remission (for use in a Medicare-approved demonstration project) ⓑ M

* **G9128** Oncology: disease status; limited to multiple myeloma, systemic disease; smouldering, stage I (for use in a Medicare-approved demonstration project) ⓑ M

* **G9129** Oncology; disease status; limited to multiple myeloma, systemic disease; stage II or higher (for use in a Medicare-approved demonstration project) ⓑ M

* **G9130** Oncology; disease status; limited to multiple myeloma, systemic disease; extent of disease unknown, staging in progress, or not listed (for use in a Medicare-approved demonstration project) ⓑ M

* **G9131** Oncology; disease status; invasive female breast cancer (does not include ductal carcinoma in situ); adenocarcinoma as predominant cell type; extent of disease unknown, staging in progress, or not listed (for use in a Medicare-approved demonstration project) ⓑ ♀ M

* **G9132** Oncology; disease status; prostate cancer, limited to adenocarcinoma; hormone-refractory/androgen-independent (e.g., rising PSA on anti-androgen therapy or post-orchiectomy); clinical metastases (for use in a Medicare-approved demonstration project) ⓑ ♂ M

* **G9133** Oncology; disease status; prostate cancer, limited to adenocarcinoma; hormone-responsive; clinical metastases or M1 at diagnosis (for use in a Medicare-approved demonstration project) ⓑ ♂ M

* **G9134** Oncology; disease status; non-Hodgkin's lymphoma, any cellular classification; stage I, II at diagnosis, not relapsed, not refractory (for use in a Medicare-approved demonstration project) ⓑ M

* **G9135** Oncology; disease status; non-Hodgkin's lymphoma, any cellular classification; stage III, IV, not relapsed, not refractory (for use in a Medicare-approved demonstration project) ⓑ M

* **G9136** Oncology; disease status; non-Hodgkin's lymphoma, transformed from original cellular diagnosis to a second cellular classification (for use in a Medicare-approved demonstration project) ⓑ M

* **G9137** Oncology; disease status; non-Hodgkin's lymphoma, any cellular classification; relapsed/refractory (for use in a Medicare-approved demonstration project) ⓑ M

* **G9138** Oncology; disease status; non-Hodgkin's lymphoma, any cellular classification; diagnostic evaluation, stage not determined, evaluation of possible relapse or non-response to therapy, or not listed (for use in a Medicare-approved demonstration project) ⓑ M

* **G9139** Oncology; disease status; chronic myelogenous leukemia, limited to Philadelphia chromosome positive and/or BCR-ABL positive; extent of disease unknown, staging in progress, not listed (for use in a Medicare-approved demonstration project) ⓑ M

* **G9140** Frontier extended stay clinic demonstration; for a patient stay in a clinic approved for the CMS demonstration project; the following measures should be present: the stay must be equal to or greater than 4 hours; weather or other conditions must prevent transfer or the case falls into a category of monitoring and observation cases that are permitted by the rules of the demonstration; there is a maximum frontier extended stay clinic (FESC) visit of 48 hours, except in the case when weather or other conditions prevent transfer; payment is made on each period up to 4 hours, after the first 4 hours ⓑ A

🐾 MIPS	Ⓠp Quantity Physician	Ⓠh Quantity Hospital	♀ Female only
♂ Male only Ⓐ Age	♿ DMEPOS	A2-Z3 ASC Payment Indicator	A-Y ASC Status Indicator Coding Clinic

Warfarin Responsiveness Testing

✳ **G9143** Warfarin responsiveness testing by genetic technique using any method, any number of specimen(s) Ⓑ ⓆⓅ Ⓠⓗ   N

This would be a once-in-a-lifetime test unless there is a reason to believe that the patient's personal genetic characteristics would change over time. (https://www.cms.gov/ ContractorLearningResources/ downloads/JA6715.pdf)

Laboratory Certification: General immunology, Hematology

Coding Clinic: 2010, Q2, P10

Outpatient IV Insulin Treatment

⊘ **G9147** Outpatient intravenous insulin treatment (OIVIT) either pulsatile or continuous, by any means, guided by the results of measurements for: respiratory quotient; and/or urine urea nitrogen (UUN); and/or arterial, venous or capillary glucose; and/or potassium concentration Ⓑ   E1

On December 23, 2009, CMS issued a national non-coverage decision on the use of OIVIT. CR 6775.

Not covered on Physician Fee Schedule

Coding Clinic: 2010, Q2, P10

Quality Assurance

✳ **G9148** National Committee for Quality Assurance - level 1 medical home Ⓑ   M

✳ **G9149** National Committee for Quality Assurance - level 2 medical home Ⓑ   M

✳ **G9150** National Committee for Quality Assurance - level 3 medical home Ⓑ   M

✳ **G9151** MAPCP demonstration - state provided services Ⓑ   M

✳ **G9152** MAPCP demonstration - community health teams Ⓑ   M

✳ **G9153** MAPCP demonstration - physician incentive pool Ⓑ   M

Wheelchair Evaluation

✳ **G9156** Evaluation for wheelchair requiring face to face visit with physician Ⓑ ⓆⓅ Ⓠⓗ   M

Cardiac Monitoring

✳ **G9157** Transesophageal doppler measurement of cardiac output (including probe placement, image acquisition, and interpretation per course of treatment) for monitoring purposes Ⓑ ⓆⓅ Ⓠⓗ   B

Bundled Payment Care Improvement

✳ **G9187** Bundled payments for care improvement initiative home visit for patient assessment performed by a qualified health care professional for individuals not considered homebound including, but not limited to, assessment of safety, falls, clinical status, fluid status, medication reconciliation/management, patient compliance with orders/plan of care, performance of activities of daily living, appropriateness of care setting; (for use only in the Medicare-approved bundled payments for care improvement initiative); may not be billed for a 30-day period covered by a transitional care management code Ⓑ ⓆⓅ Ⓠⓗ   E1

Quality Measures: Miscellaneous

MIPS ✳ **G9188** Beta-blocker therapy not prescribed, reason not given Ⓑ   M

MIPS ✳ **G9189** Beta-blocker therapy prescribed or currently being taken Ⓑ   M

MIPS ✳ **G9190** Documentation of medical reason(s) for not prescribing beta-blocker therapy (e.g., allergy, intolerance, other medical reasons) Ⓑ   M

MIPS ✳ **G9191** Documentation of patient reason(s) for not prescribing beta-blocker therapy (e.g., patient declined, other patient reasons) Ⓑ   M

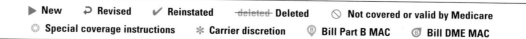

▶ New   ↻ Revised   ✔ Reinstated   ~~deleted~~ Deleted   ⊘ Not covered or valid by Medicare
Ⓢ Special coverage instructions   ✳ Carrier discretion   Ⓑ Bill Part B MAC   Ⓓ Bill DME MAC

* **G9192** Documentation of system reason(s) for not prescribing beta-blocker therapy (e.g., other reasons attributable to the health care system) ⓑ   M

* **G9212** DSM-IV-TM criteria for major depressive disorder documented at the initial evaluation ⓑ   M

* **G9213** DSM-IV-TR criteria for major depressive disorder not documented at the initial evaluation, reason not otherwise specified ⓑ   M

* **G9223** Pneumocystis jiroveci pneumonia prophylaxis prescribed within 3 months of low CD4+ cell count below 500 cells/mm3 or a CD4 percentage below 15% ⓑ   M

* **G9225** Foot exam was not performed, reason not given ⓑ   M

* **G9226** Foot examination performed (includes examination through visual inspection, sensory exam with 10-g monofilament plus testing any one of the following: vibration using 128-hz tuning fork, pinprick sensation, ankle reflexes, or vibration perception threshold, and pulse exam; report when all of the 3 components are completed) ⓑ   M

* **G9227** Functional outcome assessment documented, care plan not documented, documentation the patient is not eligible for a care plan at the time of the encounter ⓑ   M

* **G9228** Chlamydia, gonorrhea and syphilis screening results documented (report when results are present for all of the 3 screenings) ⓑ   M

* **G9229** Chlamydia, gonorrhea, and syphilis screening results not documented (patient refusal is the only allowed exception) ⓑ   M

* **G9230** Chlamydia, gonorrhea, and syphilis not screened, reason not given ⓑ   M

* **G9231** Documentation of end stage renal disease (ESRD), dialysis, renal transplant before or during the measurement period or pregnancy during the measurement period ⓑ   M

* **G9242** Documentation of viral load equal to or greater than 200 copies/ml or viral load not performed ⓑ   M

* **G9243** Documentation of viral load less than 200 copies/ml ⓑ   M

* **G9246** Patient did not have at least one medical visit in each 6 month period of the 24 month measurement period, with a minimum of 60 days between medical visits ⓑ   M

* **G9247** Patient had at least one medical visit in each 6 month period of the 24 month measurement period, with a minimum of 60 days between medical visits ⓑ   M

* **G9254** Documentation of patient discharged to home later than post-operative day 2 following CAS ⓑ   M

* **G9255** Documentation of patient discharged to home no later than post operative day 2 following CAS ⓑ   M

* **G9273** Blood pressure has a systolic value of <140 and a diastolic value of <90 ⓑ   M

* **G9274** Blood pressure has a systolic value of = 140 and a diastolic value of = 90 or systolic value <140 and diastolic value = 90 or systolic value = 140 and diastolic value <90 ⓑ   M

* **G9275** Documentation that patient is a current non-tobacco user ⓑ   M

* **G9276** Documentation that patient is a current tobacco user ⓑ   M

✳ **G9277** Documentation that the patient is on daily aspirin or anti-platelet or has documentation of a valid contraindication or exception to aspirin/anti-platelet; contraindications/exceptions include anti-coagulant use, allergy to aspirin or anti-platelets, history of gastrointestinal bleed and bleeding disorder; additionally, the following exceptions documented by the physician as a reason for not taking daily aspirin or anti-platelet are acceptable (use of non-steroidal anti-inflammatory agents, documented risk for drug interaction, uncontrolled hypertension defined as >180 systolic or >110 diastolic or gastroesophageal reflux) Ⓑ   M

✳ **G9278** Documentation that the patient is not on daily aspirin or anti-platelet regimen Ⓑ   M

✳ **G9279** Pneumococcal screening performed and documentation of vaccination received prior to discharge Ⓑ   M

✳ **G9280** Pneumococcal vaccination not administered prior to discharge, reason not specified Ⓑ   M

✳ **G9281** Screening performed and documentation that vaccination not indicated/patient refusal Ⓑ   M

✳ **G9282** Documentation of medical reason(s) for not reporting the histological type or NSCLC-NOS classification with an explanation (e.g., biopsy taken for other purposes in a patient with a history of non-small cell lung cancer or other documented medical reasons) Ⓑ   M

✳ **G9283** Non-small-cell lung cancer biopsy and cytology specimen report documents classification into specific histologic type or classified as NSCLC-NOS with an explanation Ⓑ   M

✳ **G9284** Non-small-cell lung cancer biopsy and cytology specimen report does not document classification into specific histologic type or classified as NSCLC-NOS with an explanation Ⓑ   M

✳ **G9285** Specimen site other than anatomic location of lung or is not classified as non-small-cell lung cancer Ⓑ   M

✳ **G9286** Antibiotic regimen prescribed within 10 days after onset of symptoms Ⓑ   M

✳ **G9287** Antibiotic regimen not prescribed within 10 days after onset of symptoms Ⓑ   M

✳ **G9288** Documentation of medical reason(s) for not reporting the histological type or NSCLC-NOS classification with an explanation (e.g., a solitary fibrous tumor in a person with a history of non-small cell carcinoma or other documented medical reasons) Ⓑ   M

✳ **G9289** Non-small cell lung cancer biopsy and cytology specimen report documents classification into specific histologic type or classified as NSCLC-NOS with an explanation Ⓑ   M

✳ **G9290** Non-small cell lung cancer biopsy and cytology specimen report does not document classification into specific histologic type or classified as NSCLC-NOS with an explanation Ⓑ   M

✳ **G9291** Specimen site other than anatomic location of lung, is not classified as non-small-cell lung cancer or classified as NSCLC-NOS Ⓑ   M

✳ **G9292** Documentation of medical reason(s) for not reporting PT category and a statement on thickness and ulceration and for PT1, mitotic rate (e.g., negative skin biopsies in a patient with a history of melanoma or other documented medical reasons) Ⓑ   M

✳ **G9293** Pathology report does not include the PT category and a statement on thickness and ulceration and for PT1, mitotic rate Ⓑ   M

✳ **G9294** Pathology report includes the PT category and a statement on thickness and ulceration and for PT1, mitotic rate Ⓑ   M

✳ **G9295** Specimen site other than anatomic cutaneous location Ⓑ   M

✳ **G9296** Patients with documented shared decision-making including discussion of conservative (non-surgical) therapy (e.g., NSAIDs, analgesics, weight loss, exercise, injections) prior to the procedure Ⓑ   M

✳ **G9297** Shared decision-making including discussion of conservative (non-surgical) therapy (e.g., NSAIDs, analgesics, weight loss, exercise, injections) prior to the procedure not documented, reason not given Ⓑ   M

✳ **G9298** Patients who are evaluated for venous thromboembolic and cardiovascular risk factors within 30 days prior to the procedure (e.g., history of DVT, PE, MI, arrhythmia and stroke) Ⓑ   M

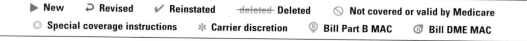

▶ New   ↻ Revised   ✔ Reinstated   ~~deleted~~ Deleted   ⊘ Not covered or valid by Medicare
Ⓢ Special coverage instructions   ✳ Carrier discretion   Ⓑ Bill Part B MAC   Ⓖ Bill DME MAC

* **G9299** Patients who are not evaluated for venous thromboembolic and cardiovascular risk factors within 30 days prior to the procedure (e.g., history of DVT, PE, MI, arrhythmia and stroke, reason not given) Ⓑ M

* **G9305** Intervention for presence of leak of endoluminal contents through an anastomosis not required Ⓑ M

* **G9306** Intervention for presence of leak of endoluminal contents through an anastomosis required Ⓑ M

* **G9307** No return to the operating room for a surgical procedure, for complications of the principal operative procedure, within 30 days of the principal operative procedure Ⓑ M

* **G9308** Unplanned return to the operating room for a surgical procedure, for complications of the principal operative procedure, within 30 days of the principal operative procedure Ⓑ M

* **G9309** No unplanned hospital readmission within 30 days of principal procedure Ⓑ M

* **G9310** Unplanned hospital readmission within 30 days of principal procedure Ⓑ M

* **G9311** No surgical site infection Ⓑ M

* **G9312** Surgical site infection Ⓑ M

* **G9313** Amoxicillin, with or without clavulanate, not prescribed as first line antibiotic at the time of diagnosis for documented reason Ⓑ M

* **G9314** Amoxicillin, with or without clavulanate, not prescribed as first line antibiotic at the time of diagnosis, reason not given Ⓑ M

* **G9315** Amoxicillin, with or without clavulanate, prescribed as a first line antibiotic at the time of diagnosis Ⓑ M

* **G9316** Documentation of patient-specific risk assessment with a risk calculator based on multi-institutional clinical data, the specific risk calculator used, and communication of risk assessment from risk calculator with the patient or family Ⓑ M

* **G9317** Documentation of patient-specific risk assessment with a risk calculator based on multi-institutional clinical data, the specific risk calculator used, and communication of risk assessment from risk calculator with the patient or family not completed Ⓑ M

* **G9318** Imaging study named according to standardized nomenclature Ⓑ M

* **G9319** Imaging study not named according to standardized nomenclature, reason not given Ⓑ M

* **G9321** Count of previous CT (any type of CT) and cardiac nuclear medicine (myocardial perfusion) studies documented in the 12-month period prior to the current study Ⓑ M

* **G9322** Count of previous CT and cardiac nuclear medicine (myocardial perfusion) studies not documented in the 12-month period prior to the current study, reason not given Ⓑ M

* **G9341** Search conducted for prior patient CT studies completed at non-affiliated external healthcare facilities or entities within the past 12-months and are available through a secure, authorized, media-free, shared archive prior to an imaging study being performed Ⓑ M

* **G9342** Search not conducted prior to an imaging study being performed for prior patient CT studies completed at non-affiliated external healthcare facilities or entities within the past 12-months and are available through a secure, authorized, media-free, shared archive, reason not given Ⓑ M

* **G9344** Due to system reasons search not conducted for DICOM format images for prior patient CT imaging studies completed at non-affiliated external healthcare facilities or entities within the past 12 months that are available through a secure, authorized, media-free, shared archive (e.g., non-affiliated external healthcare facilities or entities does not have archival abilities through a shared archival system) Ⓑ M

* **G9345** Follow-up recommendations documented according to recommended guidelines for incidentally detected pulmonary nodules (e.g., follow-up CT imaging studies needed or that no follow-up is needed) based at a minimum on nodule size and patient risk factors Ⓑ M

* **G9347** Follow-up recommendations not documented according to recommended guidelines for incidentally detected pulmonary nodules, reason not given Ⓑ M

* **G9351** More than one CT scan of the paranasal sinuses ordered or received within 90 days after diagnosis Ⓑ M

* **G9352** More than one CT scan of the paranasal sinuses ordered or received within 90 days after the date of diagnosis, reason not given Ⓑ M

* **G9353** More than one CT scan of the paranasal sinuses ordered or received within 90 days after the date of diagnosis for documented reasons (e.g., patients with complications, second CT obtained prior to surgery, other medical reasons) Ⓑ M

* **G9354** One CT scan or no CT scan of the paranasal sinuses ordered within 90 days after the date of diagnosis Ⓑ M

* **G9355** Elective delivery (without medical indication) by c-section, or early induction not performed (less than 39 weeks gestation) Ⓑ M

* **G9356** Elective delivery (without medical indication) by c-section, or early induction performed (less than 39 weeks gestation) Ⓑ M

* **G9357** Post-partum screenings, evaluations and education performed Ⓑ M

* **G9358** Post-partum screenings, evaluations and education not performed Ⓑ M

* **G9361** Medical indication for induction [delivery by cesarean birth or induction of labor (<39 weeks of gestation)] [documentation of reason(s) for elective delivery (e.g., hemorrhage and placental complications, hypertension, preeclampsia and eclampsia, rupture of membranes-premature or prolonged, maternal conditions complicating pregnancy/delivery, fetal conditions complicating pregnancy/delivery, late pregnancy, prior uterine surgery, or participation in clinical trial)] Ⓑ M

* **G9364** Sinusitis caused by, or presumed to be caused by, bacterial infection Ⓑ M

* **G9367** At least two orders for high-risk medications from the same drug class ordered Ⓑ M

* **G9368** At least two orders for high-risk medications from the same drug class not ordered Ⓑ M

* **G9380** Patient offered assistance with end of life issues during the measurement period Ⓑ M

* **G9382** Patient not offered assistance with end of life issues during the measurement period Ⓑ M

* **G9383** Patient received screening for HCV infection within the 12 month reporting period Ⓑ M

* **G9384** Documentation of medical reason(s) for not receiving annual screening for HCV infection (e.g., decompensated cirrhosis indicating advanced disease [i.e., ascites, esophageal variceal bleeding, hepatic encephalopathy], hepatocellular carcinoma, waitlist for organ transplant, limited life expectancy, other medical reasons) Ⓑ M

* **G9385** Documentation of patient reason(s) for not receiving annual screening for HCV infection (e.g., patient declined, other patient reasons) Ⓑ M

* **G9386** Screening for HCV infection not received within the 12 month reporting period, reason not given Ⓑ M

* **G9393** Patient with an initial PHQ-9 score greater than nine who achieves remission at 12 months as demonstrated by a 12 month (+/- 30 days) PHQ-9 score of less than five Ⓑ M

* **G9394** Patient who had a diagnosis of bipolar disorder or personality disorder, death, permanent nursing home resident or receiving hospice or palliative care any time during the measurement or assessment period Ⓑ M

* **G9395** Patient with an initial PHQ-9 score greater than nine who did not achieve remission at 12 months as demonstrated by a 12 month (+/- 30 days) PHQ-9 score greater than or equal to five Ⓑ M

* **G9396** Patient with an initial PHQ-9 score greater than nine who was not assessed for remission at 12 months (+/- 30 days) Ⓑ M

* **G9402** Patient received follow-up within 30 days after discharge Ⓑ M

* **G9403** Clinician documented reason patient was not able to complete 30 day follow-up from acute inpatient setting discharge (e.g., patient death prior to follow-up visit, patient non-compliant for visit follow-up) Ⓑ M

* **G9404** Patient did not receive follow-up within 30 days after discharge Ⓑ M

* **G9405** Patient received follow-up within 7 days after discharge Ⓑ M

▶ New   ↻ Revised   ✔ Reinstated   ~~deleted~~ Deleted   ⊘ Not covered or valid by Medicare
   ⊛ Special coverage instructions   * Carrier discretion   Ⓑ Bill Part B MAC   Ⓑ Bill DME MAC

* **G9406** Clinician documented reason patient was not able to complete 7 day follow-up from acute inpatient setting discharge (i.e patient death prior to follow-up visit, patient non-compliance for visit follow-up) Ⓑ M

* **G9407** Patient did not receive follow-up within 7 days after discharge Ⓑ M

* **G9408** Patients with cardiac tamponade and/or pericardiocentesis occurring within 30 days Ⓑ M

* **G9409** Patients without cardiac tamponade and/or pericardiocentesis occurring within 30 days Ⓑ M

* **G9410** Patient admitted within 180 days, status post CIED implantation, replacement, or revision with an infection requiring device removal or surgical revision Ⓑ M

* **G9411** Patient not admitted within 180 days, status post CIED implantation, replacement, or revision with an infection requiring device removal or surgical revision Ⓑ M

* **G9412** Patient admitted within 180 days, status post CIED implantation, replacement, or revision with an infection requiring device removal or surgical revision Ⓑ M

* **G9413** Patient not admitted within 180 days, status post CIED implantation, replacement, or revision with an infection requiring device removal or surgical revision Ⓑ M

* **G9414** Patient had one dose of meningococcal vaccine (serogroups a, c, w, y) on or between the patient's 11th and 13th birthdays Ⓑ M

* **G9415** Patient did not have one dose of meningococcal (serogroups a, c, w, y) vaccine on or between the patient's 11th and 13th birthdays Ⓑ M

* **G9416** Patient had one tetanus, diphtheria toxoids and acellular pertussis vaccine (Tdap) or one tetanus, diphtheria toxoids vaccine (Td) on or between the patient's 10th and 13th birthdays Ⓑ M

* **G9417** Patient did not have one tetanus, diphtheria toxoids and acellular pertussis vaccine (Tdap) on or between the patient's 10th and 13th birthdays Ⓑ M

* **G9418** Primary non-small cell lung cancer lung biopsy and cytology specimen report documents classification into specific histologic type following IASLC guidance or classified as NSCLC-NOS with an explanation Ⓑ M

* **G9419** Documentation of medical reason(s) for not including the histological type or NSCLC-NOS classification with an explanation (e.g., specimen insufficient or non-diagnostic, specimen does not contain cancer, other documented medical reasons) Ⓑ M

* **G9420** Specimen site other than anatomic location of lung or is not classified as primary non-small cell lung cancer Ⓑ M

* **G9421** Primary non-small cell lung cancer biopsy and cytology specimen report does not document classification into specific histologic type or histologic type does not follow IASLC guidance or is classified as NSCLC-NOS but without an explanation Ⓑ M

* **G9422** Primary lung carcinoma resection report documents pT category, pN category and for non-small cell lung cancer, histologic type (e.g., squamous cell carcinoma, adenocarcinoma and not NSCLC-NOS) Ⓑ M

* **G9423** Documentation of medical reason for not including pT category, pN category and histologic type [for patient with appropriate exclusion criteria (e.g., metastatic disease, benign tumors, malignant tumors other than carcinomas, inadequate surgical specimens)] Ⓑ M

* **G9424** Specimen site other than anatomic location of lung, or classified as NSCLC-NOS Ⓑ M

* **G9425** Primary lung carcinoma resection report does not document pT category, pN category and for non-small cell lung cancer, histologic type (e.g., squamous cell carcinoma, adenocarcinoma) Ⓑ M

* **G9426** Improvement in median time from ED arrival to initial ED oral or parenteral pain medication administration performed for ED admitted patients Ⓑ M

* **G9427** Improvement in median time from ED arrival to initial ED oral or parenteral pain medication administration not performed for ED admitted patients Ⓑ M

* **G9428** Pathology report includes the pT category, thickness, ulceration and mitotic rate, peripheral and deep margin status and presence or absence of microsatellitosis for invasive tumors ⑧   M

* **G9429** Documentation of medical reason(s) for not including pT category, thickness, ulceration and mitotic rate, peripheral and deep margin status and presence or absence of microsatellitosis for invasive tumors (e.g., negative skin biopsies in a patient with a history of melanoma or other documented medical reasons) ⑧ M

* **G9430** Specimen site other than anatomic cutaneous location ⑧   M

* **G9431** Pathology report does not include the pT category, thickness, ulceration and mitotic rate, peripheral and deep margin status and presence or absence of microsatellitosis for invasive tumors ⑧   M

* **G9432** Asthma well-controlled based on the ACT, C-ACT, ACQ, or ATAQ score and results documented ⑧   M

* **G9434** Asthma not well-controlled based on the ACT, C-ACT, ACQ, or ATAQ score, or specified asthma control tool not used, reason not given ⑧   M

* **G9451** Patient received one-time screening for HCV infection ⑧   M

* **G9452** Documentation of medical reason(s) for not receiving one-time screening for HCV infection (e.g., decompensated cirrhosis indicating advanced disease [i.e., ascites, esophageal variceal bleeding, hepatic encephalopathy], hepatocellular carcinoma, waitlist for organ transplant, limited life expectancy, other medical reasons) ⑧ M

* **G9453** Documentation of patient reason(s) for not receiving one-time screening for HCV infection (e.g., patient declined, other patient reasons) ⑧   M

* **G9454** One-time screening for HCV infection not received within 12 month reporting period and no documentation of prior screening for HCV infection, reason not given ⑧   M

* **G9455** Patient underwent abdominal imaging with ultrasound, contrast enhanced CT or contrast MRI for HCC ⑧   M

* **G9456** Documentation of medical or patient reason(s) for not ordering or performing screening for HCC. medical reason: comorbid medical conditions with expected survival <5 years, hepatic decompensation and not a candidate for liver transplantation, or other medical reasons; patient reasons: patient declined or other patient reasons (e.g., cost of tests, time related to accessing testing equipment) ⑧   M

* **G9457** Patient did not undergo abdominal imaging and did not have a documented reason for not undergoing abdominal imaging in the submission period ⑧   M

* **G9458** Patient documented as tobacco user and received tobacco cessation intervention (must include at least one of the following: advice given to quit smoking or tobacco use, counseling on the benefits of quitting smoking or tobacco use, assistance with or referral to external smoking or tobacco cessation support programs, or current enrollment in smoking or tobacco use cessation program) if identified as a tobacco user ⑧   M

* **G9459** Currently a tobacco non-user ⑧   M

* **G9460** Tobacco assessment or tobacco cessation intervention not performed, reason not given ⑧   M

* **G9468** Patient not receiving corticosteroids greater than or equal to 10 mg/day of prednisone equivalents for 60 or greater consecutive days or a single prescription equating to 600 mg prednisone or greater for all fills ⑧   M

* **G9470** Patients not receiving corticosteroids greater than or equal to 10 mg/day of prednisone equivalents for 60 or greater consecutive days or a single prescription equating to 600 mg prednisone or greater for all fills ⑧   M

* **G9471** Within the past 2 years, central dual-energy x-ray absorptiometry (DXA) not ordered or documented ⑧   M

* **G9473** Services performed by chaplain in the hospice setting, each 15 minutes ⑧   B

* **G9474** Services performed by dietary counselor in the hospice setting, each 15 minutes ⑧   B

* **G9475** Services performed by other counselor in the hospice setting, each 15 minutes ⑧   B

* **G9476** Services performed by volunteer in the hospice setting, each 15 minutes ⑧   B

▶ New   ↻ Revised   ✔ Reinstated   ~~deleted~~ Deleted   ⊘ Not covered or valid by Medicare
✪ Special coverage instructions   * Carrier discretion   ⑧ Bill Part B MAC   ⑧ Bill DME MAC

✻ **G9477** Services performed by care coordinator in the hospice setting, each 15 minutes Ⓑ B

✻ **G9478** Services performed by other qualified therapist in the hospice setting, each 15 minutes Ⓑ B

✻ **G9479** Services performed by qualified pharmacist in the hospice setting, each 15 minutes Ⓑ B

✻ **G9480** Admission to Medicare Care Choice Model program (MCCM) Ⓑ Qp Qh B

✻ **G9481** Remote in-home visit for the evaluation and management of a new patient for use only in the Medicare-approved comprehensive care for joint replacement model, which requires these 3 key components: a problem focused history; a problem focused examination; and straightforward medical decision making, furnished in real time using interactive audio and video technology. Counseling and coordination of care with other physicians, other qualified health care professionals or agencies are provided consistent with the nature of the problem(s) and the needs of the patient or the family or both. Usually, the presenting problem(s) are self limited or minor. Typically, 10 minutes are spent with the patient or family or both via real time, audio and video intercommunications technology Ⓑ B

✻ **G9482** Remote in-home visit for the evaluation and management of a new patient for use only in the Medicare-approved comprehensive care for joint replacement model, which requires these 3 key components: an expanded problem focused history; an expanded problem focused examination; straightforward medical decision making, furnished in real time using interactive audio and video technology. Counseling and coordination of care with other physicians, other qualified health care professionals or agencies are provided consistent with the nature of the problem(s) and the needs of the patient or the family or both. Usually, the presenting problem(s) are of low to moderate severity. Typically, 20 minutes are spent with the patient or family or both via real time, audio and video intercommunications technology Ⓑ B

✻ **G9483** Remote in-home visit for the evaluation and management of a new patient for use only in the Medicare-approved comprehensive care for joint replacement model, which requires these 3 key components: a detailed history; a detailed examination; medical decision making of low complexity, furnished in real time using interactive audio and video technology. Counseling and coordination of care with other physicians, other qualified health care professionals or agencies are provided consistent with the nature of the problem(s) and the needs of the patient or the family or both. Usually, the presenting problem(s) are of moderate severity. Typically, 30 minutes are spent with the patient or family or both via real time, audio and video intercommunications technology Ⓑ B

✻ **G9484** Remote in-home visit for the evaluation and management of a new patient for use only in the Medicare-approved comprehensive care for joint replacement model, which requires these 3 key components: a comprehensive history; a comprehensive examination; medical decision making of moderate complexity, furnished in real time using interactive audio and video technology. Counseling and coordination of care with other physicians, other qualified health care professionals or agencies are provided consistent with the nature of the problem(s) and the needs of the patient or the family or both. Usually, the presenting problem(s) are of moderate to high severity. Typically, 45 minutes are spent with the patient or family or both via real time, audio and video intercommunications technology Ⓑ B

🅜 MIPS   Qp **Quantity Physician**   Qh **Quantity Hospital**   ♀ **Female only**

♂ **Male only**   🅐 **Age**   ⅃ **DMEPOS**   A2-Z3 **ASC Payment Indicator**   A-Y **ASC Status Indicator**   Coding Clinic

✳ **G9485**   Remote in-home visit for the evaluation and management of a new patient for use only in the Medicare-approved comprehensive care for joint replacement model, which requires these 3 key components: a comprehensive history; a comprehensive examination; medical decision making of high complexity, furnished in real time using interactive audio and video technology. Counseling and coordination of care with other physicians, other qualified health care professionals or agencies are provided consistent with the nature of the problem(s) and the needs of the patient or the family or both. Usually, the presenting problem(s) are of moderate to high severity. Typically, 60 minutes are spent with the patient or family or both via real time, audio and video intercommunications technology ⑧   **B**

✳ **G9486**   Remote in-home visit for the evaluation and management of an established patient for use only in the Medicare-approved comprehensive care for joint replacement model, which requires at least 2 of the following 3 key components: a problem focused history; a problem focused examination; straightforward medical decision making, furnished in real time using interactive audio and video technology. Counseling and coordination of care with other physicians, other qualified health care professionals or agencies are provided consistent with the nature of the problem(s) and the needs of the patient or the family or both. Usually, the presenting problem(s) are self limited or minor. Typically, 10 minutes are spent with the patient or family or both via real time, audio and video intercommunications technology ⑧   **B**

✳ **G9487**   Remote in-home visit for the evaluation and management of an established patient for use only in the Medicare-approved comprehensive care for joint replacement model, which requires at least 2 of the following 3 key components: an expanded problem focused history; an expanded problem focused examination; medical decision making of low complexity, furnished in real time using interactive audio and video technology. Counseling and coordination of care with other physicians, other qualified health care professionals or agencies are provided consistent with the nature of the problem(s) and the needs of the patient or the family or both. Usually, the presenting problem(s) are of low to moderate severity. Typically, 15 minutes are spent with the patient or family or both via real time, audio and video intercommunications technology ⑧   **B**

✳ **G9488**   Remote in-home visit for the evaluation and management of an established patient for use only in the Medicare-approved comprehensive care for joint replacement model, which requires at least 2 of the following 3 key components: a detailed history; a detailed examination; medical decision making of moderate complexity, furnished in real time using interactive audio and video technology. Counseling and coordination of care with other physicians, other qualified health care professionals or agencies are provided consistent with the nature of the problem(s) and the needs of the patient or the family or both. Usually, the presenting problem(s) are of moderate to high severity. Typically, 25 minutes are spent with the patient or family or both via real time, audio and video intercommunications technology ⑧   **B**

▶ **New**   ↻ **Revised**   ✔ **Reinstated**   ~~deleted~~ **Deleted**   ⊘ **Not covered or valid by Medicare**
⊜ **Special coverage instructions**   ✳ **Carrier discretion**   ⑧ **Bill Part B MAC**   ⑧ **Bill DME MAC**

* **G9489** Remote in-home visit for the evaluation and management of an established patient for use only in the Medicare-approved comprehensive care for joint replacement model, which requires at least 2 of the following 3 key components: a comprehensive history; a comprehensive examination; medical decision making of high complexity, furnished in real time using interactive audio and video technology. Counseling and coordination of care with other physicians, other qualified health care professionals or agencies are provided consistent with the nature of the problem(s) and the needs of the patient or the family or both. Usually, the presenting problem(s) are of moderate to high severity. Typically, 40 minutes are spent with the patient or family or both via real time, audio and video intercommunications technology ⓑ B

* **G9490** Comprehensive care for joint replacement model, home visit for patient assessment performed by clinical staff for an individual not considered homebound, including, but not necessarily limited to patient assessment of clinical status, safety/fall prevention, functional status/ambulation, medication reconciliation/management, compliance with orders/plan of care, performance of activities of daily living, and ensuring beneficiary connections to community and other services. (for use only in the Medicare-approved CJR model); may not be billed for a 30 day period covered by a transitional care management code ⓑ B

* **G9497** Received instruction from the anesthesiologist or proxy prior to the day of surgery to abstain from smoking on the day of surgery ⓑ M

* **G9498** Antibiotic regimen prescribed ⓑ M

* **G9500** Radiation exposure indices documented in final report for procedure using fluoroscopy ⓑ M

* **G9501** Radiation exposure indices not documented in final report for procedure using fluoroscopy, reason not given ⓑM

* **G9502** Documentation of medical reason for not performing foot exam (i.e., patients who have had either a bilateral amputation above or below the knee, or both a left and right amputation above or below the knee before or during the measurement period) ⓑ M

* **G9504** Documented reason for not assessing Hepatitis B virus (HBV) status (e.g. patient not initiating anti-TNF therapy, patient declined) prior to initiating anti-TNF therapy ⓑ M

* **G9505** Antibiotic regimen prescribed within 10 days after onset of symptoms for documented medical reason ⓑ M

* **G9507** Documentation that the patient is on a statin medication or has documentation of a valid contraindication or exception to statin medications; contraindications/exceptions that can be defined by diagnosis codes include pregnancy during the measurement period, active liver disease, rhabdomyolysis, end stage renal disease on dialysis and heart failure; provider documented contraindications/exceptions include breastfeeding during the measurement period, woman of child-bearing age not actively taking birth control, allergy to statin, drug interaction (HIV protease inhibitors, nefazodone, cyclosporine, gemfibrozil, and danazol) and intolerance (with supporting documentation of trying a statin at least once within the last 5 years or diagnosis codes for myostitis or toxic myopathy related to drugs) ⓑM

* **G9508** Documentation that the patient is not on a statin medication ⓑ M

* **G9509** Adult patients 18 years of age or older with major depression or dysthymia who reached remission at 12 months as demonstrated by a 12 month (+/-60 days) PHQ-9 or PHQ-9m score of less than 5 ⓑ M

* **G9510** Adult patients 18 years of age or older with major depression or dysthymia who did not reach remission at twelve months as demonstrated by a twelve month (+/-60 days) PHQ-9 or PHQ-9m score of less than 5. Either PHQ-9 or PHQ-9m score was not assessed or is greater than or equal to 5 ⑧   M

* **G9511** Index event date PHQ-9 score greater than 9 documented during the 12 month denominator identification period ⑧   M

* **G9512** Individual had a PDC of 0.8 or greater ⑧   M

* **G9513** Individual did not have a PDC of 0.8 or greater ⑧   M

* **G9514** Patient required a return to the operating room within 90 days of surgery ⑧   M

* **G9515** Patient did not require a return to the operating room within 90 days of surgery ⑧   M

* **G9516** Patient achieved an improvement in visual acuity, from their preoperative level, within 90 days of surgery ⑧   M

* **G9517** Patient did not achieve an improvement in visual acuity, from their preoperative level, within 90 days of surgery, reason not given ⑧   M

* **G9518** Documentation of active injection drug use ⑧   M

* **G9519** Patient achieves final refraction (spherical equivalent) +/-1.0 diopters of their planned refraction within 90 days of surgery ⑧   M

* **G9520** Patient does not achieve final refraction (spherical equivalent) +/-1.0 diopters of their planned refraction within 90 days of surgery ⑧   M

* **G9521** Total number of emergency department visits and inpatient hospitalizations less than two in the past 12 months ⑧   M

* **G9522** Total number of emergency department visits and inpatient hospitalizations equal to or greater than two in the past 12 months or patient not screened, reason not given ⑧   M

* **G9529** Patient with minor blunt head trauma had an appropriate indication(s) for a head CT ⑧   M

* **G9530** Patient presented within a minor blunt head trauma and had a head CT ordered for trauma by an emergency care provider ⑧   M

* **G9531** Patient has documentation of ventricular shunt, brain tumor, multisystem trauma, or is currently taking an antiplatelet medication including: abciximab, anagrelide, cangrelor, cilostazol, clopidogrel, dipyridamole, eptifibatide, prasugrel, ticlopidine, ticagrelor, tirofiban, or vorapaxar ⑧   M

* **G9533** Patient with minor blunt head trauma did not have an appropriate indication(s) for a head CT ⑧   M

* **G9537** Imaging needed as part of a clinical trial; or other clinician ordered the study ⑧   M

* **G9539** Intent for potential removal at time of placement ⑧   M

* **G9540** Patient alive 3 months post procedure ⑧   M

* **G9541** Filter removed within 3 months of placement ⑧   M

* **G9542** Documented re-assessment for the appropriateness of filter removal within 3 months of placement ⑧   M

* **G9543** Documentation of at least two attempts to reach the patient to arrange a clinical re-assessment for the appropriateness of filter removal within 3 months of placement ⑧   M

* **G9544** Patients that do not have the filter removed, documented re-assessment for the appropriateness of filter removal, or documentation of at least two attempts to reach the patient to arrange a clinical re-assessment for the appropriateness of filter removal within 3 months of placement ⑧   M

* **G9547** Cystic renal lesion that is simple appearing (Bosniak I or II), or adrenal lesion less than or equal to 1.0 cm or adrenal lesion greater than 1.0 cm but less than or equal to 4.0 cm classified as likely benign by unenhanced CT or washout protocol CT, or MRI with in- and opposed-phase sequences or other equivalent institutional imaging protocols ⑧   M

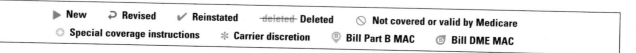

* **G9548** Final reports for imaging studies stating no follow-up imaging is recommended Ⓑ M

* **G9549** Documentation of medical reason(s) that follow-up imaging is indicated (e.g., patient has lymphadenopathy, signs of metastasis or an active diagnosis or history of cancer, and other medical reason(s)) Ⓑ M

* **G9550** Final reports for imaging studies with follow-up imaging recommended, or final reports that do not include a specific recommendation of no follow-up Ⓑ M

* **G9551** Final reports for imaging studies without an incidentally found lesion noted Ⓑ M

* **G9552** Incidental thyroid nodule <1.0 cm noted in report Ⓑ M

* **G9553** Prior thyroid disease diagnosis Ⓑ M

* **G9554** Final reports for CT, CTA, MRI or MRA of the chest or neck with follow-up imaging recommended Ⓑ M

* **G9555** Documentation of medical reason(s) for recommending follow up imaging (e.g., patient has multiple endocrine neoplasia, patient has cervical lymphadenopathy, other medical reason(s)) Ⓑ M

* **G9556** Final reports for CT, CTA, MRI or MRA of the chest or neck with follow-up imaging not recommended Ⓑ M

* **G9557** Final reports for CT, CTA, MRI or MRA studies of the chest or neck without an incidentally found thyroid nodule <1.0 cm noted or no nodule found Ⓑ M

* **G9580** Door to puncture time of 90 minutes or less Ⓑ M

* **G9582** Door to puncture time of greater than 90 minutes, no reason given Ⓑ M

* **G9593** Pediatric patient with minor blunt head trauma classified as low risk according to the pecarn Prediction Rules Ⓑ Ⓐ M

* **G9594** Patient presented with a minor blunt head trauma and had a head CT ordered for trauma by an emergency care provider Ⓑ M

* **G9595** Patient has documentation of ventricular shunt, brain tumor, or coagulopathy Ⓑ M

* **G9596** Pediatric patient had a head CT for trauma ordered by someone other than an emergency care provider, or was ordered for a reason other than trauma Ⓑ Ⓐ M

* **G9597** Pediatric patient with minor blunt head trauma not classified as low risk according to the pecarn Prediction Rules Ⓑ Ⓐ M

* **G9598** Aortic aneurysm 5.5-5.9 cm maximum diameter on centerline formatted CT or minor diameter on axial formatted CT Ⓑ M

* **G9599** Aortic aneurysm 6.0 cm or greater maximum diameter on centerline formatted CT or minor diameter on axial formatted CT Ⓑ M

* **G9603** Patient survey score improved from baseline following treatment Ⓑ M

* **G9604** Patient survey results not available Ⓑ M

* **G9605** Patient survey score did not improve from baseline following treatment Ⓑ M

* **G9606** Intraoperative cystoscopy performed to evaluate for lower tract injury Ⓑ M

* **G9607** Documented medical reasons for not performing intraoperative cystoscopy (e.g., urethral pathology precluding cystoscopy, any patient who has a congenital or acquired absence of the urethra) or in the case of patient death Ⓑ M

* **G9608** Intraoperative cystoscopy not performed to evaluate for lower tract injury Ⓑ M

* **G9609** Documentation of an order for anti-platelet agents Ⓑ M

* **G9610** Documentation of medical reason(s) in the patient's record for not ordering anti-platelet agents Ⓑ M

* **G9611** Order for anti-platelet agents was not documented in the patient's record, reason not given Ⓑ M

* **G9612** Photodocumentation of two or more cecal landmarks to establish a complete examination Ⓑ M

* **G9613** Documentation of post-surgical anatomy (e.g., right hemicolectomy, ileocecal resection, etc.) Ⓑ M

* **G9614** Photodocumentation of less than two cecal landmarks (i.e., no cecal landmarks or only one cecal landmark) to establish a complete examination Ⓑ M

* **G9621** Patient identified as an unhealthy alcohol user when screened for unhealthy alcohol use using a systematic screening method and received brief counseling Ⓑ M

* **G9622** Patient not identified as an unhealthy alcohol user when screened for unhealthy alcohol use using a systematic screening method Ⓑ M

* **G9624** Patient not screened for unhealthy alcohol use using a systematic screening method or patient did not receive brief counseling if identified as an unhealthy alcohol user Ⓑ M

* **G9625** Patient sustained bladder injury at the time of surgery or discovered subsequently up to 30 days post-surgery Ⓑ M

* **G9626** Documented medical reason for not reporting bladder injury (e.g., gynecologic or other pelvic malignancy documented, concurrent surgery involving bladder pathology, injury that occurs during urinary incontinence procedure, patient death from non-medical causes not related to surgery, patient died during procedure without evidence of bladder injury) Ⓑ M

* **G9627** Patient did not sustain bladder injury at the time of surgery nor discovered subsequently up to 30 days post-surgery Ⓑ M

* **G9628** Patient sustained bowel injury at the time of surgery or discovered subsequently up to 30 days post-surgery Ⓑ M

* **G9629** Documented medical reasons for not reporting bowel injury (e.g., gynecologic or other pelvic malignancy documented, planned (e.g., not due to an unexpected bowel injury) resection and/or re-anastomosis of bowel, or patient death from non-medical causes not related to surgery, patient died during procedure without evidence of bowel injury) Ⓑ M

* **G9630** Patient did not sustain a bowel injury at the time of surgery nor discovered subsequently up to 30 days post-surgery Ⓑ M

* **G9637** At least two orders for the same high-risk medications Ⓑ M

* **G9638** At least two orders for the same high-risk medications not ordered Ⓑ M

* **G9642** Current smoker (e.g., cigarette, cigar, pipe, e-cigarette or marijuana) Ⓑ M

* **G9643** Elective surgery Ⓑ M

* **G9644** Patients who abstained from smoking prior to anesthesia on the day of surgery or procedure Ⓑ M

* **G9645** Patients who did not abstain from smoking prior to anesthesia on the day of surgery or procedure Ⓑ M

* **G9646** Patients with 90 day MRS score of 0 to 2 Ⓑ M

* **G9648** Patients with 90 day MRS score greater than 2 Ⓑ M

* **G9649** Psoriasis assessment tool documented meeting any one of the specified benchmarks (e.g., PGA; 5-point or 6-point scale), body surface area (BSA), psoriasis area and severity index (PASI) and/or dermatology life quality index) (DLQI)) Ⓑ M

▶ New   ↻ Revised   ✓ Reinstated   deleted Deleted   ⊘ Not covered or valid by Medicare
Ⓢ Special coverage instructions   * Carrier discretion   Ⓑ Bill Part B MAC   Ⓑ Bill DME MAC

* **G9651** Psoriasis assessment tool documented not meeting any one of the specified benchmarks (e.g., (pga; 5-point or 6-point scale), body surface area (bsa), psoriasis area and severity index (pasi) and/or dermatology life quality index) (dlqi)) or psoriasis assessment tool not documented Ⓑ M

* **G9654** Monitored anesthesia care (mac) Ⓑ M

* **G9655** A transfer of care protocol or handoff tool/checklist that includes the required key handoff elements is used Ⓑ M

* **G9656** Patient transferred directly from anesthetizing location to PACU or other non-ICU location Ⓑ M

* **G9658** A transfer of care protocol or handoff tool/checklist that includes the required key handoff elements is not used Ⓑ M

* **G9659** Patients greater than 86 years of age who underwent a screening colonoscopy and did not have a history of colorectal cancer or valid medical reason for the colonoscopy, including: iron deficiency anemia, lower gastrointestinal bleeding, Crohn disease (i.e., regional enteritis), familial adenomatous polyposis, Lynch syndrome (i.e., hereditary non-polyposis colorectal cancer), inflammatory bowel disease, ulcerative colitis, abnormal finding of gastrointestinal tract, or changes in bowel habits Ⓑ M

* **G9660** Documentation of medical reason(s) for a colonoscopy performed on a patient greater than or equal to 86 years of age (e.g., iron deficiency anemia, lower gastrointestinal bleeding, Crohn disease (i.e., regional enteritis), familial history of adenomatous polyposis, Lynch syndrome (i.e., hereditary non-polyposis colorectal cancer), inflammatory bowel disease, ulcerative colitis, abnormal finding of gastrointestinal tract, or changes in bowel habits) Ⓑ M

* **G9661** Patients greater than or equal to 86 years of age who received a colonoscopy for an assessment of signs/symptoms of GI tract illness, and/or because the patient meets high risk criteria, and/or to follow-up on previously diagnosed advance lesions Ⓑ M

* **G9662** Previously diagnosed or have a diagnosis of clinical ASCVD, including ASCVD procedure Ⓑ M

* **G9663** Any ldl-c laboratory test result >=190 mg/dL Ⓑ M

* **G9664** Patients who are currently statin therapy users or received an order (prescription) for statin therapy Ⓑ M

* **G9665** Patients who are not currently statin therapy users or did not receive an order (prescription) for statin therapy Ⓑ M

* **G9674** Patients with clinical ascvd diagnosis Ⓑ M

* **G9675** Patients who have ever had a fasting or direct laboratory result of ldl-c = 190 mg/dl Ⓑ M

* **G9676** Patients aged 40 to 75 years at the beginning of the measurement period with type 1 or type 2 diabetes and with an ldl-c result of 70-189 mg/dl recorded as the highest fasting or direct laboratory test result in the measurement year or during the two years prior to the beginning of the measurement period Ⓑ M

* **G9679** This code is for onsite acute care treatment of a nursing facility resident with pneumonia; may only be billed once per day per beneficiary Ⓑ B

* **G9680** This code is for onsite acute care treatment of a nursing facility resident with CHF; may only be billed once per day per beneficiary Ⓑ B

* **G9681** This code is for onsite acute care treatment of a resident with COPD or asthma; may only be billed once per day per beneficiary Ⓑ B

* **G9682** This code is for the onsite acute care treatment a nursing facility resident with a skin infection; may only be billed once per day per beneficiary Ⓑ B

* **G9683** Facility service(s) for the onsite acute care treatment of a nursing facility resident with fluid or electrolyte disorder. (May only be billed once per day per beneficiary). This service is for a demonstration project. Ⓑ B

* **G9684** This code is for the onsite acute care treatment of a nursing facility resident for a UTI; may only be billed once per day per beneficiary Ⓑ B

* **G9685** Physician service or other qualified health care professional for the evaluation and management of a beneficiary's acute change in condition in a nursing facility. This service is for a demonstration project. Ⓑ **M**

* **G9687** Hospice services provided to patient any time during the measurement period Ⓑ **M**

* **G9688** Patients using hospice services any time during the measurement period Ⓑ **M**

* **G9689** Patient admitted for performance of elective carotid intervention Ⓑ **M**

* **G9690** Patient receiving hospice services any time during the measurement period Ⓑ **M**

* **G9691** Patient had hospice services any time during the measurement period Ⓑ **M**

* **G9692** Hospice services received by patient any time during the measurement period Ⓑ **M**

* **G9693** Patient use of hospice services any time during the measurement period Ⓑ **M**

* **G9694** Hospice services utilized by patient any time during the measurement period Ⓑ **M**

* **G9695** Long-acting inhaled bronchodilator prescribed Ⓑ **M**

* **G9696** Documentation of medical reason(s) for not prescribing a long-acting inhaled bronchodilator Ⓑ **M**

* **G9697** Documentation of patient reason(s) for not prescribing a long-acting inhaled bronchodilator Ⓑ **M**

* **G9698** Documentation of system reason(s) for not prescribing a long-acting inhaled bronchodilator Ⓑ **M**

* **G9699** Long-acting inhaled bronchodilator not prescribed, reason not otherwise specified Ⓑ **M**

* **G9700** Patients who use hospice services any time during the measurement period Ⓑ **M**

* **G9702** Patients who use hospice services any time during the measurement period Ⓑ **M**

* **G9703** Episodes where the patient is taking antibiotics (table 1) in the 30 days prior to the episode date, or had an active prescription on the episode date Ⓑ **M**

* **G9704** AJCC breast cancer stage I: T1 mic or T1a documented Ⓑ **M**

* **G9705** AJCC breast cancer stage I: T1b (tumor >0.5 cm but <=1 cm in greatest dimension) documented Ⓑ **M**

* **G9706** Low (or very low) risk of recurrence, prostate cancer Ⓑ **M**

* **G9707** Patient received hospice services any time during the measurement period Ⓑ **M**

* **G9708** Women who had a bilateral mastectomy or who have a history of a bilateral mastectomy or for whom there is evidence of a right and a left unilateral mastectomy Ⓑ **M**

* **G9709** Hospice services used by patient any time during the measurement period Ⓑ **M**

* **G9710** Patient was provided hospice services any time during the measurement period Ⓑ **M**

* **G9711** Patients with a diagnosis or past history of total colectomy or colorectal cancer Ⓑ **M**

* **G9712** Documentation of medical reason(s) for prescribing or dispensing antibiotic (e.g., intestinal infection, pertussis, bacterial infection, Lyme disease, otitis media, acute sinusitis, acute pharyngitis, acute tonsillitis, chronic sinusitis, infection of the pharynx/larynx/tonsils/adenoids, prostatitis, cellulitis/ mastoiditis/bone infections, acute lymphadenitis, impetigo, skin staph infections, pneumonia, gonococcal infections/venereal disease/syphilis, chlamydia, inflammatory diseases, female reproductive organs), infections of the kidney, cystitis/UTI, acne, HIV disease/asymptomatic HIV, cystic fibrosis, disorders of the immune system, malignancy neoplasms, chronic bronchitis, emphysema, bronchiectasis, extrinsic allergic alveolitis, chronic airway obstruction, chronic obstructive asthma, pneumoconiosis and other lung disease due to external agents, other diseases of the respiratory system, and tuberculosis Ⓑ **M**

* **G9713** Patients who use hospice services any time during the measurement period Ⓑ **M**

* **G9714** Patient is using hospice services any time during the measurement period Ⓑ **M**

▶ New ↻ Revised ✔ Reinstated ~~deleted~~ Deleted ⊘ Not covered or valid by Medicare
⊛ Special coverage instructions ✳ Carrier discretion Ⓑ Bill Part B MAC Ⓑ Bill DME MAC

* **G9715** Patients who use hospice services any time during the measurement period ⓑ M

* **G9716** BMI is documented as being outside of normal parameters, follow-up plan is not completed for documented medical reason ⓑ M

* **G9717** Documentation stating the patient has had a diagnosis of depression or has had a diagnosis bipolar disorder ⓑ M

* **G9719** Patient is not ambulatory, bed ridden, immobile, confined to chair, wheelchair bound, dependent on helper pushing wheelchair, independent in wheelchair or minimal help in wheelchair ⓑ M

* **G9720** Hospice services for patient occurred any time during the measurement period ⓑ M

* **G9721** Patient not ambulatory, bed ridden, immobile, confined to chair, wheelchair bound, dependent on helper pushing wheelchair, independent in wheelchair or minimal help in wheelchair ⓑ M

* **G9722** Documented history of renal failure or baseline serum creatinine > = 4.0 mg/dl; renal transplant recipients are not considered to have preoperative renal failure, unless, since transplantation the CR has been or is 4.0 or higher ⓑ M

* **G9723** Hospice services for patient received any time during the measurement period ⓑ M

* **G9724** Patients who had documentation of use of anticoagulant medications overlapping the measurement year ⓑ M

* **G9725** Patients who use hospice services any time during the measurement period ⓑ M

* **G9726** Patient refused to participate ⓑ M

* **G9727** Patient unable to complete the LEPF prom at initial evaluation and/or discharge due to blindness, illiteracy, severe mental incapacity or language incompatibility and an adequate proxy is not available ⓑ M

* **G9728** Patient refused to participate ⓑ M

* **G9729** Patient unable to complete the LEPF prom at initial evaluation and/or discharge due to blindness, illiteracy, severe mental incapacity or language incompatibility and an adequate proxy is not available ⓑ M

* **G9730** Patient refused to participate ⓑ M

* **G9731** Patient unable to complete the LEPF prom at initial evaluation and/or discharge due to blindness, illiteracy, severe mental incapacity or language incompatibility and an adequate proxy is not available ⓑ M

* **G9732** Patient refused to participate ⓑ M

* **G9733** Patient unable to complete the low back FS prom at initial evaluation and/or discharge due to blindness, illiteracy, severe mental incapacity or language incompatibility and an adequate proxy is not available ⓑ M

* **G9734** Patient refused to participate ⓑ M

* **G9735** Patient unable to complete the shoulder FS prom at initial evaluation and/or discharge due to blindness, illiteracy, severe mental incapacity or language incompatibility and an adequate proxy is not available ⓑ M

* **G9736** Patient refused to participate ⓑ M

* **G9737** Patient unable to complete the elbow/wrist/hand FS prom at initial evaluation and/or discharge due to blindness, illiteracy, severe mental incapacity or language incompatibility and an adequate proxy is not available ⓑ M

* **G9740** Hospice services given to patient any time during the measurement period ⓑ M

* **G9741** Patients who use hospice services any time during the measurement period ⓑ M

* **G9744** Patient not eligible due to active diagnosis of hypertension ⓑ M

* **G9745** Documented reason for not screening or recommending a follow-up for high blood pressure ⓑ M

* **G9746** Patient has mitral stenosis or prosthetic heart valves or patient has transient or reversible cause of AF (e.g., pneumonia, hyperthyroidism, pregnancy, cardiac surgery) ⓑ M

🐟 MIPS   **Qp** Quantity Physician   **Qh** Quantity Hospital   ♀ Female only

♂ Male only   **A** Age   ♿ DMEPOS   A2-Z3 ASC Payment Indicator   A-Y ASC Status Indicator   Coding Clinic

* **G9751** Patient died at any time during the 24-month measurement period Ⓑ M

* **G9752** Emergency surgery Ⓑ M

* **G9753** Documentation of medical reason for not conducting a search for DICOM format images for prior patient CT imaging studies completed at non-affiliated external healthcare facilities or entities within the past 12 months that are available through a secure, authorized, media-free, shared archive (e.g., trauma, acute myocardial infarction, stroke, aortic aneurysm where time is of the essence) Ⓑ M

* **G9754** A finding of an incidental pulmonary nodule Ⓑ M

* **G9755** Documentation of medical reason(s) for not including a recommended interval and modality for follow-up or for no follow-up, and source of recommendations (e.g., patients with unexplained fever, immunocompromised patients who are at risk for infection) Ⓑ M

* **G9756** Surgical procedures that included the use of silicone oil Ⓑ M

* **G9757** Surgical procedures that included the use of silicone oil Ⓑ M

* **G9758** Patient in hospice at any time during the measurement period Ⓑ M

* **G9760** Patients who use hospice services any time during the measurement period Ⓑ M

* **G9761** Patients who use hospice services any time during the measurement period Ⓑ M

* **G9762** Patient had at least two HPV vaccines (with at least 146 days between the two) or three HPV vaccines on or between the patient's 9th and 13th birthdays Ⓑ M

* **G9763** Patient did not have at least two HPV vaccines (with at least 146 days between the two) or three HPV vaccines on or between the patient's 9th and 13th birthdays Ⓑ M

* **G9764** Patient has been treated with systemic medication for psoriasis vulgaris Ⓑ M

* **G9765** Documentation that the patient declined change in medication or alternative therapies were unavailable, has documented contraindications, or has not been treated with systemic for at least six consecutive months (e.g., experienced adverse effects or lack of efficacy with all other therapy options) in order to achieve better disease control as measured by PGA, BSA, PASI, or DLQI Ⓑ M

* **G9766** Patients who are transferred from one institution to another with a known diagnosis of CVA for endovascular stroke treatment Ⓑ M

* **G9767** Hospitalized patients with newly diagnosed CVA considered for endovascular stroke treatment Ⓑ M

* **G9768** Patients who utilize hospice services any time during the measurement period Ⓑ M

* **G9769** Patient had a bone mineral density test in the past two years or received osteoporosis medication or therapy in the past 12 months Ⓑ M

* **G9770** Peripheral nerve block (PNB) Ⓑ M

* **G9771** At least 1 body temperature measurement equal to or greater than 35.5 degrees Celsius (or 95.9 degrees Fahrenheit) achieved within the 30 minutes immediately before or the 15 minutes immediately after anesthesia end time Ⓑ M

* **G9772** Documentation of medical reason(s) for not achieving at least 1 body temperature measurement equal to or greater than 35.5 degrees Celsius (or 95.9 degrees Fahrenheit) within the 30 minutes immediately before or the 15 minutes immediately after anesthesia end time (e.g., emergency cases, intentional hypothermia, etc.) Ⓑ M

* **G9773** At least 1 body temperature measurement equal to or greater than 35.5 degrees Celsius (or 95.9 degrees Fahrenheit) not achieved within the 30 minutes immediately before or the 15 minutes immediately after anesthesia end time, reason not given Ⓑ M

* **G9775** Patient received at least 2 prophylactic pharmacologic anti-emetic agents of different classes preoperatively and/or intraoperatively Ⓑ M

▶ **New**   ↻ **Revised**   ✔ **Reinstated**   ~~deleted~~ **Deleted**   ⊘ **Not covered or valid by Medicare**
⊛ **Special coverage instructions**   ✳ **Carrier discretion**   Ⓑ **Bill Part B MAC**   Ⓑ **Bill DME MAC**

G9776 Documentation of medical reason for not receiving at least 2 prophylactic pharmacologic anti-emetic agents of different classes preoperatively and/or intraoperatively (e.g., intolerance or other medical reason) Ⓑ M

G9777 Patient did not receive at least 2 prophylactic pharmacologic anti-emetic agents of different classes preoperatively and/or intraoperatively Ⓑ M

G9779 Patients who are breastfeeding at any time during the measurement period ⒷM

G9780 Patients who have a diagnosis of rhabdomyolysis at any time during the measurement period Ⓑ M

G9781 Documentation of medical reason(s) for not currently being a statin therapy user or receiving an order (prescription) for statin therapy (e.g., patients with statin-associated muscle symptoms, patients who are receiving palliative care or hospice care, patients with active liver disease or hepatic disease or insufficiency, and patients with end stage renal disease [ESRD]) Ⓑ M

G9782 History of or active diagnosis of familial hypercholesterolemia Ⓑ M

G9784 Pathologists/dermatopathologists providing a second opinion on a biopsy Ⓑ M

G9785 Pathology report diagnosing cutaneous basal cell carcinoma, squamous cell carcinoma, or melanoma (to include in situ disease) sent from the pathologist/dermatopathologist to the biopsying clinician for review within 7 days from the time when the tissue specimen was received by the pathologist Ⓑ M

G9786 Pathology report diagnosing cutaneous basal cell carcinoma, squamous cell carcinoma, or melanoma (to include in situ disease) was not sent from the pathologist/dermatopathologist to the biopsying clinician for review within 7 days from the time when the tissue specimen was received by the pathologist Ⓑ M

G9787 Patient alive as of the last day of the measurement year Ⓑ M

G9788 Most recent bp is less than or equal to 140/90 mm hg Ⓑ M

G9789 Blood pressure recorded during inpatient stays, emergency room visits, urgent care visits Ⓑ M

G9790 Most recent BP is greater than 140/90 mm hg, or blood pressure not documented Ⓑ M

G9791 Most recent tobacco status is tobacco free Ⓑ M

G9792 Most recent tobacco status is not tobacco free Ⓑ M

G9793 Patient is currently on a daily aspirin or other antiplatelet Ⓑ M

G9794 Documentation of medical reason(s) for not on a daily aspirin or other antiplatelet (e.g., history of gastrointestinal bleed, intra-cranial bleed, idiopathic thrombocytopenic purpura (ITP), gastric bypass or documentation of active anticoagulant use during the measurement period) ⒷM

G9795 Patient is not currently on a daily aspirin or other antiplatelet Ⓑ M

G9796 Patient is currently on a statin therapy Ⓑ M

G9797 Patient is not on a statin therapy Ⓑ M

G9805 Patients who use hospice services any time during the measurement period ⒷM

G9806 Patients who received cervical cytology or an HPV test Ⓑ M

G9807 Patients who did not receive cervical cytology or an HPV test Ⓑ M

G9812 Patient died including all deaths occurring during the hospitalization in which the operation was performed, even if after 30 days, and those deaths occurring after discharge from the hospital, but within 30 days of the procedure Ⓑ M

G9813 Patient did not die within 30 days of the procedure or during the index hospitalization Ⓑ M

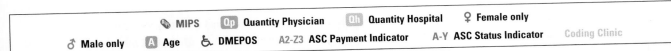

* **G9818** Documentation of sexual activity Ⓑ M

* **G9819** Patients who use hospice services any time during the measurement period ⒷM

* **G9820** Documentation of a chlamydia screening test with proper follow-up ⒷM

* **G9821** No documentation of a chlamydia screening test with proper follow-up ⒷM

* **G9822** Patient who had an endometrial ablation procedure during the year prior to the index date (exclusive of the index date) Ⓑ M

* **G9823** Endometrial sampling or hysteroscopy with biopsy and results documented during the 12 months prior to the index date (exclusive of the index date) of the endometrial ablation Ⓑ M

* **G9824** Endometrial sampling or hysteroscopy with biopsy and results not documented during the 12 months prior to the index date (exclusive of the index date) of the endometrial ablation Ⓑ M

* **G9830** HER-2/neu positive Ⓑ M

* **G9831** AJCC stage at breast cancer diagnosis = II or III Ⓑ M

* **G9832** AJCC stage at breast cancer diagnosis = I (Ia or Ib) and T-stage at breast cancer diagnosis does not equal = T1, T1a, T1b Ⓑ M

* **G9838** Patient has metastatic disease at diagnosis Ⓑ M

* **G9839** Anti-EGFR monoclonal antibody therapy Ⓑ M

* **G9840** Ras (KRas and NRas) gene mutation testing performed before initiation of anti-EGFR MoAb Ⓑ M

* **G9841** Ras (KRas and NRas) gene mutation testing not performed before initiation of anti-EGFR MoAb Ⓑ M

* **G9842** Patient has metastatic disease at diagnosis Ⓑ M

* **G9843** Ras (KRas and NRas) gene mutation Ⓑ M

* **G9844** Patient did not receive anti-EGFR monoclonal antibody therapy Ⓑ M

* **G9845** Patient received anti-EGFR monoclonal antibody therapy Ⓑ M

* **G9846** Patients who died from cancer Ⓑ M

* **G9847** Patient received systemic cancer-directed therapy in the last 14 days of life Ⓑ M

* **G9848** Patient did not receive systemic cancer-directed therapy in the last 14 days of life Ⓑ M

* **G9852** Patients who died from cancer Ⓑ M

* **G9853** Patient admitted to the ICU in the last 30 days of life Ⓑ M

* **G9854** Patient was not admitted to the ICU in the last 30 days of life Ⓑ M

* **G9858** Patient enrolled in hospice Ⓑ M

* **G9859** Patients who died from cancer Ⓑ M

* **G9860** Patient spent less than three days in hospice care Ⓑ M

* **G9861** Patient spent greater than or equal to three days in hospice care Ⓑ M

* **G9862** Documentation of medical reason(s) for not recommending at least a 10 year follow-up interval (e.g., inadequate prep, familial or personal history of colonic polyps, patient had no adenoma and age is = 66 years old, or life expectancy <10 years old, other medical reasons) Ⓑ M

* **G9868** Receipt and analysis of remote, asynchronous images for dermatologic and/or ophthalmologic evaluation, for use only in a medicare-approved cmmi model, less than 10 minutes

* **G9869** Receipt and analysis of remote, asynchronous images for dermatologic and/or ophthalmologic evaluation, for use only in a medicare-approved cmmi model, 10-20 minutes

* **G9870** Receipt and analysis of remote, asynchronous images for dermatologic and/or ophthalmologic evaluation, for use only in a medicare-approved cmmi model, more than 20 minutes

* **G9873** First Medicare diabetes prevention program (MDPP) core session was attended by an MDPP beneficiary under the MDPP expanded model (EM). A core session is an MDPP service that: (1) is furnished by an MDPP supplier during months 1 through 6 of the MDPP services period; (2) is approximately 1 hour in length; and (3) adheres to a CDC-approved DPP curriculum for core sessions. M

* **G9874** Four total Medicare diabetes prevention program (MDPP) core sessions were attended by an MDPP beneficiary under the mdpp expanded model (EM). A core session is an MDPP service that: (1) is furnished by an MDPP supplier during months 1 through 6 of the MDPP services period; (2) is approximately 1 hour in length; and (3) adheres to a CDC-approved DPP curriculum for core sessions. M

▶ New   ↻ Revised   ✔ Reinstated   ~~deleted~~ Deleted   ⊘ Not covered or valid by Medicare

⊙ Special coverage instructions   * Carrier discretion   Ⓑ Bill Part B MAC   Ⓑ Bill DME MAC

* **G9875** Nine total Medicare diabetes prevention program (MDPP) core sessions were attended by an MDPP beneficiary under the MDPP expanded model (EM). A core session is an MDPP service that: (1) is furnished by an MDPP supplier during months 1 through 6 of the MDPP services period; (2) is approximately 1 hour in length; and (3) adheres to a CDC-approved DPP curriculum for core sessions. **M**

* **G9876** Two Medicare diabetes prevention program (MDPP) core maintenance sessions (MS) were attended by an MDPP beneficiary in months (mo) 7-9 under the mdpp expanded model (EM). A core maintenance session is an MDPP service that: (1) is furnished by an MDPP supplier during months 7 through 12 of the MDPP services period; (2) is approximately 1 hour in length; and (3) adheres to a CDC-approved DPP curriculum for maintenance sessions. The beneficiary did not achieve at least 5% weight loss (WL) from his/her baseline weight, as measured by at least one in-person weight measurement at a core maintenance session in months 7-9. **M**

* **G9877** Two Medicare diabetes prevention program (MDPP) core maintenance sessions (MS) were attended by an MDPP beneficiary in months (mo) 10-12 under the MDPP expanded model (EM). A core maintenance session is an MDPP service that: (1) is furnished by an MDPP supplier during months 7 through 12 of the MDPP services period; (2) is approximately 1 hour in length; and (3) adheres to a CDC-approved DPP curriculum for maintenance sessions. The beneficiary did not achieve at least 5% weight loss (WL) from his/her baseline weight, as measured by at least one in-person weight measurement at a core maintenance session in months 10-12. **M**

* **G9878** Two Medicare diabetes prevention program (MDPP) core maintenance sessions (MS) were attended by an MDPP beneficiary in months (mo) 7-9 under the MDPP expanded model (EM). A core maintenance session is an MDPP service that: (1) is furnished by an MDPP supplier during months 7 through 12 of the MDPP services period; (2) is approximately 1 hour in length; and (3) adheres to a CDC-approved DPP curriculum for maintenance sessions. The beneficiary achieved at least 5% weight loss (WL) from his/her baseline weight, as measured by at least one in-person weight measurement at a core maintenance session in months 7-9. **M**

* **G9879** Two Medicare diabetes prevention program (MDPP) core maintenance sessions (MS) were attended by an MDPP beneficiary in months (mo) 10-12 under the MDPP expanded model (EM). A core maintenance session is an MDPP service that: (1) is furnished by an MDPP supplier during months 7 through 12 of the MDPP services period; (2) is approximately 1 hour in length; and (3) adheres to a CDC-approved DPP curriculum for maintenance sessions. The beneficiary achieved at least 5% weight loss (WL) from his/her baseline weight, as measured by at least one in-person weight measurement at a core maintenance session in months 10-12. **M**

* **G9880** The MDPP beneficiary achieved at least 5% weight loss (WL) from his/her baseline weight in months (mo) 1-12 of the MDPP services period under the MDPP expanded model (EM). This is a one-time payment available when a beneficiary first achieves at least 5% weight loss from baseline as measured by an in-person weight measurement at a core session or core maintenance session. **M**

* **G9881** The MDPP beneficiary achieved at least 9% weight loss (WL) from his/her baseline weight in months (mo) 1-24 under the MDPP expanded model (EM). This is a one-time payment available when a beneficiary first achieves at least 9% weight loss from baseline as measured by an in-person weight measurement at a core session, core maintenance session, or ongoing maintenance session. **M**

MIPS Qp Quantity Physician Qh Quantity Hospital ♀ Female only ♂ Male only A Age DMEPOS A2-Z3 ASC Payment Indicator A-Y ASC Status Indicator Coding Clinic

295

✳ **G9882** Two Medicare diabetes prevention program (MDPP) ongoing maintenance sessions (MS) were attended by an MDPP beneficiary in months (mo) 13-15 under the MDPP expanded model (EM). An ongoing maintenance session is an MDPP service that: (1) is furnished by an MDPP supplier during months 13 through 24 of the MDPP services period; (2) is approximately 1 hour in length; and (3) adheres to a CDC-approved DPP curriculum for maintenance sessions. The beneficiary maintained at least 5% weight loss (WL) from his/her baseline weight, as measured by at least one in-person weight measurement at an ongoing maintenance session in months 13-15.   M

✳ **G9883** Two Medicare diabetes prevention program (MDPP) ongoing maintenance sessions (MS) were attended by an MDPP beneficiary in months (mo) 16-18 under the MDPP expanded model (EM). An ongoing maintenance session is an MDPP service that: (1) is furnished by an MDPP supplier during months 13 through 24 of the MDPP services period; (2) is approximately 1 hour in length; and (3) adheres to a CDC-approved DPP curriculum for maintenance sessions. The beneficiary maintained at least 5% weight loss (WL) from his/her baseline weight, as measured by at least one in-person weight measurement at an ongoing maintenance session in months 16-18.   M

✳ **G9884** Two Medicare diabetes prevention program (MDPP) ongoing maintenance sessions (MS) were attended by an MDPP beneficiary in months (mo) 19-21 under the MDPP expanded model (EM). An ongoing maintenance session is an MDPP service that: (1) is furnished by an MDPP supplier during months 13 through 24 of the MDPP services period; (2) is approximately 1 hour in length; and (3) adheres to a CDC-approved DPP curriculum for maintenance sessions. The beneficiary maintained at least 5% weight loss (WL) from his/her baseline weight, as measured by at least one in-person weight measurement at an ongoing maintenance session in months 19-21.   M

✳ **G9885** Two Medicare diabetes prevention program (MDPP) ongoing maintenance sessions (MS) were attended by an MDPP beneficiary in months (mo) 22-24 under the MDPP expanded model (EM). An ongoing maintenance session is an MDPP service that: (1) is furnished by an MDPP supplier during months 13 through 24 of the MDPP services period; (2) is approximately 1 hour in length; and (3) adheres to a CDC-approved DPP curriculum for maintenance sessions. The beneficiary maintained at least 5% weight loss (WL) from his/her baseline weight, as measured by at least one in-person weight measurement at an ongoing maintenance session in months 22-24.   M

NOTE: The following codes do not imply that codes in other sections are necessarily covered.

Quality Measures: Miscellaneous

✳ **G9890** Bridge payment: a one-time payment for the first Medicare diabetes prevention program (MDPP) core session, core maintenance session, or ongoing maintenance session furnished by an MDPP supplier to an MDPP beneficiary during months 1-24 of the MDPP expanded model (EM) who has previously received MDPP services from a different MDPP supplier under the MDPP expanded model. A supplier may only receive one bridge payment per MDPP beneficiary.   M

✳ **G9891** MDPP session reported as a line-item on a claim for a payable MDPP expanded model (EM) HCPCS code for a session furnished by the billing supplier under the MDPP expanded model and counting toward achievement of the attendance performance goal for the payable MDPP expanded model HCPCS code (this code is for reporting purposes only)   M

✳ **G9890** Dilated macular exam performed, including documentation of the presence or absence of macular thickening or geographic atrophy or hemorrhage and the level of macular degeneration severity Ⓑ   M

✳ **G9891** Documentation of medical reason(s) for not performing a dilated macular examination Ⓑ   M

▶ New   ↻ Revised   ✔ Reinstated   ~~deleted~~ Deleted   ⊘ Not covered or valid by Medicare
⊛ Special coverage instructions   ✳ Carrier discretion   Ⓑ Bill Part B MAC   Ⓑ Bill DME MAC

* **G9892** Documentation of patient reason(s) for not performing a dilated macular examination Ⓑ   M

* **G9893** Dilated macular exam was not performed, reason not otherwise specified Ⓑ   M

* **G9894** Androgen deprivation therapy prescribed/administered in combination with external beam radiotherapy to the prostate Ⓑ   M

* **G9895** Documentation of medical reason(s) for not prescribing/administering androgen deprivation therapy in combination with external beam radiotherapy to the prostate (e.g., salvage therapy) Ⓑ   M

* **G9896** Documentation of patient reason(s) for not prescribing/administering androgen deprivation therapy in combination with external beam radiotherapy to the prostate Ⓑ   M

* **G9897** Patients who were not prescribed/administered androgen deprivation therapy in combination with external beam radiotherapy to the prostate, reason not given Ⓑ   M

* **G9898** Patient age 66 or older in institutional special needs plans (SNP) or residing in long-term care with pos code 32, 33, 34, 54, or 56 for more than 90 consecutive days during the measurement period Ⓑ   M

* **G9899** Screening, diagnostic, film, digital or digital breast tomosynthesis (3D) mammography results documented and reviewed Ⓑ   M

* **G9900** Screening, diagnostic, film, digital or digital breast tomosynthesis (3D) mammography results were not documented and reviewed, reason not otherwise specified Ⓑ   M

* **G9901** Patient age 66 or older in institutional special needs plans (SNP) or residing in long-term care with pos code 32, 33, 34, 54, or 56 for more than 90 consecutive days during the measurement period Ⓑ   M

* **G9902** Patient screened for tobacco use and identified as a tobacco user Ⓑ   M

* **G9903** Patient screened for tobacco use and identified as a tobacco non-user Ⓑ   M

* **G9905** Patient not screened for tobacco use Ⓑ   M

* **G9906** Patient identified as a tobacco user received tobacco cessation intervention during the measurement period or in the six months prior to the measurement period (counseling and/or pharmacotherapy) Ⓑ   M

* **G9908** Patient identified as tobacco user did not receive tobacco cessation intervention during the measurement period or in the six months prior to the measurement period (counseling and/or pharmacotherapy) Ⓑ   M

* **G9910** Patients age 66 or older in institutional special needs plans (SNP) or residing in long-term care with pos code 32, 33, 34, 54, or 56 for more than 90 consecutive days during the measurement period Ⓑ   M

* **G9911** Clinically node negative (t1n0m0 or t2n0m0) invasive breast cancer before or after neoadjuvant systemic therapy Ⓑ   M

* **G9912** Hepatitis B virus (HBV) status assessed and results interpreted prior to initiating anti-TNF (tumor necrosis factor) therapy Ⓑ   M

* **G9913** Hepatitis B virus (HBV) status not assessed and results interpreted prior to initiating anti-TNF (tumor necrosis factor) therapy, reason not otherwise specified Ⓑ   M

* **G9914** Patient receiving an anti-TNF agent Ⓑ   M

* **G9915** No record of HBV results documented Ⓑ   M

* **G9916** Functional status performed once in the last 12 months Ⓑ   M

* **G9917** Documentation of advanced stage dementia and caregiver knowledge is limited Ⓑ   M

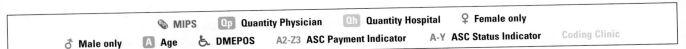

🐌 MIPS   🅠ₚ **Quantity Physician**   🅠ₕ **Quantity Hospital**   ♀ **Female only**

♂ **Male only**   Ⓐ **Age**   ♿ **DMEPOS**   A2-Z3 **ASC Payment Indicator**   A-Y **ASC Status Indicator**   Coding Clinic

* **G9918** Functional status not performed, reason not otherwise specified Ⓑ M

* **G9919** Screening performed and positive and provision of recommendations Ⓑ M

* **G9920** Screening performed and negative Ⓑ M

* **G9921** No screening performed, partial screening performed or positive screen without recommendations and reason is not given or otherwise specified Ⓑ M

* **G9922** Safety concerns screen provided and if positive then documented mitigation recommendations Ⓑ M

* **G9923** Safety concerns screen provided and negative Ⓑ M

* **G9925** Safety concerns screening not provided, reason not otherwise specified Ⓑ M

* **G9926** Safety concerns screening positive screen is without provision of mitigation recommendations, including but not limited to referral to other resources Ⓑ M

* **G9927** Documentation of system reason(s) for not prescribing an FDA-approved anticoagulation due to patient being currently enrolled in a clinical trial related to af/atrial flutter treatment Ⓑ M

* **G9928** FDA-approved anticoagulant not prescribed, reason not given Ⓑ M

* **G9929** Patient with transient or reversible cause of AF (e.g., pneumonia, hyperthyroidism, pregnancy, cardiac surgery) Ⓑ M

* **G9930** Patients who are receiving comfort care only Ⓑ M

* **G9931** Documentation of CHA2DS2-VASc risk score of 0 or 1 for men; or 0, 1, or 2 for women Ⓑ M

* **G9938** Patients age 66 or older in institutional special needs plans (SNP) or residing in long-term care with POS code 32, 33, 34, 54, or 56 for more than 90 consecutive days during the six months prior to the measurement period through December 31 of the measurement period Ⓑ M

* **G9939** Pathologist/dermatopathologist is the same clinician who performed the biopsy Ⓑ M

* **G9940** Documentation of medical reason(s) for not on a statin (e.g., pregnancy, in vitro fertilization, clomiphene rx, ESRD, cirrhosis, muscular pain and disease during the measurement period or prior year) Ⓑ M

* **G9943** Back pain was not measured by the visual analog scale (VAS) or numeric pain scale at three months (6-20 weeks) postoperatively Ⓑ M

* **G9945** Patient had cancer, acute fracture or infection related to the lumbar spine or patient had neuromuscular, idiopathic or congenital lumbar scoliosis Ⓑ M

* **G9946** Back pain was not measured by the visual analog scale (VAS) or numeric pain scale at one year (9 to 15 months) postoperatively Ⓑ M

* **G9949** Leg pain was not measured by the visual analog scale (VAS) or numeric pain scale at three months (6 to 20 weeks) postoperatively Ⓑ M

* **G9954** Patient exhibits 2 or more risk factors for post-operative vomiting Ⓑ M

* **G9955** Cases in which an inhalational anesthetic is used only for induction Ⓑ M

* **G9956** Patient received combination therapy consisting of at least two prophylactic pharmacologic anti-emetic agents of different classes preoperatively and/or intraoperatively Ⓑ M

* **G9957** Documentation of medical reason for not receiving combination therapy consisting of at least two prophylactic pharmacologic anti-emetic agents of different classes preoperatively and/or intraoperatively (e.g., intolerance or other medical reason) Ⓑ M

* **G9958** Patient did not receive combination therapy consisting of at least two prophylactic pharmacologic anti-emetic agents of different classes preoperatively and/or intraoperatively Ⓑ M

▶ **New** ↻ **Revised** ✔ **Reinstated** ~~deleted~~ **Deleted** ⊘ **Not covered or valid by Medicare**
⊛ **Special coverage instructions** ✳ **Carrier discretion** Ⓟ **Bill Part B MAC** Ⓑ **Bill DME MAC**

＊ **G9959** Systemic antimicrobials not prescribed Ⓑ M

＊ **G9960** Documentation of medical reason(s) for prescribing systemic antimicrobials Ⓑ M

＊ **G9961** Systemic antimicrobials prescribed Ⓑ M

＊ **G9962** Embolization endpoints are documented separately for each embolized vessel and ovarian artery angiography or embolization performed in the presence of variant uterine artery anatomy Ⓑ M

＊ **G9963** Embolization endpoints are not documented separately for each embolized vessel or ovarian artery angiography or embolization not performed in the presence of variant uterine artery anatomy Ⓑ M

＊ **G9964** Patient received at least one well-child visit with a PCP during the performance period Ⓑ M

＊ **G9965** Patient did not receive at least one well-child visit with a PCP during the performance period Ⓑ M

＊ **G9968** Patient was referred to another clinician or specialist during the performance period Ⓑ M

＊ **G9969** Clinician who referred the patient to another clinician received a report from the provider to whom the patient was referred Ⓑ M

＊ **G9970** Clinician who referred the patient to another clinician did not receive a report from the provider to whom the patient was referred Ⓑ M

＊ **G9974** Dilated macular exam performed, including documentation of the presence or absence of macular thickening or geographic atrophy or hemorrhage and the level of macular degeneration severity Ⓑ M

＊ **G9975** Documentation of medical reason(s) for not performing a dilated macular examination Ⓑ M

＊ **G9976** Documentation of patient reason(s) for not performing a dilated macular examination Ⓑ M

＊ **G9977** Dilated macular exam was not performed, reason not otherwise specified Ⓑ M

＊ **G9978** Remote in-home visit for the evaluation and management of a new patient for use only in a Medicare-approved bundled payments for care improvement advanced (BCPI advanced) model episode of care, which requires these 3 key components: a problem focused history; a problem focused examination; and straightforward medical decision making, furnished in real time using interactive audio and video technology. Counseling and coordination of care with other physicians, other qualified health care professionals or agencies are provided consistent with the nature of the problem(s) and the needs of the patient or the family or both. Usually, the presenting problem(s) are self limited or minor. Typically, 10 minutes are spent with the patient or family or both via real time, audio and video intercommunications technology. Ⓑ B

＊ **G9979** Remote in-home visit for the evaluation and management of a new patient for use only in a Medicare-approved bundled payments for care improvement advanced (BCPI advanced) model episode of care, which requires these 3 key components: an expanded problem focused history; an expanded problem focused examination; straightforward medical decision making, furnished in real time using interactive audio and video technology. Counseling and coordination of care with other physicians, other qualified health care professionals or agencies are provided consistent with the nature of the problem(s) and the needs of the patient or the family or both. Usually, the presenting problem(s) are of low to moderate severity. Typically, 20 minutes are spent with the patient or family or both via real time, audio and video intercommunications technology. Ⓑ B

MIPS   Qp Quantity Physician   Qh Quantity Hospital   ♀ Female only
♂ Male only   A Age   & DMEPOS   A2-Z3 ASC Payment Indicator   A-Y ASC Status Indicator   Coding Clinic

✳ **G9980** Remote in-home visit for the evaluation and management of a new patient for use only in a Medicare-approved bundled payments for care improvement advanced (BCPI advanced) model episode of care, which requires these 3 key components: a detailed history; a detailed examination; medical decision making of low complexity, furnished in real time using interactive audio and video technology. Counseling and coordination of care with other physicians, other qualified health care professionals or agencies are provided consistent with the nature of the problem(s) and the needs of the patient or the family or both. Usually, the presenting problem(s) are of moderate severity. Typically, 30 minutes are spent with the patient or family or both via real time, audio and video intercommunications technology. Ⓑ **B**

✳ **G9981** Remote in-home visit for the evaluation and management of a new patient for use only in a Medicare-approved bundled payments for care improvement advanced (BCPI advanced) model episode of care, which requires these 3 key components: a comprehensive history; a comprehensive examination; medical decision making of moderate complexity, furnished in real time using interactive audio and video technology. Counseling and coordination of care with other physicians, other qualified health care professionals or agencies are provided consistent with the nature of the problem(s) and the needs of the patient or the family or both. Usually, the presenting problem(s) are of moderate to high severity. Typically, 45 minutes are spent with the patient or family or both via real time, audio and video intercommunications technology. Ⓑ **B**

✳ **G9982** Remote in-home visit for the evaluation and management of a new patient for use only in a Medicare-approved bundled payments for care improvement advanced (BCPI advanced) model episode of care, which requires these 3 key components: a comprehensive history; a comprehensive examination; medical decision making of high complexity, furnished in real time using interactive audio and video technology. Counseling and coordination of care with other physicians, other qualified health care professionals or agencies are provided consistent with the nature of the problem(s) and the needs of the patient or the family or both. Usually, the presenting problem(s) are of moderate to high severity. Typically, 60 minutes are spent with the patient or family or both via real time, audio and video intercommunications technology. Ⓑ **B**

✳ **G9983** Remote in-home visit for the evaluation and management of an established patient for use only in a Medicare-approved bundled payments for care improvement advanced (BCPI advanced) model episode of care, which requires at least 2 of the following 3 key components: a problem focused history; a problem focused examination; straightforward medical decision making, furnished in real time using interactive audio and video technology. Counseling and coordination of care with other physicians, other qualified health care professionals or agencies are provided consistent with the nature of the problem(s) and the needs of the patient or the family or both. Usually, the presenting problem(s) are self limited or minor. Typically, 10 minutes are spent with the patient or family or both via real time, audio and video intercommunications technology. Ⓑ **B**

▶ New   ↻ Revised   ✔ Reinstated   ~~deleted~~ Deleted   ⃠ Not covered or valid by Medicare
❂ Special coverage instructions   ✳ Carrier discretion   Ⓑ Bill Part B MAC   Ⓖ Bill DME MAC

300

✳ **G9984** Remote in-home visit for the evaluation and management of an established patient for use only in a Medicare-approved bundled payments for care improvement advanced (BCPI advanced) model episode of care, which requires at least 2 of the following 3 key components: an expanded problem focused history; an expanded problem focused examination; medical decision making of low complexity, furnished in real time using interactive audio and video technology. Counseling and coordination of care with other physicians, other qualified health care professionals or agencies are provided consistent with the nature of the problem(s) and the needs of the patient or the family or both. Usually, the presenting problem(s) are of low to moderate severity. Typically, 15 minutes are spent with the patient or family or both via real time, audio and video intercommunications technology. Ⓑ B

✳ **G9985** Remote in-home visit for the evaluation and management of an established patient for use only in a Medicare-approved bundled payments for care improvement advanced (BCPI advanced) model episode of care, which requires at least 2 of the following 3 key components: a detailed history; a detailed examination; medical decision making of moderate complexity, furnished in real time using interactive audio and video technology. Counseling and coordination of care with other physicians, other qualified health care professionals or agencies are provided consistent with the nature of the problem(s) and the needs of the patient or the family or both. Usually, the presenting problem(s) are of moderate to high severity. Typically, 25 minutes are spent with the patient or family or both via real time, audio and video intercommunications technology. Ⓑ B

✳ **G9986** Remote in-home visit for the evaluation and management of an established patient for use only in a Medicare-approved bundled payments for care improvement advanced (BCPI advanced) model episode of care, which requires at least 2 of the following 3 key components: a comprehensive history; a comprehensive examination; medical decision making of high complexity, furnished in real time using interactive audio and video technology. Counseling and coordination of care with other physicians, other qualified health care professionals or agencies are provided consistent with the nature of the problem(s) and the needs of the patient or the family or both. Usually, the presenting problem(s) are of moderate to high severity. Typically, 40 minutes are spent with the patient or family or both via real time, audio and video intercommunications technology. Ⓑ B

✳ **G9987** Bundled payments for care improvement advanced (BCPI advanced) model home visit for patient assessment performed by clinical staff for an individual not considered homebound, including, but not necessarily limited to patient assessment of clinical status, safety/fall prevention, functional status/ambulation, medication reconciliation/management, compliance with orders/plan of care, performance of activities of daily living, and ensuring beneficiary connections to community and other services; for use only for a BCPI advanced model episode of care; may not be billed for a 30-day period covered by a transitional care management code. Ⓑ B

✳ **G9988** Palliative care services provided to patient any time during the measurement period M

✳ **G9990** Patient did not receive any pneumococcal conjugate or polysaccharide vaccine on or after their 60th birthday and before the end of the measurement period M

✳ **G9991** Patient received any pneumococcal conjugate or polysaccharide vaccine on or after their 60th birthday and before the end of the measurement period M

✳ **G9992** Palliative care services used by patient any time during the measurement period M

✳ **G9993** Patient was provided palliative care services any time during the measurement period M

✳ **G9994** Patient is using palliative care services any time during the measurement period M

✳ **G9995** Patients who use palliative care services any time during the measurement period M

✳ **G9996** Documentation stating the patient has received or is currently receiving palliative or hospice care M

✳ **G9997** Documentation of patient pregnancy anytime during the measurement period prior to and including the current encounter M

✳ **G9998** Documentation of medical reason(s) for an interval of less than 3 years since the last colonoscopy (e.g., last colonoscopy incomplete, last colonoscopy had inadequate prep, piecemeal removal of adenomas, last colonoscopy found greater than 10 adenomas, or patient at high risk for colon cancer [Crohn's disease, ulcerative colitis, lower gastrointestinal bleeding, personal or family history of colon cancer, hereditary colorectal cancer syndromes]) M

✳ **G9999** Documentation of system reason(s) for an interval of less than 3 years since the last colonoscopy (e.g., unable to locate previous colonoscopy report, previous colonoscopy report was incomplete) M

▶ New   ↻ Revised   ✔ Reinstated   ~~deleted~~ Deleted   ⊘ Not covered or valid by Medicare
⊛ Special coverage instructions   ✳ Carrier discretion   ⑧ Bill Part B MAC   ⑥ Bill DME MAC

BEHAVIORAL HEALTH AND/OR SUBSTANCE ABUSE TREATMENT SERVICES (H0001-H9999)

NOTE: Used by Medicaid state agencies because no national code exists to meet the reporting needs of these agencies.

⊘ **H0001** Alcohol and/or drug assessment

🏷⊘ **H0002** Behavioral health screening to determine eligibility for admission to treatment program

⊘ **H0003** Alcohol and/or drug screening; laboratory analysis of specimens for presence of alcohol and/or drugs

🏷⊘ **H0004** Behavioral health counseling and therapy, per 15 minutes

⊘ **H0005** Alcohol and/or drug services; group counseling by a clinician

⊘ **H0006** Alcohol and/or drug services; case management

⊘ **H0007** Alcohol and/or drug services; crisis intervention (outpatient)

⊘ **H0008** Alcohol and/or drug services; sub-acute detoxification (hospital inpatient)

⊘ **H0009** Alcohol and/or drug services; acute detoxification (hospital inpatient)

⊘ **H0010** Alcohol and/or drug services; sub-acute detoxification (residential addiction program inpatient)

⊘ **H0011** Alcohol and/or drug services; acute detoxification (residential addiction program inpatient)

⊘ **H0012** Alcohol and/or drug services; sub-acute detoxification (residential addiction program outpatient)

⊘ **H0013** Alcohol and/or drug services; acute detoxification (residential addiction program outpatient)

⊘ **H0014** Alcohol and/or drug services; ambulatory detoxification

⊘ **H0015** Alcohol and/or drug services; intensive outpatient (treatment program that operates at least 3 hours/day and at least 3 days/week and is based on an individualized treatment plan), including assessment, counseling; crisis intervention, and activity therapies or education

⊘ **H0016** Alcohol and/or drug services; medical/somatic (medical intervention in ambulatory setting)

⊘ **H0017** Behavioral health; residential (hospital residential treatment program), without room and board, per diem

⊘ **H0018** Behavioral health; short-term residential (non-hospital residential treatment program), without room and board, per diem

⊘ **H0019** Behavioral health; long-term residential (non-medical, non-acute care in a residential treatment program where stay is typically longer than 30 days), without room and board, per diem

⊘ **H0020** Alcohol and/or drug services; methadone administration and/or service (provision of the drug by a licensed program)

⊘ **H0021** Alcohol and/or drug training service (for staff and personnel not employed by providers)

⊘ **H0022** Alcohol and/or drug intervention service (planned facilitation)

⊘ **H0023** Behavioral health outreach service (planned approach to reach a targeted population)

⊘ **H0024** Behavioral health prevention information dissemination service (one-way direct or non-direct contact with service audiences to affect knowledge and attitude)

⊘ **H0025** Behavioral health prevention education service (delivery of services with target population to affect knowledge, attitude and/or behavior)

⊘ **H0026** Alcohol and/or drug prevention process service, community-based (delivery of services to develop skills of impactors)

⊘ **H0027** Alcohol and/or drug prevention environmental service (broad range of external activities geared toward modifying systems in order to mainstream prevention through policy and law)

⊘ **H0028** Alcohol and/or drug prevention problem identification and referral service (e.g., student assistance and employee assistance programs), does not include assessment

⊘ **H0029** Alcohol and/or drug prevention alternatives service (services for populations that exclude alcohol and other drug use, e.g., alcohol-free social events)

⊘ **H0030** Behavioral health hotline service

🏷⊘ **H0031** Mental health assessment, by non-physician

⊘ **H0032** Mental health service plan development by non-physician

⊘ **H0033** Oral medication administration, direct observation

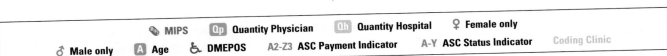

⊘ **H0034** Medication training and support, per 15 minutes

⊘ **H0035** Mental health partial hospitalization, treatment, less than 24 hours

⊘ **H0036** Community psychiatric supportive treatment, face-to-face, per 15 minutes

⊘ **H0037** Community psychiatric supportive treatment program, per diem

⊘ **H0038** Self-help/peer services, per 15 minutes

⊘ **H0039** Assertive community treatment, face-to-face, per 15 minutes

⊘ **H0040** Assertive community treatment program, per diem

⊘ **H0041** Foster care, child, non-therapeutic, per diem **A**

⊘ **H0042** Foster care, child, non-therapeutic, per month **A**

⊘ **H0043** Supported housing, per diem

⊘ **H0044** Supported housing, per month

⊘ **H0045** Respite care services, not in the home, per diem

⊘ **H0046** Mental health services, not otherwise specified

⊘ **H0047** Alcohol and/or other drug abuse services, not otherwise specified

⊘ **H0048** Alcohol and/or other drug testing: collection and handling only, specimens other than blood

⊘ **H0049** Alcohol and/or drug screening

⊘ **H0050** Alcohol and/or drug services, brief intervention, per 15 minutes

⊘ **H1000** Prenatal care, at-risk assessment ♀

⊘ **H1001** Prenatal care, at-risk enhanced service; antepartum management ♀

⊘ **H1002** Prenatal care, at-risk enhanced service; care coordination ♀

⊘ **H1003** Prenatal care, at-risk enhanced service; education ♀

⊘ **H1004** Prenatal care, at-risk enhanced service; follow-up home visit ♀

⊘ **H1005** Prenatal care, at-risk enhanced service package (includes H1001-H1004) ♀

⊘ **H1010** Non-medical family planning education, per session

⊘ **H1011** Family assessment by licensed behavioral health professional for state defined purposes

⊘ **H2000** Comprehensive multidisciplinary evaluation

⊘ **H2001** Rehabilitation program, per 1/2 day

⊘ **H2010** Comprehensive medication services, per 15 minutes

⊘ **H2011** Crisis intervention service, per 15 minutes

⊘ **H2012** Behavioral health day treatment, per hour

⊘ **H2013** Psychiatric health facility service, per diem

⊘ **H2014** Skills training and development, per 15 minutes

⊘ **H2015** Comprehensive community support services, per 15 minutes

⊘ **H2016** Comprehensive community support services, per diem

⊘ **H2017** Psychosocial rehabilitation services, per 15 minutes

⊘ **H2018** Psychosocial rehabilitation services, per diem

⊘ **H2019** Therapeutic behavioral services, per 15 minutes

⊘ **H2020** Therapeutic behavioral services, per diem

⊘ **H2021** Community-based wrap-around services, per 15 minutes

⊘ **H2022** Community-based wrap-around services, per diem

⊘ **H2023** Supported employment, per 15 minutes

⊘ **H2024** Supported employment, per diem

⊘ **H2025** Ongoing support to maintain employment, per 15 minutes

⊘ **H2026** Ongoing support to maintain employment, per diem

⊘ **H2027** Psychoeducational service, per 15 minutes

⊘ **H2028** Sexual offender treatment service, per 15 minutes

⊘ **H2029** Sexual offender treatment service, per diem

⊘ **H2030** Mental health clubhouse services, per 15 minutes

⊘ **H2031** Mental health clubhouse services, per diem

⊘ **H2032** Activity therapy, per 15 minutes

⊘ **H2033** Multisystemic therapy for juveniles, per 15 minutes **A**

⊘ **H2034** Alcohol and/or drug abuse halfway house services, per diem

⊘ **H2035** Alcohol and/or other drug treatment program, per hour

⊘ **H2036** Alcohol and/or other drug treatment program, per diem

⊘ **H2037** Developmental delay prevention activities, dependent child of client, per 15 minutes **A**

▶⊘ **H2040** Coordinated specialty care, team-based, for first episode psychosis, per month

▶⊘ **H2041** Coordinated specialty care, team-based, for first episode psychosis, per encounter

---

▶ **New**   ↻ **Revised**   ✔ **Reinstated**   ~~deleted~~ **Deleted**   ⊘ **Not covered or valid by Medicare**

✿ **Special coverage instructions**   ✳ **Carrier discretion**   Ⓑ **Bill Part B MAC**   Ⓑ **Bill DME MAC**

DRUGS OTHER THAN CHEMOTHERAPY DRUGS
(J0100–J8999)

Injection

⊘ **J0120** Injection, tetracycline, up to
250 mg Ⓑ Ⓑ Qp Qh   N1 N

     Other: Achromycin

     IOM: 100-02, 15, 50

✳ **J0121** Injection, omadacycline, 1 mg   K2 G

✳ **J0122** Injection, eravacycline, 1 mg   K2 K

✳ **J0129** Injection, abatacept, 10 mg (Code
may be used for Medicare when
drug administered under the direct
supervision of a physician, not
for use when drug is
self-administered) Ⓑ Ⓑ Qp Qh   K2 K

     Other: Orencia

⊘ **J0130** Injection, abciximab,
10 mg Ⓑ Ⓑ Qp Qh   N1 N

     Other: ReoPro

     IOM: 100-02, 15, 50

▶ ✳ **J0131** Injection, acetaminophen, not
otherwise specified,
10 mg Ⓑ Ⓑ Qp Qh   N1 N

     Other: Ofirmev, Acetaminophen

     Coding Clinic: 2012, Q1, P9

▶ ✳ **J0132** Injection, acetylcysteine,
100 mg Ⓑ Ⓑ Qp Qh   N1 N

     Other: Acetadote, Acettylcysteine

✳ **J0133** Injection, acyclovir,
5 mg Ⓑ Ⓑ Qp Qh   N1 N

▶ **J0134** Injection, acetaminophen (fresenius
kabi) not therapeutically equivalent to
J0131, 10 mg   N

     Other: Acetaminophen

✳ **J0135** Injection, adalimumab,
20 mg Ⓑ Ⓑ Qp Qh   K2 K

     Other: Humira

     IOM: 100-02, 15, 50

▶ **J0136** Injection, acetaminophen (b braun)
not therapeutically equivalent to J0131,
10 mg   N

     Other: Acetaminophen

▶ **J0137** Injection, acetaminophen (hikma) not
therapeutically equivalent to J0131,
10 mg

⊘ **J0153** Injection, adenosine, 1 mg (not to be
used to report any adenosine phosphate
compounds) Ⓑ Ⓑ Qp Qh   N1 N

     Other: Adenocard, Adenoscan

⊘ **J0171** Injection, adrenalin, epinephrine,
0.1 mg Ⓑ Ⓑ Qp Qh   N1 N

     Other: AUVI-Q, Sus-Phrine

     IOM: 100-02, 15, 50

     Coding Clinic: 2011, Q1, P8

J0172 Injection, aducanumab-avwa, 2 mg   K2 K

▶ **J0173** Injection, epinephrine (belcher) not
therapeutically equivalent to J0171,
0.1 mg   N

     Other: Epinephrine HCl

▶ **J0174** Injection, lecanemab-irmb, 1 mg

✳ **J0178** Injection, aflibercept,
1 mg Ⓑ Ⓑ Qp Qh   K2 K

     Other: Eylea

✳ **J0179** Injection, brolucizumab-dbll,
1 mg   K2 K

✳ **J0180** Injection, agalsidase beta,
1 mg Ⓑ Ⓑ Qp Qh   K2 K

     Other: Fabrazyme

     IOM: 100-02, 15, 50

✳ **J0185** Injection, aprepitant, 1 mg   G

     Other: Emend

⊘ **J0190** Injection, biperiden lactate, per
5 mg Ⓑ Ⓑ Qp Qh   E2

     Other: Akineton

     IOM: 100-02, 15, 50

⊘ **J0200** Injection, alatrofloxacin mesylate,
100 mg Ⓑ Ⓑ Qp Qh   E2

     Other: Trovan

     IOM: 100-02, 15, 50

✳ **J0202** Injection, alemtuzumab,
1 mg Ⓑ Ⓑ Qp Qh   K2 K

     Other: Lemtrada

⊘ **J0205** Injection, alglucerase, per
10 units Ⓑ Ⓑ Qp Qh   E2

     Other: Ceredase

     IOM: 100-02, 15, 50

⊘ **J0207** Injection, amifostine,
500 mg Ⓑ Ⓑ Qp Qh   K2 N

     Other: Ethyol

     IOM: 100-02, 15, 50

▶ **J0208** Injection, sodium thiosulfate, 100 mg

⊘ **J0210** Injection, methyldopate HCL, up to 250 mg Ⓑ Ⓓ Qp Qh   N1 N

Other: Aldomet

IOM: 100-02, 15, 50

✳ **J0215** Injection, alefacept, 0.5 mg Ⓑ Ⓓ Qp Qh   E2

▶ **J0216** Injection, alfentanil hydrochloride, 500 micrograms

▶ **J0218** Injection, olipudase alfa-rpcp, 1 mg

✳ **J0220** Injection, alglucosidase alfa, not otherwise specified, 10 mg Ⓑ Ⓓ Qp Qh   K2 K

Coding Clinic: 2013, Q2, P5; 2012, Q1, P9

✳ **J0221** Injection, alglucosidase alfa, (lumizyme), 10 mg Ⓑ Ⓓ Qp Qh   K2 K

Coding Clinic: 2013, Q2, P5

✳ **J0222** Injection, patisiran, 0.1 mg   K2 K

✳ **J0223** Injection, givosiran, 0.5 mg   K2

▶ ✳ **J0224** Injection, lumasiran, 0.5 mg   K2 G

Other: Oxlumo

▶ **J0225** Injection, vutrisiran, 1 mg   K2 G

Other: Amvuttra

⊘ **J0256** Injection, alpha 1-proteinase inhibitor (human), not otherwise specified, 10 mg Ⓑ Ⓓ Qp Qh   K2 K

Other: ~~Prolastin,~~ Zemaira

IOM: 100-02, 15, 50

Coding Clinic: 2012, Q1, P9

⊘ **J0257** Injection, alpha 1 proteinase inhibitor (human), (glassia), 10 mg Ⓑ Ⓓ Qp Qh   K2 K

IOM: 100-02, 15, 50

Coding Clinic: 2012, Q1, P8

⊘ **J0270** Injection, alprostadil, per 1.25 mcg (Code may be used for Medicare when drug administered under the direct supervision of a physician, not for use when drug is self-administered) Ⓑ Ⓓ Qp Qh   B

Other: Caverject, Prostaglandin E1, Prostin VR Pediatric

IOM: 100-02, 15, 50

⊘ **J0275** Alprostadil urethral suppository (Code may be used for Medicare when drug administered under the direct supervision of a physician, not for use when drug is self-administered) Ⓑ Ⓓ Qp Qh   B

Other: Muse

IOM: 100-02, 15, 50

✳ **J0278** Injection, amikacin sulfate, 100 mg Ⓑ Ⓓ Qp Qh   N1 N

⊘ **J0280** Injection, aminophylline, up to 250 mg Ⓟ Ⓑ Qp Qh   N1 N

IOM: 100-02, 15, 50

⊘ **J0282** Injection, amiodarone hydrochloride, 30 mg Ⓑ Ⓓ Qp Qh   N1 N

Other: Cordarone

IOM: 100-02, 15, 50

J0283 Injection, amiodarone hydrochloride (nexterone), 30 mg   N

⊘ **J0285** Injection, amphotericin B, 50 mg Ⓟ Ⓑ Qp Qh   N1 N

Other: ABLC, Amphocin, Fungizone

IOM: 100-02, 15, 50

⊘ **J0287** Injection, amphotericin B lipid complex, 10 mg Ⓟ Ⓑ Qp Qh   K2 K

Other: ~~Abelcet~~

IOM: 100-02, 15, 50

⊘ **J0288** Injection, amphotericin B cholesteryl sulfate complex, 10 mg Ⓟ Ⓑ Qp Qh   E2

IOM: 100-02, 15, 50

⊘ **J0289** Injection, amphotericin B liposome, 10 mg Ⓟ Ⓑ Qp Qh   K2 K

Other: AmBisome, Amphotericin B Liposome

IOM: 100-02, 15, 50

⊘ **J0290** Injection, ampicillin sodium, 500 mg Ⓟ Ⓑ Qp Qh   N1 N

Other: Omnipen-N, Polycillin-N, Totacillin-N

IOM: 100-02, 15, 50

▶ ✳ **J0291** Injection, plazomicin, 5 mg   K2 K

Other: Zemdri

⊘ **J0295** Injection, ampicillin sodium/sulbactam sodium, per 1.5 gm Ⓑ Ⓓ Qp Qh   N1 N

Other: Omnipen-N, Polycillin-N, Totacillin-N, Unasyn

IOM: 100-02, 15, 50

⊘ **J0300** Injection, amobarbital, up to 125 mg Ⓑ Ⓓ Qp Qh   K2 K

Other: Amytal

IOM: 100-02, 15, 50

⊘ **J0330** Injection, succinylcholine chloride, up to 20 mg Ⓑ Ⓓ Qp Qh   N1 N

Other: Anectine, Quelicin, Surostrin

IOM: 100-02, 15, 50

▶ New   ⟲ Revised   ✔ Reinstated   ~~deleted~~ Deleted   ⊘ Not covered or valid by Medicare
⊘ Special coverage instructions   ✳ Carrier discretion   Ⓟ Bill Part B MAC   Ⓓ Bill DME MAC

* **J0348** Injection, anidulafungin, 1 mg Ⓑ Ⓑ Qp Qh   N1 N

    Other: Eraxis

▶ **J0349** Injection, rezafungin, 1 mg

⊛ **J0350** Injection, anistreplase, per 30 units Ⓑ Ⓑ Qp Qh   E2

    Other: Eminase

    IOM: 100-02, 15, 50

⊛ **J0360** Injection, hydralazine hydrochloride, up to 20 mg Ⓑ Ⓑ Qp Qh   N1 N

    Other: Apresoline

    IOM: 100-02, 15, 50

* **J0364** Injection, apomorphine hydrochloride, 1 mg ⊙ Ⓑ Qp Qh   E2

⊛ **J0365** Injection, aprotinin, 10,000 KIU Ⓑ Ⓑ Qp Qh   E2

    IOM: 100-02, 15, 50

⊛ **J0380** Injection, metaraminol bitartrate, per 10 mg Ⓑ Ⓑ Qp Qh   N1 N

    Other: Aramine

    IOM: 100-02, 15, 50

⊛ **J0390** Injection, chloroquine hydrochloride, up to 250 mg Ⓑ Ⓑ Qp Qh   N1 N

    Benefit only for diagnosed malaria or amebiasis

    Other: Aralen

    IOM: 100-02, 15, 50

⊛ **J0395** Injection, arbutamine HCL, 1 mg Ⓑ Ⓑ Qp Qh   E2

    IOM: 100-02, 15, 50

* **J0400** Injection, aripiprazole, intramuscular, 0.25 mg ⊙ Ⓑ Qp Qh   K2 K

* **J0401** Injection, aripiprazole, extended release, 1 mg Ⓑ Ⓑ Qp Qh   K2 K

    Other: Abilify Maintena

⊛ **J0456** Injection, azithromycin, 500 mg ⊙ Ⓑ Qp Qh   N1 N

    Other: Zithromax

    IOM: 100-02, 15, 50

▶ **J0457** Injection, aztreonam

⊛ **J0461** Injection, atropine sulfate, 0.01 mg ⊙ Ⓑ Qp Qh   N1 N

    IOM: 100-02, 15, 50

⊛ **J0470** Injection, dimercaprol, per 100 mg ⊙ Ⓑ Qp Qh   K2 K

    Other: BAL In Oil

    IOM: 100-02, 15, 50

⊛ **J0475** Injection, baclofen, 10 mg Ⓑ Ⓑ Qp Qh   K2 K

    Other: Gablofen, Lioresal

    IOM: 100-02, 15, 50

⊛ **J0476** Injection, baclofen 50 mcg for intrathecal trial ⊙ Ⓑ Qp Qh   K2 K

    Other: Gablofen, Lioresal

    IOM: 100-02, 15, 50

⊛ **J0480** Injection, basiliximab, 20 mg ⊙ Ⓑ Qp Qh   K2 K

    Other: Simulect

    IOM: 100-02, 15, 50

* **J0485** Injection, belatacept, 1 mg Ⓑ Ⓑ Qp Qh   K2 K

    Other: Nulojix

* **J0490** Injection, belimumab, 10 mg Ⓑ Ⓑ Qp Qh   K2 K

    Other: Benlysta

    Coding Clinic: 2012, Q1, P9

⊛ **J0500** Injection, dicyclomine HCL, up to 20 mg ⊙ Ⓑ Qp Qh   N1 N

    Other: Antispas, Bentyl, Dibent, Dilomine, Di-Spaz, Neoquess, Or-Tyl, Spasmoject

    IOM: 100-02, 15, 50

⊛ **J0515** Injection, benztropine mesylate, per 1 mg ⊙ Ⓑ Qp Qh   N1 N

    Other: Cogentin

    IOM: 100-02, 15, 50

* **J0517** Injection, benralizumab, 1 mg   G

    Other: Fasenra

⊛ **J0520** Injection, bethanechol chloride, myotonachol or urecholine, up to 5 mg Ⓑ Ⓑ Qp Qh   E2

    IOM: 100-02, 15, 50

* **J0558** Injection, penicillin G benzathine and penicillin G procaine,100,000 units Ⓑ Ⓑ Qp Qh   N1 N

    Other: Bicillin C-R

    Coding Clinic: 2011, Q1, P8

⊛ **J0561** Injection, penicillin G benzathine, 100,000 units ⊙ Ⓑ Qp Qh   K2 K

    Other: Bicillin L-A, Permapen

    IOM: 100-02, 15, 50

    Coding Clinic: 2013: Q2, P3; 2011, Q1, P8

* **J0565** Injection, bezlotoxumab, 10 mg   K2 G

* **J0567** Injection, cerliponase alfa, 1 mg   G

    Other: Brineura

---

* **J0570** Buprenorphine implant, 74.2 mg Qp Qh K2 G

    Other: Probuphine System Kit

    Coding Clinic: 2017, Q1, P9

○ **J0571** Buprenorphine, oral, 1 mg Ⓑ Ⓖ Qp Qh E1

○ **J0572** Buprenorphine/naloxone, oral, less than or equal to 3 mg buprenorphine Ⓑ Ⓖ Qp Qh E1

○ **J0573** Buprenorphine/naloxone, oral, greater than 3 mg, but less than or equal to 6 mg buprenorphine Ⓑ Ⓖ Qp Qh E1

○ **J0574** Buprenorphine/naloxone, oral, greater than 6 mg, but less than or equal to 10 mg buprenorphine Ⓑ Ⓖ Qp Qh E1

○ **J0575** Buprenorphine/naloxone, oral, greater than 10 mg buprenorphine Ⓑ Ⓖ Qp Qh E1

* **J0583** Injection, bivalirudin, 1 mg Ⓑ Ⓖ Qp Qh N1 N

    Other: Angiomax

* **J0584** Injection, burosumab-twza 1 mg K

    Other: Crysvita

○ **J0585** Injection, onabotulinumtoxinaA, 1 unit Ⓑ Ⓖ Qp Qh K2 K

    Other: Botox, Botox Cosmetic, Oculinum

    IOM: 100-02, 15, 50

* **J0586** Injection, abobotulinumtoxinaA, 5 units Ⓑ Ⓖ Qp Qh K2 K

○ **J0587** Injection, rimabotulinumtoxinB, 100 units Ⓑ Ⓖ Qp Qh K2 K

    Other: Myobloc, Nplate

    IOM: 100-02, 15, 50

* **J0588** Injection, incobotulinumtoxin A, 1 unit Ⓑ Ⓖ Qp Qh K2 K

    Other: Xeomin

    Coding Clinic: 2012, Q1, P9

* **J0591** Injection, deoxycholic acid, 1 mg E1

○ **J0592** Injection, buprenorphine hydrochloride, 0.1 mg Ⓑ Ⓖ Qp Qh N1 N

    Other: Buprenex

    IOM: 100-02, 15, 50

* **J0593** Injection, lanadelumab-flyo, 1 mg (Code may be used for Medicare when drug administered under direct supervision of a physician, not for use when drug is self-administered) K2 K

* **J0594** Injection, busulfan, 1 mg Ⓑ Ⓖ Qp Qh K2 K

    Other: Myleran

* **J0595** Injection, butorphanol tartrate, 1 mg Ⓑ Ⓖ Qp Qh N1 N

* **J0596** Injection, C1 esterase inhibitor (recombinant), ruconest, 10 units Ⓑ Ⓖ Qp Qh K2 K

* **J0597** Injection, C-1 esterase inhibitor (human), Berinert, 10 units Ⓑ Ⓖ Qp Qh K2 K

    Coding Clinic: 2011, Q1, P7

* **J0598** Injection, C1 esterase inhibitor (human), cinryze, 10 units Ⓑ Ⓖ Qp Qh K2 K

* **J0599** Injection, c-1 esterase inhibitor (human), (haegarda), 10 units E2

    Other: Berinert

○ **J0600** Injection, edetate calcium disodium, up to 1000 mg Ⓑ Ⓖ Qp Qh K2 K

    Other: Calcium Disodium Versenate

    IOM: 100-02, 15, 50

○ **J0604** Cinacalcet, oral, 1 mg, (for ESRD on dialysis) B

○ **J0606** Injection, etelcalcetide, 0.1 mg K2 K

 ~~J0610~~ ~~Injection, calcium gluconate (fresenius kabi), per 10 ml~~ ~~N1 N~~

    ~~*Other: Kaleinate*~~

    ~~*IOM: 100-02, 15, 50*~~

 ~~J0611~~ ~~Injection, calcium gluconate (wg critical care), per 10 ml~~ ~~N~~

▶ **J0612** Injection, calcium gluconate (fresenius kabi), per 10 mg

▶ **J0613** Injection, calcium gluconate (wg critical care), per 10 mg

○ **J0620** Injection, calcium glycerophosphate and calcium lactate, per 10 ml Ⓑ Ⓖ Qp Qh N1 N

    Other: Calphosan

    MCM: 2049

    IOM: 100-02, 15, 50

○ **J0630** Injection, calcitonin (salmon), up to 400 units Ⓑ Ⓖ Qp Qh K2 K

    Other: Calcimar, Calcitonin-salmon, Miacalcin

    IOM: 100-02, 15, 50

○ **J0636** Injection, calcitriol, 0.1 mcg Ⓑ Ⓖ Qp Qh N1 N

    Non-dialysis use

    Other: Calcijex

    IOM: 100-02, 15, 50

* **J0637** Injection, caspofungin acetate, 5 mg Ⓑ Ⓖ Qp Qh K2 K

    Other: Cancidas, Caspofungin

▶ New ↻ Revised ✔ Reinstated ~~deleted~~ Deleted ⊘ Not covered or valid by Medicare
○ Special coverage instructions * Carrier discretion Ⓑ Bill Part B MAC Ⓖ Bill DME MAC

* **J0638** Injection, canakinumab, 1 mg Ⓑ Ⓒ Ⓠp Ⓠh   K2 K

Other: *Ilaris*

⊙ **J0640** Injection, leucovorin, calcium, per 50 mg Ⓑ Ⓒ Ⓠp Ⓠh   N1 N

Other: *Wellcovorin*

IOM: *100-02, 15, 50*

Coding Clinic: 2009, Q1, P10

⊙ **J0641** Injection, levoleucovorin, not otherwise specified, 0.5 mg Ⓑ Ⓒ Ⓠp Ⓠh   K2 K

Part of treatment regimen for osteosarcoma

▶ **J0665** Injection, bupivicaine, not otherwise specified, 0.5 mg

* **J0642** Injection, levoleucovorin, (khapzory), 0.5 mg   K2 G

⊙ **J0670** Injection, mepivacaine HCL, per 10 ml Ⓑ Ⓒ Ⓠp Ⓠh   N1 N

Other: *Carbocaine, Isocaine HCl, Polocaine*

IOM: *100-02, 15, 50*

J0689 Injection, cefazolin sodium (baxter), not therapeutically equivalent to J0690, 500 mg   N

⊙ **J0690** Injection, cefezolin sodium, 500 mg Ⓑ Ⓒ Ⓠp Ⓠh   N1 N

Other: *Ancef, Kefzol, Zolicef*

IOM: *100-02, 15, 50*

* **J0691** Injection, lefamulin, 1 mg   K2 N

* **J0692** Injection, cefepime ~~HCL,~~ 500 mg Ⓑ Ⓒ Ⓠp Ⓠh   N1 N

Other: *Maxipime*

⊙ **J0694** Injection, cefoxitin sodium, 1 gm Ⓑ Ⓒ Ⓠp Ⓠh   N1 N

Other: *Mefoxin*

IOM: *100-02, 15, 50,*

Cross Reference Q0090

* **J0695** Injection, ceftolozane 50 mg and tazobactam25 mg Ⓑ Ⓒ Ⓠp Ⓠh   K2 K

Other: *Zerbaxa*

⊙ **J0696** Injection, ceftriaxone sodium, per 250 mg Ⓑ Ⓒ Ⓠp Ⓠh   N1 N

Other: *Rocephin*

IOM: *100-02, 15, 50*

⊙ **J0697** Injection, sterile cefuroxime sodium, per 750 mg Ⓑ Ⓒ Ⓠp Ⓠh   N1 N

Other: *Kefurox, Zinacef*

IOM: *100-02, 15, 50*

⊙ **J0698** Injection, cefotaxime sodium, per gm Ⓑ Ⓒ Ⓠp Ⓠh   N1 N

Other: *Claforan*

IOM: *100-02, 15, 50*

⊙ **J0699** Injection, cefiderocol, 10 mg   G

J0701 Injection, cefepime hydrochloride (baxter), not therapeutically equivalent to maxipime, 500 mg   N

⊙ **J0702** Injection, betamethasone acetate 3 mg and betamethasone sodium phosphate 3 mg Ⓑ Ⓒ Ⓠp Ⓠh   N1 N

Other: *Betameth, Celestone Soluspan, Selestoject*

IOM: *100-02, 15, 50*

Coding Clinic: 2018, Q4, P6

J0703 Injection, cefepime hydrochloride (b braun), not therapeutically equivalent to maxipime, 500 mg   N

* **J0706** Injection, caffeine citrate, 5 mg Ⓑ Ⓒ Ⓠp Ⓠh   N1 N

Other: *Cafcit, Cipro IV, Ciprofloxacin*

⊙ **J0710** Injection, cephapirin sodium, up to 1 gm Ⓑ Ⓒ Ⓠp Ⓠh   E2

Other: *Cefadyl*

IOM: *100-02, 15, 50*

* **J0712** Injection, ceftaroline fosamil, 10 mg Ⓑ Ⓒ Ⓠp Ⓠh   K2 K

Other: *Teflaro*

Coding Clinic: 2012, Q1, P9

⊙ **J0713** Injection, ceftazidime, per 500 mg Ⓑ Ⓒ Ⓠp Ⓠh   N1 N

Other: *Fortaz, Tazicef*

IOM: *100-02, 15, 50*

* **J0714** Injection, ceftazidime and avibactam, 0.5 g/0.125 g Ⓑ Ⓒ Ⓠp Ⓠh   K2 K

⊙ **J0715** Injection, ceftizoxime sodium, per 500 mg Ⓑ Ⓒ Ⓠp Ⓠh   N1 N

IOM: *100-02, 15, 50*

* **J0716** Injection, centruroides immune F(ab)2, up to 120 milligrams Ⓑ Ⓒ Ⓠp Ⓠh K2 K

Other: *Anascorp*

* **J0717** Injection, certolizumab pegol, 1 mg (Code may be used for Medicare when drug administered under the direct supervision of a physician, not for use when drug is self-administered) Ⓑ Ⓒ Ⓠp Ⓠh   K2 K

Other: *Cimzia*

○ **J0720** Injection, chloramphenicol sodium succinate, up to 1 gm Ⓑ Ⓑ Qp Qh   N1 N

Other: Chloromycetin Sodium Succinate

IOM: 100-02, 15, 50

○ **J0725** Injection, chorionic gonadotropin, per 1,000 USP units Ⓑ Ⓑ Qp Qh   N1 N

Other: A.P.L., Chorex-5, Chorex-10, Chorignon, Choron-10, Chorionic Gonadotropin, Choron 10, Corgonject-5, Follutein, Glukor, Gonic, Novarel, Pregnyl, Profasi HP

IOM: 100-02, 15, 50

○ **J0735** Injection, clonidine hydrochloride (HCL), 1 mg Ⓑ Ⓑ Qp Qh   N1 N

Other: Duraclon

IOM: 100-02, 15, 50

▶ **J0736** Injection, clindamycin phosphate, 300 mg

▶ **J0737** Injection, clindamycin phosphate (baxter), not therapeutically equivalent to J0736, 300 mg

J0739 Injection, cabotegravir, 1 mg   E1

○ **J0740** Injection, cidofovir, 375 mg Ⓑ Ⓑ Qp Qh   K2 K

Other: Vistide

IOM: 100-02, 15, 50

○ **J0741** Injection, cabotegravir and rilpivirine, 2mg/3mg   K2 G

○ **J0742** Injection, imipenem 4 mg, cilastatin 4 mg and relebactam 2 mg   K2 G

○ **J0743** Injection, cilastatin sodium; imipenem, per 250 mg Ⓑ Ⓑ Qp Qh   N1 N

Other: Primaxin

IOM: 100-02, 15, 50

✳ **J0744** Injection, ciprofloxacin for intravenous infusion, 200 mg Ⓑ Ⓑ Qp Qh   N1 N

○ **J0745** Injection, codeine phosphate, per 30 mg Ⓑ Ⓑ Qp Qh   N1 N

IOM: 100-02, 15, 50

○ **J0770** Injection, colistimethate sodium, up to 150 mg Ⓑ Ⓑ Qp Qh   N1 N

Other: Coly-Mycin M

IOM: 100-02, 15, 50

✳ **J0775** Injection, collagenase, clostridium histolyticum, 0.01 mg Ⓑ Ⓑ Qp Qh   K2 K

Other: Xiaflex

Coding Clinic: 2011, Q1, P7

○ **J0780** Injection, prochlorperazine, up to 10 mg Ⓑ Ⓑ Qp Qh   N1 N

Other: Compa-Z, Compazine, Cotranzine, Ultrazine-10

IOM: 100-02, 15, 50

○ **J0791** Injection, crizanlizumab-tmca, 5 mg   K2 G

○ **J0795** Injection, corticorelin ovine triflutate, 1 mcg Ⓑ Ⓑ Qp Qh   K2 K

Other: Acthrel

IOM: 100-02, 15, 50

~~J0800~~ ~~Injection, corticotropin, up to 40 units~~   ~~K2 K~~

~~*Other: ACTH, Acthar*~~

~~*IOM: 100-02, 15, 50*~~

▶ ○ **J0801** Injection, corticotropin (acthar gel), up to 40 units   K2 K

▶ ○ **J0802** Injection, corticotropin (ani), up to 40 units   K2 K

✳ **J0834** Injection, cosyntropin, 0.25 mg Ⓑ Ⓑ Qp Qh   N1 N

✳ **J0840** Injection, crotalidae polyvalent immune fab (ovine), up to 1 gram Ⓑ Ⓑ Qp Qh   K2 K

Other: Crofab

Coding Clinic: 2012, Q1, P9

✳ **J0841** Injection, crotalidae immune f(ab')2 (equine), 120 mg   K

Other: Anavip

○ **J0850** Injection, cytomegalovirus immune globulin intravenous (human), per vial Ⓑ Ⓑ Qp Qh   K2 K

Prophylaxis to prevent cytomegalovirus disease associated with transplantation of kidney, lung, liver, pancreas, and heart.

Other: Cytogam

IOM: 100-02, 15, 50

▶ **J0874** Injection, daptomycin (baxter), not therapeutically equivalent to J0878, 1 mg

✳ **J0875** Injection, dalbavancin, 5 mg Ⓑ Ⓑ Qp Qh   K2 K

Other: Dalvance

J0877 Injection, daptomycin (hospira), not therapeutically equivalent to J0878, 1 mg   N

✳ **J0878** Injection, daptomycin, 1 mg Ⓑ Ⓑ Qp Qh   K2 K

Other: Cubicin

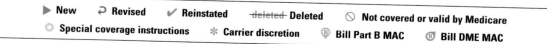

▶ New   ↻ Revised   ✔ Reinstated   ~~deleted~~ Deleted   ⊘ Not covered or valid by Medicare
○ Special coverage instructions   ✳ Carrier discretion   Ⓑ Bill Part B MAC   Ⓑ Bill DME MAC

⊘ **J0881** Injection, darbepoetin alfa, 1 mcg (non-ESRD use) Ⓑ Ⓑ Ⓠⁱ Ⓠⁱ K2 K

Other: Aranesp

⊘ **J0882** Injection, darbepoetin alfa, 1 mcg (for ESRD on dialysis) Ⓑ Ⓑ Ⓠⁱ Ⓠⁱ K2 K

Other: Aranesp

IOM: 100-02, 6, 10; 100-04, 4, 240

⊘ **J0883** Injection, argatroban, 1 mg (for non-ESRD use) Ⓠⁱ Ⓠⁱ K2 K

IOM: 100-02, 15, 50

⊘ **J0884** Injection, argatroban, 1 mg (for ESRD on dialysis) Ⓠⁱ Ⓠⁱ K2 K

IOM: 100-02, 15, 50

⊘ **J0885** Injection, epoetin alfa, (for non-ESRD use), 1000 units Ⓑ Ⓑ Ⓠⁱ Ⓠⁱ K2 K

Other: Epogen, Procrit

IOM: 100-02, 15, 50

Coding Clinic: 2006, Q2, P5

⊘ **J0887** Injection, epoetin beta, 1 mcg, (for ESRD on dialysis) Ⓑ Ⓑ Ⓠⁱ Ⓠⁱ N1 N

Other: Mircera

⊘ **J0888** Injection, epoetin beta, 1 mcg, (for non-ESRD use) Ⓑ Ⓑ Ⓠⁱ Ⓠⁱ K2 K

Other: Mircera

▶ **J0889** Daprodustat, oral, 1 mg, (for ESRD on dialysis)

✳ **J0890** Injection, peginesatide, 0.1 mg (for ESRD on dialysis) Ⓑ Ⓑ Ⓠⁱ Ⓠⁱ E1

Other: Omontys

J0891 Injection, argatroban (accord), not therapeutically equivalent to J0883, 1 mg (for non-ESRD use) K2 K

J0892 Injection, argatroban (accord), not therapeutically equivalent to J0884, 1 mg (for ESRD on dialysis) K2 K

J0893 Injection, decitabine (sun pharma) not therapeutically equivalent to J0894, 1 mg N

✳ **J0894** Injection, decitabine, 1 mg Ⓑ Ⓑ Ⓠⁱ Ⓠⁱ K2 N

Indicated for treatment of myelodysplastic syndromes (MDS)

Other: Dacogen

⊘ **J0895** Injection, deferoxamine mesylate, 500 mg Ⓑ Ⓑ Ⓠⁱ Ⓠⁱ N1 N

Other: Desferal, Desferal mesylate

IOM: 100-02, 15, 50,

Cross Reference Q0087

⊘ **J0896** Injection, luspatercept-aamt, 0.25 mg K2 G

✳ **J0897** Injection, denosumab, 1 mg Ⓥ Ⓑ Ⓑ Ⓠⁱ Ⓠⁱ K2 K

Other: Prolia, Xgeva

Coding Clinic: 2016, Q1, P5; 2012, Q1, P9

J0898 Injection, argatroban (auromedics), not therapeutically equivalent to J0883, 1 mg (for non-ESRD use) K2 K

J0899 Injection, argatroban (auromedics), not therapeutically equivalent to J0884, 1 mg (for ESRD on dialysis) K2 K

⊘ **J0945** Injection, brompheniramine maleate, per 10 mg Ⓑ Ⓥ Ⓑ Ⓠⁱ Ⓠⁱ N1 E2

Other: Codimal-A, Cophene-B, Dehist, Histaject, Nasahist B, ND Stat, Oraminic II, Sinusol-B

IOM: 100-02, 15, 50

⊘ **J1000** Injection, depo-estradiol cypionate, up to 5 mg Ⓑ Ⓑ Ⓠⁱ Ⓠⁱ N1 N

Other: DepGynogen, Depogen, Dura-Estrin, Estra-D, Estro-Cyp, Estroject LA, Estronol-LA

IOM: 100-02, 15, 50

⊘ **J1020** Injection, methylprednisolone acetate, 20 mg Ⓥ Ⓑ Ⓑ Ⓠⁱ Ⓠⁱ N1 N

Other: DepMedalone, Depoject, Depo-Medrol, Depopred, D-Med 80, Duralone, Medralone, M-Prednisol, Rep-Pred

IOM: 100-02, 15, 50

Coding Clinic: 2019, Q3, P14; 2018, Q4, P5-6; 2005, Q3, P10

⊘ **J1030** Injection, methylprednisolone acetate, 40 mg Ⓥ Ⓑ Ⓑ Ⓠⁱ Ⓠⁱ N1 N

Other: DepMedalone, Depoject, Depo-Medrol, Depropred, D-Med 80, Duralone, Medralone, M-Prednisol, Rep-Pred

IOM: 100-02, 15, 50

Coding Clinic: 2022, Q4, P15; 2019, Q3, P14; 2018, Q4, P6; 2005, Q3, P10

⊘ **J1040** Injection, methylprednisolone acetate, 80 mg Ⓥ Ⓑ Ⓑ Ⓠⁱ Ⓠⁱ N1 N

Other: DepMedalone, Depoject, Depo-Medrol, Depropred, D-Med 80, Duralone, Medralone, M-Prednisol, Rep-Pred

IOM: 100-02, 15, 50

Coding Clinic: 2018, Q4, P6

✳ **J1050** Injection, medroxyprogesterone acetate, 1 mg Ⓥ Ⓑ Ⓑ Ⓠⁱ Ⓠⁱ N1 N

Other: Depo-Provera Contraceptive

🏷 MIPS   Ⓠⁱ **Quantity Physician**   Ⓠⁱ **Quantity Hospital**   ♀ **Female only**

♂ **Male only**   Ⓐ **Age**   ♿ **DMEPOS**   A2-Z3 **ASC Payment Indicator**   A-Y **ASC Status Indicator**   Coding Clinic

⊘ **J1071** Injection, testosterone cypionate, 1 mg Qp Qh   N1 N

Other: Andro-Cyp, Andro/Fem, Andronaq-LA, Andronate, De-Comberol, DepAndro, DepAndrogyn, Depotest, Depo-Testadiol, Depo-Testosterone, Depotestrogen, Duratest, Duratestrin, Menoject LA, Testa-C, Testadiate-Depo, Testaject-LA, Test-Estro Cypionates, Testoject-LA

Coding Clinic: 2015, Q2, P7

⊘ **J1094** Injection, dexamethasone acetate, 1 mg Ⓑ Ⓓ Qp Qh   N1 N

Other: Dalalone LA, Decadron LA, Decaject LA, Dexacen-LA-8, Dexasone L.A., Dexone-LA, Solurex LA

IOM: 100-02, 15, 50

⊘ **J1095** Injection, dexamethasone 9% Ⓑ   N

✱ **J1096** Dexamethasone, lacrimal ophthalmic insert, 0.1 mg Ⓓ   K2 N

✱ **J1097** Phenylephrine 10.16 mg/ml and ketorolac 2.88 mg/ml ophthalmic irrigation solution, 1 ml Ⓑ   K2 G

⊘ **J1100** Injection, dexamethasone sodium phosphate, 1 mg Ⓟ Ⓑ Qp Qh   N1 N

Other: Dalalone, Decadron Phosphate, Decaject, Dexacen-4, Dexone, Hexadrol Phosphate, Solurex

IOM: 100-02, 15, 50

⊘ **J1110** Injection, dihydroergotamine mesylate, per 1 mg Ⓑ Ⓓ Qp Qh   K2 K

Other: D.H.E. 45

IOM: 100-02, 15, 50

⊘ **J1120** Injection, acetazolamide sodium, up to 500 mg Ⓟ Ⓑ Qp Qh   N1 N

Other: Diamox

IOM: 100-02, 15, 50

✱ **J1130** Injection, diclofenac sodium, 0.5 mg Qp Qh   K2 K

Coding Clinic: 2017, Q1, P9

⊘ **J1160** Injection, digoxin, up to 0.5 mg Ⓑ Ⓓ Qp Qh   N1 N

Other: Lanoxin

IOM: 100-02, 15, 50

⊘ **J1162** Injection, digoxin immune Fab (ovine), per vial Ⓟ Ⓓ Qp Qh   K2 K

Other: DigiFab

IOM: 100-02, 15, 50

⊘ **J1165** Injection, phenytoin sodium, per 50 mg Ⓑ Ⓓ Qp Qh   N1 N

Other: Dilantin

IOM: 100-02, 15, 50

⊘ **J1170** Injection, hydromorphone, up to 4 mg Ⓟ Ⓑ Qp Qh   N1 N

Other: Dilaudid

IOM: 100-02, 15, 50

⊘ **J1180** Injection, dyphylline, up to 500 mg Ⓑ Ⓓ Qp Qh   E2

Other: Dilor, Lufyllin

IOM: 100-02, 15, 50

⊘ **J1190** Injection, dexrazoxane hydrochloride, per 250 mg Ⓑ Ⓓ Qp Qh   K2 K

Other: Totect, Zinecard

IOM: 100-02, 15, 50

⊘ **J1200** Injection, diphenhydramine HCL, up to 50 mg Ⓑ Ⓓ Qp Qh   N1 N

Other: Bena-D, Benadryl, Benahist, Ben-Allergin, Benoject, Chlorothiazide sodium, Dihydrex, Diphenacen-50, Hyrexin-50, Nordryl, Wehdryl

IOM: 100-02, 15, 50

⊘ **J1201** Injection, cetirizine hydrochloride, 0.5 mg   K2 G

⊘ **J1205** Injection, chlorothiazide sodium, per 500 mg Ⓟ Ⓑ Qp Qh   N1 N

Other: Diuril

IOM: 100-02, 15, 50

⊘ **J1212** Injection, DMSO, dimethyl sulfoxide, 50%, 50 ml Ⓟ Ⓑ Qp Qh   K2 K

Other: Rimso-50

IOM: 100-02, 15, 50; 100-03, 4, 230.12

⊘ **J1230** Injection, methadone HCL, up to 10 mg Ⓑ Ⓓ Qp Qh   N1 N

Other: Dolophine HCl

MCM: 2049

IOM: 100-02, 15, 50

⊘ **J1240** Injection, dimenhydrinate, up to 50 mg Ⓑ Ⓓ Qp Qh   N1 N

Other: Dinate, Dommanate, Dramamine, Dramanate, Dramilin, Dramocen, Dramoject, Dymenate, Hydrate, Marmine, Wehamine

IOM: 100-02, 15, 50

⊘ **J1245** Injection, dipyridamole, per 10 mg Ⓑ Ⓓ Qp Qh   N1 N

Other: Persantine

IOM: 100-04, 15, 50; 100-04, 12, 30.6

⊘ **J1250** Injection, dobutamine HCL, per 250 mg Ⓑ Ⓓ Qp Qh   N1 N

Other: Dobutrex

IOM: 100-02, 15, 50

▶ **New** ↻ **Revised** ✔ **Reinstated** ~~deleted~~ **Deleted** ⊘ **Not covered or valid by Medicare**
⊘ **Special coverage instructions** ✱ **Carrier discretion** Ⓑ **Bill Part B MAC** Ⓓ **Bill DME MAC**

⊘ **J1260** Injection, dolasetron mesylate, 10 mg ⑧ ⑥ **Qp** **Qh**   N1 N

   Other: Anzemet

   IOM: 100-02, 15, 50

✳ **J1265** Injection, dopamine HCL, 40 mg ⑧ ⑥ **Qp** **Qh**   N1 N

✳ **J1267** Injection, doripenem, 10 mg ⑧ ⑥ **Qp** **Qh**   N1 E2

   Other: Donbax, Doribax

✳ **J1270** Injection, doxercalciferol, 1 mcg ⑧ ⑥ **Qp** **Qh**   N1 N

   Other: Hectorol

✳ **J1290** Injection, ecallantide, 1 mg ⑧ ⑥ **Qp** **Qh**   K2 K

   Other: Kalbitor

   Coding Clinic: 2011, Q1, P7

✳ **J1300** Injection, eculizumab, 10 mg ⑧ ⑥ **Qp** **Qh**   K2 K

   Other: Soliris

✳ **J1301** Injection, edaravone, 1 mg ⑧   G

   Other: Radicava

J1302 Injection, sutimlimab-jome, 10 mg K2 G

✳ **J1303** Injection, ravulizumab-cwvz, 10 mg   K2 K

✳ **J1305** Injection, evinacumab-dgnb, 5mg K2 G

J1306 Injection, inclisiran, 1 mg   K2 G

⊘ **J1320** Injection, amitriptyline HCL, up to 20 mg ⑧ ⑥ **Qp** **Qh**   N1 N

   Other: Elavil, Enovil

   IOM: 100-02, 15, 50

✳ **J1322** Injection, elosulfase alfa, 1 mg ⑧ ⑥ **Qp** **Qh**   K2 K

✳ **J1324** Injection, enfuvirtide, 1 mg ⑧ ⑥ **Qp** **Qh**   E2

⊘ **J1325** Injection, epoprostenol, 0.5 mg ⑧ ⑥ **Qp** **Qh**   N1 N

   Other: Flolan, Veletri

   IOM: 100-02, 15, 50

⊘ **J1327** Injection, eptifibatide, 5 mg ⑧ ⑥ **Qp** **Qh**   K2 N

   Other: Integrilin

   IOM: 100-02, 15, 50

⊘ **J1330** Injection, ergonovine maleate, up to 0.2 mg ⑧ ⑥ **Qp** **Qh**   N1 N

   Benefit limited to obstetrical diagnosis

   IOM: 100-02, 15, 50

✳ **J1335** Injection, ertapenem sodium, 500 mg ⑧ ⑥ **Qp** **Qh**   N1 N

   Other: Invanz

⊘ **J1364** Injection, erythromycin lactobionate, per 500 mg ⑧ ⑥ **Qp** **Qh**   K2 K

   IOM: 100-02, 15, 50

⊘ **J1380** Injection, estradiol valerate, up to 10 mg ⑧ ⑥ **Qp** **Qh**   N1 N

   Other: Delestrogen, Dioval, Duragen, Estra-L, Gynogen L.A., L.A.E. 20, Valergen

   IOM: 100-02, 15, 50

   Coding Clinic: 2011, Q1, P8

⊘ **J1410** Injection, estrogen conjugated, per 25 mg ♀ ⑧ ⑥ **Qp** **Qh**   K2 K

   Other: Premarin

   IOM: 100-02, 15, 50

▶ **J1411** Injection, etranacogene dezaparvovec-drlb, per therapeutic dose

✳ **J1426** Injection, casimersen, 10 mg   K2 G

✳ **J1427** Injection, viltolarsen, 10 mg   K2 G

✳ **J1428** Injection, eteplirsen, 10 mg   K2 G

✳ **J1429** Injection, golodirsen, 10 mg   K2 G

⊘ **J1430** Injection, ethanolamine oleate, 100 mg ⑧ ⑥ **Qp** **Qh**   K2 K

   Other: Ethamolin

   IOM: 100-02, 15, 50

⊘ **J1435** Injection, estrone, per 1 mg ⑧ ⑥ **Qp** **Qh**   E2

   Other: Estronol, Kestrone 5, Theelin Aqueous

   IOM: 100-02, 15, 50

⊘ **J1436** Injection, etidronate disodium, per 300 mg ⑧ ⑥ **Qp** **Qh**   E1

   Other: Didronel

   IOM: 100-02, 15, 50

⊘ **J1437** Injection, ferric derisomaltose, 10 mg   K2 G

⊘ **J1438** Injection, etanercept, 25 mg (Code may be used for Medicare when drug administered under the direct supervision of a physician, not for use when drug is self-administered) ♀ ⑧ ⑥ **Qp** **Qh**   K2 K

   Other: Enbrel

   IOM: 100-02, 15, 50

✳ **J1439** Injection, ferric carboxymaltose, 1 mg ⑧ ⑥ **Qp** **Qh**   K2 K

   Other: Injectafer

▶ **J1440** Fecal microbiota, live - jslm, 1 ml

⊘ **J1442** Injection, filgrastim (G-CSF), excludes biosimilars, 1 mcg ⑧ ⑥ **Qp** **Qh**   K2 K

   Other: Neupogen

✳ **J1443** Injection, ferric pyrophosphate citrate solution (triferic), 0.1 mg of iron ⑧ ⑥ **Qp** **Qh**   N1 N

🐾 **MIPS**   **Qp** **Quantity Physician**   **Qh** **Quantity Hospital**   ♀ **Female only**

♂ **Male only**   **A** **Age**   ♿ **DMEPOS**   **A2-Z3** **ASC Payment Indicator**   **A-Y** **ASC Status Indicator**   Coding Clinic

⊛ **J1444** Injection, ferric pyrophosphate citrate powder, 0.1 mg of iron ⬤ N

⊛ **J1445** Injection, ferric pyrophosphate citrate solution (triferic avnu), 0.1 mg of iron ⬤ K2 E2

⊛ **J1447** Injection, TBO-filgrastim, 1 mcg Ⓑ Ⓑ Qp Qh K2 K

Other: GRANIX

IOM: 100-02, 15, 50

⊛ **J1448** Injection, trilaciclib, 1mg K2 G

▶ **J1449** Injection, eflapegrastim-xnst, 0.1 mg

⊛ **J1450** Injection, fluconazole, 200 mg Ⓑ Ⓑ Qp Qh N1 N

Other: Diflucan

IOM: 100-02, 15, 50

⊛ **J1451** Injection, fomepizole, 15 mg Ⓑ Ⓑ Qp Qh K2 K

IOM: 100-02, 15, 50

⊛ **J1452** Injection, fomivirsen sodium, intraocular, 1.65 mg Ⓑ Ⓑ Qp Qh E2

IOM: 100-02, 15, 50

⁕ **J1453** Injection, fosaprepitant, 1 mg Ⓑ Ⓑ Qp Qh K2 K

Prevents chemotherapy-induced nausea and vomiting

Other: Emend

⁕ **J1454** Injection, fosnetupitant 235 mg and palonosetron 0.25 mg Ⓑ Ⓑ G

Other: Akynzeo and Aloxi

⊛ **J1455** Injection, foscarnet sodium, per 1000 mg Ⓑ Ⓑ Qp Qh K2 K

Other: Foscavir

IOM: 100-02, 15, 50

J1456 Injection, fosaprepitant (teva), not therapeutically equivalent to J1453, 1 mg N

⁕ **J1457** Injection, gallium nitrate, 1 mg Ⓑ Ⓑ Qp Qh E2

⁕ **J1458** Injection, galsulfase, 1 mg Ⓑ Ⓑ Qp Qh K2 K

Other: Naglazyme

⁕ **J1459** Injection, immune globulin (Privigen), intravenous, non-lyophilized (e.g., liquid), 500 mg Ⓑ Ⓑ Qp Qh K2 K

⊛ **J1460** Injection, gamma globulin, intramuscular, 1 cc Ⓑ Ⓑ Qp Qh K2 K

Other: Gammar, GamaSTAN

IOM: 100-02, 15, 50

Coding Clinic: 2011, Q1, P8

J1551 Injection, immune globulin (cutaquig), 100 mg K2 K

⁕ **J1554** Injection, immune globulin (asceniv), 500 mg K2 G

⁕ **J1555** Injection, immune globulin (cuvitru), 100 mg K2 K

⁕ **J1556** Injection, immune globulin (Bivigam), 500 mg Ⓑ Ⓑ Qp Qh K2 K

⁕ **J1557** Injection, immune globulin, (gammaplex), intravenous, non-lyophilized (e.g., liquid), 500 mg Ⓑ Ⓑ Qp Qh K2 K

Coding Clinic: 2012, Q1, P9

⁕ **J1558** Injection, immune globulin (xembify), 100 mg K2 G

⁕ **J1559** Injection, immune globulin (hizentra), 100 mg Ⓑ Ⓑ Qp Qh K2 K

Coding Clinic: 2011, Q1, P6

⊛ **J1560** Injection, gamma globulin, intramuscular, over 10 cc Ⓑ Ⓑ Qp Qh K2 K

Other: Gammar, GamaSTAN

IOM: 100-02, 15, 50

⊛ **J1561** Injection, immune globulin, (Gamunex-C/Gammaked), non-lyophilized (e.g., liquid), 500 mg Ⓑ Ⓑ Qp Qh K2 K

IOM: 100-02, 15, 50

Coding Clinic: 2012, Q1, P9

⁕ **J1562** Injection, immune globulin (Vivaglobin), 100 mg Ⓑ Ⓑ Qp Qh E2

⊛ **J1566** Injection, immune globulin, intravenous, lyophilized (e.g., powder), not otherwise specified, 500 mg Ⓑ Ⓑ Qp Qh K2 K

Other: Carimune, Gammagard S/D, Polygam

IOM: 100-02, 15, 50

⁕ **J1568** Injection, immune globulin, (Octagam), intravenous, non-lyophilized (e.g., liquid), 500 mg Ⓑ Ⓑ Qp Qh K2 K

⊛ **J1569** Injection, immune globulin, (Gammagard Liquid), non-lyophilized (e.g., liquid), 500 mg Ⓑ Ⓑ Qp Qh K2 K

IOM: 100-02, 15, 50

⊛ **J1570** Injection, ganciclovir sodium, 500 mg Ⓑ Ⓑ Qp Qh N1 N

Other: Cytovene

IOM: 100-02, 15, 50

⊛ **J1571** Injection, hepatitis B immune globulin (HepaGam B), intramuscular, 0.5 ml Ⓑ Ⓑ Qp Qh K2 K

IOM: 100-02, 15, 50

Coding Clinic: 2008, Q3, P7-8

▶ **New**   ↻ **Revised**   ✔ **Reinstated**   ~~deleted~~ **Deleted**   ⊘ **Not covered or valid by Medicare**
⊛ **Special coverage instructions**   ⁕ **Carrier discretion**   Ⓑ **Bill Part B MAC**   Ⓑ **Bill DME MAC**

⊛ **J1572** Injection, immune globulin, (flebogamma/flebogamma DIF) intravenous, non-lyophilized (e.g., liquid), 500 mg Ⓑ Ⓑ Qp Qh   K2 K

IOM: 100-02, 15, 50

✳ **J1573** Injection, hepatitis B immune globulin (HepaGam B), intravenous, 0.5 ml Ⓑ Ⓑ Qp Qh   K2 K

Coding Clinic: 2008, Q3, P8

J1574 Injection, ganciclovir sodium (exela) not therapeutically equivalent to J1570, 500 mg   N

✳ **J1575** Injection, immune globulin/ hyaluronidase (HYQVIA), 100 mg immunoglobulin Ⓑ Ⓑ Qp Qh   K2 K

▶ **J1576** Injection, immune globulin (panzyga), intravenous, non-lyophilized (e.g., liquid), 500 mg

⊛ **J1580** Injection, Garamycin, gentamicin, up to 80 mg Ⓑ Ⓑ Qp Qh   N1 N

Other: Gentamicin Sulfate, Jenamicin

IOM: 100-02, 15, 50

⊛ **J1595** Injection, glatiramer acetate, 20 mg Ⓑ Ⓑ Qp Qh   K2 K

Other: Copaxone

IOM: 100-02, 15, 50

✳ **J1599** Injection, immune globulin, intravenous, non-lyophilized (e.g., liquid), not otherwise specified, 500 mg Ⓑ Ⓑ Qp Qh   N1 N

Coding Clinic: 2011, P1, Q6

⊛ **J1600** Injection, gold sodium thiomalate, up to 50 mg Ⓑ Ⓑ Qp Qh   E2

Other: Myochrysine

IOM: 100-02, 15, 50

✳ **J1602** Injection, golimumab, 1 mg for intravenous use Ⓑ Ⓑ Qp Qh   K2 K

Other: Simponi Aria

⊛ **J1610** Injection, glucagon hydrochloride, per 1 mg Ⓑ Ⓑ Qp Qh   K2 K

Other: GlucaGen, Glucagon Emergency

IOM: 100-02, 15, 50

J1611 Injection, glucagon hydrochloride (fresenius kabi), not therapeutically equivalent to J1610, per 1 mg   K2 K

⊛ **J1620** Injection, gonadorelin hydrochloride, per 100 mcg Ⓑ Ⓑ Qp Qh   E2

Other: Factrel

IOM: 100-02, 15, 50

⊛ **J1626** Injection, granisetron hydrochloride, 100 mcg Ⓑ Ⓑ Qp Qh   N1 N

Other: Kytril

IOM: 100-02, 15, 50

✳ **J1627** Injection, granisetron, extended-release, 0.1 mg   K2 G

✳ **J1628** Injection, guselkumab, 1 mg Ⓑ Ⓑ   G

Other: Tremfya

⊛ **J1630** Injection, haloperidol, up to 5 mg Ⓑ Ⓑ Qp Qh   N1 N

Other: Haldol, Haloperidol Lactate

IOM: 100-02, 15, 50

⊛ **J1631** Injection, haloperidol decanoate, per 50 mg Ⓑ Ⓑ Qp Qh   N1 N

IOM: 100-02, 15, 50

⊛ **J1632** Injection, brexanolone, 1 mg   K2 G

⊛ **J1640** Injection, hemin, 1 mg Ⓥ Ⓑ Ⓑ Qp Qh   K2 K

Other: Panhematin

IOM: 100-02, 15, 50

⊛ **J1642** Injection, heparin sodium (heparin lock flush), per 10 units Ⓑ Ⓑ Qp Qh   N1 N

Other: Hep-Lock U/P, Vasceze

IOM: 100-02, 15, 50

J1643 Injection, heparin sodium (pfizer), not therapeutically equivalent to J1644, per 1000 units   N

⊛ **J1644** Injection, heparin sodium, per 1000 units Ⓥ Ⓑ Qp Qh   N1 N

Other: Heparin Sodium (Porcine), Liquaemin Sodium

IOM: 100-02, 15, 50

⊛ **J1645** Injection, dalteparin sodium, per 2500 IU Ⓥ Ⓑ Qp Qh   N1 N

Other: Fragmin

IOM: 100-02, 15, 50

✳ **J1650** Injection, enoxaparin sodium, 10 mg Ⓑ Ⓑ Qp Qh   N1 N

Other: Lovenox

⊛ **J1652** Injection, fondaparinux sodium, 0.5 mg Ⓥ Ⓑ Qp Qh   N1 N

Other: Arixtra

IOM: 100-02, 15, 50

✳ **J1655** Injection, tinzaparin sodium, 1000 IU Ⓑ Ⓑ Qp Qh   N1 E2

Other: Innohep

⊛ **J1670** Injection, tetanus immune globulin, human, up to 250 units Ⓑ Ⓑ Qp Qh   K2 K

Indicated for transient protection against tetanus post-exposure to tetanus (Z23).

Other: Hyper-Tet

IOM: 100-02, 15, 50

🅜 MIPS   Qp Quantity Physician   Qh Quantity Hospital   ♀ Female only
♂ Male only   Ⓐ Age   ♿ DMEPOS   A2-Z3 ASC Payment Indicator   A-Y ASC Status Indicator   Coding Clinic

⊛ **J1675** Injection, histrelin acetate, 10 mcg Ⓥ Ⓑ Qp Qh B

IOM: 100-02, 15, 50

⊛ **J1700** Injection, hydrocortisone acetate, up to 25 mg Ⓑ Ⓖ Qp Qh N1 N

Other: Hydrocortone Acetate

IOM: 100-02, 15, 50

⊛ **J1710** Injection, hydrocortisone sodium phosphate, up to 50 mg Ⓑ Ⓖ Qp Qh N1 N

Other: A-hydroCort, Hydrocortone phosphate, Solu-Cortef

IOM: 100-02, 15, 50

⊛ **J1720** Injection, hydrocortisone sodium succinate, up to 100 mg Ⓑ Ⓖ Qp Qh N1 N

Other: A-HydroCort, Solu-Cortef

IOM: 100-02, 15, 50

✳ **J1726** Injection, hydroxyprogesterone caproate (makena), 10 mg K2 K

✳ **J1729** Injection, hydroxyprogesterone caproate, not otherwise specified, 10 mg N1 N

⊛ **J1730** Injection, diazoxide, up to 300 mg Ⓑ Ⓖ Qp Qh E2

Other: Hyperstat

IOM: 100-02, 15, 50

✳ **J1738** Injection, meloxicam, 1 mg K2 G

✳ **J1740** Injection, ibandronate sodium, 1 mg Ⓑ Ⓖ Qp Qh K2 K

Other: Boniva

✳ **J1741** Injection, ibuprofen, 100 mg Ⓥ Ⓖ Qp Qh N1 N

Other: Caldolor

⊛ **J1742** Injection, ibutilide fumarate, 1 mg Ⓑ Ⓖ Qp Qh K2 K

Other: Corvert

IOM: 100-02, 15, 50

✳ **J1743** Injection, idursulfase, 1 mg Ⓑ Ⓖ Qp Qh K2 K

Other: Elaprase

✳ **J1744** Injection, icatibant, 1 mg Ⓑ Ⓖ Qp Qh K2 K

Other: Firazyr

⊛ **J1745** Injection, infliximab, excludes biosimilar, 10 mg Ⓥ Ⓑ Qp Qh K2 K

Report total number of 10 mg increments administered

For biosimilar, Inflectra, report Q5102

Other: Remicade

IOM: 100-02, 15, 50

✳ **J1746** Injection, ibalizumab-uiyk, 10 mg Ⓥ Ⓑ K

Other: Trogarzo

▶ **J1747** Injection, spesolimab-sbzo, 1 mg

⊛ **J1750** Injection, iron dextran, 50 mg Ⓥ Ⓑ Qp Qh K2 K

Other: Dexferrum, Imferon, Infed

IOM: 100-02, 15, 50

✳ **J1756** Injection, iron sucrose, 1 mg Ⓑ Ⓖ Qp Qh N1 N

Other: Venofer

⊛ **J1786** Injection, imiglucerase, 10 units Ⓑ Ⓖ Qp Qh K2 K

Other: Cerezyme

IOM: 100-02, 15, 50

Coding Clinic: 2011, Q1, P8

⊛ **J1790** Injection, droperidol, up to 5 mg Ⓑ Ⓖ Qp Qh N1 N

Other: Inapsine

IOM: 100-02, 15, 50

⊛ **J1800** Injection, propranolol HCL, up to 1 mg Ⓥ Ⓑ Qp Qh N1 N

Other: Inderal

IOM: 100-02, 15, 50

▶ **J1805** Injection, esmolol hydrochloride, 10 mg

▶ **J1806** Injection, esmolol hydrochloride (wg critical care) not therapeutically equivalent to J1805, 10 mg

⊛ **J1810** Injection, droperidol and fentanyl citrate, up to 2 ml ampule Ⓥ Ⓖ Qp Qh E1

Other: Innovar

IOM: 100-02, 15, 50

▶ **J1811** Insulin (fiasp) for administration through dme (i.e., insulin pump) per 50 units

▶ **J1812** Insulin (fiasp), per 5 units

▶ **J1813** Insulin (lyumjev) for administration through dme (i.e., insulin pump) per 50 units

▶ **J1814** Insulin (lyumjev), per 5 units

▶ New   ↻ Revised   ✔ Reinstated   ~~deleted~~ Deleted   ⊘ Not covered or valid by Medicare
⊛ Special coverage instructions   ✳ Carrier discretion   Ⓑ Bill Part B MAC   Ⓖ Bill DME MAC

⚙ **J1815** Injection, insulin, per 5 units Ⓑ Ⓑ Qp Qh N1 N

Other: Humalog, Humulin, Lantus, Novolin, Novolog

IOM: 100-02, 15, 50; 100-03, 4, 280.14

✳ **J1817** Insulin for administration through DME (i.e., insulin pump) per 50 units Ⓑ Ⓑ Qp Qh N1 N

Other: Apidra Solostar, Insulin Lispro, Humalog, Humulin, Novolin, Novolog

✳ **J1823** Injection, inebilizumab-cdon, 1 mg K2 G

✳ **J1826** Injection, interferon beta-1a, 30 mcg Ⓑ Ⓑ K2 K

Other: Avonex

Coding Clinic: 2011, Q2, P9; Q1, P8

⚙ **J1830** Injection, interferon beta-1b, 0.25 mg (Code may be used for Medicare when drug administered under the direct supervision of a physician, not for use when drug is self-administered) Ⓑ Ⓑ Qp Qh K2 N

Other: Betaseron

IOM: 100-02, 15, 50

✳ **J1833** Injection, isavuconazonium, 1 mg Ⓑ Ⓑ Qp Qh K2 K

✳ **J1835** Injection, itraconazole, 50 mg Ⓑ Ⓑ Qp Qh E2

Other: Sporanox

▶ **J1836** Injection, metronidazole, 10 mg

⚙ **J1840** Injection, kanamycin sulfate, up to 500 mg Ⓑ Ⓑ Qp Qh N1 N

Other: Kantrex, Klebcil

IOM: 100-02, 15, 50

⚙ **J1850** Injection, kanamycin sulfate, up to 75 mg Ⓑ Ⓑ Qp Qh N1 N

Other: Kantrex, Klebcil

IOM: 100-02, 15, 50

Coding Clinic: 2013; Q2, P3

⚙ **J1885** Injection, ketorolac tromethamine, per 15 mg Ⓑ Ⓑ Qp Qh N1 N

Other: Toradol

IOM: 100-02, 15, 50

⚙ **J1890** Injection, cephalothin sodium, up to 1 gram Ⓑ Ⓑ Qp Qh N1 E2

Other: Keflin

IOM: 100-02, 15, 50

▶ **J1920** Injection, labetalol hydrochloride, 5 mg

▶ **J1921** Injection, labetalol hydrochloride (hikma) not therapeutically equivalent to J1920, 5 mg

✳ **J1930** Injection, lanreotide, 1 mg Ⓑ Ⓑ Qp Qh K2 K

Treats acromegaly and symptoms caused by neuroendocrine tumors

Other: Somatuline Depot

✳ **J1931** Injection, laronidase, 0.1 mg Ⓑ Ⓑ Qp Qh K2 K

Other: Aldurazyme

J1932 Injection, lanreotide, (cipla), 1 mg K2 G

⚙ **J1940** Injection, furosemide, up to 20 mg Ⓑ Ⓑ Qp Qh N1 N

Other: Furomide M.D., Lasix

MCM: 2049

IOM: 100-02, 15, 50

▶ **J1941** Injection, furosemide (furoscix), 20 mg

✳ **J1943** Injection, aripiprazole lauroxil, (aristada initio), 1 mg K2 K

✳ **J1944** Injection, aripiprazole lauroxil, (aristada), 1 mg K2 K

⚙ **J1945** Injection, lepirudin, 50 mg Ⓑ Ⓑ Qp Qh E2

IOM: 100-02, 15, 50

⚙ **J1950** Injection, leuprolide acetate (for depot suspension), per 3.75 mg Ⓑ Ⓑ Qp Qh K2 K

Other: Lupron, Lupron Depot, Lupron Depot-Ped

IOM: 100-02, 15, 50

Coding Clinic: 2019, Q2, P11-12

✳ **J1951** Injection, leuprolide acetate for depot suspension (fensolvi), 0.25 mg K2 K

✳ **J1952** Leuprolide injectable, camcevi, 1 mg K5 G

✳ **J1953** Injection, levetiracetam, 10 mg Ⓑ Ⓑ Qp Qh N1 N

Other: Keppra

▶ **J1954** Injection, leuprolide acetate for depot suspension (cipla), 7.5 mg E2

⚙ **J1955** Injection, levocarnitine, per 1 gm Ⓑ Ⓑ Qp Qh B

Other: Carnitor

IOM: 100-02, 15, 50

⚙ **J1956** Injection, levofloxacin, 250 mg Ⓑ Ⓑ Qp Qh N1 N

Other: Levaquin

IOM: 100-02, 15, 50

⊛ **J1960** Injection, levorphanol tartrate, up to 2 mg Ⓑ Ⓑ Qp Qh   N1 N

Other: Levo-Dromoran

MCM: 2049

IOM: 100-02, 15, 50

▶ **J1961** Injection, lenacapavir, 1 mg

⊛ **J1980** Injection, hyoscyamine sulfate, up to 0.25 mg Ⓑ Ⓑ Qp Qh   N1 N

Other: Levsin

IOM: 100-02, 15, 50

⊛ **J1990** Injection, chlordiazepoxide HCL, up to 100 mg Ⓑ Ⓑ Qp Qh   N1 E2

Other: Librium

IOM: 100-02, 15, 50

⊛ **J2001** Injection, lidocaine HCL for intravenous infusion, 10 mg Ⓑ Ⓑ Qp Qh   N1 N

Other: Caine-1, Caine-2, Dilocaine, L-Caine, Lidocaine in D5W, Lidoject, Nervocaine, Nulicaine, Xylocaine

IOM: 100-02, 15, 50

Coding Clinic: 2023, Q3, P10

⊛ **J2010** Injection, lincomycin HCL, up to 300 mg Ⓑ Ⓑ Qp Qh   N1 N

Other: Lincocin

IOM: 100-02, 15, 50

✳ **J2020** Injection, linezolid, 200 mg Ⓑ Ⓑ Qp Qh   N1 N

Other: Zyvox

J2021 Injection, linezolid (hospira) not therapeutically equivalent to J2020, 200 mg   N

⊛ **J2060** Injection, lorazepam, 2 mg Ⓑ Ⓑ Qp Qh   N1 N

Other: Ativan

IOM: 100-02, 15, 50

✳ **J2062** Loxapine for inhalation, 1 mg Ⓑ Ⓑ   K

Other: Adasuve

⊛ **J2150** Injection, mannitol, 25% in 50 ml Ⓑ Ⓑ Qp Qh   N1 N

Other: Aridol

MCM: 2049

IOM: 100-02, 15, 50

✳ **J2170** Injection, mecasermin, 1 mg Ⓑ Ⓑ Qp Qh   N1 N

Other: Increlex

⊛ **J2175** Injection, meperidine hydrochloride, per 100 mg Ⓑ Ⓑ Qp Qh   N1 N

Other: Demerol

IOM: 100-02, 15, 50

⊛ **J2180** Injection, meperidine and promethazine HCL, up to 50 mg Ⓑ Ⓑ Qp Qh   N1 N

Other: Mepergan

IOM: 100-02, 15, 50

✳ **J2182** Injection, mepolizumab, 1 mg Qp Qh   K2 G

J2184 Injection, meropenem (b. braun) not therapeutically equivalent to J2185, 100 mg   N

✳ **J2185** Injection, meropenem, 100 mg Ⓑ Ⓑ Qp Qh   N1 N

Other: Merrem

✳ **J2186** Inj., meropenem, vaborbactam Ⓑ Ⓑ   G

Other: Vabomere

Medicare Statute 1833(t)

⊛ **J2210** Injection, methylergonovine maleate, up to 0.2 mg Ⓑ Ⓑ Qp Qh   N1 N

Benefit limited to obstetrical diagnoses for prevention and control of postpartum hemorrhage

Other: Methergine

IOM: 100-02, 15, 50

✳ **J2212** Injection, methylnaltrexone, 0.1 mg Ⓑ Ⓑ Qp Qh   N1 N

Other: Relistor

J2247 Injection, micafungin sodium (par pharm) not thereapeutically equivalent to J2248, 1 mg   N

✳ **J2248** Injection, micafungin sodium, 1 mg Ⓑ Ⓑ Qp Qh   N1 N

Other: Mycamine

▶ **J2249** Injection, remimazolam, 1 mg

⊛ **J2250** Injection, midazolam hydrochloride, per 1 mg Ⓑ Ⓑ Qp Qh   N1 N

Other: Versed

IOM: 100-02, 15, 50

J2251 Injection, midazolam hydrochloride (wg critical care) not therapeutically equivalent to J2250, per 1 mg   N

⊛ **J2260** Injection, milrinone lactate, 5 mg Ⓑ Ⓑ Qp Qh   N1 N

Other: Primacor

IOM: 100-02, 15, 50

▶ New   ↻ Revised   ✔ Reinstated   ~~deleted~~ Deleted   ⊘ Not covered or valid by Medicare
⊛ Special coverage instructions   ✳ Carrier discretion   Ⓑ Bill Part B MAC   Ⓑ Bill DME MAC

✳ **J2265** Injection, minocycline hydrochloride, 1 mg ⑧ ⑧ **Qp** **Qh**   K2 K

Other: Minocine

⊘ **J2270** Injection, morphine sulfate, up to 10 mg ⑧ ⑧ **Qp** **Qh**   N1 N

Other: Astramorph PF, Duramorph

IOM: 100-02, 15, 50

Coding Clinic: 2013, Q2, P4

J2272 Injection, morphine sulfate (fresenius kabi) not therapeutically equivalent to J2270, up to 10 mg   N

⊘ **J2274** Injection, morphine sulfate, preservative-free for epidural or intrathecal use, 10 mg ⑧ ⑧ **Qp** **Qh**   N1 N

Other: Duramorph, Infumorph

IOM: 100-03, 4, 280.1; 100-02, 15, 50

⊘ **J2278** Injection, ziconotide, 1 mcg ⑧ ⑧ **Qp** **Qh**   K2 K

Other: Prialt

✳ **J2280** Injection, moxifloxacin, 100 mg ⑧ ⑧ **Qp** **Qh**   N1 N

Other: Avelox

J2281 Injection, moxifloxacin (fresenius kabi) not therapeutically equivalent to J2280, 100 mg   N

⊘ **J2300** Injection, nalbuphine hydrochloride, per 10 mg ⑧ ⑧ **Qp** **Qh**   N1 N

Other: Nubain

IOM: 100-02, 15, 50

▶ **J2305** Injection, nitroglycerin, 5 mg

⊘ **J2310** Injection, naloxone hydrochloride, per 1 mg ⑧ ⑧ **Qp** **Qh**   N1 N

Other: Narcan

IOM: 100-02, 15, 50

J2311 Injection, naloxone hydrochloride (zimhi), 1 mg   N

✳ **J2315** Injection, naltrexone, depot form, 1 mg ⑧ ⑧ **Qp** **Qh**   K2 K

Other: Vivitrol

⊘ **J2320** Injection, nandrolone decanoate, up to 50 mg ⑧ ⑧ **Qp** **Qh**   K2 K

Other: Anabolin LA 100, Androlone, Deca-Durabolin, Decolone, Hybolin Decanoate, Nandrobolic LA, Neo-Durabolic

IOM: 100-02, 15, 50

Coding Clinic: 2011, Q1, P8

✳ **J2323** Injection, natalizumab, 1 mg ⑧ ⑧ **Qp** **Qh**   K2 K

Other: Tysabri

⊘ **J2325** Injection, nesiritide, 0.1 mg ⑧ ⑧ **Qp** **Qh**   K2 K

Other: Natrecor

IOM: 100-02, 15, 50

✳ **J2326** Injection, nusinersen, 0.1 mg   K2 G

Coding Clinic: 2021, Q1, P11; 2020, Q1, P11

J2327 Injection, risankizumab-rzaa, intravenous, 1 mg   K2 G

▶ **J2329** Injection, ublituximab-xiiy, 1mg

✳ **J2350** Injection, ocrelizumab, 1 mg   K2 G

✳ **J2353** Injection, octreotide, depot form for intramuscular injection, 1 mg ⑧ ⑧ **Qp** **Qh**   K2 K

Other: Sandostatin LAR Depot

✳ **J2354** Injection, octreotide, non-depot form for subcutaneous or intravenous injection, 25 mcg ⑧ ⑧ **Qp** **Qh**   N1 N

Other: Sandostatin LAR Depot

⊘ **J2355** Injection, oprelvekin, 5 mg ⑧ ⑧ **Qp** **Qh**   K2 K

Other: Neumega

IOM: 100-02, 15, 50

J2356 Injection, tezepelumab-ekko, 1 mg   K2 G

✳ **J2357** Injection, omalizumab, 5 mg ⑧ ⑧ **Qp** **Qh**   K2 K

Other: Xolair

✳ **J2358** Injection, olanzapine, long-acting, 1 mg ⑧ ⑧ **Qp** **Qh**   N1 N

Other: Zyprexa Relprevv

Coding Clinic: 2011, Q1, P6

▶ **J2359** Injection, olanzapine, 0.5 mg

⊘ **J2360** Injection, orphenadrine citrate, up to 60 mg ⑧ ⑧ **Qp** **Qh**   N1 N

Other: Antiflex, Banflex, Flexoject, Flexon, K-Flex, Myolin, Neocyten, Norflex, O-Flex, Orphenate

IOM: 100-02, 15, 50

~~J2370~~ ~~Injection, phenylephrine HCL, up to 1 ml~~   N1 N

~~Other: Neo-Synephrine~~

~~IOM: 100-02, 15, 50~~

▶ **J2371** Injection, phenylephrine hydrochloride, 20 micrograms

▶ **J2372** Injection, phenylephrine hydrochloride (biorphen), 20 micrograms

---

🐾 MIPS   **Qp** Quantity Physician   **Qh** Quantity Hospital   ♀ Female only

♂ Male only   🅐 Age   ♿ DMEPOS   A2-Z3 ASC Payment Indicator   A-Y ASC Status Indicator   Coding Clinic

J2401 Injection, chloroprocaine hydrochloride, per 1 mg   N

J2402 Injection, chloroprocaine hydrochloride (clorotekal), per 1 mg   N

▶ **J2403** Chloroprocaine hcl ophthalmic, 3% gel, 1 mg

⊘ **J2406** Injection, oritavancin (kimyrsa), 10 mg   K2 G

⊘ **J2407** Injection, oritavancin (orbactiv), 10 mg ⑧ ⓖ ⓠp ⓠh   K2 K

    Other: Orbactiv

    IOM: 100-02, 15, 50

⊘ **J2410** Injection, oxymorphone HCL, up to 1 mg ⑧ ⓖ ⓠp ⓠh   N1 E2

    Other: Numorphan, Opana

    IOM: 100-02, 15, 50

✳ **J2425** Injection, palifermin, 50 mcg ⑧ ⓖ ⓠp ⓠh   K2 K

    Other: Kepivance

↻ ✳ **J2426** Injection, paliperidone palmitate extended release, (invega sustenna) 1 mg ⑧ ⓖ ⓠp ⓠh   K2 K

    Other: Invega Sustenna

    Coding Clinic: 2011, Q1, P7

▶ **J2427** Injection, paliperidone palmitate extended release (invega hafyera, or invega trinza), 1 mg

⊘ **J2430** Injection, pamidronate disodium, per 30 mg ⑧ ⓖ ⓠp ⓠh   N1 N

    Other: Aredia

    IOM: 100-02, 15, 50

⊘ **J2440** Injection, papaverine HCL, up to 60 mg ⑧ ⓖ ⓠp ⓠh   N1 N

    IOM: 100-02, 15, 50

⊘ **J2460** Injection, oxytetracycline HCL, up to 50 mg ⑧ ⓖ ⓠp ⓠh   E2

    Other: Terramycin IM

    IOM: 100-02, 15, 50

✳ **J2469** Injection, palonosetron HCL, 25 mcg ⑧ ⓖ ⓠp ⓠh   K2 K

    Example: 0.25 mgm dose = 10 units
    Example of use is acute, delayed, nausea and vomiting due to chemotherapy

    Other: Aloxi

⊘ **J2501** Injection, paricalcitol, 1 mcg ⑧ ⓖ ⓠp ⓠh   N1 N

    Other: Zemplar

    IOM: 100-02, 15, 50

✳ **J2502** Injection, pasireotide long acting, 1 mg ⑧ ⓖ ⓠp ⓠh   K2 K

    Other: Signifor LAR

✳ **J2503** Injection, pegaptanib sodium, 0.3 mg ⑧ ⓖ ⓠp ⓠh   K2 K

    Other: Macugen

⊘ **J2504** Injection, pegademase bovine, 25 IU ⑧ ⓖ ⓠp ⓠh   K2 K

    Other: Adagen

    IOM: 100-02, 15, 50

✳ **J2506** Injection, pegfilgrastim, excludes biosimilar, 0.5 mg   K2 K

✳ **J2507** Injection, pegloticase, 1 mg ⑧ ⓖ ⓠp ⓠh   K2 K

    Other: Krystexxa

    Coding Clinic: 2012, Q1, P9

⊘ **J2510** Injection, penicillin G procaine, aqueous, up to 600,000 units ⑧ ⓖ ⓠp ⓠh   N1 N

    Other: Crysticillin, Duracillin AS, Pfizerpen AS, Wycillin

    IOM: 100-02, 15, 50

⊘ **J2513** Injection, pentastarch, 10% solution, 100 ml ⑧ ⓖ ⓠp ⓠh   E2

    IOM: 100-02, 15, 50

⊘ **J2515** Injection, pentobarbital sodium, per 50 mg ⑧ ⓖ ⓠp ⓠh   K2 K

    Other: Nembutal sodium solution

    IOM: 100-02, 15, 50

⊘ **J2540** Injection, penicillin G potassium, up to 600,000 units ⑧ ⓖ ⓠp ⓠh   N1 N

    Other: Pfizerpen-G

    IOM: 100-02, 15, 50

⊘ **J2543** Injection, piperacillin sodium/ tazobactam sodium, 1 gram/0.125 grams (1.125 grams) ⑧ ⓖ ⓠp ⓠh   N1 N

    Other: Zosyn

    IOM: 100-02, 15, 50

⊘ **J2545** Pentamidine isethionate, inhalation solution, FDA-approved final product, non-compounded, administered through DME, unit dose form, per 300 mg ⑧ ⓖ ⓠp ⓠh   B

    Other: Nebupent

✳ **J2547** Injection, peramivir, 1 mg ⑧ ⓖ ⓠp ⓠh   K2 K

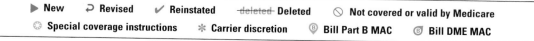

⚙ **J2550** Injection, promethazine HCL, up to 50 mg ⓟ ⓑ Qp Qh   N1 N

Administration of phenergan suppository considered part of E/M encounter

Other: Anergan, Phenazine, Phenergan, Prorex, Prothazine, V-Gan

IOM: 100-02, 15, 50

⚙ **J2560** Injection, phenobarbital sodium, up to 120 mg ⓟ ⓑ Qp Qh   N1 N

Other: Luminal Sodium

IOM: 100-02, 15, 50

▶ **J2561** Injection, phenobarbital sodium (sezaby), 1 mg

✳ **J2562** Injection, plerixafor, 1 mg ⓟ ⓑ Qp Qh   K2 K

FDA approved for non-Hodgkin lymphoma and multiple myeloma in 2008.

Other: Mozobil

⚙ **J2590** Injection, oxytocin, up to 10 units ⓑ ⓑ Qp Qh   N1 N

Other: Pitocin, Syntocinon

IOM: 100-02, 15, 50

⚙ **J2597** Injection, desmopressin acetate, per 1 mcg ⓟ ⓑ Qp Qh   K2 K

Other: DDAVP

IOM: 100-02, 15, 50

▶ **J2598** Injection, vasopressin, 1 unit

▶ **J2599** Injection, vasopressin (american regent) not therapeutically equivalent to J2598, 1 unit

⚙ **J2650** Injection, prednisolone acetate, up to 1 ml ⓟ ⓑ Qp Qh   N1 N

Other: Key-Pred, Predalone, Predcor, Predicort, Predoject

IOM: 100-02, 15, 50

⚙ **J2670** Injection, tolazoline HCL, up to 25 mg ⓟ ⓑ Qp Qh   N1 N

Other: Priscoline HCl

IOM: 100-02, 15, 50

⚙ **J2675** Injection, progesterone, per 50 mg ⓟ ⓑ Qp Qh   N1 N

Other: Gesterol 50, Progestaject

IOM: 100-02, 15, 50

⚙ **J2680** Injection, fluphenazine decanoate, up to 25 mg ⓟ ⓑ Qp Qh   N1 N

Other: Prolixin Decanoate

MCM: 2049

IOM: 100-02, 15, 50

⚙ **J2690** Injection, procainamide HCL, up to 1 gm ⓟ ⓑ Qp Qh ♀   N1 N

Benefit limited to obstetrical diagnoses

Other: Pronestyl, Prostaphlin

IOM: 100-02, 15, 50

⚙ **J2700** Injection, oxacillin sodium, up to 250 mg ⓑ ⓑ Qp Qh   N1 N

Other: Bactocill

IOM: 100-02, 15, 50

✳ **J2704** Injection, propofol, 10 mg ⓟ ⓑ Qp Qh   N1 N

Other: Diprivan

⚙ **J2710** Injection, neostigmine methylsulfate, up to 0.5 mg ⓟ ⓑ Qp Qh   N1 N

Other: Prostigmin

IOM: 100-02, 15, 50

⚙ **J2720** Injection, protamine sulfate, per 10 mg ⓟ ⓑ Qp Qh   N1 N

IOM: 100-02, 15, 50

✳ **J2724** Injection, protein C concentrate, intravenous, human, 10 IU ⓟ ⓑ Qp Qh   K2 K

Other: Ceprotin

⚙ **J2725** Injection, protirelin, per 250 mcg ⓟ ⓑ Qp Qh   E2

Other: Relefact TRH, Thypinone

IOM: 100-02, 15, 50

⚙ **J2730** Injection, pralidoxime chloride, up to 1 gm ⓟ ⓑ Qp Qh   N1 N

Other: Protopam Chloride

IOM: 100-02, 15, 50

⚙ **J2760** Injection, phentolamine mesylate, up to 5 mg ⓟ ⓑ Qp Qh   K2 K

Other: Regitine

IOM: 100-02, 15, 50

⚙ **J2765** Injection, metoclopramide HCL, up to 10 mg ⓟ ⓑ Qp Qh   N1 N

Other: Reglan

IOM: 100-02, 15, 50

⚙ **J2770** Injection, quinupristin/dalfopristin, 500 mg (150/350) ⓟ ⓑ Qp Qh   K2 K

Other: Synercid

IOM: 100-02, 15, 50

J2777 Injection, faricimab-svoa, 0.1 mg   K2 G

✳ **J2778** Injection, ranibizumab, 0.1 mg ⓟ ⓑ Qp Qh   K2 K

May be reported for exudative senile macular degeneration (wet AMD) with 67028 (RT or LT)

Other: Lucentis

🐾 MIPS	Qp Quantity Physician	Qh Quantity Hospital	♀ Female only
♂ Male only A Age ♿ DMEPOS	A2-Z3 ASC Payment Indicator	A-Y ASC Status Indicator	Coding Clinic

J2779 Injection, ranibizumab, via intravitreal implant (susvimo), 0.1 mg K2 G

○ **J2780** Injection, ranitidine hydrochloride, 25 mg Ⓥ Ⓑ Qp Qh N1 N

Other: Zantac

IOM: 100-02, 15, 50

▶ **J2781** Injection, pegcetacoplan, intravitreal, 1 mg

✳ **J2783** Injection, rasburicase, 0.5 mg Ⓑ Ⓑ Qp Qh K2 K

Other: Elitek

✳ **J2785** Injection, regadenoson, 0.1 mg Ⓑ Ⓑ Qp Qh N1 N

One billing unit equal to 0.1 mg of regadenoson

Other: Lexiscan

✳ **J2786** Injection, reslizumab, 1 mg Qp Qh K2 G

Coding Clinic: 2016, Q4, P9

✳ **J2787** Riboflavin 5'-phosphate, ophthalmic solution, up to 3 mL Ⓑ

Other: Photrexa Viscous

○ **J2788** Injection, Rho D immune globulin, human, minidose, 50 mcg (250 IU) Ⓥ Ⓑ Qp Qh N1 N

Other: HypRho-D, MicRhoGAM, Rhesonativ, RhoGam

IOM: 100-02, 15, 50

○ **J2790** Injection, Rho D immune globulin, human, full dose, 300 mcg (1500 IU) Ⓥ Ⓑ Qp Qh N1 N

Administered to pregnant female to prevent hemolistic disease of newborn. Report 90384 to private payer

Other: Gamulin Rh, Hyperrho S/D, HypRho-D, Rhesonativ, RhoGAM

IOM: 100-02, 15, 50

○ **J2791** Injection, Rho(D) immune globulin (human), (Rhophylac), intramuscular or intravenous, 100 IU Ⓥ Ⓑ Qp Qh N1 N

Agent must be billed per 100 IU in both physician office and hospital outpatient settings

Other: HypRho-D

IOM: 100-02, 15, 50

○ **J2792** Injection, Rho D immune globulin intravenous, human, solvent detergent, 100 IU Ⓥ Ⓑ Qp Qh K2 K

Other: Gamulin Rh, Hyperrho S/D, WinRHo-SDF

IOM: 100-02, 15, 50

○ **J2793** Injection, rilonacept, 1 mg Ⓑ Ⓑ Qp Qh K2 K

Other: Arcalyst

IOM: 100-02, 15, 50

✳ **J2794** Injection, risperidone (risperdal consta), 0.5 mg Ⓥ Ⓑ Qp Qh K2 K

Other: Risperdal Costa

✳ **J2795** Injection, ropivacaine hydrochloride, 1 mg Ⓥ Ⓑ Qp Qh N1 N

Other: Naropin

✳ **J2796** Injection, romiplostim, 10 mcg Ⓥ Ⓑ Qp Qh K2 K

Stimulates bone marrow megakarocytes to produce platelets (i.e., ITP)

Other: Nplate

○ **J2797** Injection, rolapitant, 0.5 mg G

Other: Varubi

✳ **J2798** Injection, risperidone, (perseris), 0.5 mg K2 G

○ **J2800** Injection, methocarbamol, up to 10 ml Ⓥ Ⓑ Qp Qh N1 N

Other: Robaxin

IOM: 100-02, 15, 50

✳ **J2805** Injection, sincalide, 5 mcg Ⓥ Ⓑ Qp Qh N1 N

Other: Kinevac

▶ **J2806** Injection, sincalide (maia) not therapeutically equivalent to J2805, 5 micrograms

○ **J2810** Injection, theophylline, per 40 mg Ⓑ Ⓑ Qp Qh N1 N

IOM: 100-02, 15, 50

○ **J2820** Injection, sargramostim (GM-CSF), 50 mcg Ⓥ Ⓑ Qp Qh K2 K

Other: Leukine, Prokine

IOM: 100-02, 15, 50

✳ **J2840** Injection, sebelipase alfa, 1 mg Qp Qh K2 G

○ **J2850** Injection, secretin, synthetic, human, 1 mcg Ⓑ Ⓑ Qp Qh K2 K

Other: Chirhostim

IOM: 100-02, 15, 50

✳ **J2860** Injection, siltuximab, 10 mg Ⓥ Ⓑ Qp Qh K2 K

○ **J2910** Injection, aurothioglucose, up to 50 mg Ⓥ Ⓑ Qp Qh E2

Other: Solganal

IOM: 100-02, 15, 50

▶ New   ↻ Revised   ✔ Reinstated   ~~deleted~~ Deleted   ⊘ Not covered or valid by Medicare
○ Special coverage instructions   ✳ Carrier discretion   Ⓑ Bill Part B MAC   Ⓑ Bill DME MAC

⊘ **J2916** Injection, sodium ferric gluconate complex in sucrose injection, 12.5 mg Ⓥ Ⓑ Qp Qh   N1 N

Other: Ferrlecit, Nulecit

IOM: 100-02, 15, 50

⊘ **J2920** Injection, methylprednisolone sodium succinate, up to 40 mg Ⓑ Ⓑ Qp Qh   N1 N

Other: A-MethaPred, Solu-Medrol

IOM: 100-02, 15, 50

⊘ **J2930** Injection, methylprednisolone sodium succinate, up to 125 mg Ⓑ Ⓑ Qp Qh   N1 N

Other: A-MethaPred, Solu-Medrol

IOM: 100-02, 15, 50

⊘ **J2940** Injection, somatrem, 1 mg Ⓑ Ⓑ Qp Qh   E2

IOM: 100-02, 15, 50,

Medicare Statute 1861s2b

⊘ **J2941** Injection, somatropin, 1 mg Ⓑ Ⓑ Qp Qh   K2 K

Other: Genotropin, Humatrope, Nutropin, Omnitrope, Saizen, Serostim, Zorbtive

IOM: 100-02, 15, 50,

Medicare Statute 1861s2b

⊘ **J2950** Injection, promazine HCL, up to 25 mg Ⓑ Ⓑ Qp Qh   N1 N

Other: Prozine-50, Sparine

IOM: 100-02, 15, 50

⊘ **J2993** Injection, reteplase, 18.1 mg Ⓑ Ⓑ Qp Qh   K2 K

Other: Retavase

IOM: 100-02, 15, 50

⊘ **J2995** Injection, streptokinase, per 250,000 IU Ⓑ Ⓑ Qp Qh   N1 N

Bill 1 unit for each 250,000 IU

Other: Kabikinase, Streptase

IOM: 100-02, 15, 50

⊘ **J2997** Injection, alteplase recombinant, 1 mg Ⓑ Ⓑ Qp Qh   K2 K

Thrombolytic agent, treatment of occluded catheters. Bill units of 1 mg administered.

Other: Activase, Cathflo Activase

IOM: 100-02, 15, 50

Coding Clinic: 2014, Q1, P4

J2998 Injection, plasminogen, human-tvmh, 1 mg   K2 K

⊘ **J3000** Injection, streptomycin, up to 1 gm Ⓑ Ⓑ Qp Qh   N1 N

IOM: 100-02, 15, 50

⊘ **J3010** Injection, fentanyl citrate, 0.1 mg Ⓥ Ⓑ Qp Qh   N1 N

Other: Sublimaze

IOM: 100-02, 15, 50

⊘ **J3030** Injection, sumatriptan succinate, 6 mg (Code may be used for Medicare when drug administered under the direct supervision of a physician, not for use when drug is self-administered) Ⓑ Ⓑ Qp Qh   N1 N

Other: Imitrex, Sumarel Dosepro

IOM: 100-02, 15, 150

✳ **J3031** Injection, fremanezumab-vfrm, 1 mg (Code may be used for Medicare when drug administered under the direct supervision of a physician, not for use when drug is self-administered)   K2 K

✳ **J3032** Injection, eptinezumab-jjmr, 1 mg   K2 G

✳ **J3060** Injection, taliglucerase alfa, 10 units Ⓑ Ⓑ Qp Qh   K2 K

Other: Elelyso

⊘ **J3070** Injection, pentazocine, 30 mg Ⓥ Ⓑ Qp Qh   K2 K

Other: Talwin

IOM: 100-02, 15, 50

✳ **J3090** Injection, tedizolid phosphate, 1 mg Ⓑ Ⓑ Qp Qh   K2 K

Other: Sivextro

✳ **J3095** Injection, televancin, 10 mg Ⓑ Ⓑ Qp Qh   K2 K

Prescribed for the treatment of adults with complicated skin and skin structure infections (cSSSI) of the following Gram-positive microorganisms: Staphylococcus aureus; Streptococcus pyogenes, Streptococcus agalactiae, Streptococcus anginosusgroup. Separately payable under the ASC payment system.

Other: Vibativ

Coding Clinic: 2011, Q1, P7

✳ **J3101** Injection, tenecteplase, 1 mg Ⓑ Ⓑ Qp Qh   K2 K

Other: TNKase

⊘ **J3105** Injection, terbutaline sulfate, up to 1 mg Ⓑ Ⓑ Qp Qh   N1 N

Other: Brethine

IOM: 100-02, 15, 50

🖋 MIPS   Qp Quantity Physician   Qh Quantity Hospital   ♀ Female only

♂ Male only   Ⓐ Age   ♿ DMEPOS   A2-Z3 ASC Payment Indicator   A-Y ASC Status Indicator   Coding Clinic

⊛ **J3110** Injection, teriparatide,
10 mcg ⑧ ⑤ **Qp** **Qh**   B

✳ **J3111** Injection, romosozumab-aqqg,
1 mg   K2 K

⊛ **J3121** Injection, testosterone enanthate,
1 mg ⑧ ⑤ **Qp** **Qh**   N1 N

*Other: Andrest 90-4, Andro L.A. 200,
Andro-Estro 90-4, Androgyn L.A,
Andropository 100, Andryl 200,
Deladumone, Deladumone OB, Delatest,
Delatestadiol, Delatestryl, Ditate-DS,
Dua-Gen L.A., Duoval P.A.,
Durathate-200, Estra-Testrin, Everone,
TEEV, Testadiate, Testone LA, Testradiol
90/4, Testrin PA, Valertest*

⊛ **J3145** Injection, testosterone undecanoate,
1 mg ⑧ ⑤ **Qp** **Qh**   K2 K

⊛ **J3230** Injection, chlorpromazine HCL,
up to 50 mg ⑧ ⑤ **Qp** **Qh**   N1 N

Other: Ormazine, Thorazine

IOM: 100-02, 15, 50

⊛ **J3240** Injection, thyrotropin alfa,
0.9 mg provided in
1.1 mg vial ⑧ ⑤ **Qp** **Qh**   K2 K

Other: Thyrogen

IOM: 100-02, 15, 50

✳ **J3241** Injection, teprotumumab-trbw,
10 mg   K2 G

✳ **J3243** Injection, tigecycline,
1 mg ⑧ ⑤ **Qp** **Qh**   K2 K

J3244 Injection, tigecycline (accord) not
therapeutically equivalent to J3243,
1 mg   N

✳ **J3245** Injection, tildrakizumab,
1 mg ⑧ ⑤   K

Other: Ilumya

✳ **J3246** Injection, tirofiban HCL,
0.25 mg ⑧ ⑤ **Qp** **Qh**   K2 N

Other: Aggrastat

⊛ **J3250** Injection, trimethobenzamide HCL,
up to 200 mg ⑧ ⑤ **Qp** **Qh**   N1 N

Other: Arrestin, Ticon, Tigan, Tiject 20

IOM: 100-02, 15, 50

⊛ **J3260** Injection, tobramycin sulfate,
up to 80 mg ⑧ ⑤ **Qp** **Qh**   N1 N

Other: Nebcin

IOM: 100-02, 15, 50

✳ **J3262** Injection, tocilizumab,
1 mg ⑧ ⑤ **Qp** **Qh**   K2 K

Indicated for the treatment of adult
patients with moderately to severely
active rheumatoid arthritis (RA) who
have had an inadequate response to
one or more tumor necrosis factor
(TNF) antagonist therapies.

Other: Actemra

Coding Clinic: 2011, Q1, P7

⊛ **J3265** Injection, torsemide,
10 mg/ml ⑧ ⑤ **Qp** **Qh**   N1 E2

Other: Demadex

IOM: 100-02, 15, 50

⊛ **J3280** Injection, thiethylperazine maleate,
up to 10 mg ⑧ ⑤ **Qp** **Qh**   E2

Other: Norzine, Torecan

IOM: 100-02, 15, 50

✳ **J3285** Injection, treprostinil,
1 mg ⑧ ⑤ **Qp** **Qh**   K2 K

Other: Remodulin

J3299 Injection, triamcinolone acetonide
(xipere), 1 mg   G

⊛ **J3300** Injection, triamcinolone
acetonide, preservative free,
1 mg ⑧ ⑤ **Qp** **Qh**   K2 K

*Other: Cenacort A-40, Kenaject-40,
Kenalog, Triam-A, Triesence, Tri-Kort,
Trilog*

⊛ **J3301** Injection, triamcinolone acetonide,
not otherwise specified,
10 mg ⑧ ⑤ **Qp** **Qh**   N1 N

*Other: Cenacort A-40, Kenaject-40,
Kenalog, Triam A, Triesence, Tri-Kort,
Trilog*

IOM: 100-02, 15, 50

Coding Clinic: 2018, Q4, P7; 2013, Q2, P4

⊛ **J3302** Injection, triamcinolone diacetate,
per 5 mg ⑧ ⑤ **Qp** **Qh**   N1 N

*Other: Amcort, Aristocort , Cenacort
Forte, Trilone*

IOM: 100-02, 15, 50

⊛ **J3303** Injection, triamcinolone hexacetonide,
per 5 mg ⑧ ⑤ **Qp** **Qh**   N1 N

Other: Aristospan

IOM: 100-02, 15, 50

⊛ **J3304** Injection, triamcinolone acetonide,
preservative-free, extended-release,
microsphere formulation, 1 mg ⑧ ⑤   G

Other: Zilretta

▶ **New**   ⮌ **Revised**   ✔ **Reinstated**   ~~deleted~~ **Deleted**   ⊘ **Not covered or valid by Medicare**
⊛ **Special coverage instructions**   ✳ **Carrier discretion**   ⑧ **Bill Part B MAC**   ⑤ **Bill DME MAC**

J3305 Injection, trimetrexate glucuronate, per 25 mg Ⓜ Ⓑ Qp Qh   E2

Other: NeuTrexin

IOM: 100-02, 15, 50

J3310 Injection, perphenazine, up to 5 mg Ⓜ Ⓑ Qp Qh   N1 N

Other: Trilafon

IOM: 100-02, 15, 50

J3315 Injection, triptorelin pamoate, 3.75 mg Ⓑ Ⓑ Qp Qh   K2 K

Other: Trelstar

IOM: 100-02, 15, 50

J3316 Injection, triptorelin, extended-release, 3.75 mg Ⓑ Ⓑ   G

Other: Trelstar, Trelstar Depot, Trelstar LA

J3320 Injection, spectinomycin dihydrochloride, up to 2 gm Ⓜ Ⓑ Qp Qh   E2

Other: Trobicin

IOM: 100-02, 15, 50

J3350 Injection, urea, up to 40 gm Ⓑ Ⓑ Qp Qh   N1 N

Other: Ureaphil

IOM: 100-02, 15, 50

J3355 Injection, urofollitropin, 75 IU Ⓑ Ⓑ Qp Qh   E2

Other: Bravelle, Metrodin

IOM: 100-02, 15, 50

*** J3357** Ustekinumab, for subcutaneous injection, 1 mg Ⓑ Ⓑ Qp Qh   K2 K

Other: Stelara

Coding Clinic: 2017, Q1, P3; 2016, Q4, P10; 2011, Q1, P7

*** J3358** Ustekinumab, for intravenous injection, 1 mg   K2 G

Cross Reference Q9989

J3360 Injection, diazepam, up to 5 mg Ⓜ Ⓑ Qp Qh   N1 N

Other: Valium, Zetran

IOM: 100-02, 15, 50

Coding Clinic: 2007, Q2, P6-7

J3364 Injection, urokinase, 5000 IU vial Ⓜ Ⓑ Qp Qh   N1 N

Other: Abbokinase

IOM: 100-02, 15, 50

J3365 Injection, IV, urokinase, 250,000 IU vial Ⓜ Ⓑ Qp Qh   E2

Other: Abbokinase

IOM: 100-02, 15, 50,

Cross Reference Q0089

J3370 Injection, vancomycin HCL, 500 mg Ⓜ Ⓑ Qp Qh   N1 N

Other: Vancocin, Vancoled

IOM: 100-02, 15, 50; 100-03, 4, 280.14

J3371 Injection, vancomycin hcl (mylan) not therapeutically equivalent to J3370, 500 mg   N

J3372 Injection, vancomycin hcl (xellia) not therapeutically equivalent to J3370, 500 mg   N

J3380 Injection, vedolizumab, 1 mg Ⓜ Ⓑ Qp Qh   K2 K

Other: Entyvio

*** J3385** Injection, velaglucerase alfa, 100 units Ⓑ Ⓑ Qp Qh   K2 K

Enzyme replacement therapy in Gaucher Disease that results from a specific enzyme deficiency in the body, caused by a genetic mutation received from both parents. Type 1 is the most prevalent Ashkenazi Jewish genetic disease, occurring in one in every 1,000.

Other: VPRIV

Coding Clinic: 2011, Q1, P7

J3396 Injection, verteporfin, 0.1 mg Ⓜ Ⓑ Qp Qh   K2 K

Other: Visudyne

IOM: 100-03, 1, 80.2; 100-03, 1, 80.3

*** J3397** Injection, vestronidase alfa-vjbk, 1 mg Ⓜ Ⓑ   K

Other: Mepsevii

*** J3398** Injection, voretigene neparvovec-rzyl, 1 billion vector genomes Ⓑ Ⓑ   G

Other: Luxturna

*** J3399** Injection, onasemnogene abeparvovec-xioi, per treatment, up to 5x10^15 vector genomes   K

J3400 Injection, triflupromazine HCL, up to 20 mg Ⓜ Ⓑ Qp Qh   E2

Other: Vesprin

IOM: 100-02, 15, 50

J3410 Injection, hydroxyzine HCL, up to 25 mg Ⓜ Ⓑ Qp Qh   N1 N

Other: Hyzine-50, Vistaject 25, Vistaril

IOM: 100-02, 15, 50

*** J3411** Injection, thiamine HCL, 100 mg Ⓑ Ⓑ Qp Qh   N1 N

Ⓜ MIPS   Qp Quantity Physician   Qh Quantity Hospital   ♀ Female only

♂ Male only   Ⓐ Age   🦽 DMEPOS   A2-Z3 ASC Payment Indicator   A-Y ASC Status Indicator   Coding Clinic

✳ **J3415** Injection, pyridoxine HCL, 100 mg Ⓠ Ⓖ Qp Qh   N1 N

⊛ **J3420** Injection, vitamin B-12 cyanocobalamin, up to 1000 mcg Ⓑ Ⓖ Qp Qh   N1 N

Medicare carriers may have local coverage decisions regarding vitamin B12 injections that provide reimbursement only for patients with certain types of anemia and other conditions.

Other: Berubigen, Betalin 12, Cobex, Redisol, Rubramin PC, Sytobex

IOM: 100-02, 15, 50; 100-03, 2, 150.6

⊛ **J3430** Injection, phytonadione (vitamin K), per 1 mg Ⓑ Ⓖ Qp Qh   N1 N

Other: AquaMephyton, Konakion, Menadione, Synkavite, Vitamin K1

IOM: 100-02, 15, 50

⊛ **J3465** Injection, voriconazole, 10 mg Ⓑ Ⓖ Qp Qh   K2 K

Other: VFEND

IOM: 100-02, 15, 50

⊛ **J3470** Injection, hyaluronidase, up to 150 units Ⓠ Ⓑ Qp Qh   N1 N

Other: Amphadase, Wydase

IOM: 100-02, 15, 50

⊛ **J3471** Injection, hyaluronidase, ovine, preservative free, per 1 USP unit (up to 999 USP units) Ⓠ Ⓑ Qp Qh   N1 N

Other: Vitrase

⊛ **J3472** Injection, hyaluronidase, ovine, preservative free, per 1000 USP units Ⓑ Ⓖ Qp Qh   N1 N

⊛ **J3473** Injection, hyaluronidase, recombinant, 1 USP unit Ⓑ Ⓖ Qp Qh   N1 N

Other: Hylenex

IOM: 100-02, 15, 50

⊛ **J3475** Injection, magnesium sulfate, per 500 mg Ⓑ Ⓖ Qp Qh   N1 N

IOM: 100-02, 15, 50

⊛ **J3480** Injection, potassium chloride, per 2 meq Ⓑ Ⓖ Qp Qh   N1 N

IOM: 100-02, 15, 50

⊛ **J3485** Injection, zidovudine, 10 mg Ⓑ Ⓖ Qp Qh   N1 N

Other: Retrovir

IOM: 100-02, 15, 50

✳ **J3486** Injection, ziprasidone mesylate, 10 mg Ⓑ Ⓖ Qp Qh   N1 N

Other: Geodon

✳ **J3489** Injection, zoledronic acid, 1 mg Ⓠ Ⓑ Qp Qh   N1 N

Other: Reclast, Zometra

⊛ **J3490** Unclassified drugs Ⓠ Ⓖ   N1 N

Bill on paper. Bill one unit. Identify drug and total dosage in "Remarks" field.

Other: Acthib, Aminocaproic Acid, Baciim, Bacitracin, Benzocaine, Bumetanide, Bupivacaine, Cefotetan, Ciprofloxacin, Cleocin Phosphate, Clindamycin, Cortisone Acetate Micronized, Definity, Diprivan, Doxy, Engerix-B, Ethanolamine, Famotidine, Ganirelix, Gonal-F, Hyaluronic Acid, Marcaine, Metronidazole, Nafcillin, Naltrexone, Ovidrel, Pegasys, Peg-Intron, Penicillin G Sodium, Propofol, Protonix, Recombivax, Rifadin, Rifampin, Sensorcaine-MPF, Smz-TMP, Sufentanil Citrate, Testopel Pellets, Testosterone, Treanda, Valcyte, Veritas Collagen Matrix

IOM: 100-02, 15, 50

Coding Clinic: 2017, Q1, P1-3, P8; 2014, Q2, P6; 2013, Q2, P3-4

⊘ **J3520** Edetate disodium, per 150 mg Ⓠ Ⓑ Qp Qh   E1

Other: Chealamide, Disotate, Endrate ethylenediamine-tetra-acetic

IOM: 100-03, 1, 20.21; 100-03, 1, 20.22

⊛ **J3530** Nasal vaccine inhalation Ⓑ Ⓖ Qp Qh   N1 N

IOM: 100-02, 15, 50

⊘ **J3535** Drug administered through a metered dose inhaler Ⓠ Ⓑ   E1

Other: Ipratropium bromide

IOM: 100-02, 15, 50

⊘ **J3570** Laetrile, amygdalin, vitamin B-17 Ⓠ Ⓖ   E1

IOM: 100-03, 1, 30.7

✳ **J3590** Unclassified biologics Ⓑ   N1 N

Bill on paper. Bill one unit. Identify drug and total dosage in "Remarks" field.

Coding Clinic: 2017, Q1, P1-3; 2016, Q4, P10

✳ **J3591** Unclassified drug or biological used for ESRD on dialysis Ⓠ   B

⊛ **J7030** Infusion, normal saline solution, 1000 cc Ⓠ Ⓑ Qp Qh   N1 N

Other: Sodium Chloride

IOM: 100-02, 15, 50

▶ New   ↻ Revised   ✔ Reinstated   ~~deleted~~ Deleted   ⊘ Not covered or valid by Medicare
⊛ Special coverage instructions   ✳ Carrier discretion   Ⓑ Bill Part B MAC   Ⓖ Bill DME MAC

⊕ **J7040** Infusion, normal saline solution, sterile (500 ml = 1 unit) Ⓑ Ⓖ Qp Qh   N1 N

Other: Sodium Chloride

IOM: 100-02, 15, 50

⊕ **J7042** 5% dextrose/normal saline (500 ml = 1 unit) Ⓑ Ⓖ Qp Qh   N1 N

Other: Dextrose-Nacl

IOM: 100-02, 15, 50

⊕ **J7050** Infusion, normal saline solution, 250 cc Ⓑ Ⓖ Qp Qh   N1 N

Other: Sodium Chloride

IOM: 100-02, 15, 50

⊕ **J7060** 5% dextrose/water (500 ml = 1 unit) Ⓑ Ⓖ Qp Qh   N1 N

IOM: 100-02, 15, 50

⊕ **J7070** Infusion, D 5 W, 1000 cc Ⓑ Ⓖ Qp Qh   N1 N

Other: Dextrose

IOM: 100-02, 15, 50

⊕ **J7100** Infusion, dextran 40, 500 ml Ⓑ Ⓖ Qp Qh   N1 N

Other: Gentran, LMD, Rheomacrodex

IOM: 100-02, 15, 50

⊕ **J7110** Infusion, dextran 75, 500 ml Ⓑ Ⓖ Qp Qh   N1 N

Other: Gentran 75

IOM: 100-02, 15, 50

⊕ **J7120** Ringer's lactate infusion, up to 1000 cc Ⓑ Ⓖ Qp Qh   N1 N

Replacement fluid or electrolytes.

Other: Potassium Chloride

IOM: 100-02, 15, 50

⊕ **J7121** 5% dextrose in lactated ringers infusion, up to 1000 cc Ⓑ Ⓖ Qp Qh   N1 N

IOM: 100-02, 15, 50

⊕ **J7131** Hypertonic saline solution, 1 ml Ⓥ Ⓑ Ⓖ Qp Qh   N1 N

IOM: 100-02, 15, 50

Coding Clinic: 2012, Q1, P9

Clotting Factors

✳ **J7168** Prothrombin complex concentrate (human), kcentra, per i.u. of factor ix activity   K2 K

✳ **J7169** Injection, coagulation factor xa (recombinant), inactivated-zhzo (andexxa), 10 mg   K2 K

✳ **J7170** Injection, emicizumab-kxwh, 0.5 mg Ⓑ   G

Other: Hemlibra

✳ **J7175** Injection, Factor X, (human), 1 IU Ⓑ Qp Qh   K2 K

Coding Clinic: 2017, Q1, P9

✳ **J7177** Injection, human fibrinogen concentrate (fibryga), 1 mg Ⓑ   K

✳ **J7178** Injection, human fibrinogen concentrate, not otherwise specified, 1 mg Ⓥ Qp Qh   K2 K

Other: Riastap

⊕ **J7179** Injection, von Willebrand factor (recombinant), (vonvendi), 1 IU VWF:RCo Ⓥ Qp Qh   K2 G

Coding Clinic: 2017, Q1, P9

✳ **J7180** Injection, factor XIII (antihemophilic factor, human), 1 IU Ⓥ Qp Qh   K2 N

Other: Corifact

Coding Clinic: 2012, Q1, P8

✳ **J7181** Injection, factor XIII a-subunit, (recombinant), per IU Ⓑ Qp Qh   K2 N

✳ **J7182** Injection, factor VIII, (antihemophilic factor, recombinant), (novoeight), per IU Ⓑ Qp Qh   K2 K

⊕ **J7183** Injection, von Willebrand factor complex (human), wilate, 1 IU VWF:RCo Ⓥ Qp Qh   K2 K

IOM: 100-02, 15, 50

Coding Clinic: 2012, Q1, P9

✳ **J7185** Injection, Factor VIII (antihemophilic factor, recombinant) (Xyntha), per IU Ⓑ Qp Qh   K2 K

⊕ **J7186** Injection, anti-hemophilic factor VIII/von Willebrand factor complex (human), per factor VIII IU Ⓥ Qp Qh   K2 K

Other: Alphanate

IOM: 100-02, 15, 50

⊕ **J7187** Injection, von Willebrand factor complex (HUMATE-P), per IU VWF:RCo Ⓑ Qp Qh   K2 K

Other: Humate-P Low Dilutent

IOM: 100-02, 15, 50

⊕ **J7188** Injection, factor VIII (antihemophilic factor, recombinant), (obizur), per IU Ⓥ Qp Qh   K2 K

IOM: 100-02, 15, 50

⊕ **J7189** Factor VIIa (anti-hemophilic factor, recombinant), (novoseven rt), per 1 mcg Ⓑ Qp Qh   K2 K

Other: NovoSeven

IOM: 100-02, 15, 50

🐾 **MIPS**   Qp **Quantity Physician**   Qh **Quantity Hospital**   ♀ **Female only**

♂ **Male only**   Ⓐ **Age**   ⅙ **DMEPOS**   A2-Z3 **ASC Payment Indicator**   A-Y **ASC Status Indicator**   Coding Clinic

⊛ **J7190** Factor VIII anti-hemophilic factor, human, per IU Ⓑ 𝗤𝗽 𝗤𝗵 K2 K

Other: Alphanate/von Willebrand factor complex, Hemofil M, Koate DVI, Koate-HP, Kogenate, Monoclate-P, Recombinate

IOM: 100-02, 15, 50

⊛ **J7191** Factor VIII, anti-hemophilic factor (porcine), per IU Ⓑ 𝗤𝗽 𝗤𝗵 E2

Other: Hyate:C, Koate-HP, Kogenate, Monoclate-P, Recombinate

IOM: 100-02, 15, 50

⊛ **J7192** Factor VIII (anti-hemophilic factor, recombinant) per IU, not otherwise specified Ⓑ 𝗤𝗽 𝗤𝗵 K2 K

Other: Advate, Helixate FS, Kogenate FS, Koate-HP, Recombinate, Xyntha

IOM: 100-02, 15, 50

⊛ **J7193** Factor IX (anti-hemophilic factor, purified, non-recombinant) per IU Ⓑ 𝗤𝗽 𝗤𝗵 K2 K

Other: AlphaNine SD, Mononine, Proplex

IOM: 100-02, 15, 50

⊛ **J7194** Factor IX, complex, per IU Ⓑ 𝗤𝗽 𝗤𝗵 K2 K

Other: Bebulin, Konyne-80, Profilnine Heat-treated, Profilnine SD, Proplex SX-T, Proplex T

IOM: 100-02, 15, 50

⊛ **J7195** Injection, Factor IX (anti-hemophilic factor, recombinant) per IU, not otherwise specified Ⓑ 𝗤𝗽 𝗤𝗵 K2 K

Other: Benefix, Profiline, Proplex T

IOM: 100-02, 15, 50

✳ **J7196** Injection, antithrombin recombinant, 50 IU Ⓑ 𝗤𝗽 𝗤𝗵 E2

Other: ATryn, Feiba VH Immuno

Coding Clinic: 2011, Q1, P6

⊛ **J7197** Anti-thrombin III (human), per IU Ⓑ 𝗤𝗽 𝗤𝗵 K2 K

Other: Thrombate III

IOM: 100-02, 15, 50

⊛ **J7198** Anti-inhibitor, per IU Ⓑ 𝗤𝗽 𝗤𝗵 K2 K

Diagnosis examples: D66 Congenital Factor VIII disorder; D67 Congenital Factor IX disorder; D68.0 VonWillebrand's disease

Other: Autoplex T, Feiba NF, Hemophilia clotting factors

IOM: 100-02, 15, 50; 100-03, 2, 110.3

⊛ **J7199** Hemophilia clotting factor, not otherwise classified Ⓑ B

Other: Autoplex T

IOM: 100-02, 15, 50; 100-03, 2, 110.3

⊛ **J7200** Injection, factor IX, (antihemophilic factor, recombinant), rixubis, per IU Ⓑ 𝗤𝗽 𝗤𝗵 K2 K

IOM: 100-02, 15, 50

⊛ **J7201** Injection, factor IX, fc fusion protein (recombinant), alprolix, 1 IU Ⓑ 𝗤𝗽 𝗤𝗵 K2 K

IOM: 100-02, 15, 50

⊛ **J7202** Injection, Factor IX, albumin fusion protein, (recombinant), idelvion, 1 IU 𝗤𝗽 𝗤𝗵 K2 G

Coding Clinic: 2016, Q4, P9

⊛ **J7203** Injection Factor IX, (antihemophilic factor, recombinant), glycopegylated, (rebinyn), 1 iu G

Other: Profilnine SD, Bebulin VH, Bebulin, Proplex T

⊛ **J7204** Injection, Factor VIII, antihemophilic factor (recombinant), (esperoct), glycopegylated-exei, per iu K2 G

⊛ **J7205** Injection, Factor VIII Fc fusion protein (recombinant), per IU Ⓑ 𝗤𝗽 𝗤𝗵 K2 K

Other: Eloctate

⊛ **J7207** Injection, Factor VIII, (antihemophilic factor, recombinant), PEGylated, 1 IU 𝗤𝗽 𝗤𝗵 K2 G

Other: Adynovate

⊛ **J7208** Injection, Factor VIII, (antihemophilic factor, recombinant), pegylated-aucl, (jivi), 1 i.u. K2 G

✳ **J7209** Injection, Factor VIII, (antihemophilic factor, recombinant), (Nuwiq), 1 IU 𝗤𝗽 𝗤𝗵 K2 G

✳ **J7210** Injection, Factor VIII, (antihemophilic factor, recombinant), (afstyla), 1 i.u. Ⓑ K2 G

✳ **J7211** Injection, Factor VIII, (antihemophilic factor, recombinant), (kovaltry), 1 i.u. Ⓑ K2 K

J7212 Factor VIIA (antihemophilic factor, recombinant)-jncw (sevenfact), 1 microgram K2 K

▶ **J7213** Injection, coagulation Factor IX (recombinant), ixinity, 1 IU

▶ **J7214** Injection, Factor VIII/von willebrand factor complex, recombinant (altuviiio), per factor VIII IU

Contraceptives

⊘ **J7294** Segesterone acetate and ethinyl estradiol 0.15mg, 0.013mg per 24 hours; yearly vaginal system, each E1

▶ New ↻ Revised ✔ Reinstated ~~deleted~~ Deleted ⊘ Not covered or valid by Medicare
⊛ Special coverage instructions ✳ Carrier discretion Ⓑ Bill Part B MAC Ⓑ Bill DME MAC

⊘ **J7295** Ethinyl estradiol and etonogestrel 0.015mg, 0.12mg per 24 hours; monthly vaginal ring, each   E1

⊘ **J7296** Levonorgestrel-releasing intrauterine contraceptive system (Kyleena), 19.5 mg ⑧ ♀   E1

Medicare Statute 1862(a)(1)

Cross Reference Q9984

⊘ **J7297** Levonorgestrel-releasing intrauterine contraceptive system (Liletta), 52 mg ⑧ [Qp] [Qh] ♀   E1

Medicare Statute 1862(a)(1)

⊘ **J7298** Levonorgestrel-releasing intrauterine contraceptive system (Mirena), 52 mg ⑧ [Qp] [Qh] ♀   E1

Medicare Statute 1862(a)(1)

Coding Clinic: 2023, Q1, P21

⊘ **J7300** Intrauterine copper contraceptive ⑧ ♀   E1

Report IUD insertion with 58300. Bill usual and customary charge.

Other: Paragard T 380 A

Medicare Statute 1862a1

⊘ **J7301** Levonorgestrel-releasing intrauterine contraceptive system (Skyla), 13.5 mg ⑧ [Qp] [Qh] ♀   E1

Medicare Statute 1862(a)(1)

⊘ **J7304** Contraceptive supply, hormone containing patch, each ⑧ ♀   E1

Only billed by Family Planning Clinics

Medicare Statute 1862.1

⊘ **J7306** Levonorgestrel (contraceptive) implant system, including implants and supplies ⑧ ♀   E1

⊘ **J7307** Etonogestrel (contraceptive) implant system, including implant and supplies ⑧ ♀   E1

Aminolevulinic Acid HCL

✳ **J7308** Aminolevulinic acid HCL for topical administration, 20%, single unit dosage form (354 mg) ⑧ [Qp] [Qh]   K2 K

Other: Levulan Kerastick

✵ **J7309** Methyl aminolevulinate (MAL) for topical administration, 16.8%, 1 gram ⑧ [Qp] [Qh]   N1 N

Other: Metvixia

Coding Clinic: 2011, Q1, P6

Ganciclovir

✵ **J7310** Ganciclovir, 4.5 mg, long-acting implant ⑧ [Qp] [Qh]   E2

IOM: 100-02, 15, 50

Ophthalmic Drugs

✳ **J7311** Injection, fluocinolone acetonide, intravitreal implant (retisert), 0.01 mg ⑧ [Qp] [Qh]   K2 K

Treatment of chronic noninfectious posterior segment uveitis

Other: Retisert

✳ **J7312** Injection, dexamethasone, intravitreal implant, 0.1 mg ⑧ [Qp] [Qh]   K2 K

To bill for Ozurdex services submit the following codes: J7312 and 67028 with the modifier -22 (for the increased work difficulty and increased risk). Indicated for the treatment of macular edema occurring after branch retinal vein occlusion (BRVO) or central retinal vein occlusion (CRVO) and non-infectious uveitis affecting the posterior segment of the eye.

Other: Ozurdex

Coding Clinic: 2011, Q1, P7

✳ **J7313** Injection, fluocinolone acetonide, intravitreal implant (iluvien), 0.01 mg ⑧ [Qp] [Qh]   K2 K

Other: Iluvien

✳ **J7314** Injection, fluocinolone acetonide, intravitreal implant (yutiq), 0.01 mg   K2 G

✳ **J7315** Mitomycin, ophthalmic, 0.2 mg ⑧ [Qp] [Qh]   N1 N

Other: Mitosol, Mutamycin

Coding Clinic: 2016, Q4, P8; 2014, Q2, P6

✳ **J7316** Injection, ocriplasmin, 0.125 mg ⑧ [Qp] [Qh]   K2 K

Other: Jetrea

Hyaluronan

✳ **J7318** Hyaluronan or derivative, durolane, for intra-articular injection, 1 mg ⑧   G

Other: Morisu

✳ **J7320** Hyaluronan or derivitive, genvisc 850, for intra-articular injection, 1 mg ⑧ [Qp] [Qh]   K2 K

🐾 **MIPS**   [Qp] **Quantity Physician**   [Qh] **Quantity Hospital**   ♀ **Female only**

♂ **Male only**   Ⓐ **Age**   ♿ **DMEPOS**   A2-Z3 **ASC Payment Indicator**   A-Y **ASC Status Indicator**   Coding Clinic

* **J7321** Hyaluronan or derivative, Hyalgan, Supartz or Visco-3, for intra-articular injection, per dose Ⓑ **Qp** **Qh**   K2 K

Therapeutic goal is to restore visco-elasticity of synovial hyaluronan, thereby decreasing pain, improving mobility and restoring natural protective functions of hyaluronan in joint

* **J7322** Hyaluronan or derivative, hymovis, for intra-articular injection, 1 mg Ⓑ **Qp** **Qh**   K2 G

* **J7323** Hyaluronan or derivative, Euflexxa, for intra-articular injection, per dose Ⓑ **Qp** **Qh**   K2 K

* **J7324** Hyaluronan or derivative, Orthovisc, for intra-articular injection, per dose Ⓑ **Qp** **Qh**   K2 K

* **J7325** Hyaluronan or derivative, Synvisc or Synvisc-One, for intra-articular injection, 1 mg Ⓑ **Qp** **Qh**   K2 K

* **J7326** Hyaluronan or derivative, Gel-One, for intra-articular injection, per dose Ⓑ **Qp** **Qh**   K2 K

Coding Clinic: 2012, Q1, P8

* **J7327** Hyaluronan or derivative, monovisc, for intra-articular injection, per dose Ⓑ **Qp** **Qh**   K2 K

* **J7328** Hyaluronan or derivative, gelsyn-3, for intra-articular injection, 0.1 mg Ⓑ **Qp** **Qh**   K2 G

* **J7329** Hyaluronan or derivative, trivisc, for intra-articular injection, 1 mg Ⓑ   E2

Miscellaneous Drugs

* **J7330** Autologous cultured chondrocytes, implant Ⓑ **Qp** **Qh**   B

Other: Carticel

Coding Clinic: 2010, Q4, P3

* **J7331** Hyaluronan or derivative, synojoynt, for intra-articular injection, 1 mg Ⓑ   K

* **J7332** Hyaluronan or derivative, triluron, for intra-articular injection, 1 mg Ⓑ   N

* **J7336** Capsaicin 8% patch, per square centimeter Ⓑ **Qp** **Qh**   K2 K

Other: Qutenza

* **J7340** Carbidopa 5 mg/levodopa 20 mg enteral suspension, 100 ml Ⓑ Ⓑ **Qp** **Qh**   K2 K

Other: Duopa

* **J7342** Instillation, ciprofloxacin otic suspension, 6 mg Ⓑ **Qp** **Qh**   K2 G

⊘ **J7345** Aminolevulinic acid HCL for topical administration, 10% gel, 10 mg Ⓑ   K2 G

* **J7351** Injection, bimatoprost, intracameral implant, 1 microgram   K2 G

* **J7352** Afamelanotide implant, 1 mg   K2 K

▶ **J7353** Anacaulase-bcdb, 8.8% gel, 1 gram

* **J7402** Mometasone furoate sinus implant, (sinuva), 10 micrograms   K2 G

Immunosuppressive Drugs (Includes Non-injectibles)

⊘ **J7500** Azathioprine, oral, 50 mg Ⓥ Ⓑ **Qp** **Qh**   N1 N

Other: Azasan, Imuran

IOM: 100-02, 15, 50

⊘ **J7501** Azathioprine, parenteral, 100 mg Ⓑ Ⓑ **Qp** **Qh**   K2 K

Other: Imuran

IOM: 100-02, 15, 50

⊘ **J7502** Cyclosporine, oral, 100 mg Ⓥ Ⓑ **Qp** **Qh**   N1 N

Other: Gengraf, Neoral, Sandimmune

IOM: 100-02, 15, 50

⊘ **J7503** Tacrolimus, extended release, (Envarsus XR), oral, 0.25 mg Ⓥ Ⓑ **Qp** **Qh**   K2 G

IOM: 100-02, 15, 50

⊘ **J7504** Lymphocyte immune globulin, antithymocyte globulin, equine, parenteral, 250 mg Ⓥ Ⓑ **Qp** **Qh**   K2 K

Other: Atgam

IOM: 100-02, 15, 50; 100-03, 2, 110.3

⊘ **J7505** Muromonab-CD3, parenteral, 5 mg Ⓥ Ⓑ **Qp** **Qh**   K2 K

Other: Monoclonal antibodies (parenteral)

IOM: 100-02, 15, 50

⊘ **J7507** Tacrolimus, immediate release, oral, 1 mg Ⓥ Ⓑ **Qp** **Qh**   N1 N

Other: Prograf

IOM: 100-02, 15, 50

⊘ **J7508** Tacrolimus, extended release, (Astagraf XL), oral, 0.1 mg Ⓥ Ⓑ **Qp** **Qh**   N1 N

IOM: 100-02, 15, 50

⊘ **J7509** Methylprednisolone oral, per 4 mg Ⓑ Ⓥ **Qp** **Qh**   N1 N

Other: Medrol

IOM: 100-02, 15, 50

⊘ **J7510** Prednisolone oral, per 5 mg Ⓥ Ⓑ **Qp** **Qh**   N1 N

Other: Delta-Cortef, Flo-Pred, Orapred

IOM: 100-02, 15, 50

▶ New   ↻ Revised   ✔ Reinstated   ~~deleted~~ Deleted   ⊘ Not covered or valid by Medicare
⊘ Special coverage instructions   * Carrier discretion   Ⓑ Bill Part B MAC   Ⓑ Bill DME MAC

* **J7511** Lymphocyte immune globulin, antithymocyte globulin, rabbit, parenteral, 25 mg ⊙ Ⓑ Ⓠp Ⓠh   K2 K

     Other: Thymoglobulin

⊛ **J7512** Prednisone, immediate release or delayed release, oral, 1 mg Ⓥ Ⓑ Ⓠp Ⓠh   N1 N

     Other: Cyclosporine

     IOM: 100-02, 15, 50

⊛ **J7513** Daclizumab, parenteral, 25 mg ⊙ Ⓑ Ⓠp Ⓠh   E2

     Other: Zenapax

     IOM: 100-02, 15, 50

* **J7515** Cyclosporine, oral, 25 mg ⊙ Ⓑ Ⓠp Ⓠh   N1 N

     Other: Gengraf, Neoral, Sandimmune

* **J7516** Cyclosporin, parenteral, 250 mg Ⓑ Ⓑ Ⓠp Ⓠh   N1 N

     Other: Sandimmune

* **J7517** Mycophenolate mofetil, oral, 250 mg ⊙ Ⓑ Ⓠp Ⓠh   N1 N

     Other: CellCept

⊛ **J7518** Mycophenolic acid, oral, 180 mg Ⓑ ⊙ Ⓠp Ⓠh   N1 N

     Other: Myfortic

     IOM: 100-04, 4, 240; 100-4, 17, 80.3.1

▶ **J7519** Injection, mycophenolate mofetil, 10 mg   N1 N

⊛ **J7520** Sirolimus, oral, 1 mg ⊙ Ⓑ Ⓠp Ⓠh   N1 N

     Other: Rapamune

     IOM: 100-02, 15, 50

⊛ **J7525** Tacrolimus, parenteral, 5 mg ⊙ ⊙ Ⓠp Ⓠh   K2 K

     Other: Prograf

     IOM: 100-02, 15, 50

⊛ **J7527** Everolimus, oral, 0.25 mg ⊙ ⊙ Ⓠp Ⓠh   N1 N

     Other: Zortress

     IOM: 100-02, 15, 50

⊛ **J7599** Immunosuppressive drug, not otherwise classified Ⓑ ⊙   N1 N

     Bill on paper. Bill one unit. Identify drug and total dosage in "Remarks" field.

     IOM: 100-02, 15, 50

Inhalation Solutions

* **J7604** Acetylcysteine, inhalation solution, compounded product, administered through DME, unit dose form, per gram Ⓑ ⊙ Ⓠp Ⓠh   M

     Other: Mucomyst (unit dose form), Mucosol

* **J7605** Arformoterol, inhalation solution, FDA approved final product, non-compounded, administered through DME, unit dose form, 15 mcg ⊙ ⊙ Ⓠp Ⓠh   M

     Maintenance treatment of bronchoconstriction in patients with chronic obstructive pulmonary disease (COPD).

     Other: Brovana

* **J7606** Formoterol fumarate, inhalation solution, FDA approved final product, non-compounded, administered through DME, unit dose form, 20 mcg ⊙ ⊙ Ⓠp Ⓠh   M

     Other: Perforomist

* **J7607** Levalbuterol, inhalation solution, compounded product, administered through DME, concentrated form, 0.5 mg ⊙ ⊙ Ⓠp Ⓠh   M

⊛ **J7608** Acetylcysteine, inhalation solution, FDA-approved final product, non-compounded, administered through DME, unit dose form, per gram ⊙ ⊙ Ⓠp Ⓠh   M

     Other: Mucomyst, Mucosol

* **J7609** Albuterol, inhalation solution, compounded product, administered through DME, unit dose, 1 mg ⊙ ⊙ Ⓠp Ⓠh   M

     Patient's home, medications—such as a albuterol when administered through a nebulizer—are considered DME and are payable under Part B.

     Other: Proventil, Ventolin, Xopenex

* **J7610** Albuterol, inhalation solution, compounded product, administered through DME, concentrated form, 1 mg ⊙ ⊙ Ⓠp Ⓠh   M

     Other: Proventil, Ventolin, Xopenex

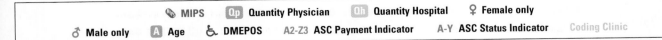

🐾 MIPS   Ⓠp **Quantity Physician**   Ⓠh **Quantity Hospital**   ♀ **Female only**

♂ **Male only**   Ⓐ **Age**   ♿ **DMEPOS**   A2-Z3 **ASC Payment Indicator**   A-Y **ASC Status Indicator**   Coding Clinic

⊛ **J7611** Albuterol, inhalation solution, FDA-approved final product, non-compounded, administered through DME, concentrated form, 1 mg Ⓑ Ⓓ Qp Qh M

Report once for each milligram administered. For example, 2 mg of concentrated albuterol (usually diluted with saline), reported with J7611×2.

Other: Proventil, Ventolin, Xopenex

⊛ **J7612** Levalbuterol, inhalation solution, FDA-approved final product, non-compounded, administered through DME, concentrated form, 0.5 mg Ⓑ Ⓓ Qp Qh M

Other: Xopenex

⊛ **J7613** Albuterol, inhalation solution, FDA-approved final product, non-compounded, administered through DME, unit dose, 1 mg Ⓑ Ⓓ Qp Qh M

Other: Accuneb, Proventil, Ventolin, Xopenex

⊛ **J7614** Levalbuterol, inhalation solution, FDA-approved final product, non-compounded, administered through DME, unit dose, 0.5 mg Ⓑ Ⓓ Qp Qh M

Other: Xopenex

✳ **J7615** Levalbuterol, inhalation solution, compounded product, administered through DME, unit dose, 0.5 mg Ⓑ Ⓓ Qp Qh M

⊛ **J7620** Albuterol, up to 2.5 mg and ipratropium bromide, up to 0.5 mg,FDA-approved final product, non-compounded, administered through DME Ⓑ Ⓓ Qp Qh M

Other: DuoNeb

✳ **J7622** Beclomethasone, inhalation solution, compounded product, administered through DME, unit dose form, per mg Ⓑ Ⓓ Qp Qh M

✳ **J7624** Betamethasone, inhalation solution, compounded product, administered through DME, unit dose form, per mg Ⓑ Ⓓ Qp Qh M

✳ **J7626** Budesonide inhalation solution, FDA-approved final product, non-compounded, administered through DME, unit dose form, up to 0.5 mg Ⓑ Ⓓ Qp Qh M

Other: Pulmicort

✳ **J7627** Budesonide, inhalation solution, compounded product, administered through DME, unit dose form, up to 0.5 mg Ⓑ Ⓓ Qp Qh M

Other: Pulmicort Respules

⊛ **J7628** Bitolterol mesylate, inhalation solution, compounded product, administered through DME, concentrated form, per milligram Ⓑ Ⓓ Qp Qh M

Other: Tornalate

⊛ **J7629** Bitolterol mesylate, inhalation solution, compounded product, administered through DME, unit dose form, per milligram Ⓑ Ⓓ Qp Qh M

Other: Tornalate

⊛ **J7631** Cromolyn sodium, inhalation solution, FDA-approved final product, non-compounded, administered through DME, unit dose form, per 10 mg Ⓑ Ⓓ Qp Qh M

Other: Intal

✳ **J7632** Cromolyn sodium, inhalation solution, compounded product, administered through DME, unit dose, per 10 mg Ⓑ Ⓓ Qp Qh M

Other: Intal

✳ **J7633** Budesonide, inhalation solution, FDA-approved final product, non-compounded, administered through DME, concentrated form, per 0.25 mg Ⓑ Ⓓ Qp Qh M

Other: Pulmicort Respules

✳ **J7634** Budesonide, inhalation solution, compounded product, administered through DME, concentrated form, per 0.25 mg Ⓑ Ⓓ Qp Qh M

Other: Pulmicort Respules

⊛ **J7635** Atropine, inhalation solution, compounded product, administered through DME, concentrated form, per milligram Ⓑ Ⓓ Qp Qh M

⊛ **J7636** Atropine, inhalation solution, compounded product, administered through DME, unit dose form, per milligram Ⓑ Ⓓ Qp Qh M

⊛ **J7637** Dexamethasone, inhalation solution, compounded product, administered through DME, concentrated form, per milligram Ⓑ Ⓓ Qp Qh M

⊛ **J7638** Dexamethasone, inhalation solution, compounded product, administered through DME, unit dose form, per milligram Ⓑ Ⓓ Qp Qh M

▶ New   ⟲ Revised   ✔ Reinstated   ~~deleted~~ Deleted   ⊘ Not covered or valid by Medicare
⊛ Special coverage instructions   ✳ Carrier discretion   Ⓑ Bill Part B MAC   Ⓓ Bill DME MAC

⊙ **J7639** Dornase alfa, inhalation solution, FDA-approved final product, non-compounded, administered through DME, unit dose form, per milligram Ⓑ Ⓑ Ⓠp Ⓠh M

Other: Pulmozyme

* **J7640** Formoterol, inhalation solution, compounded product, administered through DME, unit dose form, 12 mcg Ⓥ Ⓑ Ⓠp Ⓠh E1

* **J7641** Flunisolide, inhalation solution, compounded product, administered through DME, unit dose, per milligram Ⓥ Ⓑ Ⓠp Ⓠh M

⊙ **J7642** Glycopyrrolate, inhalation solution, compounded product, administered through DME, concentrated form, per milligram Ⓥ Ⓑ Ⓠp Ⓠh M

⊙ **J7643** Glycopyrrolate, inhalation solution, compounded product, administered through DME, unit dose form, per milligram Ⓥ Ⓑ Ⓠp Ⓠh M

⊙ **J7644** Ipratropium bromide, inhalation solution, FDA-approved final product, non-compounded, administered through DME, unit dose form, per milligram Ⓥ Ⓑ Ⓠp Ⓠh M

Other: Atrovent

* **J7645** Ipratropium bromide, inhalation solution, compounded product, administered through DME, unit dose form, per milligram Ⓑ Ⓥ Ⓠp Ⓠh M

Other: Atrovent

* **J7647** Isoetharine HCL, inhalation solution, compounded product, administered through DME, concentrated form, per milligram Ⓥ Ⓥ Ⓠp Ⓠh M

Other: Bronkosol

⊙ **J7648** Isoetharine HCL, inhalation solution, FDA-approved final product, non-compounded, administered through DME, concentrated form, per milligram Ⓥ Ⓥ Ⓠp Ⓠh M

Other: Bronkosol

⊙ **J7649** Isoetharine HCL, inhalation solution, FDA-approved final product, non-compounded, administered through DME, unit dose form, per milligram Ⓥ Ⓥ Ⓠp Ⓠh M

Other: Bronkosol

* **J7650** Isoetharine HCL, inhalation solution, compounded product, administered through DME, unit dose form, per milligram Ⓥ Ⓑ Ⓠp Ⓠh M

Other: Bronkosol

* **J7657** Isoproterenol HCL, inhalation solution, compounded product, administered through DME, concentrated form, per milligram Ⓑ Ⓑ Ⓠp Ⓠh M

Other: Isuprel

⊙ **J7658** Isoproterenol HCL inhalation solution, FDA-approved final product, non-compounded, administered through DME, concentrated form, per milligram Ⓥ Ⓑ Ⓠp Ⓠh M

Other: Isuprel

⊙ **J7659** Isoproterenol HCL, inhalation solution, FDA-approved final product, non-compounded, administered through DME, unit dose form, per milligram Ⓥ Ⓑ Ⓠp Ⓠh M

Other: Isuprel

* **J7660** Isoproterenol HCL, inhalation solution, compounded product, administered through DME, unit dose form, per milligram Ⓑ Ⓥ Ⓠp Ⓠh M

Other: Isuprel

* **J7665** Mannitol, administered through an inhaler, 5 mg Ⓥ Ⓑ Ⓠp Ⓠh N1 N

Other: Aridol

* **J7667** Metaproterenol sulfate, inhalation solution, compounded product, concentrated form, per 10 mg Ⓥ Ⓑ Ⓠp Ⓠh M

Other: Alupent, Metaprel

⊙ **J7668** Metaproterenol sulfate, inhalation solution, FDA-approved final product, non-compounded, administered through DME, concentrated form, per 10 mg Ⓥ Ⓑ Ⓠp Ⓠh M

Other: Alupent, Metaprel

⊙ **J7669** Metaproterenol sulfate, inhalation solution, FDA-approved final product, non-compounded, administered through DME, unit dose form, per 10 mg Ⓥ Ⓑ Ⓠp Ⓠh M

Other: Alupent, Metaprel

* **J7670** Metaproterenol sulfate, inhalation solution, compounded product, administered through DME, unit dose form, per 10 mg Ⓥ Ⓑ Ⓠp Ⓠh M

Other: Alupent, Metaprel

* **J7674** Methacholine chloride administered as inhalation solution through a nebulizer, per 1 mg Ⓥ Ⓥ Ⓠp Ⓠh N1 N

Other: Provocholine

🐾 **MIPS** Ⓠp **Quantity Physician** Ⓠh **Quantity Hospital** ♀ **Female only**
♂ **Male only** Ⓐ **Age** ♿ **DMEPOS** A2-Z3 **ASC Payment Indicator** A-Y **ASC Status Indicator** *Coding Clinic*

* **J7676** Pentamidine isethionate, inhalation solution, compounded product, administered through DME, unit dose form, per 300 mg ⒷⒼ **Qp** **Qh** M

Other: NebuPent, Pentam

* **J7677** Revefenacin inhalation solution, FDA-approved final product, non-compounded, administered through DME, 1 microgram M

* **J7680** Terbutaline sulfate, inhalation solution, compounded product, administered through DME, concentrated form, per milligram ⓅⒷ **Qp** **Qh** M

Other: Brethine

* **J7681** Terbutaline sulfate, inhalation solution, compounded product, administered through DME, unit dose form, per milligram ⓅⒷ **Qp** **Qh** M

Other: Brethine

* **J7682** Tobramycin, inhalation solution, FDA-approved final product, non-compounded unit dose form, administered through DME, per 300 mg ⒷⒼ **Qp** **Qh** M

Other: Bethkis, Kitabis PAK, Tobi

* **J7683** Triamcinolone, inhalation solution, compounded product, administered through DME, concentrated form, per milligram ⒷⒼ **Qp** **Qh** M

* **J7684** Triamcinolone, inhalation solution, compounded product, administered through DME, unit dose form, per milligram ⒷⒼ **Qp** **Qh** M

Other: Triamcinolone acetonide

* **J7685** Tobramycin, inhalation solution, compounded product, administered through DME, unit dose form, per 300 mg ⓅⒷⒼ **Qp** **Qh** M

Other: Tobi

* **J7686** Treprostinil, inhalation solution, FDA-approved final product, non-compounded, administered through DME, unit dose form, 1.74 mg ⓅⒷ **Qp** **Qh** M

Other: Tyvaso

Not Otherwise Classified/Specified

* **J7699** NOC drugs, inhalation solution administered through DME ⒷⒼ M

Other: Gentamicin Sulfate

* **J7799** NOC drugs, other than inhalation drugs, administered through DME ⓅⒷ N1 N

Bill on paper. Bill one unit and identify drug and total dosage in the "Remark" field.

Other: Cuvitru, Epinephrine, Mannitol, Osmitrol, Phenylephrine, Resectisol, Sodium chloride

IOM: 100-02, 15, 110.3

* **J7999** Compounded drug, not otherwise classified ⒷⒼ N1 N

Coding Clinic: 2017, Q1, P1-2; 2016, Q4, P8

* **J8498** Antiemetic drug, rectal/suppository, not otherwise specified Ⓖ B

Other: Compazine, Compro, Phenadoz, Phenergan, Prochlorperazine, Promethazine, Promethegan

Medicare Statute 1861(s)2t

⊘ **J8499** Prescription drug, oral, non chemotherapeutic, NOS ⓅⒷⒼ E1

Other: Acyclovir, Calcitrol, Cromolyn Sodium, OFEV, Valganciclovir HCL, Zovirax

IOM: 100-02, 15, 50

Coding Clinic: 2013, Q2, P4

Oral Anti-Cancer Drugs

* **J8501** Aprepitant, oral, 5 mg Ⓑ **Qp** **Qh** K2 K

Other: Emend

* **J8510** Busulfan; oral, 2 mg Ⓑ **Qp** **Qh** N1 N

Other: Myleran

IOM: 100-02, 15, 50; 100-04, 4, 240; 100-04, 17, 80.1.1

⊘ **J8515** Cabergoline, oral, 0.25 mg Ⓖ E1

IOM: 100-02, 15, 50; 100-04, 4, 240

* **J8520** Capecitabine, oral, 150 mg Ⓑ **Qp** **Qh** N1 N

Other: Xeloda

IOM: 100-02, 15, 50; 100-04, 4, 240; 100-04, 17, 80.1.1

* **J8521** Capecitabine, oral, 500 mg Ⓑ **Qp** **Qh** N1 N

Other: Xeloda

IOM: 100-02, 15, 50; 100-04, 4, 240; 100-04, 17, 80.1.1

▶ New   ↻ Revised   ✔ Reinstated   deleted Deleted   ⊘ Not covered or valid by Medicare
✣ Special coverage instructions   ✻ Carrier discretion   Ⓑ Bill Part B MAC   Ⓖ Bill DME MAC

⊘ **J8530** Cyclophosphamide; oral,
25 mg ⑧ Qp Qh   N1 N

Other: Cytoxan

*IOM: 100-02, 15, 50; 100-04, 4, 240;
100-04, 17, 80.1.1*

⊘ **J8540** Dexamethasone, oral,
0.25 mg ⑧ Qp Qh   N1 N

Other: Decadron, Dexone, Dexpak, Locort

Medicare Statute 1861(s)2t

⊘ **J8560** Etoposide; oral,
50 mg ⑧ Qp Qh   K2 K

Other: VePesid

*IOM: 100-02, 15, 50; 100-04, 4, 230.1;
100-04, 4, 240; 100-04, 17, 80.1.1*

✳ **J8562** Fludarabine phosphate, oral,
10 mg ⑧ Qp Qh   E2

Other: Fludara, Oforta

Coding Clinic: 2011, Q1, P9

⊘ **J8565** Gefitinib, oral, 250 mg ⑧   E2

Other: Iressa

⊘ **J8597** Antiemetic drug, oral, not otherwise
specified ⑧   N1 N

Medicare Statute 1861(s)2t

⊘ **J8600** Melphalan; oral,
2 mg ⑧ Qp Qh   N1 E2

Other: Alkeran

*IOM: 100-02, 15, 50; 100-04, 4, 240;
100-04, 17, 80.1.1*

⊘ **J8610** Methotrexate; oral,
2.5 mg ⑧ Qp Qh   N1 N

Other: Rheumatrex, Trexall

*IOM: 100-02, 15, 50; 100-04, 4, 240;
100-04, 17, 80.1.1*

✳ **J8650** Nabilone, oral, 1 mg ⑧ Qp Qh   E2

⊘ **J8655** Netupitant 300 mg and palonosetron
0.5 mg, oral ⑧ Qp Qh   K2 K

Other: Akynzeo

Coding Clinic: 2015, Q4, P4

⊘ **J8670** Rolapitant, oral, 1 mg Qp Qh   K2 K

Other: Varubi

⊘ **J8700** Temozolomide, oral,
5 mg ⑧ Qp Qh   N1 N

Other: Temodar

IOM: 100-02, 15, 50; 100-04, 4, 240

✳ **J8705** Topotecan, oral,
0.25 mg ⑧ Qp Qh   K2 K

Treatment for ovarian and lung
cancers, etc. Report J9350 (Topotecan,
4 mg) for intravenous version

Other: Hycamtin

⊘ **J8999** Prescription drug, oral,
chemotherapeutic, NOS ⑧   B

*Other: Anastrozole, Arimidex, Aromasin,
Droxia, Erivedge, Flutamide, Gleevec,
Hydrea, Hydroxyurea, Leukeran,
Matulane, Megestrol Acetate,
Mercaptopurine, Nolvadex, Tamoxifen
Citrate*

*IOM: 100-02, 15, 50; 100-04, 4, 250;
100-04, 17, 80.1.1; 100-04, 17, 80.1.2*

CHEMOTHERAPY DRUGS (J9000-J9999)

NOTE: These codes cover the cost of the chemotherapy drug only, not to include the administration

⊘ **J9000** Injection, doxorubicin hydrochloride,
10 mg ⑧ ⑧ Qp Qh   N1 N

Other: Adriamycin, Rubex

IOM: 100-02, 15, 50

Coding Clinic: 2007, Q4, P5

⊘ **J9015** Injection, aldesleukin, per single use
vial ⑧ ⑧ Qp Qh   K2 K

Other: Proleukin

IOM: 100-02, 15, 50

✳ **J9017** Injection, arsenic trioxide,
1 mg ⑨ ⑧ Qp Qh   K2 K

Other: Trisenox

⊘ **J9019** Injection, asparaginase (Erwinaze),
1,000 IU ⑧ ⑧ Qp Qh   K2 K

IOM: 100-02, 15, 50

⊘ **J9020** Injection, asparaginase,
not otherwise specified
10,000 units ⑨ ⑧ Qp Qh   N1 N

IOM: 100-02, 15, 50

J9021 Injection, asparaginase, recombinant,
(rylaze), 0.1 mg   K2 G

✳ **J9022** Injection, atezolizumab, 10 mg   K2 G

✳ **J9023** Injection, avelumab, 10 mg   K2 G

✳ **J9025** Injection, azacitidine,
1 mg ⑧ ⑧ Qp Qh   K2 N

✳ **J9027** Injection, clofarabine,
1 mg ⑨ ⑧ Qp Qh   K2 K

Other: Clolar

▶ **J9029** Injection, nadofaragene firadenovec-vncg, per therapeutic dose

◎ **J9030** BCG live intravesical instillation, 1 mg   K2 K

✳ **J9032** Injection, belinostat, 10 mg Ⓑ Ⓑ Qp Qh   K2 K

    Other: Beleodaq

✳ **J9033** Injection, bendamustine HCL (treanda), 1 mg Ⓑ Ⓑ Qp Qh   K2 K

    Treatment for form of non-Hodgkin's lymphoma; standard administration time is as an intravenous infusion over 30 minutes

    Other: Treanda

✳ **J9034** Injection, bendamustine HCL (bendeka), 1 mg Qp Qh   K2 G

    Coding Clinic: 2017, Q1, P10

✳ **J9035** Injection, bevacizumab, 10 mg Ⓑ Ⓑ Qp Qh   K2 K

    For malignant neoplasm of breast, considered J9207.

    Other: Avastin

    Coding Clinic: 2013, Q3, P9, Q2, P8

✳ **J9036** Injection, bendamustine hydrochloride, (belrapzo/bendamustine), 1 mg   K2 K

✳ **J9037** Injection, belantamab mafodontin-blmf, 0.5 mg   K2 G

✳ **J9039** Injection, blinatumomab, 1 mcg Ⓑ Ⓑ Qp Qh   K2 K

    Other: Blincyto

◎ **J9040** Injection, bleomycin sulfate, 15 units Ⓑ Ⓑ Qp Qh   N1 N

    Other: Blenoxane

    IOM: 100-02, 15, 50

✳ **J9041** Injection, bortezomib, 0.1 mg Ⓑ Ⓑ Qp Qh   K2 K

    Other: Velcade

✳ **J9042** Injection, brentuximab vedotin, 1 mg Ⓑ Ⓑ Qp Qh   K2 K

    Other: Adcetris

✳ **J9043** Injection, cabazitaxel, 1 mg Ⓥ Ⓑ Qp Qh   K2 K

    Other: Jevtana

    Coding Clinic: 2012, Q1, P9

◎ **J9045** Injection, carboplatin, 50 mg Ⓑ Ⓑ Qp Qh   N1 N

    Other: Paraplatin

    IOM: 100-02, 15, 50

J9046 Injection, bortezomib, (Dr. Reddy's), not therapeutically equivalent to J9041, 0.1 mg   K2 K

✳ **J9047** Injection, carfilzomib, 1 mg Ⓥ Ⓑ Qp Qh   K2 K

    Other: Kyprolis

J9048 Injection, bortezomib (fresenius kabi), not therapeutically equivalent to J9041, 0.1 mg   K2 K

J9049 Injection, bortezomib (hospira), not therapeutically equivalent to J9041, 0.1 mg   K2 K

◎ **J9050** Injection, carmustine, 100 mg Ⓑ Ⓑ Qp Qh   K2 K

    Other: BiCNU

    IOM: 100-02, 15, 50

▶ **J9051** Injection, bortezomib (maia), not therapeutically equivalent to J9041, 0.1 mg   K2 K

✳ **J9055** Injection, cetuximab, 10 mg Ⓥ Ⓑ Ⓑ Qp Qh   K2 K

    Other: Erbitux

▶ **J9056** Injection, bendamustine hydrochloride (vivimusta), 1 mg

✳ **J9057** Injection, copanlisib, 1 mg   G

    Other: Aliqopa

▶ **J9058** Injection, bendamustine hydrochloride (apotex), 1 mg

▶ **J9059** Injection, bendamustine hydrochloride (baxter), 1 mg

◎ **J9060** Injection, cisplatin, powder or solution, 10 mg Ⓑ Ⓑ Qp Qh   N1 N

    Other: Plantinol AQ

    IOM: 100-02, 15, 50

    Coding Clinic: 2013, Q2, P6; 2011, Q1, P8

✳ **J9061** Injection, amivantamab-vmjw, 2 mg K2 G

▶ **J9063** Injection, mirvetuximab soravtansine-gynx, 1 mg

▶ **J9064** Injection, cabazitaxel (sandoz), not therapeutically equivalent to J9043, 1 mg   K2 K

◎ **J9065** Injection, cladribine, per 1 mg Ⓥ Ⓑ Qp Qh   K2 K

    Other: Leustatin

    IOM: 100-02, 15, 50

◎ **J9070** Cyclophosphamide, 100 mg Ⓑ Ⓑ Qp Qh   K2 K

    Other: Cytoxan, Neosar

    IOM: 100-02, 15, 50

    Coding Clinic: 2011, Q1, P8-9

✳ **J9098** Injection, cytarabine liposome, 10 mg Ⓑ Ⓑ Qp Qh   K2 K

    Other: DepoCyt

▶ New   ↻ Revised   ✔ Reinstated   ~~deleted~~ Deleted   ⊘ Not covered or valid by Medicare
◎ Special coverage instructions   ✳ Carrier discretion   Ⓑ Bill Part B MAC   Ⓑ Bill DME MAC

⚙ **J9100** Injection, cytarabine,
100 mg ⓑ ⓑ Qp Qh N1 N

Other: Cytosar-U

IOM: 100-02, 15, 50

Coding Clinic: 2011, Q1, P9

✳ **J9118** Injection, calaspargase pegol-mknl,
10 units E2

✳ **J9119** Injection, cemiplimab-rwlc,
1 mg K2 K

⚙ **J9120** Injection, dactinomycin,
0.5 mg ⓑ ⓑ Qp Qh K2 K

Other: Cosmegen

IOM: 100-02, 15, 50

⚙ **J9130** Dacarbazine,
100 mg ⓑ ⓑ Qp Qh N1 N

Other: DTIC-Dome

IOM: 100-02, 15, 50

Coding Clinic: 2011, Q1, P9

⚙ **J9144** Injection, daratumumab, 10 mg and
hyaluronidase-fihj K2 G

⚙ **J9145** Injection, daratumumab,
10 mg Qp Qh K2 G

Other: Darzalex

IOM: 100-02, 15, 50

⚙ **J9150** Injection, daunorubicin,
10 mg ⓑ ⓑ Qp Qh K2 K

Other: Cerubidine

IOM: 100-02, 15, 50

⚙ **J9151** Injection, daunorubicin citrate,
liposomal formulation,
10 mg ⓑ ⓑ Qp Qh E2

Other: Daunoxome

IOM: 100-02, 15, 50

✳ **J9153** njection, liposomal, 1 mg daunorubicin
and 2.27 mg cytarabine G

Other: Vyxeos

✳ **J9155** Injection, degarelix,
1 mg ⓑ ⓑ Qp Qh K2 K

Report 1 unit for every 1 mg.

Other: Firmagon

✳ **J9160** Injection, denileukin diftitox,
300 mcg ⓑ ⓑ Qp Qh E2

⚙ **J9165** Injection, diethylstilbestrol
diphosphate, 250 mg ⓑ ⓑ Qp Qh E2

Other: Stilphostrol

IOM: 100-02, 15, 50

⚙ **J9171** Injection, docetaxel,
1 mg ⓑ ⓑ Qp Qh K2 K

Report 1 unit for every 1 mg.

Other: Docefrez, Taxotere

IOM: 100-02, 15, 50

Coding Clinic: 2012, Q1, P9

✳ **J9173** Injection, durvalumab, 10 mg G

Other: Imfinzi

⚙ **J9175** Injection, Elliott's B solution,
1 ml ⓑ ⓑ Qp Qh N1 N

IOM: 100-02, 15, 50

✳ **J9176** Injection, elotuzumab,
1 mg Qp Qh K2 G

Other: Empliciti

✳ **J9177** Injection, enfortumab vedotin-ejfv,
0.25 mg K2 G

✳ **J9178** Injection, epirubicin HCL,
2 mg ⓑ ⓑ Qp Qh N1 N

Other: Ellence

✳ **J9179** Injection, eribulin mesylate,
0.1 mg ⓑ ⓑ Qp Qh K2 K

Other: Halaven

⚙ **J9181** Injection, etoposide,
10 mg ⓑ ⓑ Qp Qh N1 N

Other: Etopophos, Toposar

⚙ **J9185** Injection, fludarabine phosphate,
50 mg ⓑ ⓑ Qp Qh K2 K

Other: Fludara

IOM: 100-02, 15, 50

⚙ **J9190** Injection, fluorouracil,
500 mg ⓑ ⓑ Qp Qh N1 N

Other: Adrucil

IOM: 100-02, 15, 50

▶ **J9196** Injection, gemcitabine hydrochloride
(accord), not therapeutically equivalent
to J9201, 200 mg N1 N

⚙ **J9198** Injection, gemcitabine hydrochloride,
(infugem), 100 mg K2 G

⚙ **J9200** Injection, floxuridine,
500 mg ⓑ ⓑ Qp Qh N1 N

Other: FUDR

IOM: 100-02, 15, 50

⚙ **J9201** Injection, gemcitabine
hydrochloride, not otherwise
specified, 200 mg ⓑ ⓑ Qp Qh N1 N

Other: Gemzar

IOM: 100-02, 15, 50

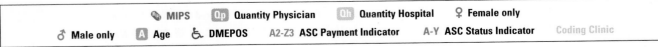

⚙ **J9202** Goserelin acetate implant, per 3.6 mg ⑧ ⑧ **Qp** **Qh** K2 K

Other: Zoladex

IOM: 100-02, 15, 50

✳ **J9203** Injection, gemtuzumab ozogamicin, 0.1 mg K2 G

✳ **J9204** Injection, mogamulizumab-kpkc, 1 mg K2 K

⚙ **J9205** Injection, irinotecan liposome, 1 mg **Qp** **Qh** K2 G

Other: ONIVYDE

IOM: 100-02, 15, 50

⚙ **J9206** Injection, irinotecan, 20 mg ⑧ ⑧ **Qp** **Qh** N1 N

Other: Camptosar

IOM: 100-02, 15, 50

✳ **J9207** Injection, ixabepilone, 1 mg ⑧ ⑧ **Qp** **Qh** K2 K

Other: Ixempra Kit

⚙ **J9208** Injection, ifosfamide, 1 gm ⑧ ⑧ **Qp** **Qh** N1 N

Other: Ifex

IOM: 100-02, 15, 50

⚙ **J9209** Injection, mesna, 200 mg ⑧ ⑧ **Qp** **Qh** N1 N

Other: Mesnex

IOM: 100-02, 15, 50

✳ **J9210** Injection, emapalumab-lzsg, 1 mg K2 K

⚙ **J9211** Injection, idarubicin hydrochloride, 5 mg ⑧ ⑧ **Qp** **Qh** K2 K

Other: Idamycin PFS

IOM: 100-02, 15, 50

⚙ **J9212** Injection, interferon alfacon-1, recombinant, 1 mcg ⑧ ⑧ **Qp** **Qh** N1 N

Other: Amgen, Infergen

IOM: 100-02, 15, 50

⚙ **J9213** Injection, interferon, alfa-2a, recombinant, 3 million units ⑧ ⑧ **Qp** **Qh** N1 N

Other: Roferon-A

IOM: 100-02, 15, 50

⚙ **J9214** Injection, interferon, alfa-2b, recombinant, 1 million units ⑧ ⑧ **Qp** **Qh** K2 K

Other: Intron-A

IOM: 100-02, 15, 50

⚙ **J9215** Injection, interferon, alfa-n3 (human leukocyte derived), 250,000 IU ⑧ ⑧ **Qp** **Qh** E2

Other: Alferon N

IOM: 100-02, 15, 50

⚙ **J9216** Injection, interferon, gamma-1B, 3 million units ⑧ ⑧ **Qp** **Qh** K2 K

Other: Actimmune

IOM: 100-02, 15, 50

⚙ **J9217** Leuprolide acetate (for depot suspension), 7.5 mg ⑧ ⑧ **Qp** **Qh** K2 K

Other: Eligard, Lupron Depot

IOM: 100-02, 15, 50

Coding Clinic: 2019, Q2, P11; 2015, Q3, P3

⚙ **J9218** Leuprolide acetate, per 1 mg ⑧ ⑧ **Qp** **Qh** K2 K

Other: Lupron

IOM: 100-02, 15, 50

Coding Clinic: 2019, Q2, P11; 2015, Q3, P3

⚙ **J9219** Leuprolide acetate implant, 65 mg ⑧ ⑧ **Qp** **Qh** E2

Other: Viadur

IOM: 100-02, 15, 50

⚙ **J9223** Injection, lurbinectedin, 0.1 mg K2 G

⚙ **J9225** Histrelin implant (Vantas), 50 mg ⑧ ⑧ **Qp** **Qh** K2 K

IOM: 100-02, 15, 50

⚙ **J9226** Histrelin implant (Supprelin LA), 50 mg ⑧ ⑧ **Qp** **Qh** K2 N

Other: Vantas

IOM: 100-02, 15, 50

⚙ **J9227** Injection, isatuximab-irfc, 10 mg K2 G

✳ **J9228** Injection, ipilimumab, 1 mg ⑧ ⑧ **Qp** **Qh** K2 K

Other: Yervoy

Coding Clinic: 2012, Q1, P9

✳ **J9229** Injection, inotuzumab ozogamicin, 0.1 mg G

Other: Besponsa

⚙ **J9230** Injection, mechlorethamine hydrochloride, (nitrogen mustard), 10 mg ⑧ ⑧ **Qp** **Qh** K2 N

Other: Mustargen

IOM: 100-02, 15, 50

⚙ **J9245** Injection, melphalan hydrochloride, not otherwise specified, 50 mg ⑧ ⑧ **Qp** **Qh** K2 K

▶ **New** ↻ **Revised** ✔ **Reinstated** ~~deleted~~ **Deleted** ⊘ **Not covered or valid by Medicare**
⚙ **Special coverage instructions** ✳ **Carrier discretion** ⑧ **Bill Part B MAC** ⑧ **Bill DME MAC**

CHEMOTHERAPY DRUGS

⊛ **J9246** Injection, melphalan (evomela), 1 mg K2 K

Other: Alkeran, Evomela

IOM: 100-02, 15, 50

⊛ **J9247** Injection, melphalan flufenamide, 1mg K2 G

⊛ **J9250** Methotrexate sodium, 5 mg ⑧ ⑧ Qp Qh N1 N

Other: Folex

IOM: 100-02, 15, 50

▶ **J9259** Injection, paclitaxel protein-bound particles (american regent) not therapeutically equivalent to J9264, 1 mg K2 K

⊛ **J9260** Methotrexate sodium, 50 mg ⑧ ⑧ Qp Qh N1 N

Other: Folex

IOM: 100-02, 15, 50

✳ **J9261** Injection, nelarabine, 50 mg ⑧ ⑧ Qp Qh K2 K

Other: Arranon

✳ **J9262** Injection, omacetaxine mepesuccinate, 0.01 mg ⑧ ⑧ Qp Qh K2 K

Other: Synribo

✳ **J9263** Injection, oxaliplatin, 0.5 mg ⑧ ⑧ Qp Qh N1 N

Eloxatin, platinum-based anticancer drug that destroys cancer cells

Other: Eloxatin

Coding Clinic: 2009, Q1, P10

✳ **J9264** Injection, paclitaxel protein-bound particles, 1 mg ⑧ ⑧ K2 K

Other: Abraxane

⊛ **J9266** Injection, pegaspargase, per single dose vial ⑧ ⑧ Qp Qh K2 K

Other: Oncaspar

IOM: 100-02, 15, 50

⊛ **J9267** Injection, paclitaxel, 1 mg ⑧ ⑧ Qp Qh N1 N

Other: Taxol

⊛ **J9268** Injection, pentostatin, 10 mg ⑧ ⑧ Qp Qh K2 K

Other: Nipent

IOM: 100-02, 15, 50

✳ **J9269** Injection, tagraxofusp-erzs, 10 micrograms K2 K

⊛ **J9270** Injection, plicamycin, 2.5 mg ⑧ ⑧ Qp Qh N1 N

Other: Mithracin

IOM: 100-02, 15, 50

✳ **J9271** Injection, pembrolizumab, 1 mg ⑧ ⑧ Qp Qh K2 K

Other: Keytruda

J9272 Injection, dostarlimab-gxly, 10 mg K2 G

J9274 Injection, tebentafusp-tebn, 1 microgram K2 G

⊛ **J9280** Injection, mitomycin, 5 mg ⑧ ⑧ Qp Qh K2 K

Other: Mitosol, Mutamycin

IOM: 100-02, 15, 50

Coding Clinic: 2016, Q4, P8; 2014, Q2, P6; 2011, Q1, P9

⊛ **J9281** Mitomycin pyelocalyceal instillation, 1 mg K2 G

✳ **J9285** Injection, olaratumab, 10 mg K2 N

⊛ **J9293** Injection, mitoxantrone hydrochloride, per 5 mg ⑧ ⑧ Qp Qh K2 K

Other: Novantrone

IOM: 100-02, 15, 50

▶ **J9294** Injection, pemetrexed (hospira) not therapeutically equivalent to J9305, 10 mg K2 K

✳ **J9295** Injection, necitumumab, 1 mg Qp Qh K2 G

Other: Portrazza

▶ **J9296** Injection, pemetrexed (accord) not therapeutically equivalent to J9305, 10 mg K2 K

▶ **J9297** Injection, pemetrexed (sandoz), not therapeutically equivalent to J9305, 10 mg K2 K

J9298 Injection, nivolumab and relatlimab-rmbw, 3 mg/1 mg K2 G

⊛ **J9299** Injection, nivolumab, 1 mg ⑧ ⑧ Qp Qh K2 K

Other: Opdivo

✳ **J9301** Injection, obinutuzumab, 10 mg ⑧ ⑧ Qp Qh K2 K

Other: Gazyva

✳ **J9302** Injection, ofatumumab, 10 mg ⑧ ⑧ Qp Qh K2 K

Other: Arzerra

Coding Clinic: 2011, Q1, P7

✳ **J9303** Injection, panitumumab, not otherwise specified, 10 mg ⑧ ⑧ Qp Qh K2 K

Other: Vectibix

✳ **J9304** Injection, pemetrexed (pemfexy), 10 mg K5 G

✳ **J9305** Injection, pemetrexed, 10 mg ⓑ ⓖ Qp Qh   K2 K

Other: Alimta

✳ **J9306** Injection, pertuzumab, 1 mg ⓑ ⓖ Qp Qh   K2 K

Other: Perjeta

✳ **J9307** Injection, pralatrexate, 1 mg ⓟ ⓑ Qp Qh   K2 K

Other: Folotyn

Coding Clinic: 2011, Q1, P7

✳ **J9308** Injection, ramucirumab, 5 mg ⓑ ⓖ Qp Qh   K2 K

Other: Cyramza

✳ **J9309** Injection, polatuzumab vedotin-piiq, 1 mg   K2 K

⊚ **J9311** Injection, rituximab 10 mg and hyaluronidase   G

Other: Rituxan

⊚ **J9312** Injection, rituximab, 10 mg   K

Other: Rituxan

✳ **J9313** Injection, moxetumomab pasudotox-tdfk, 0.01 mg   K2 K

▶ **J9314** Injection, pemetrexed (teva) not therapeutically equivalent to J9305, 10 mg   K2 K

✳ **J9316** Injection, pertuzumab, trastuzumab, and hyaluronidase-zzxf, per 10 mg   K2 G

✳ **J9317** Injection, sacituzumab govitecan-hziy, 2.5 mg   K2 G

✳ **J9318** Injection, romidepsin, non-lyophilized, 0.1 mg   K2 G

✳ **J9319** Injection, romidepsin, lyophilized, 0.1 mg   K2 G

⊚ **J9320** Injection, streptozocin, 1 gram ⓑ ⓖ Qp Qh   K2 K

Other: Zanosar

IOM: 100-02, 15, 50

▶ **J9322** Injection, pemetrexed (bluepoint) not therapeutically equivalent to J9305, 10 mg   K2 K

▶ **J9323** Injection, pemetrexed ditromethamine, 10 mg

✳ **J9325** Injection, talimogene laherparepvec, per 1 million plaque forming units Qp Qh   K2 G

Other: Imlygic

Coding Clinic: 2019, Q2, P12

✳ **J9328** Injection, temozolomide, 1 mg ⓑ ⓖ Qp Qh   K2 K

Intravenous formulation, not for oral administration

Other: Temodar

✳ **J9330** Injection, temsirolimus, 1 mg ⓟ ⓑ ⓖ Qp Qh   K2 K

Treatment for advanced renal cell carcinoma; standard administration is intravenous infusion greater than 30-60 minutes

Other: Torisel

J9331 Injection, sirolimus protein-bound particles, 1 mg   K2 G

J9332 Injection, efgartigimod alfa-fcab, 2mg   K2 G

⊚ **J9340** Injection, thiotepa, 15 mg ⓟ ⓑ Qp Qh   K2 K

Other: Tepadina, Triethylene thio Phosphoramide/T

IOM: 100-02, 15, 50

▶ **J9345** Injection, retifanlimab-dlwr, 1 mg

▶ **J9347** Injection, tremelimumab-actl, 1 mg

✳ **J9348** Injection, naxitamab-gqgk, 1 mg   K2 G

✳ **J9349** Injection, tafasitamab-cxix, 2 mg   K2 G

▶ **J9350** Injection, mosunetuzumab-axgb, 1 mg

✳ **J9351** Injection, topotecan, 0.1 mg ⓟ ⓑ Qp Qh   N1 N

Other: Hycamtin

Coding Clinic: 2011, Q1, P9

✳ **J9352** Injection, trabectedin, 0.1 mg Qp Qh   K2 G

Other: Yondelis

✳ **J9353** Injection, margetuximab-cmkb, 5 mg   K2 G

✳ **J9354** Injection, ado-trastuzumab emtansine, 1 mg ⓑ ⓖ Qp Qh   K2 K

Other: Kadcyla

✳ **J9355** Injection, trastuzumab, excludes biosimilar, 10 mg ⓟ ⓑ Qp Qh   K2 K

Other: Herceptin

✳ **J9356** Injection, trastuzumab, 10 mg and hyaluronidase-oysk   K2 K

⊚ **J9357** Injection, valrubicin, intravesical, 200 mg ⓑ ⓖ Qp Qh   K2 K

Other: Valstar

IOM: 100-02, 15, 50

⊚ **J9358** Injection, fam-trastuzumab deruxtecan-nxki, 1 mg   K2 G

▶ New   ↻ Revised   ✔ Reinstated   ~~deleted~~ Deleted   ⊘ Not covered or valid by Medicare
⊚ Special coverage instructions   ✳ Carrier discretion   ⓑ Bill Part B MAC   ⓖ Bill DME MAC

⊘ **J9360** Injection, vinblastine sulfate,
1 mg Ⓑ Ⓑ 〔Qp〕 〔Qh〕 N1 N

Other: Alkaban-AQ, Velban, Velsar

IOM: 100-02, 15, 50

⊘ **J9370** Vincristine sulfate,
1 mg Ⓑ Ⓑ 〔Qp〕 〔Qh〕 N1 N

Other: Oncovin, Vincasar PFS

IOM: 100-02, 15, 50

Coding Clinic: 2011, Q1, P9

✳ **J9371** Injection, vincristine sulfate liposome,
1 mg Ⓑ Ⓑ 〔Qp〕 〔Qh〕 K2 K

▶ **J9380** Injection, teclistamab-cqyv, 0.5 mg

▶ **J9381** Injection, teplizumab-mzwv, 5 mcg

⊘ **J9390** Injection, vinorelbine tartrate,
10 mg Ⓑ Ⓑ 〔Qp〕 〔Qh〕 N1 N

Other: Navelbine

IOM: 100-02, 15, 50

J9393 Injection, fulvestrant (teva) not
therapeutically equivalent to J9395,
25 mg K2 K

J9394 Injection, fulvestrant (fresenius
kabi) not therapeutically equivalent
to J9395, 25 mg K2 K

✳ **J9395** Injection, fulvestrant,
25 mg Ⓑ Ⓑ 〔Qp〕 〔Qh〕 K2 K

Other: Faslodex

✳ **J9400** Injection, ziv-aflibercept,
1 mg Ⓑ Ⓑ 〔Qp〕 〔Qh〕 K2 K

Other: Zaltrap

⊘ **J9600** Injection, porfimer sodium,
75 mg Ⓑ Ⓑ 〔Qp〕 〔Qh〕 K2 K

Other: Photofrin

IOM: 100-02, 15, 50

⊘ **J9999** Not otherwise classified, antineoplastic
drugs Ⓑ Ⓑ N1 N

Bill on paper, bill one unit, and identify
drug and total dosage in "Remarks"
field. Include invoice of cost or NDC
number in "Remarks" field.

Other: Imlygic, Yondelis

IOM: 100-02, 15, 50; 100-03, 2, 110.2

Coding Clinic: 2017, Q1, P3; 2013, Q2, P3

TEMPORARY CODES ASSIGNED TO DME REGIONAL CARRIERS (K0000-K9999)

NOTE: This section contains national codes assigned by CMS on a temporary basis and for the exclusive use of the durable medical equipment regional carriers (DMERC).

Wheelchairs and Accessories

✳ **K0001** Standard wheelchair ⑧ [Qp] [Qh] ♿ Y
Capped rental

✳ **K0002** Standard hemi (low seat) wheelchair ⑧ [Qp] [Qh] ♿ Y
Capped rental

✳ **K0003** Lightweight wheelchair ⑧ [Qp] [Qh] ♿ Y
Capped rental

✳ **K0004** High strength, lightweight wheelchair ⑧ [Qp] [Qh] ♿ Y
Capped rental

✳ **K0005** Ultralightweight wheelchair ⑧ [Qp] [Qh] ♿ Y
Capped rental. Inexpensive and routinely purchased DME

✳ **K0006** Heavy duty wheelchair ⑧ [Qp] [Qh] ♿ Y
Capped rental

✳ **K0007** Extra heavy duty wheelchair ⑧ [Qp] [Qh] ♿ Y
Capped rental

⊚ **K0008** Custom manual wheelchair/base ⑧ [Qh] Y

✳ **K0009** Other manual wheelchair/base ⑧ [Qp] [Qh] ♿ Y
Not otherwise classified

✳ **K0010** Standard - weight frame motorized/power wheelchair ⑧ ♿ Y
Capped rental. Codes K0010-K0014 are not for manual wheelchairs with add-on power packs. Use the appropriate code for the manual wheelchair base provided (K0001-K0009) and code K0460.

✳ **K0011** Standard - weight frame motorized/power wheelchair with programmable control parameters for speed adjustment, tremor dampening, acceleration control and braking ⑧ ♿Y
Capped rental. A patient who requires a power wheelchair usually is totally nonambulatory and has severe weakness of the upper extremities due to a neurologic or muscular disease/condition.

✳ **K0012** Lightweight portable motorized/power wheelchair ⑧ ♿ Y
Capped rental

⊚ **K0013** Custom motorized/power wheelchair base ⑧ [Qh] Y

✳ **K0014** Other motorized/power wheelchair base ⑧ Y
Capped rental

✳ **K0015** Detachable, non-adjustable height armrest, replacement only, each ⑧ [Qp] [Qh] ♿ Y
Inexpensive and routinely purchased DME

✳ **K0017** Detachable, adjustable height armrest, base, replacement only, each ⑧ [Qp] [Qh] ♿ Y
Inexpensive and routinely purchased DME

✳ **K0018** Detachable, adjustable height armrest, upper portion, replacement only, each ⑧ [Qp] [Qh] ♿ Y
Inexpensive and routinely purchased DME

✳ **K0019** Arm pad, replacement only, each ⑧ [Qp] [Qh] ♿ Y
Inexpensive and routinely purchased DME

✳ **K0020** Fixed, adjustable height armrest, pair ⑧ [Qp] [Qh] ♿ Y
Inexpensive and routinely purchased DME

✳ **K0037** High mount flip-up footrest, each ⑧ [Qp] [Qh] ♿ Y
Inexpensive and routinely purchased DME

✳ **K0038** Leg strap, each ⑧ [Qp] [Qh] ♿ Y
Inexpensive and routinely purchased DME

✳ **K0039** Leg strap, H style, each ⑧ [Qp] [Qh] ♿ Y
Inexpensive and routinely purchased DME

✳ **K0040** Adjustable angle footplate, each ⑧ [Qp] [Qh] ♿ Y
Inexpensive and routinely purchased DME

✳ **K0041** Large size footplate, each ⑧ [Qp] [Qh] ♿ Y
Inexpensive and routinely purchased DME

✳ **K0042** Standard size footplate, replacement only, each ⑧ [Qp] [Qh] ♿ Y
Inexpensive and routinely purchased DME

▶ New   ⟳ Revised   ✔ Reinstated   ~~deleted~~ Deleted   ⊘ Not covered or valid by Medicare
⊚ Special coverage instructions   ✳ Carrier discretion   ⑧ Bill Part B MAC   ⑧ Bill DME MAC

* **K0043** Footrest, lower extension tube, replacement only, each ⑧ Qp Qh ૐ Y

Inexpensive and routinely purchased DME

* **K0044** Footrest, upper hanger bracket, replacement only, each ⑧ Qp Qh ૐ Y

Inexpensive and routinely purchased DME

* **K0045** Footrest, complete assembly, replacement only, each ⑧ Qp Qh ૐ Y

Inexpensive and routinely purchased DME

* **K0046** Elevating legrest, lower extension tube, replacement only, each ⑧ Qp Qh ૐ Y

Inexpensive and routinely purchased DME

* **K0047** Elevating legrest, upper hanger bracket, replacement only, each ⑧ Qp Qh ૐ Y

Inexpensive and routinely purchased DME

* **K0050** Ratchet assembly, replacement only ⑧ Qp Qh ૐ Y

Inexpensive and routinely purchased DME

* **K0051** Cam release assembly, footrest or legrests, replacement only, each ⑧ Qp Qh ૐ Y

Inexpensive and routinely purchased DME

* **K0052** Swing-away, detachable footrests, replacement only, each ⑧ Qp Qh ૐ Y

Inexpensive and routinely purchased DME

* **K0053** Elevating footrests, articulating (telescoping), each ⑧ Qp Qh ૐ Y

Inexpensive and routinely purchased DME

* **K0056** Seat height less than 17" or equal to or greater than 21" for a high strength, lightweight, or ultralightweight wheelchair ⑧ Qp Qh ૐ Y

Inexpensive and routinely purchased DME

* **K0065** Spoke protectors, each ⑧ Qp Qh ૐ Y

Inexpensive and routinely purchased DME

* **K0069** Rear wheel assembly, complete, with solid tire, spokes or molded, replacement only, each ⑧ Qp Qh ૐ Y

Inexpensive and routinely purchased DME

* **K0070** Rear wheel assembly, complete, with pneumatic tire, spokes or molded, replacement only, each ⑧ Qp Qh ૐ Y

Inexpensive and routinely purchased DME

* **K0071** Front caster assembly, complete, with pneumatic tire, replacement only, each ⑧ Qp Qh ૐ Y

Caster assembly includes a caster fork (E2396), wheel rim, and tire. Inexpensive and routinely purchased DME

* **K0072** Front caster assembly, complete, with semi-pneumatic tire, replacement only, each ⑧ Qp Qh ૐ Y

Inexpensive and routinely purchased DME

* **K0073** Caster pin lock, each ⑧ Qp Qh ૐ Y

Inexpensive and routinely purchased DME

* **K0077** Front caster assembly, complete, with solid tire, replacement only, each ⑧ Qp Qh ૐ Y

* **K0098** Drive belt for power wheelchair, replacement only ⑧ ૐ Y

Inexpensive and routinely purchased DME

* **K0105** IV hanger, each ⑧ Qp Qh ૐ Y

Inexpensive and routinely purchased DME

* **K0108** Wheelchair component or accessory, not otherwise specified ⑧ Y

⊘ **K0195** Elevating leg rests, pair (for use with capped rental wheelchair base) ⑧ Qp Qh Y

Medically necessary replacement items are covered if rollabout chair or transport chair covered

IOM: 100-03, 4, 280.1

Infusion Pump, Supplies, and Batteries

⊘ **K0455** Infusion pump used for uninterrupted parenteral administration of medication (e.g., epoprostenol or treprostinol) ⑧ Qp Qh ૐ Y

An EIP may also be referred to as an external insulin pump, ambulatory pump, or mini-infuser. CMN/DIF required. Frequent and substantial service DME.

IOM: 100-03, 1, 50.3

Figure 18 Infusion pump.

⊛ **K0462** Temporary replacement for patient owned equipment being repaired, any type ⑧ Qp Qh   Y

Only report for maintenance and service for an item for which initial claim was paid. The term power mobility device (PMD) includes power operated vehicles (POVs) and power wheelchairs (PWCs). Not otherwise classified.

IOM: 100-04, 20, 40.1

⊛ **K0552** Supplies for external non-insulin drug infusion pump, syringe type cartridge, sterile, each ⑧ Qh &   Y

Supplies

IOM: 100-03, 1, 50.3

✳ **K0601** Replacement battery for external infusion pump owned by patient, silver oxide, 1.5 volt, each ⑧ Qh &   Y

Inexpensive and routinely purchased DME

✳ **K0602** Replacement battery for external infusion pump owned by patient, silver oxide, 3 volt, each ⑧ Qp Qh &   Y

Inexpensive and routinely purchased DME

✳ **K0603** Replacement battery for external infusion pump owned by patient, alkaline, 1.5 volt, each ⑧ Qh &   Y

Inexpensive and routinely purchased DME

✳ **K0604** Replacement battery for external infusion pump owned by patient, lithium, 3.6 volt, each ⑧ Qh &   Y

Inexpensive and routinely purchased DME

✳ **K0605** Replacement battery for external infusion pump owned by patient, lithium, 4.5 volt, each ⑧ Qp Qh &   Y

Inexpensive and routinely purchased DME

Defibrillator and Accessories

✳ **K0606** Automatic external defibrillator, with integrated electrocardiogram analysis, garment type ⑧ Qp Qh &   Y

Capped rental

✳ **K0607** Replacement battery for automated external defibrillator, garment type only, each ⑧ Qp Qh &   Y

Inexpensive and routinely purchased DME

✳ **K0608** Replacement garment for use with automated external defibrillator, each ⑧ Qp Qh &   Y

Inexpensive and routinely purchased DME

✳ **K0609** Replacement electrodes for use with automated external defibrillator, garment type only, each ⑧ Qp Qh &   Y

Supplies

Miscellaneous

✳ **K0669** Wheelchair accessory, wheelchair seat or back cushion, does not meet specific code criteria or no written coding verification from DME PDAC ⑧   Y

Inexpensive and routinely purchased DME

✳ **K0672** Addition to lower extremity orthosis, removable soft interface, all components, replacement only, each ⑧ Qp &   A

Prosthetics/Orthotics

✳ **K0730** Controlled dose inhalation drug delivery system ⑧ Qp Qh &   Y

Inexpensive and routinely purchased DME

✳ **K0733** Power wheelchair accessory, 12 to 24 amp hour sealed lead acid battery, each (e.g., gel cell, absorbed glassmat) ⑧ Qp Qh &   Y

Inexpensive and routinely purchased DME

✳ **K0738** Portable gaseous oxygen system, rental; home compressor used to fill portable oxygen cylinders; includes portable containers, regulator, flowmeter, humidifier, cannula or mask, and tubing ⑧ Qp Qh &   Y

Oxygen and oxygen equipment

✳ **K0739** Repair or nonroutine service for durable medical equipment other than oxygen equipment requiring the skill of a technician, labor component, per 15 minutes ⑧ ⑧   Y

⊘ **K0740** Repair or nonroutine service for oxygen equipment requiring the skill of a technician, labor component, per 15 minutes ⑧ Qp Qh   E1

✳ **K0743** Suction pump, home model, portable, for use on wounds ⑧ Qp Qh   Y

✳ **K0744** Absorptive wound dressing for use with suction pump, home model, portable, pad size 16 square inches or less ⑧ Qp   A

▶ New   ⟲ Revised   ✔ Reinstated   ~~deleted~~ Deleted   ⊘ Not covered or valid by Medicare
⊛ Special coverage instructions   ✳ Carrier discretion   ⑧ Bill Part B MAC   ⑧ Bill DME MAC

* **K0745** Absorptive wound dressing for use with suction pump, home model, portable, pad size more than 16 square inches but less than or equal to 48 square inches ⑧ Qp   A

* **K0746** Absorptive wound dressing for use with suction pump, home model, portable, pad size greater than 48 square inches ⑧ Qp   A

Power Mobility Devices

* **K0800** Power operated vehicle, group 1 standard, patient weight capacity up to and including 300 pounds ⑧ Qp Qh ♿   Y

  Power mobility device (PMD) includes power operated vehicles (POVs) and power wheelchairs (PWCs). Inexpensive and routinely purchased DME

* **K0801** Power operated vehicle, group 1 heavy duty, patient weight capacity 301 to 450 pounds ⑧ Qp Qh ♿   Y

  Inexpensive and routinely purchased DME

* **K0802** Power operated vehicle, group 1 very heavy duty, patient weight capacity 451 to 600 pounds ⑧ Qp Qh ♿   Y

  Inexpensive and routinely purchased DME

* **K0806** Power operated vehicle, group 2 standard, patient weight capacity up to and including 300 pounds ⑧ Qp Qh ♿   Y

  Inexpensive and routinely purchased DME

* **K0807** Power operated vehicle, group 2 heavy duty, patient weight capacity 301 to 450 pounds ⑧ Qp Qh ♿   Y

  Inexpensive and routinely purchased DME

* **K0808** Power operated vehicle, group 2 very heavy duty, patient weight capacity 451 to 600 pounds ⑧ Qp Qh ♿   Y

  Inexpensive and routinely purchased DME

* **K0812** Power operated vehicle, not otherwise classified ⑧ Qp Qh   Y

  Not otherwise classified.

* **K0813** Power wheelchair, group 1 standard, portable, sling/solid seat and back, patient weight capacity up to and including 300 pounds ⑧ Qp Qh ♿   Y

  Capped rental

* **K0814** Power wheelchair, group 1 standard, portable, captains chair, patient weight capacity up to and including 300 pounds ⑧ Qp Qh ♿   Y

  Capped rental

* **K0815** Power wheelchair, group 1 standard, sling/solid seat and back, patient weight capacity up to and including 300 pounds ⑧ Qp Qh ♿   Y

  Capped rental

* **K0816** Power wheelchair, group 1 standard, captains chair, patient weight capacity up to and including 300 pounds ⑧ Qp Qh ♿   Y

  Capped rental

* **K0820** Power wheelchair, group 2 standard, portable, sling/solid seat/back, patient weight capacity up to and including 300 pounds ⑧ Qp Qh ♿   Y

  Capped rental

* **K0821** Power wheelchair, group 2 standard, portable, captains chair, patient weight capacity up to and including 300 pounds ⑧ Qp Qh ♿   Y

  Capped rental

* **K0822** Power wheelchair, group 2 standard, sling/solid seat/back, patient weight capacity up to and including 300 pounds ⑧ Qp Qh ♿   Y

  Capped rental

* **K0823** Power wheelchair, group 2 standard, captains chair, patient weight capacity up to and including 300 pounds ⑧ Qp Qh ♿   Y

  Capped rental

* **K0824** Power wheelchair, group 2 heavy duty, sling/solid seat/back, patient weight capacity 301 to 450 pounds ⑧ Qp Qh ♿   Y

  Capped rental

* **K0825** Power wheelchair, group 2 heavy duty, captains chair, patient weight capacity 301 to 450 pounds ⑧ Qp Qh ♿   Y

  Capped rental

* **K0826** Power wheelchair, group 2 very heavy duty, sling/solid seat/back, patient weight capacity 451 to 600 pounds ⑧ Qp Qh ♿   Y

  Capped rental

* **K0827** Power wheelchair, group 2 very heavy duty, captains chair, patient weight capacity 451 to 600 pounds ⑧ Qp Qh ♿   Y

  Capped rental

* **K0828** Power wheelchair, group 2 extra heavy duty, sling/solid seat/back, patient weight capacity 601 pounds or more Ⓑ Qp Qh ♿ Y

  Capped rental

* **K0829** Power wheelchair, group 2 extra heavy duty, captains chair, patient weight 601 pounds or more Ⓑ Qp Qh ♿ Y

  Capped rental

* **K0830** Power wheelchair, group 2 standard, seat elevator, sling/solid seat/back, patient weight capacity up to and including 300 pounds Ⓑ Qp Qh Y

  Capped rental

* **K0831** Power wheelchair, group 2 standard, seat elevator, captains chair, patient weight capacity up to and including 300 pounds Ⓑ Qp Qh Y

* **K0835** Power wheelchair, group 2 standard, single power option, sling/solid seat/back, patient weight capacity up to and including 300 pounds Ⓑ Qp Qh ♿ Y

  Capped rental

* **K0836** Power wheelchair, group 2 standard, single power option, captains chair, patient weight capacity up to and including 300 pounds Ⓑ Qp Qh ♿ Y

  Capped rental

* **K0837** Power wheelchair, group 2 heavy duty, single power option, sling/solid seat/back, patient weight capacity 301 to 450 pounds Ⓑ Qp Qh ♿ Y

  Capped rental

* **K0838** Power wheelchair, group 2 heavy duty, single power option, captains chair, patient weight capacity 301 to 450 pounds Ⓑ Qp Qh ♿ Y

  Capped rental

* **K0839** Power wheelchair, group 2 very heavy duty, single power option, sling/solid seat/back, patient weight capacity 451 to 600 pounds Ⓑ Qp Qh ♿ Y

  Capped rental

* **K0840** Power wheelchair, group 2 extra heavy duty, single power option, sling/solid seat/back, patient weight capacity 601 pounds or more Ⓑ Qp Qh Y

  Capped rental

* **K0841** Power wheelchair, group 2 standard, multiple power option, sling/solid seat/back, patient weight capacity up to and including 300 pounds Ⓑ Qp Qh Y

  Capped rental

* **K0842** Power wheelchair, group 2 standard, multiple power option, captains chair, patient weight capacity up to and including 300 pounds Ⓑ Qp Qh ♿ Y

  Capped rental

* **K0843** Power wheelchair, group 2 heavy duty, multiple power option, sling/solid seat/back, patient weight capacity 301 to 450 pounds Ⓑ Qp Qh ♿ Y

  Capped rental

* **K0848** Power wheelchair, group 3 standard, sling/solid seat/back, patient weight capacity up to and including 300 pounds Ⓑ Qp Qh ♿ Y

  Capped rental

* **K0849** Power wheelchair, group 3 standard, captains chair, patient weight capacity up to and including 300 pounds Ⓑ Qp Qh ♿ Y

  Capped rental

* **K0850** Power wheelchair, group 3 heavy duty, sling/solid seat/back, patient weight capacity 301 to 450 pounds Ⓑ Qp Qh ♿ Y

  Capped rental

* **K0851** Power wheelchair, group 3 heavy duty, captains chair, patient weight capacity 301 to 450 pounds Ⓑ Qp Qh ♿ Y

  Capped rental

* **K0852** Power wheelchair, group 3 very heavy duty, sling/solid seat/back, patient weight capacity 451 to 600 pounds Ⓑ Qp Qh ♿ Y

  Capped rental

* **K0853** Power wheelchair, group 3 very heavy duty, captains chair, patient weight capacity 451 to 600 pounds Ⓑ Qp Qh ♿ Y

  Capped rental

* **K0854** Power wheelchair, group 3 extra heavy duty, sling/solid seat/back, patient weight capacity 601 pounds or more Ⓑ Qp Qh ♿ Y

  Capped rental

* **K0855** Power wheelchair, group 3 extra heavy duty, captains chair, patient weight capacity 601 pounds or more Ⓑ Qp Qh ♿ Y

  Capped rental

* **K0856** Power wheelchair, group 3 standard, single power option, sling/solid seat/back, patient weight capacity up to and including 300 pounds Ⓑ Qp Qh ♿ Y

  Capped rental

* **K0857** Power wheelchair, group 3 standard, single power option, captains chair, patient weight capacity up to and including 300 pounds Ⓑ Qp Qh ♿ Y

  Capped rental

* **K0858** Power wheelchair, group 3 heavy duty, single power option, sling/solid seat/back, patient weight 301 to 450 pounds Ⓑ Qp Qh ♿   Y

Capped rental

* **K0859** Power wheelchair, group 3 heavy duty, single power option, captains chair, patient weight capacity 301 to 450 pounds Ⓑ Qp Qh ♿   Y

Capped rental

* **K0860** Power wheelchair, group 3 very heavy duty, single power option, sling/solid seat/back, patient weight capacity 451 to 600 pounds Ⓑ Qp Qh ♿   Y

Capped rental

* **K0861** Power wheelchair, group 3 standard, multiple power option, sling/solid seat/back, patient weight capacity up to and including 300 pounds Ⓑ Qp Qh ♿ Y

Capped rental

* **K0862** Power wheelchair, group 3 heavy duty, multiple power option, sling/solid seat/back, patient weight capacity 301 to 450 pounds Ⓑ Qp Qh ♿   Y

Capped rental

* **K0863** Power wheelchair, group 3 very heavy duty, multiple power option, sling/solid seat/back, patient weight capacity 451 to 600 pounds Ⓑ Qp Qh ♿   Y

Capped rental

* **K0864** Power wheelchair, group 3 extra heavy duty, multiple power option, sling/solid seat/back, patient weight capacity 601 pounds or more Ⓑ Qp Qh ♿   Y

Capped rental

* **K0868** Power wheelchair, group 4 standard, sling/solid seat/back, patient weight capacity up to and including 300 pounds Ⓑ Qp Qh   Y

Capped rental

* **K0869** Power wheelchair, group 4 standard, captains chair, patient weight capacity up to and including 300 pounds Ⓑ Qp Qh   Y

Capped rental

* **K0870** Power wheelchair, group 4 heavy duty, sling/solid seat/back, patient weight capacity 301 to 450 pounds Ⓑ Qp Qh   Y

Capped rental

* **K0871** Power wheelchair, group 4 very heavy duty, sling/solid seat/back, patient weight capacity 451 to 600 pounds Ⓑ Qp Qh   Y

Capped rental

* **K0877** Power wheelchair, group 4 standard, single power option, sling/solid seat/back, patient weight capacity up to and including 300 pounds Ⓑ Qp Qh   Y

Capped rental

* **K0878** Power wheelchair, group 4 standard, single power option, captains chair, patient weight capacity up to and including 300 pounds Ⓑ Qp Qh   Y

Capped rental

* **K0879** Power wheelchair, group 4 heavy duty, single power option, sling/solid seat/back, patient weight capacity 301 to 450 pounds Ⓑ Qp Qh   Y

* **K0880** Power wheelchair, group 4 very heavy duty, single power option, sling/solid seat/back, patient weight 451 to 600 pounds Ⓑ Qp Qh   Y

Capped rental

* **K0884** Power wheelchair, group 4 standard, multiple power option, sling/solid seat/back, patient weight capacity up to and including 300 pounds Ⓑ Qp Qh   Y

Capped rental

* **K0885** Power wheelchair, group 4 standard, multiple power option, captains chair, patient weight capacity up to and including 300 pounds Ⓑ Qp Qh   Y

Capped rental

* **K0886** Power wheelchair, group 4 heavy duty, multiple power option, sling/solid seat/back, patient weight capacity 301 to 450 pounds Ⓑ Qp Qh   Y

Capped rental

* **K0890** Power wheelchair, group 5 pediatric, single power option, sling/solid seat/back, patient weight capacity up to and including 125 pounds Ⓑ Qp Qh A   Y

Capped rental

* **K0891** Power wheelchair, group 5 pediatric, multiple power option, sling/solid seat/back, patient weight capacity up to and including 125 pounds Ⓑ Qp Qh A   Y

Capped rental

* **K0898** Power wheelchair, not otherwise classified Ⓑ Qp Qh   Y

* **K0899** Power mobility device, not coded by DME PDAC or does not meet criteria Ⓑ   Y

Customized DME: Other than Wheelchair

⊚ **K0900** Customized durable medical equipment, other than wheelchair Ⓑ Qp Qh   Y

Devices

✳ **K1001** Electronic positional obstructive sleep apnea treatment, with sensor, includes all components and accessories, any type Ⓑ   Y

⊘ **K1002** Cranial electrotherapy stimulation (CES) system, any type Ⓑ ♿   Y

✳ **K1003** Whirlpool tub, walk-in, portable Ⓓ   E1

↻ ✳ **K1004** Low frequency ultrasonic diathermy treatment device for home use Ⓑ   E1

✳ **K1005** Disposable collection and storage bag for breast milk, any size, any type, each Ⓑ   Y

✳ **K1006** Suction pump, home model, portable or stationary, electric, any type, for use with external urine management system   Y

✳ **K1007** Bilateral hip, knee, ankle, foot device, powered, includes pelvic component, single or double upright(s), knee joints any type, with or without ankle joints any type, includes all components and accessories, motors, microprocessors, sensors   Y

✳ **K1009** Speech volume modulation system, any type, including all components and accessories   Y

✳ **K1013** Enema tube, with or without adapter, any type, replacement only, each   E1

✳ **K1014** Addition, endoskeletal knee-shin system, 4 bar linkage or multiaxial, fluid swing and stance phase control ♿   Y

✳ **K1015** Foot, adductus positioning device, adjustable   Y

✳ **K1016** Transcutaneous electrical nerve stimulator for electrical stimulation of the trigeminal nerve ♿   Y

✳ **K1017** Monthly supplies for use of device coded at K1016 ♿   Y

✳ **K1018** External upper limb tremor stimulator of the peripheral nerves of the wrist ♿   Y

↻ ✳ **K1019** Supplies and accessories for external upper limb tremor stimulator of the peripheral nerves of the wrist   Y

✳ **K1020** Non-invasive vagus nerve stimulator ♿   Y

✳ **K1021** Exsufflation belt, includes all supplies and accessories   Y

✳ **K1022** Addition to lower extremity prosthesis, endoskeletal, knee disarticulation, above knee, hip disarticulation, positional rotation unit, any type ♿   Y

✳ **K1023** Distal transcutaneous electrical nerve stimulator, stimulates peripheral nerves of the upper arm   E1

✳ **K1024** Non-pneumatic compression controller with sequential calibrated gradient pressure ♿   Y

✳ **K1025** Non-pneumatic sequential compression garment, full arm ♿   Y

✳ **K1026** Mechanical allergen particle barrier/inhalation filter, cream, nasal, topical   Y

✳ **K1027** Oral device/appliance used to reduce upper airway collapsibility, without fixed mechanical hinge, custom fabricated, includes fitting and adjustment   Y

▶ ⊚ **K1028** Power source and control electronics unit for oral device/appliance for neuromuscular electrical stimulation of the tongue muscle, controlled by phone application   E1

Self-administered test

K1030 External recharging system for battery (internal) for use with implanted cardiac contractility modulation generator, replacement only   Y

K1031 Non-pneumatic compression controller without calibrated gradient pressure   Y

K1032 Non-pneumatic sequential compression garment, full leg   Y

K1033 Non-pneumatic sequential compression garment, half leg   Y

K1034 Provision of covid-19 test, nonprescription self-administered and self-collected use, FDA approved, authorized or cleared, one test count   A

▶ **K1035** Molecular diagnostic test reader, nonprescription self-administered and self-collected use, FDA approved, authorized or cleared

▶ **K1036** Supplies and accessories (e.g., transducer) for low frequency ultrasonic diathermy treatment device, per month

---

▶ **New**   ↻ **Revised**   ✔ **Reinstated**   ~~deleted~~ **Deleted**   ⊘ **Not covered or valid by Medicare**   ⊚ **Special coverage instructions**   ✳ **Carrier discretion**   Ⓑ **Bill Part B MAC**   Ⓓ **Bill DME MAC**

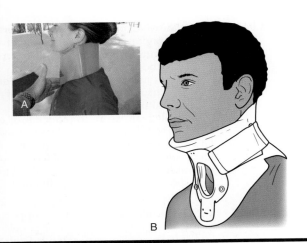

Figure 19 (A) Flexible cervical collar. (B) Adjustable cervical collar.

ORTHOTICS & DEVICES (L0112-L4631)

NOTE: DMEPOS fee schedule https://www.cms.gov/Medicare/Medicare-Fee-for-Service-Payment/DMEPOSFeeSched/DMEPOS-Fee-Schedule.html

Cervical Orthotics

* **L0112** Cranial cervical orthosis, congenital torticollis type, with or without soft interface material, adjustable range of motion joint, custom fabricated ⑬ Qp Qh &   A

* **L0113** Cranial cervical orthosis, torticollis type, with or without joint, with or without soft interface material, prefabricated, includes fitting and adjustment ⑬ Qp Qh &   A

* **L0120** Cervical, flexible, non-adjustable, prefabricated, off-the-shelf (foam collar) ⑬ Qp Qh &   A

  Cervical orthoses including soft and rigid devices may be used as nonoperative management for cervical trauma

* **L0130** Cervical, flexible, thermoplastic collar, molded to patient ⑬ Qp Qh &   A

* **L0140** Cervical, semi-rigid, adjustable (plastic collar) ⑬ Qp Qh &   A

* **L0150** Cervical, semi-rigid, adjustable molded chin cup (plastic collar with mandibular/occipital piece) ⑬ Qp Qh &   A

* **L0160** Cervical, semi-rigid, wire frame occipital/mandibular support, prefabricated, off-the-shelf ⑬ Qp Qh &   A

* **L0170** Cervical, collar, molded to patient model ⑬ Qp Qh &   A

* **L0172** Cervical, collar, semi-rigid thermoplastic foam, two-piece, prefabricated, off-the-shelf ⑬ Qp Qh &   A

* **L0174** Cervical, collar, semi-rigid, thermoplastic foam, two piece with thoracic extension, prefabricated, off-the-shelf ⑬ Qp Qh &   A

Multiple Post Collar: Cervical

* **L0180** Cervical, multiple post collar, occipital/mandibular supports, adjustable ⑬ Qp Qh &   A

* **L0190** Cervical, multiple post collar, occipital/mandibular supports, adjustable cervical bars (SOMI, Guilford, Taylor types) ⑬ Qp Qh &   A

* **L0200** Cervical, multiple post collar, occipital/mandibular supports, adjustable cervical bars, and thoracic extension ⑬ Qp Qh &   A

Thoracic Rib Belt

* **L0220** Thoracic, rib belt, custom fabricated ⑬ Qp Qh &   A

Thoracic-Lumbar-Sacral Orthotics

* **L0450** TLSO, flexible, provides trunk support, upper thoracic region, produces intracavitary pressure to reduce load on the intervertebral disks with rigid stays or panel(s), includes shoulder straps and closures, prefabricated, off-the-shelf ⑬ Qp Qh &   A

  Used to immobilize specified area of spine, and is generally worn under clothing

* **L0452** TLSO, flexible, provides trunk support, upper thoracic region, produces intracavitary pressure to reduce load on the intervertebral disks with rigid stays or panel(s), includes shoulder straps and closures, custom fabricated ⑬ Qp Qh &   A

Figure 20 Thoracic-lumbar-sacral-orthosis (TLSO).

✳ **L0454** TLSO flexible, provides trunk support, extends from sacrococcygeal junction to above T-9 vertebra, restricts gross trunk motion in the sagittal plane, produces intracavitary pressure to reduce load on the intervertebral disks with rigid stays or panel(s), includes shoulder straps and closures, prefabricated item that has been trimmed, bent, molded, assembled, or otherwise customized to fit a specific patient by an individual with expertise Ⓑ Qp Qh ♿   A

Used to immobilize specified areas of spine; and is generally designed to be worn under clothing; not specifically designed for patients in wheelchairs

✳ **L0455** TLSO, flexible, provides trunk support, extends from sacrococcygeal junction to above T-9 vertebra, restricts gross trunk motion in the sagittal plane, produces intracavitary pressure to reduce load on the intervertebral disks with rigid stays or panel(s), includes shoulder straps and closures, prefabricated, off-the-shelf Ⓑ Qp Qh ♿   A

✳ **L0456** TLSO, flexible, provides trunk support, thoracic region, rigid posterior panel and soft anterior apron, extends from the sacrococcygeal junction and terminates just inferior to the scapular spine, restricts gross trunk motion in the sagittal plane, produces intracavitary pressure to reduce load on the intervertebral disks, includes straps and closures, prefabricated item that has been trimmed, bent, molded, assembled, or otherwise customized to fit a specific patient by an individual with expertise Ⓑ Qp Qh ♿   A

✳ **L0457** TLSO, flexible, provides trunk support, thoracic region, rigid posterior panel and soft anterior apron, extends from the sacrococcygeal junction and terminates just inferior to the scapular spine, restricts gross trunk motion in the sagittal plane, produces intracavitary pressure to reduce load on the intervertebral disks, includes straps and closures, prefabricated, off-the-shelf Ⓑ Qp Qh ♿   A

✳ **L0458** TLSO, triplanar control, modular segmented spinal system, two rigid plastic shells, posterior extends from the sacrococcygeal junction and terminates just inferior to the scapular spine, anterior extends from the symphysis pubis to the xiphoid, soft liner, restricts gross trunk motion in the sagittal, coronal, and transverse planes, lateral strength is provided by overlapping plastic and stabilizing closures, includes straps and closures, prefabricated, includes fitting and adjustment Ⓑ Qp Qh ♿   A

To meet Medicare's definition of body jacket, orthosis has to have rigid plastic shell that circles trunk with overlapping edges and stabilizing closures, and entire circumference of shell must be made of same rigid material.

▶ **New**   ⟲ **Revised**   ✔ **Reinstated**   ~~deleted~~ **Deleted**   ⊘ **Not covered or valid by Medicare**
⊙ **Special coverage instructions**   ✳ **Carrier discretion**   Ⓑ **Bill Part B MAC**   Ⓑ **Bill DME MAC**

L0454 – L0458 ORTHOTICS & DEVICES

350

✳ **L0460** TLSO, triplanar control, modular segmented spinal system, two rigid plastic shells, posterior extends from the sacrococcygeal junction and terminates just inferior to the scapular spine, anterior extends from the symphysis pubis to the sternal notch, soft liner, restricts gross trunk motion in the sagittal, coronal, and transverse planes, lateral strength is provided by overlapping plastic and stabilizing closures, includes straps and closures, prefabricated item that has been trimmed, bent, molded, assembled, or otherwise customized to fit a specific patient by an individual with expertise ⑧ Qp Qh ⑤   A

✳ **L0462** TLSO, triplanar control, modular segmented spinal system, three rigid plastic shells, posterior extends from the sacrococcygeal junction and terminates just inferior to the scapular spine, anterior extends from the symphysis pubis to the sternal notch, soft liner, restricts gross trunk motion in the sagittal, coronal, and transverse planes, lateral strength is provided by overlapping plastic and stabilizing closures, includes straps and closures, prefabricated, includes fitting and adjustment ⑧ Qp Qh ⑤   A

✳ **L0464** TLSO, triplanar control, modular segmented spinal system, four rigid plastic shells, posterior extends from sacrococcygeal junction and terminates just inferior to scapular spine, anterior extends from symphysis pubis to the sternal notch, soft liner, restricts gross trunk motion in sagittal, coronal, and transverse planes, lateral strength is provided by overlapping plastic and stabilizing closures, includes straps and closures, prefabricated, includes fitting and adjustment ⑧ Qp Qh ⑤   A

✳ **L0466** TLSO, sagittal control, rigid posterior frame and flexible soft anterior apron with straps, closures and padding, restricts gross trunk motion in sagittal plane, produces intracavitary pressure to reduce load on intervertebral disks, prefabricated item that has been trimmed, bent, molded, assembled, or otherwise customized to fit a specific patient by an individual with expertise ⑧ Qp Qh ⑤   A

✳ **L0467** TLSO, sagittal control, rigid posterior frame and flexible soft anterior apron with straps, closures and padding, restricts gross trunk motion in sagittal plane, produces intracavitary pressure to reduce load on intervertebral disks, prefabricated, off-the-shelf ⑧ Qp Qh ⑤   A

✳ **L0468** TLSO, sagittal-coronal control, rigid posterior frame and flexible soft anterior apron with straps, closures and padding, extends from sacrococcygeal junction over scapulae, lateral strength provided by pelvic, thoracic, and lateral frame pieces, restricts gross trunk motion in sagittal, and coronal planes, produces intracavitary pressure to reduce load on intervertebral disks, prefabricated item that has been trimmed, bent, molded, assembled, or otherwise customized to fit a specific patient by an individual with expertise ⑧ Qp Qh ⑤   A

✳ **L0469** TLSO, sagittal-coronal control, rigid posterior frame and flexible soft anterior apron with straps, closures and padding, extends from sacrococcygeal junction over scapulae, lateral strength provided by pelvic, thoracic, and lateral frame pieces, restricts gross trunk motion in sagittal and coronal planes, produces intracavitary pressure to reduce load on intervertebral disks, prefabricated, off-the-shelf ⑧ Qp Qh ⑤   A

✳ **L0470** TLSO, triplanar control, rigid posterior frame and flexible soft anterior apron with straps, closures and padding, extends from sacrococcygeal junction to scapula, lateral strength provided by pelvic, thoracic, and lateral frame pieces, rotational strength provided by subclavicular extensions, restricts gross trunk motion in sagittal, coronal, and transverse planes, provides intracavitary pressure to reduce load on the intervertebral disks, includes fitting and shaping the frame, prefabricated, includes fitting and adjustment ⑧ Qp Qh ♿   A

✳ **L0472** TLSO, triplanar control, hyperextension, rigid anterior and lateral frame extends from symphysis pubis to sternal notch with two anterior components (one pubic and one sternal), posterior and lateral pads with straps and closures, limits spinal flexion, restricts gross trunk motion in sagittal, coronal, and transverse planes, includes fitting and shaping the frame, prefabricated, includes fitting and adjustment ⑧ Qp Qh ♿   A

✳ **L0480** TLSO, triplanar control, one piece rigid plastic shell without interface liner, with multiple straps and closures, posterior extends from sacrococcygeal junction and terminates just inferior to scapular spine, anterior extends from symphysis pubis to sternal notch, anterior or posterior opening, restricts gross trunk motion in sagittal, coronal, and transverse planes, includes a carved plaster or CAD-CAM model, custom fabricated ⑧ Qp Qh ♿   A

✳ **L0482** TLSO, triplanar control, one piece rigid plastic shell with interface liner, multiple straps and closures, posterior extends from sacrococcygeal junction and terminates just inferior to scapular spine, anterior extends from symphysis pubis to sternal notch, anterior or posterior opening, restricts gross trunk motion in sagittal, coronal, and transverse planes, includes a carved plaster or CAD-CAM model, custom fabricated ⑧ Qp Qh ♿   A

✳ **L0484** TLSO, triplanar control, two piece rigid plastic shell without interface liner, with multiple straps and closures, posterior extends from sacrococcygeal junction and terminates just inferior to scapular spine, anterior extends from symphysis pubis to sternal notch, lateral strength is enhanced by overlapping plastic, restricts gross trunk motion in the sagittal, coronal, and transverse planes, includes a carved plaster or CAD-CAM model, custom fabricated ⑧ Qp Qh ♿   A

✳ **L0486** TLSO, triplanar control, two piece rigid plastic shell with interface liner, multiple straps and closures, posterior extends from sacrococcygeal junction and terminates just inferior to scapular spine, anterior extends from symphysis pubis to sternal notch, lateral strength is enhanced by overlapping plastic, restricts gross trunk motion in the sagittal, coronal, and transverse planes, includes a carved plaster or CAD-CAM model, custom fabricated ⑧ Qp Qh ♿   A

✳ **L0488** TLSO, triplanar control, one piece rigid plastic shell with interface liner, multiple straps and closures, posterior extends from sacrococcygeal junction and terminates just inferior to scapular spine, anterior extends from symphysis pubis to sternal notch, anterior or posterior opening, restricts gross trunk motion in sagittal, coronal, and transverse planes, prefabricated, includes fitting and adjustment ⑧ Qp Qh ♿   A

Figure 21   Thoracic-lumbar-sacral orthosis (TLSO) Jewett flexion control.

▶ New	↻ Revised	✔ Reinstated	~~deleted~~ Deleted	⊘ Not covered or valid by Medicare
⊛ Special coverage instructions	✳ Carrier discretion	⑧ Bill Part B MAC	⑧ Bill DME MAC	

* **L0490** TLSO, sagittal-coronal control, one piece rigid plastic shell, with overlapping reinforced anterior, with multiple straps and closures, posterior extends from sacrococcygeal junction and terminates at or before the T-9 vertebra, anterior extends from symphysis pubis to xiphoid, anterior opening, restricts gross trunk motion in sagittal and coronal planes, prefabricated, includes fitting and adjustment ⑧ Qp Qh ċ A

* **L0491** TLSO, sagittal-coronal control, modular segmented spinal system, two rigid plastic shells, posterior extends from the sacrococcygeal junction and terminates just inferior to the scapular spine, anterior extends from the symphysis pubis to the xiphoid, soft liner, restricts gross trunk motion in the sagittal and coronal planes, lateral strength is provided by overlapping plastic and stabilizing closures, includes straps and closures, prefabricated, includes fitting and adjustment ⑧ Qp Qh ċ A

* **L0492** TLSO, sagittal-coronal control, modular segmented spinal system, three rigid plastic shells, posterior extends from the sacrococcygeal junction and terminates just inferior to the scapular spine, anterior extends from the symphysis pubis to the xiphoid, soft liner, restricts gross trunk motion in the sagittal and coronal planes, lateral strength is provided by overlapping plastic and stabilizing closures, includes straps and closures, prefabricated, includes fitting and adjustment ⑧ Qp Qh ċ A

Sacroilliac Orthotics

* **L0621** Sacroiliac orthosis, flexible, provides pelvic-sacral support, reduces motion about the sacroiliac joint, includes straps, closures, may include pendulous abdomen design, prefabricated, off-the-shelf ⑧ Qp Qh ċ A

* **L0622** Sacroiliac orthosis, flexible, provides pelvic-sacral support, reduces motion about the sacroiliac joint, includes straps, closures, may include pendulous abdomen design, custom fabricated ⑧ Qp Qh ċ A

Type of custom-fabricated device for which impression of specific body part is made (e.g., by means of plaster cast, or CAD-CAM [computer-aided design] technology); impression then used to make specific patient model

* **L0623** Sacroiliac orthosis, provides pelvic-sacral support, with rigid or semi-rigid panels over the sacrum and abdomen, reduces motion about the sacroiliac joint, includes straps, closures, may include pendulous abdomen design, prefabricated, off-the-shelf ⑧ Qp Qh ċ A

* **L0624** Sacroiliac orthosis, provides pelvic-sacral support, with rigid or semi-rigid panels placed over the sacrum and abdomen, reduces motion about the sacroiliac joint, includes straps, closures, may include pendulous abdomen design, custom fabricated ⑧ Qp Qh ċ A

Custom fitted

Lumbar Orthotics

* **L0625** Lumbar orthosis, flexible, provides lumbar support, posterior extends from L-1 to below L-5 vertebra, produces intracavitary pressure to reduce load on the intervertebral discs, includes straps, closures, may include pendulous abdomen design, shoulder straps, stays, prefabricated, off-the-shelf ⑧ Qp Qh ċ A

* **L0626** Lumbar orthosis, sagittal control, with rigid posterior panel(s), posterior extends from L-1 to below L-5 vertebra, produces intracavitary pressure to reduce load on the intervertebral discs, includes straps, closures, may include padding, stays, shoulder straps, pendulous abdomen design, prefabricated item that has been trimmed, bent, molded, assembled, or otherwise customized to fit a specific patient by an individual with expertise ⑧ Qp Qh ċ A

✳ **L0627** Lumbar orthosis, sagittal control, with rigid anterior and posterior panels, posterior extends from L-1 to below L-5 vertebra, produces intracavitary pressure to reduce load on the intervertebral discs, includes straps, closures, may include padding, shoulder straps, pendulous abdomen design, prefabricated item that has been trimmed, bent, molded, assembled, or otherwise customized to fit a specific patient by an individual with expertise ⑧ Qp Qh ⛨   A

Figure 22 Lumbar-sacral orthosis.

Lumbar-Sacral Orthotics

✳ **L0628** Lumbar-sacral orthosis, flexible, provides lumbo-sacral support, posterior extends from sacrococcygeal junction to T-9 vertebra, produces intracavitary pressure to reduce load on the intervertebral discs, includes straps, closures, may include stays, shoulder straps, pendulous abdomen design, prefabricated, off-the-shelf ⑧ Qp Qh ⛨   A

✳ **L0629** Lumbar-sacral orthosis, flexible, provides lumbo-sacral support, posterior extends from sacrococcygeal junction to T-9 vertebra, produces intracavitary pressure to reduce load on the intervertebral discs, includes straps, closures, may include stays, shoulder straps, pendulous abdomen design, custom fabricated ⑧ Qp Qh ⛨   A

    Custom fitted

✳ **L0630** Lumbar-sacral orthosis, sagittal control, with rigid posterior panel(s), posterior extends from sacrococcygeal junction to T-9 vertebra, produces intracavitary pressure to reduce load on the intervertebral discs, includes straps, closures, may include padding, stays, shoulder straps, pendulous abdomen design, prefabricated item that has been trimmed, bent, molded, assembled, or otherwise customized to fit a specific patient by an individual with expertise ⑧ Qp Qh ⛨   A

✳ **L0631** Lumbar-sacral orthosis, sagittal control, with rigid anterior and posterior panels, posterior extends from sacrococcygeal junction to T-9 vertebra, produces intracavitary pressure to reduce load on the intervertebral discs, includes straps, closures, may include padding, shoulder straps, pendulous abdomen design, prefabricated item that has been trimmed, bent, molded, assembled, or otherwise customized to fit a specific patient by an individual with expertise ⑧ Qp Qh ⛨   A

✳ **L0632** Lumbar-sacral orthosis, sagittal control, with rigid anterior and posterior panels, posterior extends from sacrococcygeal junction to T-9 vertebra, produces intracavitary pressure to reduce load on the intervertebral discs, includes straps, closures, may include padding, shoulder straps, pendulous abdomen design, custom fabricated ⑧ Qp Qh ⛨   A

    Custom fitted

✳ **L0633** Lumbar-sacral orthosis, sagittal-coronal control, with rigid posterior frame/panel(s), posterior extends from sacrococcygeal junction to T-9 vertebra, lateral strength provided by rigid lateral frame/panels, produces intracavitary pressure to reduce load on intervertebral discs, includes straps, closures, may include padding, stays, shoulder straps, pendulous abdomen design, prefabricated item that has been trimmed, bent, molded, assembled, or otherwise customized to fit a specific patient by an individual with expertise ⑧ Qp Qh ⛨   A

▶ New   ⟳ Revised   ✔ Reinstated   ~~deleted~~ Deleted   ⊘ Not covered or valid by Medicare

✪ Special coverage instructions   ✳ Carrier discretion   ⑧ Bill Part B MAC   ⑧ Bill DME MAC

* **L0634** Lumbar-sacral orthosis, sagittal-coronal control, with rigid posterior frame/panel(s), posterior extends from sacrococcygeal junction to T-9 vertebra, lateral strength provided by rigid lateral frame/panel(s), produces intracavitary pressure to reduce load on intervertebral discs, includes straps, closures, may include padding, stays, shoulder straps, pendulous abdomen design, custom fabricated ⑧ Qp Qh ♿   A

Custom fitted

* **L0635** Lumbar-sacral orthosis, sagittal-coronal control, lumbar flexion, rigid posterior frame/panel(s), lateral articulating design to flex the lumbar spine, posterior extends from sacrococcygeal junction to T-9 vertebra, lateral strength provided by rigid lateral frame/panel(s), produces intracavitary pressure to reduce load on intervertebral discs, includes straps, closures, may include padding, anterior panel, pendulous abdomen design, prefabricated, includes fitting and adjustment ⑧ Qp Qh ♿   A

* **L0636** Lumbar sacral orthosis, sagittal-coronal control, lumbar flexion, rigid posterior frame/panels, lateral articulating design to flex the lumbar spine, posterior extends from sacrococcygeal junction to T-9 vertebra, lateral strength provided by rigid lateral frame/panels, produces intracavitary pressure to reduce load on intervertebral discs, includes straps, closures, may include padding, anterior panel, pendulous abdomen design, custom fabricated ⑧ Qp Qh ♿   A

Custom fitted

* **L0637** Lumbar-sacral orthosis, sagittal-coronal control, with rigid anterior and posterior frame/panels, posterior extends from sacrococcygeal junction to T-9 vertebra, lateral strength provided by rigid lateral frame/panels, produces intracavitary pressure to reduce load on intervertebral discs, includes straps, closures, may include padding, shoulder straps, pendulous abdomen design, prefabricated item that has been trimmed, bent, molded, assembled, or otherwise customized to fit a specific patient by an individual with expertise ⑧ Qp Qh ♿   A

* **L0638** Lumbar-sacral orthosis, sagittal-coronal control, with rigid anterior and posterior frame/panels, posterior extends from sacrococcygeal junction to T-9 vertebra, lateral strength provided by rigid lateral frame/panels, produces intracavitary pressure to reduce load on intervertebral discs, includes straps, closures, may include padding, shoulder straps, pendulous abdomen design, custom fabricated ⑧ Qp Qh ♿   A

* **L0639** Lumbar-sacral orthosis, sagittal-coronal control, rigid shell(s)/panel(s), posterior extends from sacrococcygeal junction to T-9 vertebra, anterior extends from symphysis pubis to xyphoid, produces intracavitary pressure to reduce load on the intervertebral discs, overall strength is provided by overlapping rigid material and stabilizing closures, includes straps, closures, may include soft interface, pendulous abdomen design, prefabricated item that has been trimmed, bent, molded, assembled, or otherwise customized to fit a specific patient by an individual with expertise ⑧ Qp Qh ♿   A

Characterized by rigid plastic shell that encircles trunk with overlapping edges and stabilizing closures and provides high degree of immobility

* **L0640** Lumbar-sacral orthosis, sagittal-coronal control, rigid shell(s)/panel(s), posterior extends from sacrococcygeal junction to T-9 vertebra, anterior extends from symphysis pubis to xyphoid, produces intracavitary pressure to reduce load on the intervertebral discs, overall strength is provided by overlapping rigid material and stabilizing closures, includes straps, closures, may include soft interface, pendulous abdomen design, custom fabricated ⑧ Qp Qh ♿   A

Custom fitted

Lumbar Orthotics

* **L0641** Lumbar orthosis, sagittal control, with rigid posterior panel(s), posterior extends from L-1 to below L-5 vertebra, produces intracavitary pressure to reduce load on the intervertebral discs, includes straps, closures, may include padding, stays, shoulder straps, pendulous abdomen design, prefabricated, off-the-shelf ⑧ Qp Qh ♿   A

* **L0642** Lumbar orthosis, sagittal control, with rigid anterior and posterior panels, posterior extends from L-1 to below L-5 vertebra, produces intracavitary pressure to reduce load on the intervertebral discs, includes straps, closures, may include padding, shoulder straps, pendulous abdomen design, prefabricated, off-the-shelf ⑬ **Qp** **Qh** 🦽   A

Lumbar-Sacral Orthotics

* **L0643** Lumbar-sacral orthosis, sagittal control, with rigid posterior panel(s), posterior extends from sacrococcygeal junction to T-9 vertebra, produces intracavitary pressure to reduce load on the intervertebral discs, includes straps, closures, may include padding, stays, shoulder straps, pendulous abdomen design, prefabricated, off-the-shelf ⑬ **Qp** **Qh** 🦽   A

* **L0648** Lumbar-sacral orthosis, sagittal control, with rigid anterior and posterior panels, posterior extends from sacrococcygeal junction to T-9 vertebra, produces intracavitary pressure to reduce load on the intervertebral discs, includes straps, closures, may include padding, shoulder straps, pendulous abdomen design, prefabricated, off-the-shelf ⑬ **Qp** **Qh** 🦽   A

* **L0649** Lumbar-sacral orthosis, sagittal-coronal control, with rigid posterior frame/panel(s), posterior extends from sacrococcygeal junction to T-9 vertebra, lateral strength provided by rigid lateral frame/panels, produces intracavitary pressure to reduce load on intervertebral discs, includes straps, closures, may include padding, stays, shoulder straps, pendulous abdomen design, prefabricated, off-the-shelf ⑬ **Qp** **Qh** 🦽   A

* **L0650** Lumbar-sacral orthosis, sagittal-coronal control, with rigid anterior and posterior frame/panel(s), posterior extends from sacrococcygeal junction to T-9 vertebra, lateral strength provided by rigid lateral frame/panel(s), produces intracavitary pressure to reduce load on intervertebral discs, includes straps, closures, may include padding, shoulder straps, pendulous abdomen design, prefabricated, off-the-shelf ⑬ **Qp** **Qh** 🦽   A

* **L0651** Lumbar-sacral orthosis, sagittal-coronal control, rigid shell(s)/panel(s), posterior extends from sacrococcygeal junction to T-9 vertebra, anterior extends from symphysis pubis to xyphoid, produces intracavitary pressure to reduce load on the intervertebral discs, overall strength is provided by overlapping rigid material and stabilizing closures, includes straps, closures, may include soft interface, pendulous abdomen design, prefabricated, off-the-shelf ⑬ **Qp** **Qh** 🦽   A

Cervical-Thoracic-Lumbar-Sacral

* **L0700** Cervical-thoracic-lumbar-sacral-orthoses (CTLSO), anterior-posterior-lateral control, molded to patient model (Minerva type) ⑬ **Qp** **Qh** 🦽   A

* **L0710** CTLSO, anterior-posterior-lateral-control, molded to patient model, with interface material (Minerva type) ⑬ **Qp** **Qh** 🦽   A

HALO Procedure

* **L0810** HALO procedure, cervical halo incorporated into jacket vest ⑬ **Qp** **Qh** 🦽   A

* **L0820** HALO procedure, cervical halo incorporated into plaster body jacket ⑬ **Qp** **Qh** 🦽   A

* **L0830** HALO procedure, cervical halo incorporated into Milwaukee type orthosis ⑬ **Qp** **Qh** 🦽   A

* **L0859** Addition to HALO procedure, magnetic resonance image compatible systems, rings and pins, any material ⑬ **Qp** **Qh** 🦽   A

* **L0861** Addition to HALO procedure, replacement liner/interface material ⑬ **Qp** **Qh** 🦽   A

Figure 23 Halo device.

▶ New   ⟲ Revised   ✔ Reinstated   ̶d̶e̶l̶e̶t̶e̶d̶ Deleted   ⊘ Not covered or valid by Medicare   ⊙ Special coverage instructions   ✳ Carrier discretion   ⑬ Bill Part B MAC   Ⓑ Bill DME MAC

L0642 – L0861   ORTHOTICS & DEVICES

356

Additions to Spinal Orthotics

NOTE: TLSO - Thoraci-lumbar-sacral orthoses/ Spinal orthoses may be prefabricated, prefitted, or custom fabricated. Conservative treatment for back pain may include the use of spinal orthoses.

Figure 24 Milwaukee CTLSO.

✳ **L0970**	TLSO, corset front ⓑ Qp Qh ⅖	A
✳ **L0972**	LSO, corset front ⓑ Qp Qh ⅖	A
✳ **L0974**	TLSO, full corset ⓑ Qp Qh ⅖	A
✳ **L0976**	LSO, full corset ⓑ Qp Qh ⅖	A
✳ **L0978**	Axillary crutch extension ⓑ Qp Qh ⅖	A
✳ **L0980**	Peroneal straps, prefabricated, off-the-shelf, pair ⓑ Qp Qh ⅖	A
✳ **L0982**	Stocking supporter grips, prefabricated, off-the-shelf, set of four (4) ⓑ Qp Qh ⅖	A
	Convenience item	
✳ **L0984**	Protective body sock, prefabricated, off-the-shelf, each ⓑ Qp Qh ⅖	A
	Garment made of cloth or similar material that is worn under spinal orthosis and is not primarily medical in nature	
✳ **L0999**	Addition to spinal orthosis, not otherwise specified ⓑ	A

Orthotic Devices: Scoliosis Procedures

NOTE: Orthotic care of scoliosis differs from other orthotic care in that the treatment is more dynamic in nature and uses ongoing continual modification of the orthosis to the patient's changing condition. This coding structure uses the proper names, or eponyms, of the procedures because they have historic and universal acceptance in the profession. It should be recognized that variations to the basic procedures described by the founders/ developers are accepted in various medical and orthotic practices throughout the country. All procedures include a model of patient when indicated.

✳ **L1000**	Cervical-thoracic-lumbar-sacral orthosis (CTLSO) (Milwaukee), inclusive of furnishing initial orthosis, including model ⓑ Qp Qh ⅖	A
✳ **L1001**	Cervical thoracic lumbar sacral orthosis, immobilizer, infant size, prefabricated, includes fitting and adjustment ⓑ Qp Qh ⅖	A
✳ **L1005**	Tension based scoliosis orthosis and accessory pads, includes fitting and adjustment ⓑ Qp Qh ⅖	A
✳ **L1010**	Addition to cervical-thoracic-lumbar-sacral orthosis (CTLSO) or scoliosis orthosis, axilla sling ⓑ Qp Qh ⅖	A
✳ **L1020**	Addition to CTLSO or scoliosis orthosis, kyphosis pad ⓑ Qp Qh ⅖	A
✳ **L1025**	Addition to CTLSO or scoliosis orthosis, kyphosis pad, floating ⓑ Qp Qh ⅖	A
✳ **L1030**	Addition to CTLSO or scoliosis orthosis, lumbar bolster pad ⓑ Qp Qh ⅖	A
✳ **L1040**	Addition to CTLSO or scoliosis orthosis, lumbar or lumbar rib pad ⓑ Qp Qh ⅖	A
✳ **L1050**	Addition to CTLSO or scoliosis orthosis, sternal pad ⓑ Qp Qh ⅖	A
✳ **L1060**	Addition to CTLSO or scoliosis orthosis, thoracic pad ⓑ Qp Qh ⅖	A
✳ **L1070**	Addition to CTLSO or scoliosis orthosis, trapezius sling ⓑ Qp Qh ⅖	A
✳ **L1080**	Addition to CTLSO or scoliosis orthosis, outrigger ⓑ Qp Qh ⅖	A
✳ **L1085**	Addition to CTLSO or scoliosis orthosis, outrigger, bilateral with vertical extensions ⓑ Qp Qh ⅖	A
✳ **L1090**	Addition to CTLSO or scoliosis orthosis, lumbar sling ⓑ Qp Qh ⅖	A
✳ **L1100**	Addition to CTLSO or scoliosis orthosis, ring flange, plastic or leather ⓑ Qp Qh ⅖	A
✳ **L1110**	Addition to CTLSO or scoliosis orthosis, ring flange, plastic or leather, molded to patient model ⓑ Qp Qh ⅖	A
✳ **L1120**	Addition to CTLSO, scoliosis orthosis, cover for upright, each ⓑ Qp Qh ⅖	A

🅜 MIPS	Qp Quantity Physician	Qh Quantity Hospital	♀ Female only
♂ Male only	A Age	⅖ DMEPOS	A2-Z3 ASC Payment Indicator · A-Y ASC Status Indicator · Coding Clinic

Thoracic-Lumbar-Sacral (Low Profile)

* **L1200** Thoracic-lumbar-sacral-orthosis (TLSO), inclusive of furnishing initial orthosis only Ⓑ Qp Qh 🦽   A

* **L1210** Addition to TLSO, (low profile), lateral thoracic extension Ⓑ Qp Qh 🦽   A

* **L1220** Addition to TLSO, (low profile), anterior thoracic extension Ⓑ Qp Qh 🦽   A

* **L1230** Addition to TLSO, (low profile), Milwaukee type superstructure Ⓑ Qp Qh 🦽   A

* **L1240** Addition to TLSO, (low profile), lumbar derotation pad Ⓑ Qp Qh 🦽   A

* **L1250** Addition to TLSO, (low profile), anterior ASIS pad Ⓑ Qp Qh 🦽   A

* **L1260** Addition to TLSO, (low profile), anterior thoracic derotation pad Ⓑ Qp Qh 🦽   A

* **L1270** Addition to TLSO, (low profile), abdominal pad Ⓑ Qp Qh 🦽   A

* **L1280** Addition to TLSO, (low profile), rib gusset (elastic), each Ⓑ Qp Qh 🦽   A

* **L1290** Addition to TLSO, (low profile), lateral trochanteric pad Ⓑ Qp Qh 🦽   A

Other Scoliosis Procedures

* **L1300** Other scoliosis procedure, body jacket molded to patient model Ⓑ Qp Qh 🦽   A

* **L1310** Other scoliosis procedure, postoperative body jacket Ⓑ Qp Qh 🦽   A

* **L1499** Spinal orthosis, not otherwise specified Ⓑ Qp Qh   A

Orthotic Devices: Lower Limb (L1600-L3649)

NOTE: the procedures in L1600-L2999 are considered as base or basic procedures and may be modified by listing procedure from the Additions Sections and adding them to the base procedure.

Hip: Flexible

* **L1600** Hip orthosis, abduction control of hip joints, flexible, frejka type with cover, prefabricated item that has been trimmed, bent, molded, assembled, or otherwise customized to fit a specific patient by an individual with expertise Ⓑ Qp Qh 🦽   A

* **L1610** Hip orthosis, abduction control of hip joints, flexible, (frejka cover only), prefabricated item that has been trimmed, bent, molded, assembled, or otherwise customized to fit a specific patient by an individual with expertise Ⓑ Qp Qh 🦽   A

* **L1620** Hip orthosis, abduction control of hip joints, flexible, (Pavlik harness), prefabricated item that has been trimmed, bent, molded, assembled, or otherwise customized to fit a specific patient by an individual with expertise Ⓑ Qp Qh 🦽   A

* **L1630** Hip orthosis, abduction control of hip joints, semi-flexible (Von Rosen type), custom-fabricated Ⓑ Qp Qh 🦽   A

* **L1640** Hip orthosis, abduction control of hip joints, static, pelvic band or spreader bar, thigh cuffs, custom-fabricated Ⓑ Qp Qh 🦽   A

* **L1650** Hip orthosis, abduction control of hip joints, static, adjustable, (Ilfeld type), prefabricated, includes fitting and adjustment Ⓑ Qp Qh 🦽   A

* **L1652** Hip orthosis, bilateral thigh cuffs with adjustable abductor spreader bar, adult size, prefabricated, includes fitting and adjustment, any type Ⓑ Qp Qh A 🦽   A

* **L1660** Hip orthosis, abduction control of hip joints, static, plastic, prefabricated, includes fitting and adjustment Ⓑ Qp Qh 🦽   A

* **L1680** Hip orthosis, abduction control of hip joints, dynamic, pelvic control, adjustable hip motion control, thigh cuffs (Rancho hip action type), custom fabrication Ⓑ Qp Qh 🦽   A

▶ * **L1681** Hip orthosis, bilateral hip joints and thigh cuffs, adjustable flexion, extension, abduction control of hip joint, postoperative hip abduction type, prefabricated item that has been trimmed, bent, molded, assembled, or otherwise customized to fit a specific patient by an individual with expertise   A

* **L1685** Hip orthosis, abduction control of hip joint, postoperative hip abduction type, custom fabricated Ⓑ Qp Qh 🦽   A

* **L1686** Hip orthosis, abduction control of hip joint, postoperative hip abduction type, prefabricated, includes fitting and adjustment Ⓑ Qp Qh 🦽   A

* **L1690** Combination, bilateral, lumbo-sacral, hip, femur orthosis providing adduction and internal rotation control, prefabricated, includes fitting and adjustment Ⓑ Qp Qh 🦽   A

▶ New   ⟲ Revised   ✔ Reinstated   ~~deleted~~ Deleted   ⊘ Not covered or valid by Medicare
✪ Special coverage instructions   * Carrier discretion   Ⓑ Bill Part B MAC   Ⓓ Bill DME MAC

358

L1200 – L1690 ORTHOTICS & DEVICES

Figure 25 Thoracic-hip-knee-ankle orthosis (THKAO).

Figure 27 Knee orthosis.

Legg Perthes

* **L1700** Legg-Perthes orthosis (Toronto type), custom-fabricated Ⓑ Qp Qh ⅙ A

* **L1710** Legg-Perthes orthosis (Newington type), custom-fabricated Ⓑ Qp Qh ⅙ A

* **L1720** Legg-Perthes orthosis, trilateral (Tachdjian type), custom-fabricated Ⓑ Qp Qh ⅙ A

* **L1730** Legg-Perthes orthosis (Scottish Rite type), custom-fabricated Ⓑ Qp Qh ⅙ A

* **L1755** Legg-Perthes orthosis (Patten bottom type), custom-fabricated Ⓑ Qp Qh ⅙ A

Knee (KO)

* **L1810** Knee orthosis, elastic with joints, prefabricated item that has been trimmed, bent, molded, assembled, or otherwise customized to fit a specific patient by an individual with expertise Ⓑ Qp Qh ⅙ A

* **L1812** Knee orthosis, elastic with joints, prefabricated, off-the-shelf Ⓑ Qp Qh ⅙ A

* **L1820** Knee orthosis, elastic with condylar pads and joints, with or without patellar control, prefabricated, includes fitting and adjustment Ⓑ Qp Qh ⅙ A

* **L1830** Knee orthosis, immobilizer, canvas longitudinal, prefabricated, off-the-shelf Ⓑ Qp Qh ⅙ A

* **L1831** Knee orthosis, locking knee joint(s), positional orthosis, prefabricated, includes fitting and adjustment Ⓑ Qp Qh ⅙ A

* **L1832** Knee orthosis, adjustable knee joints (unicentric or polycentric), positional orthosis, rigid support, prefabricated item that has been trimmed, bent, molded, assembled, or otherwise customized to fit a specific patient by an individual with expertise Ⓑ Qp Qh ⅙ A

* **L1833** Knee orthosis, adjustable knee joints (unicentric or polycentric), positional orthosis, rigid support, prefabricated, off-the-shelf Ⓑ Qp Qh ⅙ A

* **L1834** Knee orthosis, without knee joint, rigid, custom-fabricated Ⓑ Qp Qh ⅙ A

* **L1836** Knee orthosis, rigid, without joint(s), includes soft interface material, prefabricated, off-the-shelf Ⓑ Qp Qh ⅙ A

* **L1840** Knee orthosis, derotation, medial-lateral, anterior cruciate ligament, custom fabricated Ⓑ Qp Qh ⅙ A

* **L1843** Knee orthosis, single upright, thigh and calf, with adjustable flexion and extension joint (unicentric or polycentric), medial-lateral and rotation control, with or without varus/valgus adjustment, prefabricated item that has been trimmed, bent, molded, assembled, or otherwise customized to fit a specific patient by an individual with expertise Ⓑ Qp Qh ⅙ A

Figure 26 Hip orthosis.

* **L1844** Knee orthosis, single upright, thigh and calf, with adjustable flexion and extension joint (unicentric or polycentric), medial-lateral and rotation control, with or without varus/ valgus adjustment, custom fabricated Ⓑ Qp Qh ♿ A

* **L1845** Knee orthosis, double upright, thigh and calf, with adjustable flexion and extension joint (unicentric or polycentric), medial-lateral and rotation control, with or without varus/valgus adjustment, prefabricated item that has been trimmed, bent, molded, assembled, or otherwise customized to fit a specific patient by an individual with expertise Ⓑ Qp Qh ♿ A

* **L1846** Knee orthrosis, double upright, thigh and calf, with adjustable flexion and extension joint (unicentric or polycentric), medial-lateral and rotation control, with or without varus/ valgus adjustment, custom fabricated Ⓑ Qp Qh ♿ A

* **L1847** Knee orthosis, double upright with adjustable joint, with inflatable air support chamber(s), prefabricated item that has been trimmed, bent, molded, assembled, or otherwise customized to fit a specific patient by an individual with expertise Ⓑ Qp Qh ♿ A

* **L1848** Knee orthosis, double upright with adjustable joint, with inflatable air support chamber(s), prefabricated, off-the-shelf Ⓑ Qp Qh ♿ A

* **L1850** Knee orthosis, Swedish type, prefabricated, off-the-shelf Ⓑ Qp Qh ♿ A

* **L1851** Knee orthosis (KO), single upright, thigh and calf, with adjustable flexion and extension joint (unicentric or polycentric), medial-lateral and rotation control, with or without varus/valgus adjustment, prefabricated, off-the-shelf Qp Qh ♿ A

* **L1852** Knee orthosis (KO), double upright, thigh and calf, with adjustable flexion and extension joint (unicentric or polycentric), medial-lateral and rotation control, with or without varus/valgus adjustment, prefabricated, off-the-shelf Qp Qh ♿ A

* **L1860** Knee orthosis, modification of supracondylar prosthetic socket, custom fabricated (SK) Ⓑ Qp Qh ♿ A

Ankle-Foot (AFO)

* **L1900** Ankle foot orthosis (AFO), spring wire, dorsiflexion assist calf band, custom-fabricated Ⓑ Qp Qh ♿ A

* **L1902** Ankle orthosis, ankle gauntlet or similiar, with or without joints, prefabricated, off-the-shelf Ⓑ Qp Qh ♿ A

* **L1904** Ankle orthosis, ankle gauntlet or similiar, with or without joints, custom fabricated Ⓑ Qp Qh ♿ A

* **L1906** Ankle foot orthosis, multiligamentus ankle support, prefabricated, off-the-shelf Ⓑ Qp Qh ♿ A

* **L1907** Ankle orthosis, supramalleolar with straps, with or without interface/pads, custom fabricated Ⓑ Qp Qh ♿ A

* **L1910** Ankle foot orthosis, posterior, single bar, clasp attachment to shoe counter, prefabricated, includes fitting and adjustment Ⓑ Qp Qh ♿ A

* **L1920** Ankle foot orthosis, single upright with static or adjustable stop (Phelps or Perlstein type), custom fabricated Ⓑ Qp Qh ♿ A

* **L1930** Ankle foot orthosis, plastic or other material, prefabricated, includes fitting and adjustment Ⓑ Qp Qh ♿ A

* **L1932** Ankle foot orthosis, rigid anterior tibial section, total carbon fiber or equal material, prefabricated, includes fitting and adjustment Ⓑ Qp Qh ♿ A

* **L1940** Ankle foot orthosis, plastic or other material, custom fabricated Ⓑ Qp Qh ♿ A

* **L1945** Ankle foot orthosis, plastic, rigid anterior tibial section (floor reaction), custom fabricated Ⓑ Qp Qh ♿ A

* **L1950** Ankle foot orthosis, spiral (Institute of Rehabilitation Medicine type), plastic, custom fabricated Ⓑ Qp Qh ♿ A

* **L1951** Ankle foot orthosis, spiral (Institute of Rehabilitative Medicine type), plastic or other material, prefabricated, includes fitting and adjustment Ⓑ Qp Qh ♿ A

* **L1960** Ankle foot orthosis, posterior solid ankle, plastic, custom fabricated Ⓑ Qp Qh ♿ A

* **L1970** Ankle foot orthosis, plastic, with ankle joint, custom fabricated Ⓑ Qp Qh ♿ A

* **L1971** Ankle foot orthosis, plastic or other material with ankle joint, prefabricated, includes fitting and adjustment Ⓑ Qp Qh ♿ A

▶ New   ↻ Revised   ✔ Reinstated   ~~deleted~~ Deleted   ⊘ Not covered or valid by Medicare
⊛ Special coverage instructions   * Carrier discretion   Ⓑ Bill Part B MAC   Ⓑ Bill DME MAC

Figure 28 Ankle-foot orthosis (AFO).

Figure 29 Knee-ankle-foot orthosis (KAFO).

* **L1980** Ankle foot orthosis, single upright free plantar dorsiflexion, solid stirrup, calf band/cuff (single bar 'BK' orthosis), custom fabricated ⑬ Qp Qh ♿   A

* **L1990** Ankle foot orthosis, double upright free plantar dorsiflexion, solid stirrup, calf band/cuff (double bar 'BK' orthosis), custom fabricated ⑬ Qp Qh ♿   A

Hip-Knee-Ankle-Foot (or Any Combination)

NOTE: L2000, L2020, and L2036 are base procedures to be used with any knee joint. L2010 and L2030 are to be used only with no knee joint.

* **L2000** Knee ankle foot orthosis, single upright, free knee, free ankle, solid stirrup, thigh and calf bands/cuffs (single bar 'AK' orthosis), custom-fabricated ⑬ Qp Qh ♿   A

* **L2005** Knee ankle foot orthosis, any material, single or double upright, stance control, automatic lock and swing phase release, any type activation; includes ankle joint, any type, custom fabricated ⑬ Qp Qh ♿   A

* **L2006** Knee ankle foot device, any material, single or double upright, swing and/or stance phase microprocessor control with adjustability, includes all components (e.g., sensors, batteries, charger), any type activation, with or without ankle joint(s), custom fabricated   A

* **L2010** Knee ankle foot orthosis, single upright, free ankle, solid stirrup, thigh and calf bands/cuffs (single bar 'AK' orthosis), without knee joint, custom-fabricated ⑬ Qp Qh ♿   A

* **L2020** Knee ankle foot orthosis, double upright, free knee, free ankle, solid stirrup, thigh and calf bands/cuffs (double bar 'AK' orthosis), custom fabricated ⑬ Qp Qh ♿   A

* **L2030** Knee ankle foot orthosis, double upright, free ankle, solid stirrup, thigh and calf bands/cuffs (double bar 'AK' orthosis), without knee joint, custom fabricated ⑬ Qp Qh ♿   A

* **L2034** Knee ankle foot orthosis, full plastic, single upright, with or without free motion knee, medial lateral rotation control, with or without free motion ankle, custom fabricated ⑬ Qp Qh ♿   A

* **L2035** Knee ankle foot orthosis, full plastic, static (pediatric size), without free motion ankle, prefabricated, includes fitting and adjustment ⑬ Qp Qh Ⓐ ♿   A

* **L2036** Knee ankle foot orthosis, full plastic, double upright, with or without free motion knee, with or without free motion ankle, custom fabricated ⑬ Qp Qh ♿   A

* **L2037** Knee ankle foot orthosis, full plastic, single upright, with or without free motion knee, with or without free motion ankle, custom fabricated ⑬ Qp Qh ♿   A

* **L2038** Knee ankle foot orthosis, full plastic, with or without free motion knee, multi-axis ankle, custom fabricated ⑬ Qp Qh ♿   A

Torsion Control: Hip-Knee-Ankle-Foot (TLSO)

* **L2040** Hip knee ankle foot orthosis, torsion control, bilateral rotation straps, pelvic band/belt, custom fabricated ⑬ Qp Qh ♿   A

Figure 30 Hip-knee-ankle-foot orthosis (HKAFO).

* **L2050** Hip knee ankle foot orthosis, torsion control, bilateral torsion cables, hip joint, pelvic band/belt, custom fabricated ⑧ **Qp** **Qh**   A

* **L2060** Hip knee ankle foot orthosis, torsion control, bilateral torsion cables, ball bearing hip joint, pelvic band/belt, custom fabricated ⑧ **Qp** **Qh**   A

* **L2070** Hip knee ankle foot orthosis, torsion control, unilateral rotation straps, pelvic band/belt, custom fabricated ⑧ **Qp** **Qh**   A

* **L2080** Hip knee ankle foot orthosis, torsion control, unilateral torsion cable, hip joint, pelvic band/belt, custom fabricated ⑧ **Qp** **Qh**   A

* **L2090** Hip knee ankle foot orthosis, torsion control, unilateral torsion cable, ball bearing hip joint, pelvic band/belt, custom fabricated ⑧ **Qp** **Qh**   A

Fracture Orthotics: Ankle-Foot and Knee-Ankle-Foot

* **L2106** Ankle foot orthosis, fracture orthosis, tibial fracture cast orthosis, thermoplastic type casting material, custom fabricated ⑧ **Qp** **Qh**   A

* **L2108** Ankle foot orthosis, fracture orthosis, tibial fracture cast orthosis, custom fabricated ⑧ **Qp** **Qh**   A

* **L2112** Ankle foot orthosis, fracture orthosis, tibial fracture orthosis, soft, prefabricated, includes fitting and adjustment ⑧ **Qp** **Qh**   A

* **L2114** Ankle foot orthosis, fracture orthosis, tibial fracture orthosis, semi-rigid, prefabricated, includes fitting and adjustment ⑧ **Qp** **Qh**   A

* **L2116** Ankle foot orthosis, fracture orthosis, tibial fracture orthosis, rigid, prefabricated, includes fitting and adjustment ⑧ **Qp** **Qh**   A

* **L2126** Knee ankle foot orthosis, fracture orthosis, femoral fracture cast orthosis, thermoplastic type casting material, custom fabricated ⑧ **Qp** **Qh**   A

* **L2128** Knee ankle foot orthosis, fracture orthosis, femoral fracture cast orthosis, custom fabricated ⑧ **Qp** **Qh**   A

* **L2132** Knee ankle foot orthosis, femoral fracture cast orthosis, soft, prefabricated, includes fitting and adjustment ⑧ **Qp** **Qh**   A

* **L2134** Knee ankle foot orthosis, femoral fracture cast orthosis, semi-rigid, prefabricated, includes fitting and adjustment ⑧ **Qp** **Qh**   A

* **L2136** Knee ankle foot orthosis, fracture orthosis, femoral fracture cast orthosis, rigid, prefabricated, includes fitting and adjustment ⑧ **Qp** **Qh**   A

Additions to Fracture Orthotics

* **L2180** Addition to lower extremity fracture orthosis, plastic shoe insert with ankle joints ⑧ **Qp** **Qh**   A

* **L2182** Addition to lower extremity fracture orthosis, drop lock knee joint ⑧ **Qp** **Qh**   A

* **L2184** Addition to lower extremity fracture orthosis, limited motion knee joint ⑧ **Qp** **Qh**   A

* **L2186** Addition to lower extremity fracture orthosis, adjustable motion knee joint, Lerman type ⑧ **Qp** **Qh**   A

* **L2188** Addition to lower extremity fracture orthosis, quadrilateral brim ⑧ **Qp** **Qh**   A

* **L2190** Addition to lower extremity fracture orthosis, waist belt ⑧ **Qp** **Qh**   A

* **L2192** Addition to lower extremity fracture orthosis, hip joint, pelvic band, thigh flange, and pelvic belt ⑧ **Qp** **Qh**   A

Additions to Lower Extremity Orthotics

* **L2200** Addition to lower extremity, limited ankle motion, each joint ⑧ **Qp** **Qh**   A

* **L2210** Addition to lower extremity, dorsiflexion assist (plantar flexion resist), each joint ⑧ **Qp** **Qh**   A

* **L2220** Addition to lower extremity, dorsiflexion and plantar flexion assist/resist, each joint ⑧ **Qp** **Qh**   A

* **L2230** Addition to lower extremity, split flat caliper stirrups and plate attachment ⑧ **Qp** **Qh**   A

▶ New   ↻ Revised   ✔ Reinstated   ~~deleted~~ Deleted   ⊘ Not covered or valid by Medicare
⊛ Special coverage instructions   * Carrier discretion   ⑧ Bill Part B MAC   ⑧ Bill DME MAC

✳ **L2232** Addition to lower extremity orthosis, rocker bottom for total contact ankle foot orthosis, for custom fabricated orthosis only Ⓑ Qp Qh ♿   A

✳ **L2240** Addition to lower extremity, round caliper and plate attachment Ⓑ Qp Qh ♿   A

✳ **L2250** Addition to lower extremity, foot plate, molded to patient model, stirrup attachment Ⓑ Qp Qh ♿   A

✳ **L2260** Addition to lower extremity, reinforced solid stirrup (Scott-Craig type) Ⓑ Qp Qh ♿   A

✳ **L2265** Addition to lower extremity, long tongue stirrup Ⓑ Qp Qh ♿   A

✳ **L2270** Addition to lower extremity, varus/valgus correction ('T') strap, padded/lined or malleolus pad Ⓑ Qp Qh ♿   A

✳ **L2275** Addition to lower extremity, varus/valgus correction, plastic modification, padded/lined Ⓑ Qp Qh ♿   A

✳ **L2280** Addition to lower extremity, molded inner boot Ⓑ Qp Qh ♿   A

✳ **L2300** Addition to lower extremity, abduction bar (bilateral hip involvement), jointed, adjustable Ⓑ Qp Qh ♿   A

✳ **L2310** Addition to lower extremity, abduction bar-straight Ⓑ Qp Qh ♿   A

✳ **L2320** Addition to lower extremity, non-molded lacer, for custom fabricated orthosis only Ⓑ Qp Qh ♿   A

✳ **L2330** Addition to lower extremity, lacer molded to patient model, for custom fabricated orthosis only Ⓑ Qp Qh ♿   A

Used whether closure is lacer or Velcro

✳ **L2335** Addition to lower extremity, anterior swing band Ⓑ Qp Qh ♿   A

✳ **L2340** Addition to lower extremity, pre-tibial shell, molded to patient model Ⓑ Qp Qh ♿   A

✳ **L2350** Addition to lower extremity, prosthetic type (BK) socket, molded to patient model, (used for 'PTB' and 'AFO' orthoses) Ⓑ Qp Qh ♿   A

✳ **L2360** Addition to lower extremity, extended steel shank Ⓑ Qp Qh ♿   A

✳ **L2370** Addition to lower extremity, Patten bottom Ⓑ Qp Qh ♿   A

✳ **L2375** Addition to lower extremity, torsion control, ankle joint and half solid stirrup Ⓑ Qp Qh ♿   A

✳ **L2380** Addition to lower extremity, torsion control, straight knee joint, each joint Ⓑ Qp Qh ♿   A

✳ **L2385** Addition to lower extremity, straight knee joint, heavy duty, each joint Ⓑ Qp ♿   A

✳ **L2387** Addition to lower extremity, polycentric knee joint, for custom fabricated knee ankle foot orthosis, each joint Ⓑ Qp ♿   A

✳ **L2390** Addition to lower extremity, offset knee joint, each joint Ⓑ Qp ♿   A

✳ **L2395** Addition to lower extremity, offset knee joint, heavy duty, each joint Ⓑ Qp ♿   A

✳ **L2397** Addition to lower extremity orthosis, suspension sleeve Ⓑ Qp ♿   A

Additions to Straight Knee or Offset Knee Joints

✳ **L2405** Addition to knee joint, drop lock, each Ⓑ Qp ♿   A

✳ **L2415** Addition to knee lock with integrated release mechanism (bail, cable, or equal), any material, each joint Ⓑ Qp ♿   A

✳ **L2425** Addition to knee joint, disc or dial lock for adjustable knee flexion, each joint Ⓑ Qp ♿   A

✳ **L2430** Addition to knee joint, ratchet lock for active and progressive knee extension, each joint Ⓑ Qp ♿   A

✳ **L2492** Addition to knee joint, lift loop for drop lock ring Ⓑ Qp ♿   A

Additions to Thigh/Weight Bearing Gluteal/Ischial Weight Bearing

✳ **L2500** Addition to lower extremity, thigh/weight bearing, gluteal/ischial weight bearing, ring Ⓑ Qp Qh ♿   A

✳ **L2510** Addition to lower extremity, thigh/weight bearing, quadri-lateral brim, molded to patient model Ⓑ Qp Qh ♿   A

✳ **L2520** Addition to lower extremity, thigh/weight bearing, quadri-lateral brim, custom fitted Ⓑ Qp Qh ♿   A

✳ **L2525** Addition to lower extremity, thigh/weight bearing, ischial containment/narrow M-L brim molded to patient model Ⓑ Qp Qh ♿   A

✳ **L2526** Addition to lower extremity, thigh/weight bearing, ischial containment/narrow M-L brim, custom fitted Ⓑ Qp Qh ♿   A

✳ **L2530** Addition to lower extremity, thigh-weight bearing, lacer, non-molded Ⓑ Qp Qh ♿   A

♿ MIPS   Qp Quantity Physician   Qh Quantity Hospital   ♀ Female only
♂ Male only   A Age   ♿ DMEPOS   A2-Z3 ASC Payment Indicator   A-Y ASC Status Indicator   Coding Clinic

* **L2540** Addition to lower extremity, thigh/weight bearing, lacer, molded to patient model ⑧ Qp Qh ♿   A

* **L2550** Addition to lower extremity, thigh/weight bearing, high roll cuff ⑧ Qp Qh ♿   A

Additions to Pelvic and Thoracic Control

* **L2570** Addition to lower extremity, pelvic control, hip joint, Clevis type two position joint, each ⑧ Qp Qh ♿   A

* **L2580** Addition to lower extremity, pelvic control, pelvic sling ⑧ Qp Qh ♿   A

* **L2600** Addition to lower extremity, pelvic control, hip joint, Clevis type, or thrust bearing, free, each ⑧ Qp Qh ♿   A

* **L2610** Addition to lower extremity, pelvic control, hip joint, Clevis or thrust bearing, lock, each ⑧ Qp Qh ♿   A

* **L2620** Addition to lower extremity, pelvic control, hip joint, heavy duty, each ⑧ Qp Qh ♿   A

* **L2622** Addition to lower extremity, pelvic control, hip joint, adjustable flexion, each ⑧ Qp Qh ♿   A

* **L2624** Addition to lower extremity, pelvic control, hip joint, adjustable flexion, extension, abduction control, each ⑧ Qp Qh ♿   A

* **L2627** Addition to lower extremity, pelvic control, plastic, molded to patient model, reciprocating hip joint and cables ⑧ Qp Qh ♿   A

* **L2628** Addition to lower extremity, pelvic control, metal frame, reciprocating hip joint and cables ⑧ Qp Qh ♿   A

* **L2630** Addition to lower extremity, pelvic control, band and belt, unilateral ⑧ Qp Qh ♿   A

* **L2640** Addition to lower extremity, pelvic control, band and belt, bilateral ⑧ Qp Qh ♿   A

* **L2650** Addition to lower extremity, pelvic and thoracic control, gluteal pad, each ⑧ Qp Qh ♿   A

* **L2660** Addition to lower extremity, thoracic control, thoracic band ⑧ Qp Qh ♿   A

* **L2670** Addition to lower extremity, thoracic control, paraspinal uprights ⑧ Qp Qh ♿   A

* **L2680** Addition to lower extremity, thoracic control, lateral support uprights ⑧ Qp Qh ♿   A

General Additions

* **L2750** Addition to lower extremity orthosis, plating chrome or nickel, per bar ⑧ Qp ♿   A

* **L2755** Addition to lower extremity orthosis, high strength, lightweight material, all hybrid lamination/prepreg composite, per segment, for custom fabricated orthosis only ⑧ Qp ♿   A

* **L2760** Addition to lower extremity orthosis, extension, per extension, per bar (for lineal adjustment for growth) ⑧ Qp ♿   A

* **L2768** Orthotic side bar disconnect device, per bar ⑧ Qp ♿   A

* **L2780** Addition to lower extremity orthosis, non-corrosive finish, per bar ⑧ Qp ♿   A

* **L2785** Addition to lower extremity orthosis, drop lock retainer, each ⑧ Qp ♿   A

* **L2795** Addition to lower extremity orthosis, knee control, full kneecap ⑧ Qp Qh ♿   A

* **L2800** Addition to lower extremity orthosis, knee control, knee cap, medial or lateral pull, for use with custom fabricated orthosis only ⑧ Qp Qh ♿   A

* **L2810** Addition to lower extremity orthosis, knee control, condylar pad ⑧ Qp ♿   A

* **L2820** Addition to lower extremity orthosis, soft interface for molded plastic, below knee section ⑧ Qp Qh ♿   A

  Only report if soft interface provided, either leather or other material

* **L2830** Addition to lower extremity orthosis, soft interface for molded plastic, above knee section ⑧ Qp Qh ♿   A

* **L2840** Addition to lower extremity orthosis, tibial length sock, fracture or equal, each ⑧ Qp ♿   A

* **L2850** Addition to lower extremity orthosis, femoral length sock, fracture or equal, each ⑧ Qp ♿   A

* ⊘ **L2861** Addition to lower extremity joint, knee or ankle, concentric adjustable torsion style mechanism for custom fabricated orthotics only, each ⑧ Qp Qh   E1

* **L2999** Lower extremity orthoses, not otherwise specified ⑧   A

▶ New   ↻ Revised   ✔ Reinstated   ~~deleted~~ Deleted   ⊘ Not covered or valid by Medicare
⊛ Special coverage instructions   * Carrier discretion   ⑧ Bill Part B MAC   ⑧ Bill DME MAC

Figure 31 Foot inserts.

Figure 32 Arch support.

Foot (Orthopedic Shoes) (L3000-L3649)

Inserts

⊛ **L3000** Foot, insert, removable, molded to patient model, 'UCB' type, Berkeley shell, each ⓑ Qp Qh �   A

If both feet casted and supplied with an orthosis, bill L3000-LT and L3000-RT

IOM: 100-02, 15, 290

⊛ **L3001** Foot, insert, removable, molded to patient model, Spenco, each ⓑ Qp Qh �   A

IOM: 100-02, 15, 290

⊛ **L3002** Foot, insert, removable, molded to patient model, Plastazote or equal, each ⓑ Qp Qh �   A

IOM: 100-02, 15, 290

⊛ **L3003** Foot, insert, removable, molded to patient model, silicone gel, each ⓑ Qp Qh �   A

IOM: 100-02, 15, 290

⊛ **L3010** Foot, insert, removable, molded to patient model, longitudinal arch support, each ⓑ Qp Qh �   A

IOM: 100-02, 15, 290

⊛ **L3020** Foot, insert, removable, molded to patient model, longitudinal/metatarsal support, each ⓑ Qp Qh �   A

IOM: 100-02, 15, 290

⊛ **L3030** Foot, insert, removable, formed to patient foot, each ⓑ Qp Qh �   A

IOM: 100-02, 15, 290

✳ **L3031** Foot, insert/plate, removable, addition to lower extremity orthosis, high strength, lightweight material, all hybrid lamination/prepreg composite, each ⓑ Qp Qh �   A

Arch Support, Removable, Premolded

⊛ **L3040** Foot, arch support, removable, premolded, longitudinal, each ⓑ Qp Qh �   A

IOM: 100-02, 15, 290

⊛ **L3050** Foot, arch support, removable, premolded, metatarsal, each ⓑ Qp Qh �   A

IOM: 100-02, 15, 290

⊛ **L3060** Foot, arch support, removable, premolded, longitudinal/metatarsal, each ⓑ Qp Qh �   A

IOM: 100-02, 15, 290

Arch Support, Non-removable, Attached to Shoe

⊛ **L3070** Foot, arch support, non-removable attached to shoe, longitudinal, each ⓑ Qp Qh �   A

IOM: 100-02, 15, 290

⊛ **L3080** Foot, arch support, non-removable attached to shoe, metatarsal, each ⓑ Qp Qh �   A

IOM: 100-02, 15, 290

⊛ **L3090** Foot, arch support, non-removable attached to shoe, longitudinal/metatarsal, each ⓑ Qp Qh �   A

IOM: 100-02, 15, 290

⊛ **L3100** Hallus-valgus night dynamic splint, prefabricated, off-the-shelf ⓑ Qp Qh �   A

IOM: 100-02, 15, 290

Figure 33 Hallux valgus splint.

ORTHOTICS & DEVICES   **L3000 – L3100**

Abduction and Rotation Bars

⊛ **L3140** Foot, abduction rotation bar, including shoes Ⓑ **Qp** **Qh** ♿ A
IOM: 100-02, 15, 290

⊛ **L3150** Foot, abduction rotation bar, without shoes Ⓑ **Qp** **Qh** ♿ A
IOM: 100-02, 15, 290

✳ **L3160** Foot, adjustable shoe-styled positioning device Ⓑ **Qp** **Qh** A

⊛ **L3170** Foot, plastic, silicone or equal, heel stabilizer, prefabricated, off-the-shelf, each Ⓑ **Qp** **Qh** ♿ A
IOM: 100-02, 15, 290

Orthopedic Footwear

⊛ **L3201** Orthopedic shoe, oxford with supinator or pronator, infant Ⓑ **A** A
IOM: 100-02, 15, 290

⊛ **L3202** Orthopedic shoe, oxford with supinator or pronator, child Ⓑ **A** A
IOM: 100-02, 15, 290

⊛ **L3203** Orthopedic shoe, oxford with supinator or pronator, junior Ⓑ **A** A
IOM: 100-02, 15, 290

⊛ **L3204** Orthopedic shoe, hightop with supinator or pronator, infant Ⓑ **A** A
IOM: 100-02, 15, 290

⊛ **L3206** Orthopedic shoe, hightop with supinator or pronator, child Ⓑ **A** A
IOM: 100-02, 15, 290

⊛ **L3207** Orthopedic shoe, hightop with supinator or pronator, junior Ⓑ **A** A
IOM: 100-02, 15, 290

⊛ **L3208** Surgical boot, infant, each Ⓑ **A** A
IOM: 100-02, 15, 100

Figure 34 Molded custom shoe.

⊛ **L3209** Surgical boot, each, child Ⓑ **A** A
IOM: 100-02, 15, 100

⊛ **L3211** Surgical boot, each, junior Ⓑ **A** A
IOM: 100-02, 15, 100

⊛ **L3212** Benesch boot, pair, infant Ⓑ **A** A
IOM: 100-02, 15, 100

⊛ **L3213** Benesch boot, pair, child Ⓑ **A** A
IOM: 100-02, 15, 100

⊛ **L3214** Benesch boot, pair, junior Ⓑ **A** A
IOM: 100-02, 15, 100

⊘ **L3215** Orthopedic footwear, ladies' shoe, oxford, each Ⓑ **Qp** **Qh** ♀ E1
Medicare Statute 1862a8

⊘ **L3216** Orthopedic footwear, ladies' shoe, depth inlay, each Ⓑ **Qp** **Qh** ♀ E1
Medicare Statute 1862a8

⊘ **L3217** Orthopedic footwear, ladies' shoe, hightop, depth inlay, each Ⓑ **Qp** **Qh** ♀ E1
Medicare Statute 1862a8

⊘ **L3219** Orthopedic footwear, men's shoe, oxford, each Ⓑ **Qp** **Qh** ♂ E1
Medicare Statute 1862a8

⊘ **L3221** Orthopedic footwear, men's shoe, depth inlay, each Ⓑ **Qp** **Qh** ♂ E1
Medicare Statute 1862a8

⊘ **L3222** Orthopedic footwear, men's shoe, hightop, depth inlay, each Ⓑ **Qp** **Qh** ♂ E1
Medicare Statute 1862a8

⊛ **L3224** Orthopedic footwear, ladies' shoe, oxford, used as an integral part of a brace (orthosis) Ⓑ **Qp** **Qh** ♀ ♿ A
IOM: 100-02, 15, 290

⊛ **L3225** Orthopedic footwear, men's shoe, oxford, used as an integral part of a brace (orthosis) Ⓑ **Qp** **Qh** ♂ ♿ A
IOM: 100-02, 15, 290

⊛ **L3230** Orthopedic footwear, custom shoe, depth inlay, each Ⓑ **Qp** **Qh** A
IOM: 100-02, 15, 290

⊛ **L3250** Orthopedic footwear, custom molded shoe, removable inner mold, prosthetic shoe, each Ⓑ **Qp** **Qh** A
IOM: 100-02, 15, 290

⊛ **L3251** Foot, shoe molded to patient model, silicone shoe, each Ⓑ **Qp** **Qh** A
IOM: 100-02, 15, 290

▶ New   ↺ Revised   ✔ Reinstated   deleted Deleted   ⊘ Not covered or valid by Medicare
⊛ Special coverage instructions   ✳ Carrier discretion   Ⓥ Bill Part B MAC   Ⓑ Bill DME MAC

○ **L3252** Foot, shoe molded to patient model, Plastazote (or similar), custom fabricated, each Ⓑ Qp Qh   A
IOM: 100-02, 15, 290

○ **L3253** Foot, molded shoe Plastazote (or similar), custom fitted, each Ⓑ Qp Qh   A
IOM: 100-02, 15, 290

○ **L3254** Non-standard size or width Ⓑ   A
IOM: 100-02, 15, 290

○ **L3255** Non-standard size or length Ⓑ   A
IOM: 100-02, 15, 290

○ **L3257** Orthopedic footwear, additional charge for split size Ⓑ   A
IOM: 100-02, 15, 290

○ **L3260** Surgical boot/shoe, each Ⓑ   E1
IOM: 100-02, 15, 100

✳ **L3265** Plastazote sandal, each Ⓑ   A

Shoe Lifts

○ **L3300** Lift, elevation, heel, tapered to metatarsals, per inch Ⓑ Qp   A
IOM: 100-02, 15, 290

○ **L3310** Lift, elevation, heel and sole, Neoprene, per inch Ⓑ Qp &   A
IOM: 100-02, 15, 290

○ **L3320** Lift, elevation, heel and sole, cork, per inch Ⓑ Qp   A
IOM: 100-02, 15, 290

○ **L3330** Lift, elevation, metal extension (skate) Ⓑ Qp Qh &   A
IOM: 100-02, 15, 290

○ **L3332** Lift, elevation, inside shoe, tapered, up to one-half inch Ⓑ Qp Qh &   A
IOM: 100-02, 15, 290

○ **L3334** Lift, elevation, heel, per inch Ⓑ Qp &   A
IOM: 100-02, 15, 290

Shoe Wedges

○ **L3340** Heel wedge, SACH Ⓑ Qp Qh &   A
IOM: 100-02, 15, 290

○ **L3350** Heel wedge Ⓑ Qp Qh &   A
IOM: 100-02, 15, 290

○ **L3360** Sole wedge, outside sole Ⓑ Qp Qh & A
IOM: 100-02, 15, 290

○ **L3370** Sole wedge, between sole Ⓑ Qp Qh &   A
IOM: 100-02, 15, 290

○ **L3380** Clubfoot wedge Ⓑ Qp Qh &   A
IOM: 100-02, 15, 290

○ **L3390** Outflare wedge Ⓑ Qp Qh &   A
IOM: 100-02, 15, 290

○ **L3400** Metatarsal bar wedge, rocker Ⓑ Qp Qh &   A
IOM: 100-02, 15, 290

○ **L3410** Metatarsal bar wedge, between sole Ⓑ Qp Qh &   A
IOM: 100-02, 15, 290

○ **L3420** Full sole and heel wedge, between sole Ⓑ Qp Qh &   A
IOM: 100-02, 15, 290

Shoe Heels

○ **L3430** Heel, counter, plastic reinforced Ⓑ Qp Qh &   A
IOM: 100-02, 15, 290

○ **L3440** Heel, counter, leather reinforced Ⓑ Qp Qh &   A
IOM: 100-02, 15, 290

○ **L3450** Heel, SACH cushion type Ⓑ Qp Qh &   A
IOM: 100-02, 15, 290

○ **L3455** Heel, new leather, standard Ⓑ Qp Qh &   A
IOM: 100-02, 15, 290

○ **L3460** Heel, new rubber, standard Ⓑ Qp Qh &   A
IOM: 100-02, 15, 290

○ **L3465** Heel, Thomas with wedge Ⓑ Qp Qh &   A
IOM: 100-02, 15, 290

○ **L3470** Heel, Thomas extended to ball Ⓑ Qp Qh &   A
IOM: 100-02, 15, 290

○ **L3480** Heel, pad and depression for spur Ⓑ Qp Qh &   A
IOM: 100-02, 15, 290

○ **L3485** Heel, pad, removable for spur Ⓑ Qp Qh   A
IOM: 100-02, 15, 290

Orthopedic Shoe Additions: Other

○ **L3500** Orthopedic shoe addition, insole, leather Ⓑ Qp Qh &   A
IOM: 100-02, 15, 290

⊛ **L3510** Orthopedic shoe addition, insole, rubber ⑧ Qp Qh ᕃ   A

IOM: 100-02, 15, 290

⊛ **L3520** Orthopedic shoe addition, insole, felt covered with leather ⑧ Qp Qh ᕃ   A

IOM: 100-02, 15, 290

⊛ **L3530** Orthopedic shoe addition, sole, half ⑧ Qp Qh ᕃ   A

IOM: 100-02, 15, 290

⊛ **L3540** Orthopedic shoe addition, sole, full ⑧ Qp Qh ᕃ   A

IOM: 100-02, 15, 290

⊛ **L3550** Orthopedic shoe addition, toe tap standard ⑧ Qp Qh ᕃ   A

IOM: 100-02, 15, 290

⊛ **L3560** Orthopedic shoe addition, toe tap, horseshoe ⑧ Qp Qh ᕃ   A

IOM: 100-02, 15, 290

⊛ **L3570** Orthopedic shoe addition, special extension to instep (leather with eyelets) ⑧ Qp Qh ᕃ   A

IOM: 100-02, 15, 290

⊛ **L3580** Orthopedic shoe addition, convert instep to Velcro closure ⑧ Qp Qh ᕃ   A

IOM: 100-02, 15, 290

⊛ **L3590** Orthopedic shoe addition, convert firm shoe counter to soft counter ⑧ Qp Qh ᕃ   A

IOM: 100-02, 15, 290

⊛ **L3595** Orthopedic shoe addition, March bar ⑧ Qp Qh ᕃ   A

IOM: 100-02, 15, 290

Transfer or Replacement

⊛ **L3600** Transfer of an orthosis from one shoe to another, caliper plate, existing ⑧ Qp Qh ᕃ   A

IOM: 100-02, 15, 290

⊛ **L3610** Transfer of an orthosis from one shoe to another, caliper plate, new ⑧ Qp Qh ᕃ   A

IOM: 100-02, 15, 290

⊛ **L3620** Transfer of an orthosis from one shoe to another, solid stirrup, existing ⑧ Qp Qh ᕃ   A

IOM: 100-02, 15, 290

⊛ **L3630** Transfer of an orthosis from one shoe to another, solid stirrup, new ⑧ Qp Qh ᕃ   A

IOM: 100-02, 15, 290

⊛ **L3640** Transfer of an orthosis from one shoe to another, Dennis Browne splint (Riveton), both shoes ⑧ Qp Qh ᕃ   A

IOM: 100-02, 15, 290

⊛ **L3649** Orthopedic shoe, modification, addition or transfer, not otherwise specified ⑧   A

IOM: 100-02, 15, 290

Orthotic Devices: Upper Limb

NOTE: The procedures in this section are considered as base or basic procedures and may be modified by listing procedures from the Additions section and adding them to the base procedure.

Shoulder

✳ **L3650** Shoulder orthosis, figure of eight design abduction restrainer, prefabricated, off-the-shelf ⑧ Qp Qh ᕃ   A

✳ **L3660** Shoulder orthosis, figure of eight design abduction restrainer, canvas and webbing, prefabricated, off-the-shelf ⑧ Qp Qh ᕃ   A

✳ **L3670** Shoulder orthosis, acromio/clavicular (canvas and webbing type), prefabricated, off-the-shelf ⑧ Qp Qh ᕃ   A

✳ **L3671** Shoulder orthosis, shoulder joint design, without joints, may include soft interface, straps, custom fabricated, includes fitting and adjustment ⑧ Qp Qh ᕃ   A

✳ **L3674** Shoulder orthosis, abduction positioning (airplane design), thoracic component and support bar, with or without nontorsion joint/turnbuckle, may include soft interface, straps, custom fabricated, includes fitting and adjustment ⑧ Qp Qh ᕃ   A

✳ **L3675** Shoulder orthosis, vest type abduction restrainer, canvas webbing type or equal, prefabricated, off-the-shelf ⑧ Qp Qh ᕃ   A

⊛ **L3677** Shoulder orthosis, shoulder joint design, without joints, may include soft interface, straps, prefabricated item that has been trimmed, bent, molded, assembled, or otherwise customized to fit a specific patient by an individual with expertise ⑧ Qp Qh   A

✳ **L3678** Shoulder orthosis, shoulder joint design, without joints, may include soft interface, straps, prefabricated, off-the-shelf ⑧ Qp Qh   A

Figure 35 Elbow orthoses.

Elbow

✳ **L3702** Elbow orthosis, without joints, may include soft interface, straps, custom fabricated, includes fitting and adjustment Ⓑ Qp Qh ♿   A

✳ **L3710** Elbow orthosis, elastic with metal joints, prefabricated, off-the-shelf Ⓑ Qp Qh ♿   A

✳ **L3720** Elbow orthosis, double upright with forearm/arm cuffs, free motion, custom fabricated Ⓑ Qp Qh ♿   A

✳ **L3730** Elbow orthosis, double upright with forearm/arm cuffs, extension/flexion assist, custom fabricated Ⓑ Qp Qh ♿   A

✳ **L3740** Elbow orthosis, double upright with forearm/arm cuffs, adjustable position lock with active control, custom fabricated Ⓑ Qp Qh ♿   A

✳ **L3760** Elbow orthosis (EO), with adjustable position locking joint(s), prefabricated, item that has been trimmed, bent, molded, assembled, or otherwise customized to fit a specific patient by an individual with expertise Ⓑ Qp Qh ♿   A

✳ **L3761** Elbow orthosis (EO), with adjustable position locking joint(s), prefabricated, off-the-shelf ♿   A

✳ **L3762** Elbow orthosis, rigid, without joints, includes soft interface material, prefabricated, off-the-shelf Ⓑ Qp Qh ♿   A

✳ **L3763** Elbow wrist hand orthosis, rigid, without joints, may include soft interface, straps, custom fabricated, includes fitting and adjustment Ⓑ Qp Qh ♿   A

✳ **L3764** Elbow wrist hand orthosis, includes one or more nontorsion joints, elastic bands, turnbuckles, may include soft interface, straps, custom fabricated, includes fitting and adjustment Ⓑ Qp Qh ♿   A

✳ **L3765** Elbow wrist hand finger orthosis, rigid, without joints, may include soft interface, straps, custom fabricated, includes fitting and adjustment Ⓑ Qp Qh ♿   A

✳ **L3766** Elbow wrist hand finger orthosis, includes one or more nontorsion joints, elastic bands, turnbuckles, may include soft interface, straps, custom fabricated, includes fitting and adjustment Ⓑ Qp Qh ♿   A

Wrist-Hand-Finger Orthosis (WHFO)

✳ **L3806** Wrist hand finger orthosis, includes one or more nontorsion joint(s), turnbuckles, elastic bands/springs, may include soft interface material, straps, custom fabricated, includes fitting and adjustment Ⓑ Qp Qh ♿   A

✳ **L3807** Wrist hand finger orthosis, without joint(s), prefabricated item that has been trimmed, bent, molded, assembled, or otherwise customized to fit a specific patient by an individual with expertise Ⓑ Qp Qh ♿   A

✳ **L3808** Wrist hand finger orthosis, rigid without joints, may include soft interface material; straps, custom fabricated, includes fitting and adjustment Ⓑ Qp Qh ♿   A

✳ **L3809** Wrist hand finger orthosis, without joint(s), prefabricated, off-the-shelf, any type Ⓑ Qp Qh ♿   A

⊘ **L3891** Addition to upper extremity joint, wrist or elbow, concentric adjustable torsion style mechanism for custom fabricated orthotics only, each Ⓑ Qp Qh   E1

✳ **L3900** Wrist hand finger orthosis, dynamic flexor hinge, reciprocal wrist extension/flexion, finger flexion/extension, wrist or finger driven, custom fabricated Ⓑ Qp Qh ♿   A

✳ **L3901** Wrist hand finger orthosis, dynamic flexor hinge, reciprocal wrist extension/flexion, finger flexion/extension, cable driven, custom fabricated Ⓑ Qp Qh ♿   A

✳ **L3904** Wrist hand finger orthosis, external powered, electric, custom fabricated Ⓑ Qp Qh ♿   A

⬥ MIPS	Qp **Quantity Physician**	Qh **Quantity Hospital**	♀ **Female only**
♂ **Male only**	Ⓐ **Age**	♿ **DMEPOS** A2-Z3 **ASC Payment Indicator**	A-Y **ASC Status Indicator** Coding Clinic

Other Upper Extremity Orthotics

* **L3905** Wrist hand orthosis, includes one or more nontorsion joints, elastic bands, turnbuckles, may include soft interface, straps, custom fabricated, includes fitting and adjustment Ⓑ Qp Qh ♿ A

* **L3906** Wrist hand orthosis, without joints, may include soft interface, straps, custom fabricated, includes fitting and adjustment Ⓑ Qp Qh ♿ A

* **L3908** Wrist hand orthosis, wrist extension control cock-up, non-molded, prefabricated, off-the-shelf Ⓑ Qp Qh ♿ A

* **L3912** Hand finger orthosis (HFO), flexion glove with elastic finger control, prefabricated, off-the-shelf Ⓑ Qp Qh ♿ A

* **L3913** Hand finger orthosis, without joints, may include soft interface, straps, custom fabricated, includes fitting and adjustment Ⓑ Qp Qh ♿ A

* **L3915** Wrist hand orthosis, includes one or more nontorsion joint(s), elastic bands, turnbuckles, may include soft interface, straps, prefabricated item that has been trimmed, bent, molded, assembled, or otherwise customized to fit a specific patient by an individual with expertise Ⓑ Qp Qh ♿ A

* **L3916** Wrist hand orthosis, includes one or more nontorsion joint(s), elastic bands, turnbuckles, may include soft interface, straps, prefabricated, off-the-shelf Ⓑ Qp Qh ♿ A

* **L3917** Hand orthosis, metacarpal fracture orthosis, prefabricated item that has been trimmed, bent, molded, assembled, or otherwise customized to fit a specific patient by an individual with expertise Ⓑ Qp Qh ♿ A

* **L3918** Hand orthosis, metacarpal fracture orthosis, prefabricated, off-the-shelf Ⓑ Qp Qh ♿ A

* **L3919** Hand orthosis, without joints, may include soft interface, straps, custom fabricated, includes fitting and adjustment Ⓑ Qp Qh ♿ A

* **L3921** Hand finger orthosis, includes one or more nontorsion joints, elastic bands, turnbuckles, may include soft interface, straps, custom fabricated, includes fitting and adjustment Ⓑ Qp Qh ♿ A

* **L3923** Hand finger orthosis, without joints, may include soft interface, straps, prefabricated item that has been trimmed, bent, molded, assembled, or otherwise customized to fit a specific patient by an individual with expertise Ⓑ Qp Qh ♿ A

* **L3924** Hand finger orthosis, without joints, may include soft interface, straps, prefabricated, off-the-shelf Ⓑ Qp Qh ♿ A

* **L3925** Finger orthosis, proximal interphalangeal (PIP)/distal interphalangeal (DIP), non torsion joint/spring, extension/flexion, may include soft interface material, prefabricated, off-the-shelf Ⓑ Qp Qh ♿ A

* **L3927** Finger orthosis, proximal interphalangeal (PIP)/distal interphalangeal (DIP), without joint/spring, extension/flexion (e.g., static or ring type), may include soft interface material, prefabricated, off-the-shelf Ⓑ Qp Qh ♿ A

* **L3929** Hand finger orthosis, includes one or more nontorsion joint(s), turnbuckles, elastic bands/springs, may include soft interface material, straps, prefabricated item that has been trimmed, bent, molded, assembled, or otherwise customized to fit a specific patient by an individual with expertise Ⓑ Qp Qh ♿ A

* **L3930** Hand finger orthosis, includes one or more nontorsion joint(s), turnbuckles, elastic bands/springs, may include soft interface material, straps, prefabricated, off-the-shelf Ⓑ Qp Qh ♿ A

* **L3931** Wrist hand finger orthosis, includes one or more nontorsion joint(s), turnbuckles, elastic bands/springs, may include soft interface material, straps, prefabricated, includes fitting and adjustment Ⓑ Qp Qh ♿ A

* **L3933** Finger orthosis, without joints, may include soft interface, custom fabricated, includes fitting and adjustment Ⓑ Qp Qh ♿ A

* **L3935** Finger orthosis, nontorsion joint, may include soft interface, custom fabricated, includes fitting and adjustment Ⓑ Qp Qh ♿ A

* **L3956** Addition of joint to upper extremity orthosis, any material, per joint Ⓑ Qp ♿ A

Shoulder-Elbow-Wrist-Hand Orthotics (SEWHO) (L3960-L3973)

* **L3960** Shoulder elbow wrist hand orthosis, abduction positioning, airplane design, prefabricated, includes fitting and adjustment ⓑ Qp Qh   A

* **L3961** Shoulder elbow wrist hand orthosis, shoulder cap design, without joints, may include soft interface, straps, custom fabricated, includes fitting and adjustment ⓑ Qp Qh   A

* **L3962** Shoulder elbow wrist hand orthosis, abduction positioning, Erb's palsy design, prefabricated, includes fitting and adjustment ⓑ Qp Qh   A

* **L3967** Shoulder elbow wrist hand orthosis, abduction positioning (airplane design), thoracic component and support bar, without joints, may include soft interface, straps, custom fabricated, includes fitting and adjustment ⓑ Qp Qh &   A

* **L3971** Shoulder elbow wrist hand orthosis, shoulder cap design, includes one or more nontorsion joints, elastic bands, turnbuckles, may include soft interface, straps, custom fabricated, includes fitting and adjustment ⓑ Qp Qh &   A

* **L3973** Shoulder elbow wrist hand orthosis, abduction positioning (airplane design), thoracic component and support bar, includes one or more nontorsion joints, elastic bands, turnbuckles, may include soft interface, straps, custom fabricated, includes fitting and adjustment ⓑ Qp Qh &   A

Shoulder-Elbow-Wrist-Hand-Finger Orthotics

* **L3975** Shoulder elbow wrist hand finger orthosis, shoulder cap design, without joints, may include soft interface, straps, custom fabricated, includes fitting and adjustment ⓑ Qp Qh &   A

* **L3976** Shoulder elbow wrist hand finger orthosis, abduction positioning (airplane design), thoracic component and support bar, without joints, may include soft interface, straps, custom fabricated, includes fitting and adjustment ⓑ Qp Qh &   A

* **L3977** Shoulder elbow wrist hand finger orthosis, shoulder cap design, includes one or more nontorsion joints, elastic bands, turnbuckles, may include soft interface, straps, custom fabricated, includes fitting and adjustment ⓑ Qp Qh &   A

* **L3978** Shoulder elbow wrist hand finger orthosis, abduction positioning (airplane design), thoracic component and support bar, includes one or more nontorsion joints, elastic bands, turnbuckles, may include soft interface, straps, custom fabricated, includes fitting and adjustment ⓑ Qp Qh &   A

Fracture Orthorics

* **L3980** Upper extremity fracture orthosis, humeral, prefabricated, includes fitting and adjustment ⓑ Qp Qh &   A

* **L3981** Upper extremity fracture orthosis, humeral, prefabricated, includes shoulder cap design, with or without joints, forearm section, may include soft interface, straps, includes fitting and adjustments ⓑ Qp Qh &   A

* **L3982** Upper extremity fracture orthosis, radius/ulnar, prefabricated, includes fitting and adjustment ⓑ Qp Qh &   A

* **L3984** Upper extremity fracture orthosis, wrist, prefabricated, includes fitting and adjustment ⓑ Qp Qh &   A

* **L3995** Addition to upper extremity orthosis, sock, fracture or equal, each ⓑ Qp &   A

* **L3999** Upper limb orthosis, not otherwise specified ⓑ   A

Repairs

* **L4000** Replace girdle for spinal orthosis (CTLSO or SO) ⓑ Qp Qh &   A

* **L4002** Replacement strap, any orthosis, includes all components, any length, any type ⓑ Qp &   A

* **L4010** Replace trilateral socket brim ⓑ Qp Qh &   A

* **L4020** Replace quadrilateral socket brim, molded to patient model ⓑ Qp Qh &   A

* **L4030** Replace quadrilateral socket brim, custom fitted ⓑ Qp Qh &   A

* **L4040** Replace molded thigh lacer, for custom fabricated orthosis only ⓑ Qp Qh &   A

* **L4045** Replace non-molded thigh lacer, for custom fabricated orthosis only ⓑ Qp Qh &   A

* **L4050** Replace molded calf lacer, for custom fabricated orthosis only ⓑ Qp Qh &   A

🅜 MIPS   Qp Quantity Physician   Qh Quantity Hospital   ♀ Female only

♂ Male only   A Age   & DMEPOS   A2-Z3 ASC Payment Indicator   A-Y ASC Status Indicator   Coding Clinic

* **L4055** Replace non-molded calf lacer, for custom fabricated orthosis only Ⓑ Qp Qh   A

* **L4060** Replace high roll cuff Ⓑ Qp Qh ♿   A

* **L4070** Replace proximal and distal upright for KAFO Ⓑ Qp Qh ♿   A

* **L4080** Replace metal bands KAFO, proximal thigh Ⓑ Qp Qh ♿   A

* **L4090** Replace metal bands KAFO-AFO, calf or distal thigh Ⓑ Qp ♿   A

* **L4100** Replace leather cuff KAFO, proximal thigh Ⓑ Qp Qh ♿   A

* **L4110** Replace leather cuff KAFO-AFO, calf or distal thigh Ⓑ Qp ♿   A

* **L4130** Replace pretibial shell Ⓑ Qp Qh ♿   A

⊛ **L4205** Repair of orthotic device, labor component, per 15 minutes Ⓑ Qp   A

   IOM: 100-02, 15, 110.2

⊛ **L4210** Repair of orthotic device, repair or replace minor parts Ⓑ Qp Qh   A

   IOM: 100-02, 15, 110.2; 100-02, 15, 120

Ancillary Orthotic Services

* **L4350** Ankle control orthosis, stirrup style, rigid, includes any type interface (e.g., pneumatic, gel), prefabricated, off-the-shelf Ⓑ Qp Qh ♿   A

* **L4360** Walking boot, pneumatic and/or vacuum, with or without joints, with or without interface material, prefabricated item that has been trimmed, bent, molded, assembled, or otherwise customized to fit a specific patient by an individual with expertise Ⓑ Qp Qh ♿   A

   Noncovered when walking boots used primarily to relieve pressure, especially on sole of foot, or are used for patients with foot ulcers

* **L4361** Walking boot, pneumatic and/or vacuum, with or without joints, with or without interface material, prefabricated, off-the-shelf Ⓑ Qp Qh ♿   A

* **L4370** Pneumatic full leg splint, prefabricated, off-the-shelf Ⓑ Qp Qh ♿   A

* **L4386** Walking boot, non-pneumatic, with or without joints, with or without interface material, prefabricated item that has been trimmed, bent, molded, assembled, or otherwise customized to fit a specific patient by an individual with expertise Ⓑ Qp Qh ♿   A

* **L4387** Walking boot, non-pneumatic, with or without joints, with or without interface material, prefabricated, off-the-shelf Ⓑ Qp Qh ♿   A

* **L4392** Replacement, soft interface material, static AFO Ⓑ Qp Qh ♿   A

* **L4394** Replace soft interface material, foot drop splint Ⓑ Qp Qh ♿   A

* **L4396** Static or dynamic ankle foot orthosis, including soft interface material, adjustable for fit, for positioning, may be used for minimal ambulation, prefabricated item that has been trimmed, bent, molded, assembled, or otherwise customized to fit a specific patient by an individual with expertise Ⓑ Qp Qh ♿   A

* **L4397** Static or dynamic ankle foot orthosis, including soft interface material, adjustable for fit, for positioning, may be used for minimal ambulation, prefabricated, off-the-shelf Ⓑ Qp Qh ♿   A

* **L4398** Foot drop splint, recumbent positioning device, prefabricated, off-the-shelf Ⓑ Qp Qh ♿   A

* **L4631** Ankle foot orthosis, walking boot type, varus/valgus correction, rocker bottom, anterior tibial shell, soft interface, custom arch support, plastic or other material, includes straps and closures, custom fabricated Ⓑ Qp Qh ♿   A

▶ **New**   ↺ **Revised**   ✔ **Reinstated**   ~~deleted~~ **Deleted**   ⊘ **Not covered or valid by Medicare**   ⊛ **Special coverage instructions**   * **Carrier discretion**   Ⓑ **Bill Part B MAC**   Ⓑ **Bill DME MAC**

Figure 36 Partial foot.

PROSTHETICS (L5000-L9999)

Lower Limb (L5000-L5999)

NOTE: The procedures in this section are considered as base or basic procedures and may be modified by listing items/procedures or special materials from the Additions section and adding them to the base procedure.

Partial Foot

⊘ **L5000** Partial foot, shoe insert with longitudinal arch, toe filler Ⓑ Ⓠp Ⓠh ♿   A

IOM: 100-02, 15, 290

⊘ **L5010** Partial foot, molded socket, ankle height, with toe filler Ⓑ Ⓠp Ⓠh ♿   A

IOM: 100-02, 15, 290

⊘ **L5020** Partial foot, molded socket, tibial tubercle height, with toe filler Ⓑ Ⓠp Ⓠh ♿   A

IOM: 100-02, 15, 290

Ankle

✳ **L5050** Ankle, Symes, molded socket, SACH foot Ⓑ Ⓠp Ⓠh ♿   A

✳ **L5060** Ankle, Symes, metal frame, molded leather socket, articulated ankle/foot Ⓑ Ⓠp Ⓠh ♿   A

Figure 37 Ankle Symes.

Below Knee

✳ **L5100** Below knee, molded socket, shin, SACH foot Ⓑ Ⓠp Ⓠh ♿   A

✳ **L5105** Below knee, plastic socket, joints and thigh lacer, SACH foot Ⓑ Ⓠp Ⓠh ♿   A

Knee Disarticulation

✳ **L5150** Knee disarticulation (or through knee), molded socket, external knee joints, shin, SACH foot Ⓑ Ⓠp Ⓠh ♿   A

✳ **L5160** Knee disarticulation (or through knee), molded socket, bent knee configuration, external knee joints, shin, SACH foot Ⓑ Ⓠp Ⓠh ♿   A

Above Knee

✳ **L5200** Above knee, molded socket, single axis constant friction knee, shin, SACH foot Ⓑ Ⓠp Ⓠh ♿   A

✳ **L5210** Above knee, short prosthesis, no knee joint ('stubbies'), with foot blocks, no ankle joints, each Ⓑ Ⓠp Ⓠh ♿   A

✳ **L5220** Above knee, short prosthesis, no knee joint ('stubbies'), with articulated ankle/foot, dynamically aligned, each Ⓑ Ⓠp Ⓠh ♿   A

✳ **L5230** Above knee, for proximal femoral focal deficiency, constant friction knee, shin, SACH foot Ⓑ Ⓠp Ⓠh ♿   A

Hip Disarticulation

✳ **L5250** Hip disarticulation, Canadian type; molded socket, hip joint, single axis constant friction knee, shin, SACH foot Ⓑ Ⓠp Ⓠh ♿   A

✳ **L5270** Hip disarticulation, tilt table type; molded socket, locking hip joint, single axis constant friction knee, shin, SACH foot Ⓑ Ⓠp Ⓠh ♿   A

Figure 38 Above knee.

Hemipelvectomy

∗ **L5280** Hemipelvectomy, Canadian type; molded socket, hip joint, single axis constant friction knee, shin, SACH foot ⑧ Qp Qh ⅄   A

Endoskeletal

∗ **L5301** Below knee, molded socket, shin, SACH foot, endoskeletal system ⑧ Qp Qh ⅄   A

∗ **L5312** Knee disarticulation (or through knee), molded socket, single axis knee, pylon, sach foot, endoskeletal system ⑧ Qp Qh ⅄   A

∗ **L5321** Above knee, molded socket, open end, SACH foot, endoskeletal system, single axis knee ⑧ Qp Qh ⅄   A

∗ **L5331** Hip disarticulation, Canadian type, molded socket, endoskeletal system, hip joint, single axis knee, SACH foot ⑧ Qp Qh ⅄   A

∗ **L5341** Hemipelvectomy, Canadian type, molded socket, endoskeletal system, hip joint, single axis knee, SACH foot ⑧ Qp Qh ⅄   A

Immediate Postsurgical or Early Fitting Procedures

∗ **L5400** Immediate post surgical or early fitting, application of initial rigid dressing, including fitting, alignment, suspension, and one cast change, below knee ⑧ Qp Qh ⅄   A

∗ **L5410** Immediate post surgical or early fitting, application of initial rigid dressing, including fitting, alignment and suspension, below knee, each additional cast change and realignment ⑧ Qp Qh ⅄   A

∗ **L5420** Immediate post surgical or early fitting, application of initial rigid dressing, including fitting, alignment and suspension and one cast change 'AK' or knee disarticulation ⑧ Qp Qh ⅄   A

∗ **L5430** Immediate postsurgical or early fitting, application of initial rigid dressing, including fitting, alignment, and suspension, 'AK' or knee disarticulation, each additional cast change and realignment ⑧ Qp Qh ⅄   A

∗ **L5450** Immediate post surgical or early fitting, application of non-weight bearing rigid dressing, below knee ⑧ Qp Qh ⅄   A

∗ **L5460** Immediate post surgical or early fitting, application of non-weight bearing rigid dressing, above knee ⑧ Qp Qh ⅄   A

Initial Prosthesis

∗ **L5500** Initial, below knee 'PTB' type socket, non-alignable system, pylon, no cover, SACH foot, plaster socket, direct formed ⑧ Qp Qh ⅄   A

∗ **L5505** Initial, above knee-knee disarticulation, ischial level socket, non-alignable system, pylon, no cover, SACH foot, plaster socket, direct formed ⑧ Qp Qh ⅄   A

Preparatory Prosthesis

∗ **L5510** Preparatory, below knee 'PTB' type socket, non-alignable system, pylon, no cover, SACH foot, plaster socket, molded to model ⑧ Qp Qh ⅄   A

∗ **L5520** Preparatory, below knee 'PTB' type socket, non-alignable system, pylon, no cover, SACH foot, thermoplastic or equal, direct formed ⑧ Qp Qh ⅄   A

∗ **L5530** Preparatory, below knee 'PTB' type socket, non-alignable system, pylon, no cover, SACH foot, thermoplastic or equal, molded to model ⑧ Qp Qh ⅄ A

∗ **L5535** Preparatory, below knee 'PTB' type socket, non-alignable system, no cover, SACH foot, prefabricated, adjustable open end socket ⑧ Qp Qh ⅄   A

∗ **L5540** Preparatory, below knee 'PTB' type socket, non-alignable system, pylon, no cover, SACH foot, laminated socket, molded to model ⑧ Qp Qh ⅄   A

∗ **L5560** Preparatory, above knee - knee disarticulation, ischial level socket, non-alignable system, pylon, no cover, SACH foot, plaster socket, molded to model ⑧ Qp Qh ⅄   A

∗ **L5570** Preparatory, above knee - knee disarticulation, ischial level socket, non-alignable system, pylon, no cover, SACH foot, thermoplastic or equal, direct formed ⑧ Qp Qh ⅄   A

∗ **L5580** Preparatory, above knee - knee disarticulation, ischial level socket, non-alignable system, pylon, no cover, SACH foot, thermoplastic or equal, molded to model ⑧ Qp Qh ⅄   A

∗ **L5585** Preparatory, above knee - knee disarticulation, ischial level socket, non-alignable system, pylon, no cover, SACH foot, prefabricated adjustable open end socket ⑧ Qp Qh ⅄   A

▶ New   ⟳ Revised   ✔ Reinstated   deleted Deleted   ⊘ Not covered or valid by Medicare   ⊛ Special coverage instructions   ∗ Carrier discretion   ⑧ Bill Part B MAC   ⑧ Bill DME MAC

L5280 – L5585   PROSTHETICS

374

* **L5590** Preparatory, above knee - knee disarticulation, ischial level socket, non-alignable system, pylon, no cover, SACH foot, laminated socket, molded to model ⑧ Qp Qh ♿   A

* **L5595** Preparatory, hip disarticulation-hemipelvectomy, pylon, no cover, SACH foot, thermoplastic or equal, molded to patient model ⑧ Qp Qh ♿   A

* **L5600** Preparatory, hip disarticulation-hemipelvectomy, pylon, no cover, SACH foot, laminated socket, molded to patient model ⑧ Qp Qh ♿   A

Additions to Lower Extremity

* **L5610** Addition to lower extremity, endoskeletal system, above knee, hydracadence system ⑧ Qp Qh ♿   A

* **L5611** Addition to lower extremity, endoskeletal system, above knee-knee disarticulation, 4 bar linkage, with friction swing phase control ⑧ Qp Qh ♿   A

* **L5613** Addition to lower extremity, endoskeletal system, above knee-knee disarticulation, 4 bar linkage, with hydraulic swing phase control ⑧ Qp Qh ♿   A

* **L5614** Addition to lower extremity, exoskeletal system, above knee-knee disarticulation, 4 bar linkage, with pneumatic swing phase control ⑧ Qp Qh ♿   A

* **L5616** Addition to lower extremity, endoskeletal system, above knee, universal multiplex system, friction swing phase control ⑧ Qp Qh ♿   A

* **L5617** Addition to lower extremity, quick change self-aligning unit, above knee or below knee, each ⑧ Qp Qh ♿   A

Additions to Test Sockets

* **L5618** Addition to lower extremity, test socket, Symes ⑧ Qp ♿   A

* **L5620** Addition to lower extremity, test socket, below knee ⑧ Qp ♿   A

* **L5622** Addition to lower extremity, test socket, knee disarticulation ⑧ Qp ♿   A

* **L5624** Addition to lower extremity, test socket, above knee ⑧ Qp ♿   A

* **L5626** Addition to lower extremity, test socket, hip disarticulation ⑧ Qp Qh ♿   A

* **L5628** Addition to lower extremity, test socket, hemipelvectomy ⑧ Qp Qh ♿   A

Additions to Socket Variations

* **L5629** Addition to lower extremity, below knee, acrylic socket ⑧ Qp Qh ♿   A

* **L5630** Addition to lower extremity, Symes type, expandable wall socket ⑧ Qp Qh ♿   A

* **L5631** Addition to lower extremity, above knee or knee disarticulation, acrylic socket ⑧ Qp Qh ♿   A

* **L5632** Addition to lower extremity, Symes type, 'PTB' brim design socket ⑧ Qp Qh ♿   A

* **L5634** Addition to lower extremity, Symes type, posterior opening (Canadian) socket ⑧ Qp Qh ♿   A

* **L5636** Addition to lower extremity, Symes type, medial opening socket ⑧ Qp Qh ♿   A

* **L5637** Addition to lower extremity, below knee, total contact ⑧ Qp Qh ♿   A

* **L5638** Addition to lower extremity, below knee, leather socket ⑧ Qp Qh ♿   A

* **L5639** Addition to lower extremity, below knee, wood socket ⑧ Qp Qh ♿   A

* **L5640** Addition to lower extremity, knee disarticulation, leather socket ⑧ Qp Qh ♿   A

* **L5642** Addition to lower extremity, above knee, leather socket ⑧ Qp Qh ♿   A

* **L5643** Addition to lower extremity, hip disarticulation, flexible inner socket, external frame ⑧ Qp Qh ♿   A

* **L5644** Addition to lower extremity, above knee, wood socket ⑧ Qp Qh ♿   A

* **L5645** Addition to lower extremity, below knee, flexible inner socket, external frame ⑧ Qp Qh ♿   A

* **L5646** Addition to lower extremity, below knee, air, fluid, gel or equal, cushion socket ⑧ Qp Qh ♿   A

* **L5647** Addition to lower extremity, below knee, suction socket ⑧ Qp Qh ♿   A

* **L5648** Addition to lower extremity, above knee, air, fluid, gel or equal, cushion socket ⑧ Qp Qh ♿   A

* **L5649** Addition to lower extremity, ischial containment/narrow M-L socket ⑧ Qp Qh ♿   A

* **L5650** Additions to lower extremity, total contact, above knee or knee disarticulation socket ⑧ Qp Qh ♿   A

MIPS	Qp Quantity Physician	Qh Quantity Hospital	♀ Female only
♂ Male only	A Age ♿ DMEPOS	A2-Z3 ASC Payment Indicator	A-Y ASC Status Indicator Coding Clinic

* **L5651** Addition to lower extremity, above knee, flexible inner socket, external frame ⑧ Qp Qh ⅋ A

* **L5652** Addition to lower extremity, suction suspension, above knee or knee disarticulation socket ⑧ Qp Qh ⅋ A

* **L5653** Addition to lower extremity, knee disarticulation, expandable wall socket ⑧ Qp Qh ⅋ A

Additions to Socket Insert and Suspension

* **L5654** Addition to lower extremity, socket insert, Symes, (Kemblo, Pelite, Aliplast, Plastazote or equal) ⑧ Qp Qh ⅋ A

* **L5655** Addition to lower extremity, socket insert, below knee (Kemblo, Pelite, Aliplast, Plastazote or equal) ⑧ Qp Qh ⅋ A

* **L5656** Addition to lower extremity, socket insert, knee disarticulation (Kemblo, Pelite, Aliplast, Plastazote or equal) ⑧ Qp Qh ⅋ A

* **L5658** Addition to lower extremity, socket insert, above knee (Kemblo, Pelite, Aliplast, Plastazote or equal) ⑧ Qp Qh ⅋ A

* **L5661** Addition to lower extremity, socket insert, multi-durometer Symes ⑧ Qp Qh ⅋ A

* **L5665** Addition to lower extremity, socket insert, multi-durometer, below knee ⑧ Qp Qh ⅋ A

* **L5666** Addition to lower extremity, below knee, cuff suspension ⑧ Qp Qh ⅋ A

* **L5668** Addition to lower extremity, below knee, molded distal cushion ⑧ Qp Qh ⅋ A

* **L5670** Addition to lower extremity, below knee, molded supracondylar suspension ('PTS' or similar) ⑧ Qp Qh ⅋ A

* **L5671** Addition to lower extremity, below knee/above knee suspension locking mechanism (shuttle, lanyard or equal), excludes socket insert ⑧ Qp Qh ⅋ A

* **L5672** Addition to lower extremity, below knee, removable medial brim suspension ⑧ Qp Qh ⅋ A

* **L5673** Addition to lower extremity, below knee/above knee, custom fabricated from existing mold or prefabricated, socket insert, silicone gel, elastomeric or equal, for use with locking mechanism ⑧ Qp ⅋ A

* **L5676** Additions to lower extremity, below knee, knee joints, single axis, pair ⑧ Qp Qh ⅋ A

* **L5677** Additions to lower extremity, below knee, knee joints, polycentric, pair ⑧ Qp Qh ⅋ A

* **L5678** Additions to lower extremity, below knee, joint covers, pair ⑧ Qp Qh ⅋ A

* **L5679** Addition to lower extremity, below knee/above knee, custom fabricated from existing mold or prefabricated, socket insert, silicone gel, elastomeric or equal, not for use with locking mechanism ⑧ Qp ⅋ A

* **L5680** Addition to lower extremity, below knee, thigh lacer, non-molded ⑧ Qp Qh ⅋ A

* **L5681** Addition to lower extremity, below knee/above knee, custom fabricated socket insert for congenital or atypical traumatic amputee, silicone gel, elastomeric or equal, for use with or without locking mechanism, initial only (for other than initial, use code L5673 or L5679) ⑧ Qp Qh ⅋ A

* **L5682** Addition to lower extremity, below knee, thigh lacer, gluteal/ischial, molded ⑧ Qp Qh ⅋ A

* **L5683** Addition to lower extremity, below knee/above knee, custom fabricated socket insert for other than congenital or atypical traumatic amputee, silicone gel, elastomeric, or equal, for use with or without locking mechanism, initial only (for other than initial, use code L5673 or L5679) ⑧ Qp Qh ⅋ A

* **L5684** Addition to lower extremity, below knee, fork strap ⑧ Qp Qh ⅋ A

* **L5685** Addition to lower extremity prosthesis, below knee, suspension/sealing sleeve, with or without valve, any material, each ⑧ Qp ⅋ A

* **L5686** Addition to lower extremity, below knee, back check (extension control) ⑧ Qp Qh ⅋ A

* **L5688** Addition to lower extremity, below knee, waist belt, webbing ⑧ Qp Qh ⅋ A

* **L5690** Addition to lower extremity, below knee, waist belt, padded and lined ⑧ Qp Qh ⅋ A

* **L5692** Addition to lower extremity, above knee, pelvic control belt, light ⑧ Qp Qh ⅋ A

* **L5694** Addition to lower extremity, above knee, pelvic control belt, padded and lined ⑧ Qp Qh ⅋ A

▶ New   ↻ Revised   ✔ Reinstated   ~~deleted~~ Deleted   ⊘ Not covered or valid by Medicare
⊛ Special coverage instructions   * Carrier discretion   ⑧ Bill Part B MAC   ⑤ Bill DME MAC

* **L5695** Addition to lower extremity, above knee, pelvic control, sleeve suspension, neoprene or equal, each Ⓑ Qp Qh ♿   A

* **L5696** Addition to lower extremity, above knee or knee disarticulation, pelvic joint Ⓑ Qp Qh ♿   A

* **L5697** Addition to lower extremity, above knee or knee disarticulation, pelvic band Ⓑ Qp Qh ♿   A

* **L5698** Addition to lower extremity, above knee or knee disarticulation, Silesian bandage Ⓑ Qp Qh ♿   A

* **L5699** All lower extremity prostheses, shoulder harness Ⓑ Qp Qh ♿   A

Replacement Sockets

* **L5700** Replacement, socket, below knee, molded to patient model Ⓑ Qp Qh ♿   A

* **L5701** Replacement, socket, above knee/knee disarticulation, including attachment plate, molded to patient model Ⓑ Qp Qh ♿   A

* **L5702** Replacement, socket, hip disarticulation, including hip joint, molded to patient model Ⓑ Qp Qh ♿   A

* **L5703** Ankle, Symes, molded to patient model, socket without solid ankle cushion heel (SACH) foot, replacement only Ⓑ Qp Qh ♿   A

Protective Covers

* **L5704** Custom shaped protective cover, below knee Ⓑ Qp Qh ♿   A

* **L5705** Custom shaped protective cover, above knee Ⓑ Qp Qh ♿   A

* **L5706** Custom shaped protective cover, knee disarticulation Ⓑ Qp Qh ♿   A

* **L5707** Custom shaped protective cover, hip disarticulation Ⓑ Qp Qh ♿   A

Additions to Exoskeletal–Knee-Shin System

* **L5710** Addition, exoskeletal knee-shin system, single axis, manual lock Ⓑ Qp Qh ♿   A

* **L5711** Additions exoskeletal knee-shin system, single axis, manual lock, ultra-light material Ⓑ Qp Qh ♿   A

* **L5712** Addition, exoskeletal knee-shin system, single axis, friction swing and stance phase control (safety knee) Ⓑ Qp Qh ♿   A

* **L5714** Addition, exoskeletal knee-shin system, single axis, variable friction swing phase control Ⓑ Qp Qh ♿   A

* **L5716** Addition, exoskeletal knee-shin system, polycentric, mechanical stance phase lock Ⓑ Qp Qh ♿   A

* **L5718** Addition, exoskeletal knee-shin system, polycentric, friction swing and stance phase control Ⓑ Qp Qh ♿   A

* **L5722** Addition, exoskeletal knee-shin system, single axis, pneumatic swing, friction stance phase control Ⓑ Qp Qh ♿   A

* **L5724** Addition, exoskeletal knee-shin system, single axis, fluid swing phase control Ⓑ Qp Qh ♿   A

* **L5726** Addition, exoskeletal knee-shin system, single axis, external joints, fluid swing phase control Ⓑ Qp Qh ♿   A

* **L5728** Addition, exoskeletal knee-shin system, single axis, fluid swing and stance phase control Ⓑ Qp Qh ♿   A

* **L5780** Addition, exoskeletal knee-shin system, single axis, pneumatic/hydra pneumatic swing phase control Ⓑ Qp Qh ♿   A

Vacuum Pumps

* **L5781** Addition to lower limb prosthesis, vacuum pump, residual limb volume management and moisture evacuation system Ⓑ Qp Qh ♿   A

* **L5782** Addition to lower limb prosthesis, vacuum pump, residual limb volume management and moisture evacuation system, heavy duty Ⓑ Qp Qh ♿   A

Component Modification

* **L5785** Addition, exoskeletal system, below knee, ultra-light material (titanium, carbon fiber, or equal) Ⓑ Qp Qh ♿ A

* **L5790** Addition, exoskeletal system, above knee, ultra-light material (titanium, carbon fiber, or equal) Ⓑ Qp Qh ♿ A

* **L5795** Addition, exoskeletal system, hip disarticulation, ultra-light material (titanium, carbon fiber, or equal) Ⓑ Qp Qh ♿   A

Endoskeletal

* **L5810** Addition, endoskeletal knee-shin system, single axis, manual lock Ⓑ Qp Qh ♿   A

* **L5811** Addition, endoskeletal knee-shin system, single axis, manual lock, ultralight material Ⓑ Qp Qh ♿   A

---

* **L5812** Addition, endoskeletal knee-shin system, single axis, friction swing and stance phase control (safety knee) ⑧ Qp Qh ⑤   A

* **L5814** Addition, endoskeletal knee-shin system, polycentric, hydraulic swing phase control, mechanical stance phase lock ⑧ Qp Qh ⑤   A

* **L5816** Addition, endoskeletal knee-shin system, polycentric, mechanical stance phase lock ⑧ Qp Qh ⑤   A

* **L5818** Addition, endoskeletal knee-shin system, polycentric, friction swing, and stance phase control ⑧ Qp Qh ⑤   A

* **L5822** Addition, endoskeletal knee-shin system, single axis, pneumatic swing, friction stance phase control ⑧ Qp Qh ⑤   A

* **L5824** Addition, endoskeletal knee-shin system, single axis, fluid swing phase control ⑧ Qp Qh ⑤   A

* **L5826** Addition, endoskeletal knee-shin system, single axis, hydraulic swing phase control, with miniature high activity frame ⑧ Qp Qh ⑤   A

* **L5828** Addition, endoskeletal knee-shin system, single axis, fluid swing and stance phase control ⑧ Qp Qh ⑤   A

* **L5830** Addition, endoskeletal knee-shin system, single axis, pneumatic/swing phase control ⑧ Qp Qh ⑤   A

* **L5840** Addition, endoskeletal knee/shin system, 4-bar linkage or multiaxial, pneumatic swing phase control ⑧ Qp Qh ⑤   A

* **L5845** Addition, endoskeletal, knee-shin system, stance flexion feature, adjustable ⑧ Qp Qh ⑤   A

* **L5848** Addition to endoskeletal, knee-shin system, fluid stance extension, dampening feature, with or without adjustability ⑧ Qp Qh ⑤   A

* **L5850** Addition, endoskeletal system, above knee or hip disarticulation, knee extension assist ⑧ Qp Qh ⑤   A

* **L5855** Addition, endoskeletal system, hip disarticulation, mechanical hip extension assist ⑧ Qp Qh ⑤   A

* **L5856** Addition to lower extremity prosthesis, endoskeletal knee-shin system, microprocessor control feature, swing and stance phase; includes electronic sensor(s), any type ⑧ Qp Qh ⑤   A

* **L5857** Addition to lower extremity prosthesis, endoskeletal knee-shin system, microprocessor control feature, swing phase only; includes electronic sensor(s), any type ⑧ Qp Qh ⑤   A

* **L5858** Addition to lower extremity prosthesis, endoskeletal knee shin system, microprocessor control feature, stance phase only, includes electronic sensor(s), any type ⑧ Qp Qh ⑤   A

* **L5859** Addition to lower extremity prosthesis, endoskeletal knee-shin system, powered and programmable flexion/extension assist control, includes any type motor(s) ⑧ Qp Qh ⑤   A

* **L5910** Addition, endoskeletal system, below knee, alignable system ⑧ Qp Qh ⑤   A

* **L5920** Addition, endoskeletal system, above knee or hip disarticulation, alignable system ⑧ Qp Qh ⑤   A

* **L5925** Addition, endoskeletal system, above knee, knee disarticulation or hip disarticulation, manual lock ⑧ Qp Qh ⑤   A

* **L5930** Addition, endoskeletal system, high activity knee control frame ⑧ Qp Qh ⑤   A

* **L5940** Addition, endoskeletal system, below knee, ultra-light material (titanium, carbon fiber or equal) ⑧ Qp Qh ⑤   A

* **L5950** Addition, endoskeletal system, above knee, ultra-light material (titanium, carbon fiber or equal) ⑧ Qp Qh ⑤   A

* **L5960** Addition, endoskeletal system, hip disarticulation, ultra-light material (titanium, carbon fiber, or equal) ⑧ Qp Qh ⑤   A

* **L5961** Addition, endoskeletal system, polycentric hip joint, pneumatic or hydraulic control, rotation control, with or without flexion, and/or extension control ⑧ Qp Qh ⑤   A

* **L5962** Addition, endoskeletal system, below knee, flexible protective outer surface covering system ⑧ Qp Qh ⑤   A

* **L5964** Addition, endoskeletal system, above knee, flexible protective outer surface covering system ⑧ Qp Qh ⑤   A

* **L5966** Addition, endoskeletal system, hip disarticulation, flexible protective outer surface covering system ⑧ Qp Qh ⑤   A

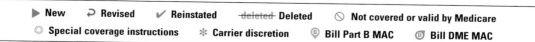

▶ New   ↻ Revised   ✔ Reinstated   ~~deleted~~ Deleted   ⊘ Not covered or valid by Medicare
✪ Special coverage instructions   * Carrier discretion   ⑧ Bill Part B MAC   ⑧ Bill DME MAC

Additions to Ankle and/or Foot

* **L5968** Addition to lower limb prosthesis, multiaxial ankle with swing phase active dorsiflexion feature ⑧ Qp Qh ♿   A

* **L5969** Addition, endoskeletal ankle-foot or ankle system, power assist, includes any type motor(s) ⑧ Qp Qh   A

* **L5970** All lower extremity prostheses, foot, external keel, SACH foot ⑧ Qp Qh ♿   A

* **L5971** All lower extremity prosthesis, solid ankle cushion keel (SACH) foot, replacement only ⑧ Qp Qh ♿   A

* **L5972** All lower extremity prostheses (foot, flexible keel) ⑧ Qp Qh ♿   A

* **L5973** Endoskeletal ankle foot system, microprocessor controlled feature, dorsiflexion and/or plantar flexion control, includes power source ⑧ Qh ♿   A

* **L5974** All lower extremity prostheses, foot, single axis ankle/foot ⑧ Qp Qh ♿   A

* **L5975** All lower extremity prostheses, combination single axis ankle and flexible keel foot ⑧ Qp Qh ♿   A

* **L5976** All lower extremity prostheses, energy storing foot (Seattle Carbon Copy II or equal) ⑧ Qp Qh ♿   A

* **L5978** All lower extremity prostheses, foot, multiaxial ankle/foot ⑧ Qp Qh ♿   A

* **L5979** All lower extremity prostheses, multiaxial ankle, dynamic response foot, one piece system ⑧ Qp Qh ♿   A

* **L5980** All lower extremity prostheses, flex foot system ⑧ Qp Qh ♿   A

* **L5981** All lower extremity prostheses, flexwalk system or equal ⑧ Qp Qh ♿   A

* **L5982** All exoskeletal lower extremity prostheses, axial rotation unit ⑧ Qp Qh ♿   A

* **L5984** All endoskeletal lower extremity prostheses, axial rotation unit, with or without adjustability ⑧ Qp Qh ♿   A

* **L5985** All endoskeletal lower extremity prostheses, dynamic prosthetic pylon ⑧ Qp Qh ♿   A

* **L5986** All lower extremity prostheses, multiaxial rotation unit ('MCP' or equal) ⑧ Qp Qh ♿   A

* **L5987** All lower extremity prostheses, shank foot system with vertical loading pylon ⑧ Qp Qh ♿   A

* **L5988** Addition to lower limb prosthesis, vertical shock reducing pylon feature ⑧ Qp Qh ♿   A

* **L5990** Addition to lower extremity prosthesis, user adjustable heel height ⑧ Qp Qh ♿   A

▶ * **L5991** Addition to lower extremity prostheses, osseointegrated external prosthetic connector   A

* **L5999** Lower extremity prosthesis, not otherwise specified ⑧   A

Upper Limb (L6000-L7600)

NOTE: The procedures in L6000-L6599 are considered as base or basic procedures and may be modified by listing procedures from the additions sections. The base procedures include only standard friction wrist and control cable system unless otherwise specified.

Partial Hand

* **L6000** Partial hand, thumb remaining ⑧ Qp Qh ♿   A

* **L6010** Partial hand, little and/or ring finger remaining ⑧ Qp Qh ♿   A

* **L6020** Partial hand, no finger remaining ⑧ Qp Qh ♿   A

* **L6026** Transcarpal/metacarpal or partial hand disarticulation prosthesis, external power, self-suspended, inner socket with removable forearm section, electrodes and cables, two batteries, charger, myoelectric control of terminal device, excludes terminal device(s) ⑧ Qp Qh ♿   A

Figure 39   Partial hand.

Wrist Disarticulation

* **L6050** Wrist disarticulation, molded socket, flexible elbow hinges, triceps pad Ⓑ 𝗤𝗽 𝗤𝗵 ♿   A

* **L6055** Wrist disarticulation, molded socket with expandable interface, flexible elbow hinges, triceps pad Ⓑ 𝗤𝗽 𝗤𝗵 ♿   A

Below Elbow

* **L6100** Below elbow, molded socket, flexible elbow hinge, triceps pad Ⓑ 𝗤𝗽 𝗤𝗵 ♿   A

* **L6110** Below elbow, molded socket, (Muenster or Northwestern suspension types) Ⓑ 𝗤𝗽 𝗤𝗵 ♿   A

* **L6120** Below elbow, molded double wall split socket, step-up hinges, half cuff Ⓑ 𝗤𝗽 𝗤𝗵 ♿   A

* **L6130** Below elbow, molded double wall split socket, stump activated locking hinge, half cuff Ⓑ 𝗤𝗽 𝗤𝗵 ♿   A

Elbow Disarticulation

* **L6200** Elbow disarticulation, molded socket, outside locking hinge, forearm Ⓑ 𝗤𝗽 𝗤𝗵 ♿   A

* **L6205** Elbow disarticulation, molded socket with expandable interface, outside locking hinges, forearm Ⓑ 𝗤𝗽 𝗤𝗵 ♿   A

Above Elbow

* **L6250** Above elbow, molded double wall socket, internal locking elbow, forearm Ⓑ 𝗤𝗽 𝗤𝗵 ♿   A

Shoulder Disarticulation

* **L6300** Shoulder disarticulation, molded socket, shoulder bulkhead, humeral section, internal locking elbow, forearm Ⓑ 𝗤𝗽 𝗤𝗵 ♿   A

* **L6310** Shoulder disarticulation, passive restoration (complete prosthesis) Ⓑ 𝗤𝗽 𝗤𝗵 ♿   A

* **L6320** Shoulder disarticulation, passive restoration (shoulder cap only) Ⓑ 𝗤𝗽 𝗤𝗵 ♿   A

Interscapular Thoracic

* **L6350** Interscapular thoracic, molded socket, shoulder bulkhead, humeral section, internal locking elbow, forearm Ⓑ 𝗤𝗽 𝗤𝗵 ♿   A

* **L6360** Interscapular thoracic, passive restoration (complete prosthesis) Ⓑ 𝗤𝗽 𝗤𝗵 ♿   A

* **L6370** Interscapular thoracic, passive restoration (shoulder cap only) Ⓑ 𝗤𝗽 𝗤𝗵 ♿   A

Immediate and Early Postsurgical Procedures

* **L6380** Immediate post surgical or early fitting, application of initial rigid dressing, including fitting alignment and suspension of components, and one cast change, wrist disarticulation or below elbow Ⓑ 𝗤𝗽 𝗤𝗵 ♿   A

* **L6382** Immediate post surgical or early fitting, application of initial rigid dressing including fitting alignment and suspension of components, and one cast change, elbow disarticulation or above elbow Ⓑ 𝗤𝗽 𝗤𝗵 ♿   A

* **L6384** Immediate post surgical or early fitting, application of initial rigid dressing including fitting alignment and suspension of components, and one cast change, shoulder disarticulation or interscapular thoracic Ⓑ 𝗤𝗽 𝗤𝗵 ♿ A

* **L6386** Immediate post surgical or early fitting, each additional cast change and realignment Ⓑ 𝗤𝗽 𝗤𝗵 ♿   A

* **L6388** Immediate post surgical or early fitting, application of rigid dressing only Ⓑ 𝗤𝗽 𝗤𝗵 ♿   A

Molded Socket

* **L6400** Below elbow, molded socket, endoskeletal system, including soft prosthetic tissue shaping Ⓑ 𝗤𝗽 𝗤𝗵 ♿   A

* **L6450** Elbow disarticulation, molded socket, endoskeletal system, including soft prosthetic tissue shaping Ⓑ 𝗤𝗽 𝗤𝗵 ♿   A

* **L6500** Above elbow, molded socket, endoskeletal system, including soft prosthetic tissue shaping Ⓑ 𝗤𝗽 𝗤𝗵 ♿   A

* **L6550** Shoulder disarticulation, molded socket, endoskeletal system, including soft prosthetic tissue shaping Ⓑ 𝗤𝗽 𝗤𝗵 ♿   A

* **L6570** Interscapular thoracic, molded socket, endoskeletal system, including soft prosthetic tissue shaping Ⓑ 𝗤𝗽 𝗤𝗵 ♿   A

▶ New   ↻ Revised   ✔ Reinstated   ~~deleted~~ Deleted   ⊘ Not covered or valid by Medicare
⊛ Special coverage instructions   ✲ Carrier discretion   Ⓑ Bill Part B MAC   Ⓑ Bill DME MAC

Preparatory Prosthetic

⁎ **L6580**   Preparatory, wrist disarticulation or below elbow, single wall plastic socket, friction wrist, flexible elbow hinges, figure of eight harness, humeral cuff, Bowden cable control, USMC or equal pylon, no cover, molded to patient model ⑧ Qp Qh ⅙   A

⁎ **L6582**   Preparatory, wrist disarticulation or below elbow, single wall socket, friction wrist, flexible elbow hinges, figure of eight harness, humeral cuff, Bowden cable control, USMC or equal pylon, no cover, direct formed ⑧ Qp Qh ⅙   A

⁎ **L6584**   Preparatory, elbow disarticulation or above elbow, single wall plastic socket, friction wrist, locking elbow, figure of eight harness, fair lead cable control, USMC or equal pylon, no cover, molded to patient model ⑧ Qp Qh ⅙   A

⁎ **L6586**   Preparatory, elbow disarticulation or above elbow, single wall socket, friction wrist, locking elbow, figure of eight harness, fair lead cable control, USMC or equal pylon, no cover, direct formed ⑧ Qp Qh ⅙   A

⁎ **L6588**   Preparatory, shoulder disarticulation or interscapular thoracic, single wall plastic socket, shoulder joint, locking elbow, friction wrist, chest strap, fair lead cable control, USMC or equal pylon, no cover, molded to patient model ⑧ Qp Qh ⅙   A

⁎ **L6590**   Preparatory, shoulder disarticulation or interscapular thoracic, single wall socket, shoulder joint, locking elbow, friction wrist, chest strap, fair lead cable control, USMC or equal pylon, no cover, direct formed ⑧ Qp Qh ⅙   A

Additions to Upper Limb

NOTE: The following procedures/modifications/components may be added to other base procedures. The items in this section should reflect the additional complexity of each modification procedure, in addition to base procedure, at the time of the original order.

⁎ **L6600**   Upper extremity additions, polycentric hinge, pair ⑧ Qp Qh ⅙   A

⁎ **L6605**   Upper extremity additions, single pivot hinge, pair ⑧ Qp Qh ⅙   A

⁎ **L6610**   Upper extremity additions, flexible metal hinge, pair ⑧ Qp Qh ⅙   A

⁎ **L6611**   Addition to upper extremity prosthesis, external powered, additional switch, any type ⑧ Qp Qh ⅙   A

⁎ **L6615**   Upper extremity addition, disconnect locking wrist unit ⑧ Qp Qh ⅙   A

⁎ **L6616**   Upper extremity addition, additional disconnect insert for locking wrist unit, each ⑧ Qp Qh ⅙   A

⁎ **L6620**   Upper extremity addition, flexion/extension wrist unit, with or without friction ⑧ Qp Qh ⅙   A

⁎ **L6621**   Upper extremity prosthesis addition, flexion/extension wrist with or without friction, for use with external powered terminal device ⑧ Qp Qh ⅙   A

⁎ **L6623**   Upper extremity addition, spring assisted rotational wrist unit with latch release ⑧ Qp Qh ⅙   A

⁎ **L6624**   Upper extremity addition, flexion/extension and rotation wrist unit ⑧ Qp Qh ⅙   A

⁎ **L6625**   Upper extremity addition, rotation wrist unit with cable lock ⑧ Qp Qh ⅙   A

⁎ **L6628**   Upper extremity addition, quick disconnect hook adapter, Otto Bock or equal ⑧ Qp Qh ⅙   A

⁎ **L6629**   Upper extremity addition, quick disconnect lamination collar with coupling piece, Otto Bock or equal ⑧ Qp Qh ⅙   A

⁎ **L6630**   Upper extremity addition, stainless steel, any wrist ⑧ Qp Qh ⅙   A

⁎ **L6632**   Upper extremity addition, latex suspension sleeve, each ⑧ Qp Qh ⅙   A

⁎ **L6635**   Upper extremity addition, lift assist for elbow ⑧ Qp Qh ⅙   A

⁎ **L6637**   Upper extremity addition, nudge control elbow lock ⑧ Qp Qh ⅙   A

⁎ **L6638**   Upper extremity addition to prosthesis, electric locking feature, only for use with manually powered elbow ⑧ Qp Qh ⅙   A

⁎ **L6640**   Upper extremity additions, shoulder abduction joint, pair ⑧ Qp Qh ⅙   A

Figure 40   Upper extremity addition.

🖎 MIPS	Qp **Quantity Physician**	Qh **Quantity Hospital**	♀ **Female only**
♂ **Male only** A **Age** ⅙ **DMEPOS**	A2-Z3 **ASC Payment Indicator**	A-Y **ASC Status Indicator**	Coding Clinic

* **L6641** Upper extremity addition, excursion amplifier, pulley type ⑧ Qp Qh & A
* **L6642** Upper extremity addition, excursion amplifier, lever type ⑧ Qp Qh & A
* **L6645** Upper extremity addition, shoulder flexion-abduction joint, each ⑧ Qp Qh & A
* **L6646** Upper extremity addition, shoulder joint, multipositional locking, flexion, adjustable abduction friction control, for use with body powered or external powered system ⑧ Qp Qh & A
* **L6647** Upper extremity addition, shoulder lock mechanism, body powered actuator ⑧ Qp Qh & A
* **L6648** Upper extremity addition, shoulder lock mechanism, external powered actuator ⑧ Qp Qh & A
* **L6650** Upper extremity addition, shoulder universal joint, each ⑧ Qp Qh & A
* **L6655** Upper extremity addition, standard control cable, extra ⑧ Qp & A
* **L6660** Upper extremity addition, heavy duty control cable ⑧ Qp & A
* **L6665** Upper extremity addition, Teflon, or equal, cable lining ⑧ Qp & A
* **L6670** Upper extremity addition, hook to hand, cable adapter ⑧ Qp Qh & A
* **L6672** Upper extremity addition, harness, chest or shoulder, saddle type ⑧ Qp Qh & A
* **L6675** Upper extremity addition, harness, (e.g., figure of eight type), single cable design ⑧ Qp Qh & A
* **L6676** Upper extremity addition, harness, (e.g., figure of eight type), dual cable design ⑧ Qp Qh & A
* **L6677** Upper extremity addition, harness, triple control, simultaneous operation of terminal device and elbow ⑧ Qp Qh & A
* **L6680** Upper extremity addition, test socket, wrist disarticulation or below elbow ⑧ Qp & A
* **L6682** Upper extremity addition, test socket, elbow disarticulation or above elbow ⑧ Qp & A
* **L6684** Upper extremity addition, test socket, shoulder disarticulation or interscapular thoracic ⑧ Qp & A
* **L6686** Upper extremity addition, suction socket ⑧ Qp Qh & A
* **L6687** Upper extremity addition, frame type socket, below elbow or wrist disarticulation ⑧ Qp Qh & A
* **L6688** Upper extremity addition, frame type socket, above elbow or elbow disarticulation ⑧ Qp Qh & A

* **L6689** Upper extremity addition, frame type socket, shoulder disarticulation ⑧ Qp Qh & A
* **L6690** Upper extremity addition, frame type socket, interscapular-thoracic ⑧ Qp Qh & A
* **L6691** Upper extremity addition, removable insert, each ⑧ Qp & A
* **L6692** Upper extremity addition, silicone gel insert or equal, each ⑧ Qp & A
* **L6693** Upper extremity addition, locking elbow, forearm counterbalance ⑧ Qp Qh & A
* **L6694** Addition to upper extremity prosthesis, below elbow/above elbow, custom fabricated from existing mold or prefabricated, socket insert, silicone gel, elastomeric or equal, for use with locking mechanism ⑧ Qp Qh & A
* **L6695** Addition to upper extremity prosthesis, below elbow/above elbow, custom fabricated from existing mold or prefabricated, socket insert, silicone gel, elastomeric or equal, not for use with locking mechanism ⑧ Qp Qh & A
* **L6696** Addition to upper extremity prosthesis, below elbow/above elbow, custom fabricated socket insert for congenital or atypical traumatic amputee, silicone gel, elastomeric or equal, for use with or without locking mechanism, initial only (for other than initial, use code L6694 or L6695) ⑧ Qp Qh & A
* **L6697** Addition to upper extremity prosthesis, below elbow/above elbow, custom fabricated socket insert for other than congenital or atypical traumatic amputee, silicone gel, elastomeric or equal, for use with or without locking mechanism, initial only (for other than initial, use code L6694 or L6695) ⑧ Qp Qh & A
* **L6698** Addition to upper extremity prosthesis, below elbow/above elbow, lock mechanism, excludes socket insert ⑧ Qp Qh & A

Terminal Devices (L6703-L6882)

* **L6703** Terminal device, passive hand/mitt, any material, any size ⑧ Qp Qh & A
* **L6704** Terminal device, sport/recreational/work attachment, any material, any size ⑧ Qp Qh & A
* **L6706** Terminal device, hook, mechanical, voluntary opening, any material, any size, lined or unlined ⑧ Qp Qh & A
* **L6707** Terminal device, hook, mechanical, voluntary closing, any material, any size, lined or unlined ⑧ Qp Qh & A

▶ New   ↻ Revised   ✔ Reinstated   deleted Deleted   ⊘ Not covered or valid by Medicare
⊙ Special coverage instructions   * Carrier discretion   ⑧ Bill Part B MAC   ⑧ Bill DME MAC

* **L6708** Terminal device, hand, mechanical, voluntary opening, any material, any size ⑧ Qp Qh &   A

* **L6709** Terminal device, hand, mechanical, voluntary closing, any material, any size ⑧ Qp Qh &   A

* **L6711** Terminal device, hook, mechanical, voluntary opening, any material, any size, lined or unlined, pediatric ⑧ Qp Qh A &   A

* **L6712** Terminal device, hook, mechanical, voluntary closing, any material, any size, lined or unlined, pediatric ⑧ Qp Qh A &   A

* **L6713** Terminal device, hand, mechanical, voluntary opening, any material, any size, pediatric ⑧ Qp Qh A &   A

* **L6714** Terminal device, hand, mechanical, voluntary closing, any material, any size, pediatric ⑧ Qp Qh A &   A

* **L6715** Terminal device, multiple articulating digit, includes motor(s), initial issue or replacement ⑧ Qp Qh &   A

* **L6721** Terminal device, hook or hand, heavy duty, mechanical, voluntary opening, any material, any size, lined or unlined ⑧ Qp Qh &   A

* **L6722** Terminal device, hook or hand, heavy duty, mechanical, voluntary closing, any material, any size, lined or unlined ⑧ Qp Qh &   A

○ **L6805** Addition to terminal device, modifier wrist unit ⑧ Qp Qh &   A

IOM: 100-02, 15, 120; 100-04, 3, 10.4

○ **L6810** Addition to terminal device, precision pinch device ⑧ Qp Qh &   A

IOM: 100-02, 15, 120; 100-04, 3, 10.4

* **L6880** Electric hand, switch or myoelectric controlled, independently articulating digits, any grasp pattern or combination of grasp patterns, includes motor(s) ⑧ Qp Qh &   A

* **L6881** Automatic grasp feature, addition to upper limb electric prosthetic terminal device ⑧ Qp Qh &   A

○ **L6882** Microprocessor control feature, addition to upper limb prosthetic terminal device ⑧ Qp Qh &   A

IOM: 100-02, 15, 120; 100-04, 3, 10.4

Replacement Sockets

* **L6883** Replacement socket, below elbow/wrist disarticulation, molded to patient model, for use with or without external power ⑧ Qp Qh &   A

* **L6884** Replacement socket, above elbow/elbow disarticulation, molded to patient model, for use with or without external power ⑧ Qp Qh &   A

* **L6885** Replacement socket, shoulder disarticulation/interscapular thoracic, molded to patient model, for use with or without external power ⑧ Qp Qh &   A

Hand Restoration

* **L6890** Addition to upper extremity prosthesis, glove for terminal device, any material, prefabricated, includes fitting and adjustment ⑧ Qp Qh &   A

* **L6895** Addition to upper extremity prosthesis, glove for terminal device, any material, custom fabricated ⑧ Qp Qh &   A

* **L6900** Hand restoration (casts, shading and measurements included), partial hand, with glove, thumb or one finger remaining ⑧ Qp Qh &   A

* **L6905** Hand restoration (casts, shading and measurements included), partial hand, with glove, multiple fingers remaining ⑧ Qp Qh &   A

* **L6910** Hand restoration (casts, shading and measurements included), partial hand, with glove, no fingers remaining ⑧ Qp Qh &   A

* **L6915** Hand restoration (shading, and measurements included), replacement glove for above ⑧ Qp Qh &   A

External Power

* **L6920** Wrist disarticulation, external power, self-suspended inner socket, removable forearm shell, Otto Bock or equal switch, cables, two batteries and one charger, switch control of terminal device ⑧ Qp Qh &   A

Figure 41 Terminal devices, hand and hook.

🐾 MIPS   Qp **Quantity Physician**   Qh **Quantity Hospital**   ♀ **Female only**   ♂ **Male only**   A **Age**   & **DMEPOS**   A2-Z3 **ASC Payment Indicator**   A-Y **ASC Status Indicator**   Coding Clinic

* **L6925** Wrist disarticulation, external power, self-suspended inner socket, removable forearm shell, Otto Bock or equal electrodes, cables, two batteries and one charger, myoelectronic control of terminal device Ⓑ Qp Qh ⛴   A

* **L6930** Below elbow, external power, self-suspended inner socket, removable forearm shell, Otto Bock or equal switch, cables, two batteries and one charger, switch control of terminal device Ⓑ Qp Qh ⛴   A

* **L6935** Below elbow, external power, self-suspended inner socket, removable forearm shell, Otto Bock or equal electrodes, cables, two batteries and one charger, myoelectronic control of terminal device Ⓑ Qp Qh ⛴   A

* **L6940** Elbow disarticulation, external power, molded inner socket, removable humeral shell, outside locking hinges, forearm, Otto Bock or equal switch, cables, two batteries and one charger, switch control of terminal device Ⓑ Qp Qh ⛴   A

* **L6945** Elbow disarticulation, external power, molded inner socket, removable humeral shell, outside locking hinges, forearm, Otto Bock or equal electrodes, cables, two batteries and one charger, myoelectronic control of terminal device Ⓑ Qp Qh ⛴   A

* **L6950** Above elbow, external power, molded inner socket, removable humeral shell, internal locking elbow, forearm, Otto Bock or equal switch, cables, two batteries and one charger, switch control of terminal device Ⓑ Qp Qh ⛴   A

* **L6955** Above elbow, external power, molded inner socket, removable humeral shell, internal locking elbow, forearm, Otto Bock or equal electrodes, cables, two batteries and one charger, myoelectronic control of terminal device Ⓑ Qp Qh ⛴   A

* **L6960** Shoulder disarticulation, external power, molded inner socket, removable shoulder shell, shoulder bulkhead, humeral section, mechanical elbow, forearm, Otto Bock or equal switch, cables, two batteries and one charger, switch control of terminal device Ⓑ Qp Qh ⛴   A

* **L6965** Shoulder disarticulation, external power, molded inner socket, removable shoulder shell, shoulder bulkhead, humeral section, mechanical elbow, forearm, Otto Bock or equal electrodes, cables, two batteries and one charger, myoelectronic control of terminal device Ⓑ Qp Qh ⛴   A

* **L6970** Interscapular-thoracic, external power, molded inner socket, removable shoulder shell, shoulder bulkhead, humeral section, mechanical elbow, forearm, Otto Bock or equal switch, cables, two batteries and one charger, switch control of terminal device Ⓑ Qp Qh ⛴   A

* **L6975** Interscapular-thoracic, external power, molded inner socket, removable shoulder shell, shoulder bulkhead, humeral section, mechanical elbow, forearm, Otto Bock or equal electrodes, cables, two batteries and one charger, myoelectronic control of terminal device Ⓑ Qp Qh ⛴   A

Additions to Electronic Hand or Hook

* **L7007** Electric hand, switch or myoelectric controlled, adult Ⓑ Qp Qh A ⛴   A

* **L7008** Electric hand, switch or myoelectric controlled, pediatric Ⓑ Qp Qh A ⛴   A

* **L7009** Electric hook, switch or myoelectric controlled, adult Ⓑ Qp Qh A ⛴   A

* **L7040** Prehensile actuator, switch controlled Ⓑ Qp Qh ⛴   A

* **L7045** Electric hook, switch or myoelectric controlled, pediatric Ⓑ Qp Qh A ⛴   A

Additions to Electronic Elbow

* **L7170** Electronic elbow, Hosmer or equal, switch controlled Ⓑ Qp Qh ⛴   A

* **L7180** Electronic elbow, microprocessor sequential control of elbow and terminal device Ⓑ Qp Qh ⛴   A

* **L7181** Electronic elbow, microprocessor simultaneous control of elbow and terminal device Ⓑ Qp Qh ⛴   A

* **L7185** Electronic elbow, adolescent, Variety Village or equal, switch controlled Ⓑ Qp Qh ⛴   A

* **L7186** Electronic elbow, child, Variety Village or equal, switch controlled Ⓑ Qp Qh A ⛴   A

* **L7190** Electronic elbow, adolescent, Variety Village or equal, myoelectronically controlled Ⓑ Qp Qh ⛴   A

* **L7191** Electronic elbow, child, Variety Village or equal, myoelectronically controlled Ⓑ Qp Qh A ⛴   A

Wrist

* **L7259** Electronic wrist rotator, any type Ⓑ Qp Qh ⛴   A

▶ **New**   ↻ **Revised**   ✓ **Reinstated**   ~~deleted~~ **Deleted**   ⊘ **Not covered or valid by Medicare**

✻ **Special coverage instructions**   * **Carrier discretion**   Ⓑ **Bill Part B MAC**   Ⓓ **Bill DME MAC**

Figure 42 Electronic elbow.

Battery Components

 ✳ **L7360** Six volt battery, each ⑧ Qp ♿ A

 ✳ **L7362** Battery charger, six volt, each ⑧ Qp Qh ♿ A

 ✳ **L7364** Twelve volt battery, each ⑧ Qp ♿ A

 ✳ **L7366** Battery charger, twelve volt, each ⑧ Qp Qh ♿ A

 ✳ **L7367** Lithium ion battery, rechargeable, replacement ⑧ Qp ♿ A

 ✳ **L7368** Lithium ion battery charger, replacement only ⑧ Qp Qh ♿ A

Additions

 ✳ **L7400** Addition to upper extremity prosthesis, below elbow/wrist disarticulation, ultralight material (titanium, carbon fiber or equal) ⑧ Qp Qh ♿ A

 ✳ **L7401** Addition to upper extremity prosthesis, above elbow disarticulation, ultralight material (titanium, carbon fiber or equal) ⑧ Qp Qh ♿ A

 ✳ **L7402** Addition to upper extremity prosthesis, shoulder disarticulation/interscapular thoracic, ultralight material (titanium, carbon fiber or equal) ⑧ Qp Qh ♿ A

 ✳ **L7403** Addition to upper extremity prosthesis, below elbow/wrist disarticulation, acrylic material ⑧ Qp Qh ♿ A

 ✳ **L7404** Addition to upper extremity prosthesis, above elbow disarticulation, acrylic material ⑧ Qp Qh ♿ A

 ✳ **L7405** Addition to upper extremity prosthesis, shoulder disarticulation/ interscapular thoracic, acrylic material ⑧ Qp Qh ♿ A

Other/Repair

 ✳ **L7499** Upper extremity prosthesis, not otherwise specified ⑧ A

 ⊘ **L7510** Repair of prosthetic device, repair or replace minor parts ⑨ ⑩ Qp Qh A

 IOM: 100-02, 15, 110.2; 100-02, 15, 120; 100-04, 32, 100

 ✳ **L7520** Repair prosthetic device, labor component, per 15 minutes ⑧ ⑧ A

 ⊘ **L7600** Prosthetic donning sleeve, any material, each ⑧ E1

 Medicare Statute 1862(1)(a)

General

Prosthetic Socket Insert

 ✳ **L7700** Gasket or seal, for use with prosthetic socket insert, any type, each ♿ A

Penile Prosthetics

 ⊘ **L7900** Male vacuum erection system ⑧ Qp Qh ♂ E1

 Medicare Statute 1834a

 ⊘ **L7902** Tension ring, for vacuum erection device, any type, replacement only, each ⑧ Qp Qh E1

 Medicare Statute 1834a

Breast Prosthetics

 ◎ **L8000** Breast prosthesis, mastectomy bra, without integrated breast prosthesis form, any size, any type ⑧ Qp ♀ ♿ A

 IOM: 100-02, 15, 120

 ◎ **L8001** Breast prosthesis, mastectomy bra, with integrated breast prosthesis form, unilateral, any size, any type ⑧ Qp ♀ ♿ A

 IOM: 100-02, 15, 120

 ◎ **L8002** Breast prosthesis, mastectomy bra, with integrated breast prosthesis form, bilateral, any size, any type ⑧ Qp ♀ ♿ A

 IOM: 100-02, 15, 120

 ◎ **L8010** Breast prosthesis, mastectomy sleeve ⑧ ♀ A

 IOM: 100-02, 15, 120

 ◎ **L8015** External breast prosthesis garment, with mastectomy form, post mastectomy ⑧ Qp ♀ ♿ A

 IOM: 100-02, 15, 120

 ◎ **L8020** Breast prosthesis, mastectomy form ⑧ Qp ♀ ♿ A

 IOM: 100-02, 15, 120

🅡 MIPS	Qp Quantity Physician	Qh Quantity Hospital	♀ Female only
♂ Male only	A Age	♿ DMEPOS	A2-Z3 ASC Payment Indicator A-Y ASC Status Indicator Coding Clinic

PROSTHETICS L7360 – L8020

385

⊛ **L8030** Breast prosthesis, silicone or equal, without integral adhesive Ⓑ Qp Qh ♀ &   A

IOM: 100-02, 15, 120

⊛ **L8031** Breast prosthesis, silicone or equal, with integral adhesive Ⓑ Qp Qh &   A

IOM: 100-02, 15, 120

✳ **L8032** Nipple prosthesis, prefabricated, reusable, any type, each Ⓑ Qp Qh &   A

✳ **L8033** Nipple prosthesis, custom fabricated, reusable, any material, any type, each   A

⊛ **L8035** Custom breast prosthesis, post mastectomy, molded to patient model Ⓑ Qp Qh ♀ &   A

IOM: 100-02, 15, 120

✳ **L8039** Breast prosthesis, not otherwise specified Ⓑ Qp Qh ♀   A

Nasal, Orbital, Auricular Prostherics

✳ **L8040** Nasal prosthesis, provided by a non-physician Ⓑ Qp Qh &   A

✳ **L8041** Midfacial prosthesis, provided by a non-physician Ⓑ Qp Qh &   A

✳ **L8042** Orbital prosthesis, provided by a non-physician Ⓑ Qp Qh &   A

✳ **L8043** Upper facial prosthesis, provided by a non-physician Ⓑ Qp Qh &   A

✳ **L8044** Hemi-facial prosthesis, provided by a non-physician Ⓑ Qp Qh &   A

✳ **L8045** Auricular prosthesis, provided by a non-physician Ⓑ Qp Qh &   A

✳ **L8046** Partial facial prosthesis, provided by a non-physician Ⓑ Qp Qh &   A

✳ **L8047** Nasal septal prosthesis, provided by a non-physician Ⓑ Qp Qh &   A

✳ **L8048** Unspecified maxillofacial prosthesis, by report, provided by a non-physician Ⓑ Qp Qh   A

✳ **L8049** Repair or modification of maxillofacial prosthesis, labor component, 15 minute increments, provided by a non-physician Ⓑ Qp   A

Trusses

⊛ **L8300** Truss, single with standard pad Ⓑ Qp Qh &   A

IOM: 100-02, 15, 120; 100-03, 4, 280.11; 100-03, 4, 280.12; 100-04, 4, 240

⊛ **L8310** Truss, double with standard pads Ⓑ Qp Qh &   A

IOM: 100-02, 15, 120; 100-03, 4, 280.11; 100-03, 4, 280.12; 100-04, 4, 240

⊛ **L8320** Truss, addition to standard pad, water pad Ⓑ Qp Qh &   A

IOM: 100-02, 15, 120; 100-03, 4, 280.11; 100-03, 4, 280.12; 100-04, 4, 240

⊛ **L8330** Truss, addition to standard pad, scrotal pad Ⓑ Qp Qh ♂ &   A

IOM: 100-02, 15, 120; 100-03, 4, 280.11; 100-03, 4, 280.12; 100-04, 4, 240

Prosthetic Socks

⊛ **L8400** Prosthetic sheath, below knee, each Ⓑ Qp &   A

IOM: 100-02, 15, 200

⊛ **L8410** Prosthetic sheath, above knee, each Ⓑ Qp &   A

IOM: 100-02, 15, 200

⊛ **L8415** Prosthetic sheath, upper limb, each Ⓑ Qp &   A

IOM: 100-02, 15, 200

✳ **L8417** Prosthetic sheath/sock, including a gel cushion layer, below knee or above knee, each Ⓑ Qp &   A

Figure 44 (A) Nasal prosthesis, (B) Auricular prosthesis.

Figure 43 Implant breast prosthesis.

▶ **New**   ↻ **Revised**   ✔ **Reinstated**   ~~deleted~~ **Deleted**   ⊘ **Not covered or valid by Medicare**

⊛ **Special coverage instructions**   ✳ **Carrier discretion**   Ⓑ **Bill Part B MAC**   Ⓑ **Bill DME MAC**

L8420 Prosthetic sock, multiple ply, below knee, each Ⓑ Qp A

IOM: 100-02, 15, 200

L8430 Prosthetic sock, multiple ply, above knee, each Ⓑ Qp A

IOM: 100-02, 15, 200

L8435 Prosthetic sock, multiple ply, upper limb, each Ⓑ Qp A

IOM: 100-02, 15, 200

L8440 Prosthetic shrinker, below knee, each Ⓑ Qp A

IOM: 100-02, 15, 200

L8460 Prosthetic shrinker, above knee, each Ⓑ Qp A

IOM: 100-02, 15, 200

L8465 Prosthetic shrinker, upper limb, each Ⓑ Qp A

IOM: 100-02, 15, 200

L8470 Prosthetic sock, single ply, fitting, below knee, each Ⓑ Qp A

IOM: 100-02, 15, 200

L8480 Prosthetic sock, single ply, fitting, above knee, each Ⓑ Qp A

IOM: 100-02, 15, 200

L8485 Prosthetic sock, single ply, fitting, upper limb, each Ⓑ Qp A

IOM: 100-02, 15, 200

Unlisted

L8499 Unlisted procedure for miscellaneous prosthetic services Ⓑ Ⓑ A

Prosthetic Implants (L8500-L9900)

Larynx, Tracheoesophageal

L8500 Artificial larynx, any type Ⓑ Qp Qh A

IOM: 100-02, 15, 120; 100-03, 1, 50.2; 100-04, 4, 240

L8501 Tracheostomy speaking valve Ⓑ Qp Qh A

IOM: 100-03, 1, 50.4

L8505 Artificial larynx replacement battery/accessory, any type Ⓑ A

L8507 Tracheo-esophageal voice prosthesis, patient inserted, any type, each Ⓑ Qp Qh A

L8509 Tracheo-esophageal voice prosthesis, inserted by a licensed health care provider, any type Ⓑ Ⓑ Qp Qh A

L8510 Voice amplifier Ⓑ Qp Qh A

IOM: 100-03, 1, 50.2

L8511 Insert for indwelling tracheoesophageal prosthesis, with or without valve, replacement only, each Ⓑ Ⓑ Qp Qh A

L8512 Gelatin capsules or equivalent, for use with tracheoesophageal voice prosthesis, replacement only, per 10 Ⓑ Ⓑ A

L8513 Cleaning device used with tracheoesophageal voice prosthesis, pipet, brush, or equal, replacement only, each Ⓑ Ⓑ A

L8514 Tracheoesophageal puncture dilator, replacement only, each Ⓑ Ⓑ Qp Qh A

L8515 Gelatin capsule, application device for use with tracheoesophageal voice prosthesis, each Ⓑ Ⓑ Qp Qh A

Breast

L8600 Implantable breast prosthesis, silicone or equal Ⓑ Qp Qh ♀ N1 N

IOM: 100-02, 15, 120; 100-3, 2, 140.2

Bulking Agents

L8603 Injectable bulking agent, collagen implant, urinary tract, 2.5 ml syringe, includes shipping and necessary supplies Ⓑ N1 N

Bill on paper, acquisition cost invoice required

IOM: 100-03, 4, 280.1

L8604 Injectable bulking agent, dextranomer/hyaluronic acid copolymer implant, urinary tract, 1 ml, includes shipping and necessary supplies Ⓑ Qp Qh N1 N

L8605 Injectable bulking agent, dextranomer/hyaluronic acid copolymer implant, anal canal, 1 ml, includes shipping and necessary supplies Ⓑ Qp Qh N1 N

L8606 Injectable bulking agent, synthetic implant, urinary tract, 1 ml syringe, includes shipping and necessary supplies Ⓑ Qp Qh N1 N

Bill on paper, acquisition cost invoice required

IOM: 100-03, 4, 280.1

L8607 Injectable bulking agent for vocal cord medialization, 0.1 ml, includes shipping and necessary supplies Ⓑ Qp Qh N1 N

IOM: 100-03, 4, 280.1

Eye and Ear

L8608 Miscellaneous external component, supply or accessory for use with the Argus II retinal prosthesis system N

L8609 Artificial cornea Ⓑ Qp Qh N1 N

⚙ **L8610** Ocular implant ⒷⓆⓅⓆⒽ ♿ N1 N
IOM: 100-02, 15, 120

⚙ **L8612** Aqueous shunt ⒷⓆⓅⓆⒽ ♿ N1 N
IOM: 100-02, 15, 120
Cross Reference Q0074

⚙ **L8613** Ossicula implant ⒷⓆⓅⓆⒽ ♿ N1 N
IOM: 100-02, 15, 120

⚙ **L8614** Cochlear device, includes all internal and external components ⚙ⓆⓅⓆⒽ ♿ N1 N
IOM: 100-02, 15, 120; 100-03, 1, 50.3

⚙ **L8615** Headset/headpiece for use with cochlear implant device, replacement ⚙ⓆⓅⓆⒽ ♿ A
IOM: 100-03, 1, 50.3

⚙ **L8616** Microphone for use with cochlear implant device, replacement ⚙ⓆⓅⓆⒽ ♿ A
IOM: 100-03, 1, 50.3

⚙ **L8617** Transmitting coil for use with cochlear implant device, replacement ⚙ⓆⓅⓆⒽ ♿ A
IOM: 100-03, 1, 50.3

⚙ **L8618** Transmitter cable for use with cochlear implant device or auditory osseointegrated device, replacement ⚙ⓆⓅⓆⒽ ♿ A
IOM: 100-03, 1, 50.3

⚙ **L8619** Cochlear implant, external speech processor and controller, integrated system, replacement ⚙ⓆⓅⓆⒽ ♿ A
IOM: 100-03, 1, 50.3

✱ **L8621** Zinc air battery for use with cochlear implant device and auditory osseointegrated sound processors, replacement, each ⚙ⓆⓅⓆⒽ ♿ A

✱ **L8622** Alkaline battery for use with cochlear implant device, any size, replacement, each ⚙ⓆⓅⓆⒽ ♿ A

✱ **L8623** Lithium ion battery for use with cochlear implant device speech processor, other than ear level, replacement, each Ⓑ ♿ A

✱ **L8624** Lithium ion battery for use with cochlear implant or auditory osseointegrated device speech processor, ear level, replacement, each Ⓑ ♿ A

⚙ **L8625** External recharging system for battery for use with cochlear implant or auditory osseointegrated device, replacement only, each ♿ A
IOM: 103-03, PART 1, 50.3

⚙ **L8627** Cochlear implant, external speech processor, component, replacement ⒷⓆⓅⓆⒽ ♿ A
IOM: 103-03, PART 1, 50.3

⚙ **L8628** Cochlear implant, external controller component, replacement ⒷⓆⓅⓆⒽ ♿ A
IOM: 103-03, PART 1, 50.3

⚙ **L8629** Transmitting coil and cable, integrated, for use with cochlear implant device, replacement ⒷⓆⓅⓆⒽ ♿ A
IOM: 103-03, PART 1, 50.3

Hand and Foot

⚙ **L8630** Metacarpophalangeal joint implant Ⓑ ♿ N1 N
IOM: 100-02, 15, 120

⚙ **L8631** Metacarpal phalangeal joint replacement, two or more pieces, metal (e.g., stainless steel or cobalt chrome), ceramic-like material (e.g., pyrocarbon), for surgical implantation (all sizes, includes entire system) ⒷⓆⓅⓆⒽ ♿ N1 N
IOM: 100-02, 15, 120

⚙ **L8641** Metatarsal joint implant ⒷⓆⓅⓆⒽ ♿ N1 N
IOM: 100-02, 15, 120

⚙ **L8642** Hallux implant ⚙ⓆⓅⓆⒽ ♿ N1 N
May be billed by ambulatory surgical center or surgeon
IOM: 100-02, 15, 120
Cross Reference Q0073

⚙ **L8658** Interphalangeal joint spacer, silicone or equal, each ⒷⓆⓅⓆⒽ ♿ N1 N
IOM: 100-02, 15, 120

⚙ **L8659** Interphalangeal finger joint replacement, 2 or more pieces, metal (e.g., stainless steel or cobalt chrome), ceramic-like material (e.g., pyrocarbon) for surgical implantation, any size Ⓑ ⓆⓅⓆⒽ ♿ N1 N
IOM: 100-02, 15, 120

Vascular

⚙ **L8670** Vascular graft material, synthetic, implant ⒷⓆⓅⓆⒽ ♿ N1 N
IOM: 100-02, 15, 120

Neurostimulator

▶ **L8678** Electrical stimulator supplies (external) for use with implantable neurostimulator, per month

⚙ **L8679** Implantable neurostimulator, pulse generator, any type ⒷⓆⓅⓆⒽ ♿ N1 N
IOM: 100-03, 4, 280.4

⊘ **L8680** Implantable neurostimulator electrode, each ⒷⓆⒽ E1
Related CPT codes: 43647, 63650, 63655, 64553, 64555, 64560, 64561, 64565, 64573, 64575, 64577, 64580, 64581.

▶ New ↻ Revised ✔ Reinstated deleted Deleted ⊘ Not covered or valid by Medicare
⚙ Special coverage instructions ✱ Carrier discretion Ⓑ Bill Part B MAC Ⓓ Bill DME MAC

⊚ **L8681** Patient programmer (external) for use with implantable programmable neurostimulator pulse generator, replacement only Ⓑ Qp Qh ♿ A

IOM: 100-03, 4, 280.4

⊚ **L8682** Implantable neurostimulator radiofrequency receiver Ⓑ Qp Qh ♿ N1 N

IOM: 100-03, 4, 280.4

⊚ **L8683** Radiofrequency transmitter (external) for use with implantable neurostimulator radiofrequency receiver Ⓑ Qp Qh ♿ A

IOM: 100-03, 4, 280.4

⊚ **L8684** Radiofrequency transmitter (external) for use with implantable sacral root neurostimulator receiver for bowel and bladder management, replacement Ⓑ Qp Qh ♿ A

IOM: 100-03, 4, 280.4

⊘ **L8685** Implantable neurostimulator pulse generator, single array, rechargeable, includes extension Ⓑ Qp Qh E1

Related CPT codes: 61885, 64590, 63685.

⊘ **L8686** Implantable neurostimulator pulse generator, single array, non-rechargeable, includes extension Ⓑ Qp Qh E1

Related CPT codes: 61885, 64590, 63685.

⊘ **L8687** Implantable neurostimulator pulse generator, dual array, rechargeable, includes extension Ⓑ Qp Qh E1

Related CPT codes: 64590, 63685, 61886.

⊘ **L8688** Implantable neurostimulator pulse generator, dual array, non-rechargeable, includes extension Ⓑ Qp Qh E1

Related CPT codes: 61885, 64590, 63685.

⊚ **L8689** External recharging system for battery (internal) for use with implantable neurostimulator, replacement only Ⓑ Qp Qh ♿ A

IOM: 100-03, 4, 280.4

Figure 45 Metacarpophalangeal implant.

Miscellaneous Orthotic and Prosthetic Components, Services, and Supplies

✳ **L8690** Auditory osseointegrated device, includes all internal and external components Ⓑ Qp Qh ♿ N1 N

Related CPT codes: 69714, 69715, 69717, 69718.

✳ **L8691** Auditory osseointegrated device, external sound processor, excludes transducer/actuator, replacement only, each Ⓑ Qp Qh ♿ A

⊘ **L8692** Auditory osseointegrated device, external sound processor, used without osseointegration, body worn, includes headband or other means of external attachment Ⓑ Qp Qh E1

Medicare Statute 1862(a)(7)

✳ **L8693** Auditory osseointegrated device abutment, any length, replacement only Ⓑ Qp Qh ♿ A

✳ **L8694** Auditory osseointegrated device, transducer/actuator, replacement only, each ♿ A

⊚ **L8695** External recharging system for battery (external) for use with implantable neurostimulator, replacement only Ⓑ Qp Qh ♿ A

IOM: 100-03, 4, 280.4

⊚ **L8696** Antenna (external) for use with implantable diaphragmatic/phrenic nerve stimulation device, replacement, each Ⓑ Qp Qh ♿ A

⊚ **L8698** Miscellaneous component, supply or accessory for use with total artificial heart system Ⓑ A

✳ **L8699** Prosthetic implant, not otherwise specified Ⓑ N1 N

✳ **L8701** Elbow, wrist, hand device, powered, with single or double upright(s), any type joint(s), includes microprocessor, sensors, all components and accessories Ⓖ A

✳ **L8702** Elbow, wrist, hand, finger device, powered, with single or double upright(s), any type joint(s), includes microprocessor, sensors, all components and accessories Ⓖ A

✳ **L9900** Orthotic and prosthetic supply, accessory, and/or service component of another HCPCS "L" code Ⓗ Ⓖ N1 N

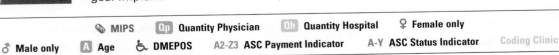

🐾 **MIPS**   Qp **Quantity Physician**   Qh **Quantity Hospital**   ♀ **Female only**

♂ **Male only**   A **Age**   ♿ **DMEPOS**   A2-Z3 **ASC Payment Indicator**   A-Y **ASC Status Indicator**   Coding Clinic

OTHER MEDICAL SERVICES (M0000-M0301)

⚙ **M0001** Advancing cancer care MIPS value pathways   **M**

⚙ **M0002** Optimal care for kidney health MIPS value pathways   **M**

⚙ **M0003** Optimal care for patients with episodic neurological conditions MIPS value pathways   **M**

⚙ **M0004** Supportive care for neurodegenerative conditions MIPS value pathways   **M**

⚙ **M0005** Promoting wellness MIPS value pathways   **M**

▶ **M0010** Enhancing oncology model (EOM) monthly enhanced oncology services (MEOS) payment for EOM enhanced services

⊘ **M0075** Cellular therapy Ⓑ   **E1**

⊘ **M0076** Prolotherapy Ⓑ   **E1**

Prolotherapy stimulates production of new ligament tissue. Not covered by Medicare.

⊘ **M0100** Intragastric hypothermia using gastric freezing Ⓑ   **E1**

⊘ **M0201** Covid-19 vaccine administration inside a patient's home; reported only once per individual home per date of service when only covid-19 vaccine administration is performed at the patient's home   **S**

M0222 Intravenous injection, bebtelovimab, includes injection and post administration monitoring   **S**

M0223 Intravenous injection, bebtelovimab, includes injection and post administration monitoring in the home or residence; this includes a beneficiary's home that has been made provider-based to the hospital during the covid-19 public health emergency   **S**

⊘ **M0240** Intravenous infusion or subcutaneous injection, casirivimab and imdevimab includes infusion or injection, and post administration monitoring, subsequent repeat doses   **S**

⊘ **M0241** Intravenous infusion or subcutaneous injection, casirivimab and imdevimab includes infusion or injection, and post administration monitoring in the home or residence; this includes a beneficiary's home that has been made provider-based to the hospital during the covid-19 public health emergency, subsequent repeat doses   **S**

⊘ **M0243** Intravenous infusion or subcutaneous injection, casirivimab and imdevimab includes infusion and post administration monitoring   **S**

Coding Clinic: 2022, Q2, P9

⊘ **M0244** Intravenous infusion or subcutaneous injection, casirivimab and imdevimab includes infusion or injection, and post administration monitoring in the home or residence; this includes a beneficiary's home that has been made provider-based to the hospital during the covid-19 public health emergency   **S**

⊘ **M0245** Intravenous infusion, bamlanivimab and etesevimab, includes infusion and post administration monitoring   **S**

⊘ **M0246** AIntravenous infusion, bamlanivimab and etesevimab, includes infusion and post administration monitoring in the home or residence; this includes a beneficiary's home that has been made provider based to the hospital during the covid 19 public health emergency   **S**

⊘ **M0247** Intravenous infusion, sotrovimab, includes infusion and post administration monitoring   **S**

⊘ **M0248** Intravenous infusion, sotrovimab, includes infusion and post administration monitoring in the home or residence; this includes a beneficiary's home that has been made provider-based to the hospital during the covid-19 public health emergency   **S**

⊘ **M0249** Intravenous infusion, tocilizumab, for hospitalized adults and pediatric patients (2 years of age and older) with covid-19 who are receiving systemic corticosteroids and require supplemental oxygen, non-invasive or invasive mechanical ventilation, or extracorporeal membrane oxygenation (ecmo) only, includes infusion and post administration monitoring, first dose   **S**

⊘ **M0250** Intravenous infusion, tocilizumab, for hospitalized adults and pediatric patients (2 years of age and older) with covid-19 who are receiving systemic corticosteroids and require supplemental oxygen, non-invasive or invasive mechanical ventilation, or extracorporeal membrane oxygenation (ecmo) only, includes infusion and post administration monitoring, second dose   **S**

⊘ **M0300** IV chelation therapy (chemical endarterectomy) Ⓑ   **E1**

⊘ **M0301** Fabric wrapping of abdominal aneurysm Ⓑ   **E1**

Treatment for abdominal aneurysms that involves wrapping aneurysms with cellophane or fascia lata. Fabric wrapping of abdominal aneurysms is not a covered Medicare procedure.

✳ **M1003** TB screening performed and results interpreted within twelve months prior to initiation of first-time biologic and/or immune response modifier therapy ⓟ **M**

▶ New   ↻ Revised   ✔ Reinstated   deleted Deleted   ⊘ Not covered or valid by Medicare

⚙ Special coverage instructions   ✳ Carrier discretion   ⓟ Bill Part B MAC   Ⓑ Bill DME MAC

* **M1004** Documentation of medical reason for not screening for TB or interpreting results (i.e., patient positive for TB and documentation of past treatment; patient who has recently completed a course of anti-TB therapy) Ⓑ   M

* **M1005** TB screening not performed or results not interpreted, reason not given Ⓑ   M

* **M1006** Disease activity not assessed, reason not given Ⓑ   M

* **M1007** >=50% of total number of a patient's outpatient RA encounters assessed Ⓑ   M

* **M1008** <50% of total number of a patient's outpatient RA encounters assessed Ⓑ   M

* **M1009** Discharge/discontinuation of the episode of care documented in the medical record Ⓑ   M

* **M1010** Discharge/discontinuation of the episode of care documented in the medical record Ⓑ   M

* **M1011** Discharge/discontinuation of the episode of care documented in the medical record Ⓑ   M

* **M1012** Discharge/discontinuation of the episode of care documented in the medical record Ⓑ   M

* **M1013** Discharge/discontinuation of the episode of care documented in the medical record Ⓑ   M

* **M1014** Discharge/discontinuation of the episode of care documented in the medical record Ⓑ   M

* **M1016** Female patients unable to bear children Ⓑ   M

* **M1018** Patients with an active diagnosis or history of cancer (except basal cell and squamous cell skin carcinoma), patients who are heavy tobacco smokers, lung cancer screening patients Ⓑ   M

* **M1019** Adolescent patients 12 to 17 years of age with major depression or dysthymia who reached remission at twelve months as demonstrated by a twelve month (+/-60 days) PHQ-9 or PHQ-9m score of less than five Ⓑ   M

* **M1020** Adolescent patients 12 to 17 years of age with major depression or dysthymia who did not reach remission at twelve months as demonstrated by a twelve month (+/-60 days) PHQ-9 or PHQ-9m score of less than 5. Either PHQ-9 or PHQ-9m score was not assessed or is greater than or equal to 5 Ⓑ   M

* **M1021** Patient had only urgent care visits during the performance period Ⓑ   M

* **M1027** Imaging of the head (CT or MRI) was obtained Ⓑ   M

* **M1028** Documentation of patients with primary headache diagnosis and imaging other than CT or MRI obtained Ⓑ   M

* **M1029** Imaging of the head (CT or MRI) was not obtained, reason not given Ⓑ   M

* **M1032** Adults currently taking pharmacotherapy for OUD Ⓑ   M

* **M1034** Adults who have at least 180 days of continuous pharmacotherapy with a medication prescribed for OUD without a gap of more than seven days Ⓑ   M

* **M1035** Adults who are deliberately phased out of medication assisted treatment (MAT) prior to 180 days of continuous treatment Ⓑ   M

* **M1036** Adults who have not had at least 180 days of continuous pharmacotherapy with a medication prescribed for oud without a gap of more than seven days Ⓑ   M

* **M1037** Patients with a diagnosis of lumbar spine region cancer at the time of the procedure Ⓑ   M

* **M1038** Patients with a diagnosis of lumbar spine region fracture at the time of the procedure Ⓑ   M

* **M1039** Patients with a diagnosis of lumbar spine region infection at the time of the procedure Ⓑ   M

* **M1040** Patients with a diagnosis of lumbar idiopathic or congenital scoliosis Ⓑ   M

* **M1041** Patient had cancer, acute fracture or infection related to the lumbar spine or patient had neuromuscular, idiopathic or congenital lumbar scoliosis Ⓑ   M

* **M1043** Functional status was not measured by the Oswestry Disability Index (ODI version 2.1a) at one year (9 to 15 months) postoperatively Ⓑ   M

* **M1045** Functional status measured by the Oxford Knee Score (OKS) at one year (9 to 15 months) postoperatively was greater than or equal to 37 or knee injury and osteoarthritis outcome score joint replacement (Koos, jr.) was greater than or equal to 71 Ⓑ   M

* **M1046** Functional status the Oxford Knee Score (OKS) at one year (9 to 15 months) postoperatively was less than 37 or the knee injury and osteoarthritis outcome score joint replacement (Koos, jr.) was less than 71 postoperatively Ⓑ   M

* **M1049** Functional status was not measured by the Oswestry Disability Index (ODI version 2.1a) at three months (6 to 20 weeks) postoperatively Ⓑ   M

* **M1051** Patient had cancer, acute fracture or infection related to the lumbar spine or patient had neuromuscular, idiopathic or congenital lumbar scoliosis Ⓑ   M

🦝 **MIPS**   🅾🅿 **Quantity Physician**   🅾🅷 **Quantity Hospital**   ♀ **Female only**

♂ **Male only**   🅰 **Age**   ♿ **DMEPOS**   A2-Z3 **ASC Payment Indicator**   A-Y **ASC Status Indicator**   Coding Clinic

✳ **M1052** Leg pain was not measured by the Visual Analog Scale (VAS) or numeric pain scale at one year (9 to 15 months) postoperatively ⑧   M

✳ **M1054** Patient had only urgent care visits during the performance period ⑧   M

✳ **M1055** Aspirin or another antiplatelet therapy used ⑧   M

✳ **M1056** Prescribed anticoagulant medication during the performance period, history of GI bleeding, history of intracranial bleeding, bleeding disorder and specific provider documented reasons: allergy to aspirin or anti-platelets, use of non-steroidal anti-inflammatory agents, drug-drug interaction, uncontrolled hypertension >180/110 mmhg or gastroesophageal reflux disease ⑧   M

✳ **M1057** Aspirin or another antiplatelet therapy not used, reason not given ⑧   M

✳ **M1058** Patient was a permanent nursing home resident at any time during the performance period ⑧   M

✳ **M1059** Patient was in hospice or receiving palliative care at any time during the performance period ⑧   M

✳ **M1060** Patient died prior to the end of the performance period ⑧   M

✳ **M1067** Hospice services for patient provided any time during the measurement period ⑧   M

✳ **M1068** Adults who are not ambulatory ⑧   M

✳ **M1069** Patient screened for future fall risk ⑧ M

✳ **M1070** Patient not screened for future fall risk, reason not given ⑧   M

✳ **M1072** Radiation therapy for anal cancer under the radiation oncology model, 90 day episode, professional component

✳ **M1073** Radiation therapy for anal cancer under the radiation oncology model, 90 day episode, technical component

✳ **M1074** Radiation therapy for bladder cancer under the radiation oncology model, 90 day episode, professional component

✳ **M1075** Radiation therapy for bladder cancer under the radiation oncology model, 90 day episode, technical component

✳ **M1076** Radiation therapy for bone metastases under the radiation oncology model, 90 day episode, professional component

✳ **M1077** Radiation therapy for bone metastases under the radiation oncology model, 90 day episode, technical component

✳ **M1078** Radiation therapy for brain metastases under the radiation oncology model, 90 day episode, professional component

✳ **M1079** Radiation therapy for brain metastases under the radiation oncology model, 90 day episode, technical component

✳ **M1080** Radiation therapy for breast cancer under the radiation oncology model, 90 day episode, professional component

✳ **M1081** Radiation therapy for breast cancer under the radiation oncology model, 90 day episode, technical component

✳ **M1082** Radiation therapy for cervical cancer under the radiation oncology model, 90 day episode, professional component

✳ **M1083** Radiation therapy for cervical cancer under the radiation oncology model, 90 day episode, technical component

✳ **M1084** Radiation therapy for cns tumors under the radiation oncology model, 90 day episode, professional component

✳ **M1085** Radiation therapy for cns tumors under the radiation oncology model, 90 day episode, technical component

✳ **M1086** Radiation therapy for colorectal cancer under the radiation oncology model, 90 day episode, professional component

✳ **M1087** Radiation therapy for colorectal cancer under the radiation oncology model, 90 day episode, technical component

✳ **M1088** Radiation therapy for head and neck cancer under the radiation oncology model, 90 day episode, professional component

✳ **M1089** Radiation therapy for head and neck cancer under the radiation oncology model, 90 day episode, technical component

✳ **M1094** Radiation therapy for lung cancer under the radiation oncology model, 90 day episode, professional component

✳ **M1095** Radiation therapy for lung cancer under the radiation oncology model, 90 day episode, technical component

✳ **M1096** Radiation therapy for lymphoma under the radiation oncology model, 90 day episode, professional component

✳ **M1097** Radiation therapy for lymphoma under the radiation oncology model, 90 day episode, technical component

✳ **M1098** Radiation therapy for pancreatic cancer under the radiation oncology model, 90 day episode, professional component

✳ **M1099** Radiation therapy for pancreatic cancer under the radiation oncology model, 90 day episode, technical component

▶ New   ↻ Revised   ✔ Reinstated   ~~deleted~~ Deleted   ⊘ Not covered or valid by Medicare
◉ Special coverage instructions   ✳ Carrier discretion   Ⓑ Bill Part B MAC   ⑧ Bill DME MAC

* **M1100** Radiation therapy for prostate cancer under the radiation oncology model, 90 day episode, professional component

* **M1101** Radiation therapy for prostate cancer under the radiation oncology model, 90 day episode, technical component

* **M1102** Radiation therapy for upper GI cancer under the radiation oncology model, 90 day episode, professional componentt

* **M1103** Radiation therapy for upper GI cancer under the radiation oncology model, 90 day episode, technical component

* **M1104** Radiation therapy for uterine cancer under the radiation oncology model, 90 day episode, professional component

* **M1105** Radiation therapy for uterine cancer under the radiation oncology model, 90 day episode, technical component

* **M1106** The start of an episode of care documented in the medical record ⑧ M

* **M1107** Documentation stating patient has a diagnosis of a degenerative neurological condition such as ALS, MS, or Parkinson's diagnosed at any time before or during the episode of care ⑧ M

* **M1108** Ongoing care not clinically indicated because the patient needed a home program only, referred to another provider or facility, consultation only, as documented in the medical record ⑧ M

* **M1109** Ongoing care not medically possible because the patient was discharged early due to specific medical events, documented in the medical record, such as the patient became hospitalized or scheduled for surgery ⑧ M

* **M1110** Ongoing care not possible because the patient self-discharged early (e.g., financial or insurance reasons, transportation problems, or reason unknown) ⑧ M

* **M1111** The start of an episode of care documented in the medical record ⑧ M

* **M1112** Documentation stating patient has a diagnosis of a degenerative neurological condition such as ALS, MS, or Parkinson's diagnosed at any time before or during the episode of care ⑧ M

* **M1113** Ongoing care not clinically indicated because the patient needed a home program only, referred to another provider or facility, consultation only, as documented in the medical record ⑧ M

* **M1114** Ongoing care not medically possible because the patient was discharged early due to specific medical events, documented in the medical record such as the patient becomes hospitalized or scheduled for surgery ⑧ M

* **M1115** Ongoing care not possible because the patient self-discharged early (e.g., financial or insurance reasons, transportation problems, or reason unknown) ⑧ M

* **M1116** The start of an episode of care documented in the medical record ⑧ M

* **M1117** Documentation stating patient has a diagnosis of a degenerative neurological condition such as ALS, MS, or Parkinson's diagnosed at any time before or during the episode of care ⑧ M

* **M1118** Ongoing care not clinically indicated because the patient needed a home program only, referred to another provider or facility, consultation only, as documented in the medical record ⑧ M

* **M1119** Ongoing care not medically possible because the patient was discharged early due to specific medical events, documented in the medical record such as the patient becomes hospitalized or scheduled for surgery ⑧ M

* **M1120** Ongoing care not possible because the patient self-discharged early (e.g., financial or insurance reasons, transportation problems, or reason unknown) ⑧ M

* **M1121** The start of an episode of care documented in the medical record ⑧ M

* **M1122** Documentation stating patient has a diagnosis of a degenerative neurological condition such as ALS, MS, or Parkinson's diagnosed at any time before or during the episode of care ⑧ M

* **M1123** Ongoing care not clinically indicated because the patient needed a home program only, referred to another provider or facility, consultation only, as documented in the medical record ⑧ M

* **M1124** Ongoing care not medically possible because the patient was discharged early due to specific medical events, documented in the medical record such as the patient becomes hospitalized or scheduled for surgery ⑧ M

🐾 MIPS **Qp** Quantity Physician **Qh** Quantity Hospital ♀ Female only

♂ **Male only**   Age   DMEPOS A2-Z3 ASC Payment Indicator A-Y ASC Status Indicator Coding Clinic

393

* **M1125** Ongoing care not possible because the patient self-discharged early (e.g., financial or insurance reasons, transportation problems, or reason unknown) ⑧   M

* **M1126** The start of an episode of care documented in the medical record ⑧ M

* **M1127** Documentation stating patient has a diagnosis of a degenerative neurological condition such as ALS, MS, or Parkinson's diagnosed at any time before or during the episode of care ⑧   M

* **M1128** Ongoing care not clinically indicated because the patient needed a home program only, referred to another provider or facility, consultation only, as documented in the medical record ⑧   M

* **M1129** Ongoing care not medically possible because the patient was discharged early due to specific medical events, documented in the medical record such as the patient becomes hospitalized or scheduled for surgery ⑧   M

* **M1130** Ongoing care not possible because the patient self-discharged early (e.g., financial or insurance reasons, transportation problems, or reason unknown) ⑧   M

* **M1131** Documentation stating patient has a diagnosis of a degenerative neurological condition such as ALS, MS, or Parkinson's diagnosed at any time before or during the episode of care ⑧   M

* **M1132** Ongoing care not clinically indicated because the patient needed a home program only, referred to another provider or facility, consultation only, as documented in the medical record ⑧   M

* **M1133** Ongoing care not due to specific medical events, documented in the medical record such as the patient becomes hospitalized or scheduled for surgery ⑧   M

* **M1134** Ongoing care not possible because the patient self-discharged early (e.g., financial or insurance reasons, transportation problems, or reason unknown) ⑧   M

* **M1135** The start of an episode of care documented in the medical record ⑧   M

* **M1141** Functional status was not measured by the Oxford Knee Score (OKS) or the knee injury and osteoarthritis outcome score joint replacement (Koos, jr.) at one year (9 to 15 months) postoperatively ⑧   M

* **M1142** Emergent cases ⑧   M

* **M1143** Initiated episode of rehabilitation therapy, medical, or chiropractic care for neck impairment ⑧   M

* **M1145** Most favored nation (MFN) model drug add-on amount, per dose, (do not bill with line items that have the JW modifier)   K

* **M1146** Ongoing care not clinically indicated because the patient needed a home program only, referral to another provider or facility, or consultation only, as documented in the medical record   M

* **M1147** Ongoing care not medically possible because the patient was discharged early due to specific medical events, documented in the medical record, such as the patient became hospitalized or scheduled for surgery   M

* **M1148** Ongoing care not possible because the patient self-discharged early (e.g., financial or insurance reasons, transportation problems, or reason unknown)   M

* **M1149** Patient unable to complete the neck fs prom at initial evaluation and/or discharge due to blindness, illiteracy, severe mental incapacity or language incompatibility, and an adequate proxy is not available   M

⊛ **M1150** Left ventricular ejection fraction (LVEF) less than or equal to 40% or documentation of moderately or severely depressed left ventricular systolic function   M

⊛ **M1151** Patients with a history of heart transplant or with a left ventricular assist device (LVAD)   M

⊛ **M1152** Patients with a history of heart transplant or with a left ventricular assist device (LVAD)   M

⊛ **M1153** Patient with diagnosis of osteoporosis on date of encounter   M

⊛ **M1154** Hospice services provided to patient any time during the measurement period   M

⊛ **M1155** Patient had anaphylaxis due to the pneumococcal vaccine any time during or before the measurement period   M

⊛ **M1156** Patient received active chemotherapy any time during the measurement period   M

▶ New   ↻ Revised   ✔ Reinstated   ~~deleted~~ Deleted   ⊘ Not covered or valid by Medicare
⊛ Special coverage instructions   * Carrier discretion   ⑧ Bill Part B MAC   ⑧ Bill DME MAC

⚙ **M1157** Patient received bone marrow transplant any time during the measurement period M

⚙ **M1158** Patient had history of immunocompromising conditions prior to or during the measurement period M

⚙ **M1159** Hospice services provided to patient any time during the measurement period M

⚙ **M1160** Patient had anaphylaxis due to the meningococcal vaccine any time on or before the patient's 13th birthday M

⚙ **M1161** Patient had anaphylaxis due to the tetanus, diphtheria, or pertussis vaccine any time on or before the patient's 13th birthday M

⚙ **M1162** Patient had encephalitis due to the tetanus, diphtheria, or pertussis vaccine any time on or before the patient's 13th birthday M

⚙ **M1163** Patient had anaphylaxis due to the HPV vaccine any time on or before the patient's 13th birthday M

⚙ **M1164** Patients with dementia any time during the patient's history through the end of the measurement period M

⚙ **M1165** Patients who use hospice services any time during the measurement period M

⚙ **M1166** Pathology report for tissue specimens produced from wide local excisions or re-excisions M

⚙ **M1167** In hospice or using hospice services during the measurement period M

⚙ **M1168** Patient received an influenza vaccine on or between July 1 of the year prior to the measurement period and June 30 of the measurement period M

⚙ **M1169** Documentation of medical reason(s) for not administering influenza vaccine (e.g., prior anaphylaxis due to the influenza vaccine) M

⚙ **M1170** Patient did not receive an influenza vaccine on or between July 1 of the year prior to the measurement period and June 30 of the measurement period M

⚙ **M1171** Patient received at least one TD vaccine or one Tdap vaccine between nine years prior to the encounter and the end of the measurement period M

⚙ **M1172** Documentation of medical reason(s) for not administering TD or Tdap vaccine (e.g., prior anaphylaxis due to the TD or Tdap vaccine or history of encephalopathy within seven days after a previous dose of a TD-containing vaccine) M

⚙ **M1173** Patient did not receive at least one TD vaccine or one Tdap vaccine between nine years prior to the encounter and the end of the measurement period M

⚙ **M1174** Patient received at least one dose of the herpes zoster live vaccine or two doses of the herpes zoster recombinant vaccine (at least 28 days apart) anytime on or after the patient's 50th birthday before or during the measurement period M

⚙ **M1175** Documentation of medical reason(s) for not administering zoster vaccine (e.g., prior anaphylaxis due to the zoster vaccine) M

⚙ **M1176** Patient did not receive at least one dose of the herpes zoster live vaccine or two doses of the herpes zoster recombinant vaccine (at least 28 days apart) anytime on or after the patient's 50th birthday before or during the measurement period M

⚙ **M1177** Patient received any pneumococcal conjugate or polysaccharide vaccine on or after their 60th birthday and before the end of the measurement period M

⚙ **M1178** Documentation of medical reason(s) for not administering pneumococcal vaccine (e.g., prior anaphylaxis due to the pneumococcal vaccine) M

⚙ **M1179** Patient did not receive any pneumococcal conjugate or polysaccharide vaccine, on or after their 60th birthday and before or during measurement period M

⚙ **M1180** Patients on immune checkpoint inhibitor therapy M

⚙ **M1181** Grade 2 or above diarrhea and/or grade 2 or above colitis M

⚙ **M1182** Patients not eligible due to pre-existing inflammatory bowel disease (IBD) (e.g., ulcerative colitis, Crohn's disease) M

⚙ **M1183** Documentation of immune checkpoint inhibitor therapy held and corticosteroids or immunosuppressants prescribed or administered M

⚙ **M1184** Documentation of medical reason(s) for not prescribing or administering corticosteroid or immunosuppressant treatment (e.g., allergy, intolerance, infectious etiology, pancreatic insufficiency, hyperthyroidism, prior bowel surgical interventions, Celiac disease, receiving other medication, awaiting diagnostic workup results for alternative etiologies, other medical reasons/contraindication) M

⊗ **M1185** Documentation of immune checkpoint inhibitor therapy not held and/or corticosteroids or immunosuppressants prescribed or administered was not performed, reason not given   **M**

⊗ **M1186** Patients who have an order for or are receiving hospice or palliative care   **M**

⊗ **M1187** Patients with a diagnosis of end stage renal disease (ESRD)   **M**

⊗ **M1188** Patients with a diagnosis of chronic kidney disease (CKD) stage 5   **M**

⊗ **M1189** Documentation of a kidney health evaluation defined by an estimated glomerular filtration rate (EGFR) and urine albumin-creatinine ratio (UACR) performed   **M**

⊗ **M1190** Documentation of a kidney health evaluation was not performed or defined by an estimated glomerular filtration rate (EGFR) and urine albumin-creatinine ratio (UACR)   **M**

⊗ **M1191** Hospice services provided to patient any time during the measurement period   **M**

⊗ **M1192** Patients with an existing diagnosis of squamous cell carcinoma of the esophagus   **M**

⊗ **M1193** Surgical pathology reports that contain impression or conclusion of or recommendation for testing of MMR by immunohistochemistry, MSI by DNA-based testing status, or both   **M**

⊗ **M1194** Documentation of medical reason(s) surgical pathology reports did not contain impression or conclusion of or recommendation for testing of MMR by immunohistochemistry, MSI by DNA-based testing status, or both tests were not included (e.g., patient will not be treated with checkpoint inhibitor therapy, no residual carcinoma is present in the sample [tissue exhausted or status post neoadjuvant treatment], insufficient tumor for testing)   **M**

⊗ **M1195** Surgical pathology reports that do not contain impression or conclusion of or recommendation for testing of MMR by immunohistochemistry, MSI by DNA-based testing status, or both, reason not given   **M**

⊗ **M1196** Initial (index visit) numeric rating scale (NRS), visual rating scale (VRS), or itchyquant assessment score of greater than or equal to 4   **M**

⊗ **M1197** Itch severity assessment score is reduced by 2 or more points from the initial (index) assessment score to the follow-up visit score   **M**

⊗ **M1198** Itch severity assessment score was not reduced by at least 2 points from initial (index) score to the follow-up visit score or assessment was not completed during the follow-up encounter   **M**

⊗ **M1199** Patients receiving RRT   **M**

⊗ **M1200** Ace inhibitor (ace-i) or ARB therapy prescribed during the measurement period   **M**

⊗ **M1201** Documentation of medical reason(s) for not prescribing ace inhibitor (ace-i) or ARB therapy during the measurement period (e.g., pregnancy, history of angioedema to ace-i, other allergy to ace-i and ARB, hyperkalemia, or history of hyperkalemia while on ace-i or ARB therapy, acute kidney injury due to ace-i or ARB therapy), other medical reasons)   **M**

⊗ **M1202** Documentation of patient reason(s) for not prescribing ace inhibitor or ARB therapy during the measurement period, (e.g., patient declined, other patient reasons)   **M**

⊗ **M1203** Ace inhibitor or ARB therapy not prescribed during the measurement period, reason not given   **M**

⊗ **M1204** Initial (index visit) numeric rating scale (NRS), visual rating scale (VRS), or itchyquant assessment score of greater than or equal to 4   **M**

⊗ **M1205** Itch severity assessment score is reduced by 2 or more points from the initial (index) assessment score to the follow-up visit score   **M**

⊗ **M1206** Itch severity assessment score was not reduced by at least 2 points from initial (index) score to the follow-up visit score or assessment was not completed during the follow-up encounter   **M**

⊗ **M1207** Number of patients screened for food insecurity, housing instability, transportation needs, utility difficulties, and interpersonal safety   **M**

⊗ **M1208** Number of patients not screened for food insecurity, housing instability, transportation needs, utility difficulties, and interpersonal safety   **M**

⊗ **M1209** At least two orders for high-risk medications from the same drug class, (table 4), not ordered   **M**

⊗ **M1210** At least two orders for high-risk medications from the same drug class, (table 4), not ordered   **M**

▶ **New**   ↻ **Revised**   ✓ **Reinstated**   ~~deleted~~ **Deleted**   ⊘ **Not covered or valid by Medicare**
⊗ **Special coverage instructions**   ✳ **Carrier discretion**   Ⓑ **Bill Part B MAC**   Ⓓ **Bill DME MAC**

LABORATORY SERVICES (P0000-P9999)

Chemistry and Toxicology Tests

⚙ **P2028** Cephalin floculation, blood Ⓑ Qp Qh   A

This code appears on a CMS list of codes that represent obsolete and unreliable tests and procedures. Verify before reporting.

IOM: 100-03, 4, 300.1

⚙ **P2029** Congo red, blood Ⓑ Qp Qh   A

This code appears on a CMS list of codes that represent obsolete and unreliable tests and procedures. Verify before reporting.

IOM: 100-03, 4, 300.1

⊘ **P2031** Hair analysis (excluding arsenic) Ⓑ   E1

IOM: 100-03, 4, 300.1

⚙ **P2033** Thymol turbidity, blood Ⓑ Qp Qh   A

This code appears on a CMS list of codes that represent obsolete and unreliable tests and procedures. Verify before reporting.

IOM: 100-03, 4, 300.1

⚙ **P2038** Mucoprotein, blood (seromucoid) (medical necessity procedure) Ⓑ Qp Qh   A

This code appears on a CMS list of codes that represent obsolete and unreliable tests and procedures. Verify before reporting.

IOM: 100-03, 4, 300.1

Pathology Screening Tests

⚙ **P3000** Screening Papanicolaou smear, cervical or vaginal, up to three smears, by technician under physician supervision Ⓑ Qp Qh ♀   A

Co-insurance and deductible waived

Assign for Pap smear ordered for screening purposes only, conventional method, performed by technician

IOM: 100-03, 3, 190.2,

Laboratory Certification: Cytology

⚙ **P3001** Screening Papanicolaou smear, cervical or vaginal, up to three smears, requiring interpretation by physician Ⓑ Qp Qh ♀   B

Co-insurance and deductible waived

Report professional component for Pap smears requiring physician interpretation. There are CPT codes assigned for diagnostic Paps, such as, 88141; HCPCS are for screening Paps.

IOM: 100-03, 3, 190.2

Laboratory Certification: Cytology

Microbiology Tests

⊘ **P7001** Culture, bacterial, urine; quantitative, sensitivity study Ⓑ   E1

Cross Reference CPT

Laboratory Certification: Bacteriology

Miscellaneous Pathology

⚙ **P9010** Blood (whole), for transfusion, per unit Ⓑ Qp Qh   R

Blood furnished on an outpatient basis, subject to Medicare Part B blood deductible; applicable to first 3 pints of whole blood or equivalent units of packed red cells in calendar year

IOM: 100-01, 3, 20.5; 100-02, 1, 10

⚙ **P9011** Blood, split unit Ⓑ Qp Qh   R

Reports all splitting activities of any blood component

IOM: 100-01, 3, 20.5; 100-02, 1, 10

⚙ **P9012** Cryoprecipitate, each unit Ⓑ Qp Qh   R

IOM: 100-01, 3, 20.5; 100-02, 1, 10

⚙ **P9016** Red blood cells, leukocytes reduced, each unit Ⓑ Qp Qh   R

IOM: 100-01, 3, 20.5; 100-02, 1, 10

⚙ **P9017** Fresh frozen plasma (single donor), frozen within 8 hours of collection, each unit Ⓑ Qp Qh   R

IOM: 100-01, 3, 20.5; 100-02, 1, 10

⚙ **P9019** Platelets, each unit Ⓑ Qp Qh   R

IOM: 100-01, 3, 20.5; 100-02, 1, 10

⚙ **P9020** Platelet rich plasma, each unit Ⓑ Qp Qh   R

IOM: 100-01, 3, 20.5; 100-02, 1, 10

⚙ **P9021** Red blood cells, each unit Ⓑ Qp Qh   R

IOM: 100-01, 3, 20.5; 100-02, 1, 10

🏵 MIPS	Qp Quantity Physician	Qh Quantity Hospital	♀ Female only
♂ Male only	A Age	♿ DMEPOS A2-Z3 ASC Payment Indicator	A-Y ASC Status Indicator Coding Clinic

⊚ **P9022** Red blood cells, washed, each
unit Ⓑ Qp Qh
R
IOM: 100-01, 3, 20.5; 100-02, 1, 10

⊚ **P9023** Plasma, pooled multiple donor, solvent/
detergent treated, frozen, each
unit Ⓑ Qp Qh
R
IOM: 100-01, 3, 20.5; 100-02, 1, 10

⊚ **P9025** Plasma, cryoprecipitate reduced,
pathogen reduced, each unit
R

⊚ **P9026** Cryoprecipitated fibrinogen complex,
pathogen reduced, each unit
R

⊚ **P9031** Platelets, leukocytes reduced, each
unit Ⓑ Qp Qh
R
IOM: 100-01, 3, 20.5; 100-02, 1, 10

⊚ **P9032** Platelets, irradiated, each
unit Ⓑ Qp Qh
R
IOM: 100-01, 3, 20.5; 100-02, 1, 10

⊚ **P9033** Platelets, leukocytes reduced,
irradiated, each unit Ⓑ Qp Qh
R
IOM: 100-01, 3, 20.5; 100-02, 1, 10

⊚ **P9034** Platelets, pheresis,
each unit Ⓑ Qp Qh
R
IOM: 100-01, 3, 20.5; 100-02, 1, 10

⊚ **P9035** Platelets, pheresis, leukocytes reduced,
each unit Ⓑ Qp Qh
R
IOM: 100-01, 3, 20.5; 100-02, 1, 10

⊚ **P9036** Platelets, pheresis, irradiated, each
unit Ⓑ Qp Qh
R
IOM: 100-01, 3, 20.5; 100-02, 1, 10

⊚ **P9037** Platelets, pheresis, leukocytes reduced,
irradiated, each unit Ⓑ Qp Qh
R
IOM: 100-01, 3, 20.5; 100-02, 1, 10

⊚ **P9038** Red blood cells, irradiated, each
unit Ⓑ Qp Qh
R
IOM: 100-01, 3, 20.5; 100-02, 1, 10

⊚ **P9039** Red blood cells, deglycerolized, each
unit Ⓑ Qp Qh
R
IOM: 100-01, 3, 20.5; 100-02, 1, 10

⊚ **P9040** Red blood cells, leukocytes reduced,
irradiated, each unit Ⓑ Qp Qh
R
IOM: 100-01, 3, 20.5; 100-02, 1, 10

✳ **P9041** Infusion, albumin (human), 5%,
50 ml Ⓑ Qp Qh
K2 K

⊚ **P9043** Infusion, plasma protein fraction
(human), 5%, 50 ml Ⓑ Qp Qh
R
IOM: 100-01, 3, 20.5; 100-02, 1, 10

⊚ **P9044** Plasma, cryoprecipitate reduced,
each unit Ⓑ Qp Qh
R
IOM: 100-01, 3, 20.5; 100-02, 1, 10

✳ **P9045** Infusion, albumin (human), 5%,
250 ml Ⓑ Qp Qh
K2 K

✳ **P9046** Infusion, albumin (human), 25%,
20 ml Ⓑ Qp Qh
K2 K

✳ **P9047** Infusion, albumin (human), 25%,
50 ml Ⓑ Qp Qh
K2 K

✳ **P9048** Infusion, plasma protein fraction
(human), 5%, 250 ml Ⓑ Qp Qh
R

✳ **P9050** Granulocytes, pheresis, each
unit Ⓑ Qp Qh
E2

⊚ **P9051** Whole blood or red blood cells,
leukocytes reduced, CMV-negative,
each unit Ⓑ Qp Qh
R
Medicare Statute 1833(t)

⊚ **P9052** Platelets, HLA-matched leukocytes
reduced, apheresis/pheresis, each
unit Ⓑ Qp Qh
R
Medicare Statute 1833(t)

⊚ **P9053** Platelets, pheresis, leukocytes reduced,
CMV-negative, irradiated, each
unit Ⓑ Qp Qh
R

Freezing and thawing are reported
separately, see Transmittal 1487
(Hospital outpatient)

Medicare Statute 1833(t)

⊚ **P9054** Whole blood or red blood cells,
leukocytes reduced, frozen, deglycerol,
washed, each unit Ⓑ Qp Qh
R
Medicare Statute 1833(t)

⊚ **P9055** Platelets, leukocytes reduced, CMV-
negative, apheresis/pheresis, each
unit Ⓑ Qp Qh
R
Medicare Statute 1833(t)

⊚ **P9056** Whole blood, leukocytes reduced,
irradiated, each unit Ⓑ Qp Qh
R
Medicare Statute 1833(t)

⊚ **P9057** Red blood cells, frozen/deglycerolized/
washed, leukocytes reduced, irradiated,
each unit Ⓑ Qp Qh
R
Medicare Statute 1833(t)

⊚ **P9058** Red blood cells, leukocytes reduced,
CMV-negative, irradiated, each
unit Ⓑ Qp Qh
R
Medicare Statute 1833(t)

⊚ **P9059** Fresh frozen plasma between
8-24 hours of collection, each
unit Ⓑ Qp Qh
R
Medicare Statute 1833(t)

⊚ **P9060** Fresh frozen plasma, donor retested,
each unit Ⓑ Qp Qh
R
Medicare Statute 1833(t)

▶ New ↻ Revised ✔ Reinstated ~~deleted~~ Deleted ⊘ Not covered or valid by Medicare
⊚ Special coverage instructions ✳ Carrier discretion Ⓑ Bill Part B MAC Ⓑ Bill DME MAC

P9070 Plasma, pooled multiple donor, pathogen reduced, frozen, each unit Ⓑ Qp Qh   R

Medicare Statute 1833(T)

P9071 Plasma (single donor), pathogen reduced, frozen, each unit Ⓑ Qp Qh   R

IOM: 100-01, 3, 20.5; 100-02, 1, 10

Medicare Statute 1833T

P9073 Platelets, pheresis, pathogen-reduced, each unit   R

IOM: 100-01, 3, 20.5; 100-02, 1, 10

Medicare Statute 1833T

✱ **P9099** Blood component or product not otherwise classified   E2

P9100 Pathogen(s) test for platelets   S

IOM: 100-03, 4, 300.1

Travel Allowance for Specimen Collection

P9603 Travel allowance one way in connection with medically necessary laboratory specimen collection drawn from home bound or nursing home bound patient; prorated miles actually traveled Ⓑ Qp Qh   A

Fee for clinical laboratory travel (P9603) is $1.025 per mile for CY2015.

IOM: 100-04, 16, 60

P9604 Travel allowance one way in connection with medically necessary laboratory specimen collection drawn from home bound or nursing home bound patient; prorated trip charge Ⓑ Qp Qh   A

For CY2010, the fee for clinical laboratory travel is $10.30 per flat rate trip for CY2015.

IOM: 100-04, 16, 60

Catheterization for Specimen Collection

P9612 Catheterization for collection of specimen, single patient, all places of service Ⓑ Qp Qh   A

NCCI edits indicate that when 51701 is comprehensive or is a Column 1 code, P9612 cannot be reported. When the catheter insertion is a component of another procedure, do not report straight catheterization separately.

IOM: 100-04, 16, 60

Coding Clinic: 2007, Q3, P7

P9615 Catheterization for collection of specimen(s) (multiple patients) Ⓑ Qp Qh   N

IOM: 100-04, 16, 60

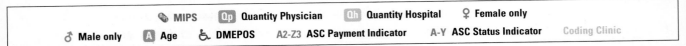

TEMPORARY CODES ASSIGNED BY CMS (Q0000-Q9999)

Cardiokymography

⊘ **Q0035** Cardiokymography ⑧ **Qp** **Qh** Q1

Report modifier 26 if professional component only

IOM: 100-03, 1, 20.24

Infusion Therapy

⊘ **Q0081** Infusion therapy, using other than chemotherapeutic drugs, per visit ⑧ **Qh** B

IV piggyback only assigned one time per patient encounter per day. Report for hydration or the intravenous administration of antibiotics, anti-emetics, or analgesics. Bill on paper. Requires a report.

IOM: 100-03, 4, 280.14

Coding Clinic: 2004, Q2, P11; Q1, P5, 8; 2002, Q2, P10; Q1, P7

Chemotherapy Administration

✳ **Q0083** Chemotherapy administration by other than infusion technique only (e.g., subcutaneous, intramuscular, push), per visit ⑧ **Qh** B

Coding Clinic: 2002, Q1, P7

⊘ **Q0084** Chemotherapy administration by infusion technique only, per visit ⑧ **Qh** B

IOM: 100-03, 4, 280.14

Coding Clinic: 2004, Q2, P11; 2002, Q1, P7

✳ **Q0085** Chemotherapy administration by both infusion technique and other technique(s) (e.g., subcutaneous, intramuscular, push), per visit ⑧ **Qh** B

Coding Clinic: 2002, Q1, P7

Smear Preparation

⊘ **Q0091** Screening Papanicolaou smear; obtaining, preparing and conveyance of cervical or vaginal smear to laboratory ⑧ **Qp** **Qh** ♀ S

Medicare does not cover comprehensive preventive medicine services; however, services described by G0101 and Q0091 (only for Medicare patients) are covered. Includes the services necessary to procure and transport the specimen to the laboratory.

IOM: 100-03, 3, 190.2

Coding Clinic: 2002, Q4, P8

Portable X-ray Setup

⊘ **Q0092** Set-up portable x-ray equipment ⑧ N

IOM: 100-04, 13, 90

Miscellaneous Lab Services

✳ **Q0111** Wet mounts, including preparations of vaginal, cervical or skin specimens ⑧ **Qp** **Qh** A

Laboratory Certification: Bacteriology, Mycology, Parasitology

✳ **Q0112** All potassium hydroxide (KOH) preparations ⑧ **Qp** **Qh** A

Laboratory Certification: Mycology

✳ **Q0113** Pinworm examinations ⑧ **Qp** **Qh** A

Laboratory Certification: Parasitology

✳ **Q0114** Fern test ⑧ **Qp** **Qh** ♀ A

Laboratory Certification: Routine chemistry

✳ **Q0115** Post-coital direct, qualitative examinations of vaginal or cervical mucous ⑧ **Qp** **Qh** ♀ A

Laboratory Certification: Hematology

Drugs

✳ **Q0138** Injection, ferumoxytol, for treatment of iron deficiency anemia, 1 mg (non-ESRD use) ⑧ **Qp** **Qh** K2 K

Feraheme is FDA approved for chronic kidney disease.

Other: Feraheme

▶ **New**   ⮌ **Revised**   ✔ **Reinstated**   ~~deleted~~ **Deleted**   ⊘ **Not covered or valid by Medicare**
⊘ **Special coverage instructions**   ✳ **Carrier discretion**   ⑧ **Bill Part B MAC**   ⓓ **Bill DME MAC**

✳ **Q0139** Injection, ferumoxytol, for treatment of iron deficiency anemia, 1 mg (for ESRD on dialysis) Ⓑ Qp Qh K2 K

Other: Feraheme

⊘ **Q0144** Azithromycin dihydrate, oral, capsules/powder, 1 gm Ⓑ Ⓑ Qp Qh E1

Other: Zithromax, Zmax

✳ **Q0161** Chlorpromazine hydrochloride, 5 mg, oral, FDA approved prescription anti-emetic, for use as a complete therapeutic substitute for an IV anti-emetic at the time of chemotherapy treatment, not to exceed a 48 hour dosage regimen Ⓑ Qp Qh N1 N

❁ **Q0162** Ondansetron 1 mg, oral, FDA-approved prescription anti-emetic, for use as a complete therapeutic substitute for an iv anti-emetic at the time of chemotherapy treatment, not to exceed a 48 hour dosage regimen Ⓑ Qp Qh N1 N

Other: Zofran

Medicare Statute 4557

Coding Clinic: 2012, Q1, P9

❁ **Q0163** Diphenhydramine hydrochloride, 50 mg, oral, FDA approved prescription anti-emetic, for use as a complete therapeutic substitute for an IV anti-emetic at time of chemotherapy treatment not to exceed a 48 hour dosage regimen Ⓑ Qp Qh N1 N

Other: Alercap, Alertab, Allergy Relief Medicine, Allermax, Anti-Hist, Antihistamine, Banophen, Complete Allergy Medication, Complete Allergy medicine, Diphedryl, Diphenhist, Diphenhydramine, Dormin Sleep Aid, Genahist, Geridryl, Good Sense Antihistamine Allergy Relief, Good Sense Nighttime Sleep Aid, Mediphedryl, Night Time Sleep Aid, Nytol Quickcaps, Nytol Quickgels maximum strength, Quality Choice Sleep Aid, Quality Choice Rest Simply, Rapidpaq Dicopanol, Rite Aid Allergy, Serabrina La France, Siladryl Allergy, Silphen, Simply Sleep, Sleep Tabs, Sleepinal, Sominex, Twilite, Valu-Dryl Allergy

Medicare Statute 4557

Coding Clinic: 2012, Q2, P10

❁ **Q0164** Prochlorperazine maleate, 5 mg, oral, FDA approved prescription anti-emetic, for use as a complete therapeutic substitute for an IV anti-emetic at the time of chemotherapy treatment, not to exceed a 48 hour dosage regimen Ⓑ Qp Qh N1 N

Other: Compazine

Medicare Statute 4557

Coding Clinic: 2012, Q2, P10

❁ **Q0166** Granisetron hydrochloride, 1 mg, oral, FDA approved prescription anti-emetic, for use as a complete therapeutic substitute for an IV anti-emetic at the time of chemotherapy treatment, not to exceed a 24 hour dosage regimen Ⓑ Qp Qh N1 N

Other: Kytril

Medicare Statute 4557

Coding Clinic: 2012, Q2, P10

❁ **Q0167** Dronabinol, 2.5 mg, oral, FDA approved prescription anti-emetic, for use as a complete therapeutic substitute for an IV anti-emetic at the time of chemotherapy treatment, not to exceed a 48 hour dosage regimen Ⓑ Qp Qh N1 N

Other: Marinol

Medicare Statute 4557

Coding Clinic: 2012, Q2, P10

❁ **Q0169** Promethazine hydrochloride, 12.5 mg, oral, FDA approved prescription anti-emetic, for use as a complete therapeutic substitute for an IV anti-emetic at the time of chemotherapy treatment, not to exceed a 48 hour dosage regimen Ⓑ Qp Qh N1 N

Other: Anergan, Chlorpromazine, Hydroxyzine Pamoate, Phenazine, Phenergan, Prorex, Prothazine, V-Gan

Medicare Statute 4557

Coding Clinic: 2012, Q2, P10

❁ **Q0173** Trimethobenzamide hydrochloride, 250 mg, oral, FDA approved prescription anti-emetic, for use as a complete therapeutic substitute for an IV anti-emetic at the time of chemotherapy treatment, not to exceed a 48 hour dosage regimen Ⓑ Qp Qh N1 N

Other: Arrestin, Ticon, Tigan, Tiject

Medicare Statute 4557

Coding Clinic: 2012, Q2, P10

○ **Q0174** Thiethylperazine maleate, 10 mg, oral, FDA approved prescription anti-emetic, for use as a complete therapeutic substitute for an IV anti-emetic at the time of chemotherapy treatment, not to exceed a 48 hour dosage regimen Ⓑ **Qp** **Qh** E2

Other: Torecan

Medicare Statute 4557

Coding Clinic: 2012, Q2, P10

○ **Q0175** Perphenazine, 4 mg, oral, FDA approved prescription anti-emetic, for use as a complete therapeutic substitute for an IV anti-emetic at the time of chemotherapy treatment, not to exceed a 48 hour dosage regimen Ⓑ **Qp** **Qh** N1 N

Medicare Statute 4557

Coding Clinic: 2012, Q2, P10

○ **Q0177** Hydroxyzine pamoate, 25 mg, oral, FDA approved prescription anti-emetic, for use as a complete therapeutic substitute for an IV anti-emetic at the time of chemotherapy treatment, not to exceed a 48 hour dosage regimen Ⓑ **Qp** **Qh** N1 N

Other: Vistaril

Medicare Statute 4557

Coding Clinic: 2012, Q2, P10

○ **Q0180** Dolasetron mesylate, 100 mg, oral, FDA approved prescription anti-emetic, for use as a complete therapeutic substitute for an IV anti-emetic at the time of chemotherapy treatment, not to exceed a 24 hour dosage regimen Ⓑ **Qp** **Qh** N1 N

Other: Anzemet

Medicare Statute 4557

Coding Clinic: 2012, Q2, P10

○ **Q0181** Unspecified oral dosage form, FDA approved prescription anti-emetic, for use as a complete therapeutic substitute for a IV anti-emetic at the time of chemotherapy treatment, not to exceed a 48 hour dosage regimen Ⓑ N1 N

Medicare Statute 4557

Coding Clinic: 2012, Q2, P10

Q0221 Injection, tixagevimab and cilgavimab, for the pre-exposure prophylaxis only, for certain adults and pediatric individuals (12 years of age and older weighing at least 40kg) with no known sars-cov-2 exposure, who either have moderate to severely compromised immune systems or for whom vaccination with any available covid-19 vaccine is not recommended due to a history of severe adverse reaction to a covid-19 vaccine(s) and/or covid-19 vaccine component(s), 600 mg L1 L

Q0222 Injection, bebtelovimab, 175 mg L1 K

○ **Q0240** Injection, casirivimab and imdevimab, 600 mg L1 L

○ **Q0243** Injection, Casirivimab and Imdevimab, 2400 mg K2 L

○ **Q0244** Injection, casirivimab and imdevimab, 1200 mg L1 L

○ **Q0245** Injection, bamlanivimab and etesevimab, 2100 mg L1 L

○ **Q0247** Injection, sotrovimab, 500 mg L1 L

○ **Q0249** Injection, tocilizumab, for hospitalized adults and pediatric patients (2 years of age and older) with covid-19 who are receiving systemic corticosteroids and require supplemental oxygen, non-invasive or invasive mechanical ventilation, or extracorporeal L1 L

Ventricular Assist Devices

○ **Q0477** Power module patient cable for use with electric or electric/pneumatic ventricular assist device, replacement only Ⓠ ♿ A

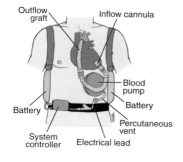

Outflow graft
Inflow cannula
Blood pump
Battery
Battery
System controller
Electrical lead
Percutaneous vent

Figure 46 Ventricular assist device.

▶ New ↻ Revised ✔ Reinstated ~~deleted~~ Deleted ⊘ Not covered or valid by Medicare
○ Special coverage instructions ✳ Carrier discretion Ⓑ Bill Part B MAC Ⓑ Bill DME MAC

Q0478 Power adapter for use with electric or electric/pneumatic ventricular assist device, vehicle type Ⓑ Qp Qh ♿ A

CMS has determined the reasonable useful lifetime is one year. Add modifier RA to claims to report when battery is replaced because it was lost, stolen, or irreparably damaged.

Q0479 Power module for use with electric or electric/pneumatic ventricular assist device, replacememnt only Ⓑ Qp Qh ♿ A

CMS has determined the reasonable useful lifetime is one year. Add modifier RA in cases where the battery is being replaced because it was lost, stolen, or irreparably damaged.

Q0480 Driver for use with pneumatic ventricular assist device, replacement only Ⓑ Qp Qh ♿ A

Q0481 Microprocessor control unit for use with electric ventricular assist device, replacement only Ⓑ Qp Qh ♿ A

Q0482 Microprocessor control unit for use with electric/pneumatic combination ventricular assist device, replacement only Ⓑ Qp Qh ♿ A

Q0483 Monitor/display module for use with electric ventricular assist device, replacement only Ⓑ Qp Qh ♿ A

Q0484 Monitor/display module for use with electric or electric/pneumatic ventricular assist device, replacement only Ⓑ Qp Qh ♿ A

Q0485 Monitor control cable for use with electric ventricular assist device, replacement only Ⓑ Qp Qh ♿ A

Q0486 Monitor control cable for use with electric/pneumatic ventricular assist device, replacement only Ⓑ Qp Qh ♿ A

Q0487 Leads (pneumatic/electrical) for use with any type electric/pneumatic ventricular assist device, replacement only Ⓑ Qp Qh ♿ A

Q0488 Power pack base for use with electric ventricular assist device, replacement only Ⓑ Qp Qh A

Q0489 Power pack base for use with electric/pneumatic ventricular assist device, replacement only Ⓑ Qp Qh A

Q0490 Emergency power source for use with electric ventricular assist device, replacement only Ⓑ Qp Qh ♿ A

Q0491 Emergency power source for use with electric/pneumatic ventricular assist device, replacement only Ⓑ Qp Qh ♿ A

Q0492 Emergency power supply cable for use with electric ventricular assist device, replacement only Ⓑ Qp Qh ♿ A

Q0493 Emergency power supply cable for use with electric/pneumatic ventricular assist device, replacement only Ⓑ Qp Qh ♿ A

Q0494 Emergency hand pump for use with electric or electric/pneumatic ventricular assist device, replacement only Ⓑ Qp Qh ♿ A

Q0495 Battery/power pack charger for use with electric or electric/pneumatic ventricular assist device, replacement only Ⓑ Qp Qh ♿ A

Q0496 Battery, other than lithium-ion, for use with electric or electric/pneumatic ventricular assist device, replacement only Ⓑ ♿ A

Reasonable useful lifetime is 6 months (CR3931).

Q0497 Battery clips for use with electric or electric/pneumatic ventricular assist device, replacement only Ⓑ Qp Qh ♿ A

Q0498 Holster for use with electric or electric/pneumatic ventricular assist device, replacement only Ⓑ Qp Qh ♿ A

Q0499 Belt/vest/bag for use to carry external peripheral components of any type ventricular assist device, replacement only Ⓑ Qp Qh ♿ A

Q0500 Filters for use with electric or electric/pneumatic ventricular assist device, replacement only Ⓑ ♿ A

Q0501 Shower cover for use with electric or electric/pneumatic ventricular assist device, replacement only Ⓑ Qp Qh ♿ A

Q0502 Mobility cart for pneumatic ventricular assist device, replacement only Ⓑ Qp Qh ♿ A

Q0503 Battery for pneumatic ventricular assist device, replacement only, each Ⓑ Qp Qh ♿ A

Reasonable useful lifetime is 6 months (CR3931).

Q0504 Power adapter for pneumatic ventricular assist device, replacement only, vehicle type Ⓑ Qp Qh ♿ A

Q0506 Battery, lithium-ion, for use with electric or electric/pneumatic, ventricular assist device, replacement only Ⓑ Qp Qh ♿ A

Reasonable useful lifetime is 12 months. Add -RA for replacement if lost, stolen, or irreparable damage.

Q0507 Miscellaneous supply or accessory for use with an external ventricular assist device Ⓑ Qp Qh A

Q0508 Miscellaneous supply or accessory for use with an implanted ventricular assist device Ⓑ Qp Qh A

🐍 MIPS Qp Quantity Physician Qh Quantity Hospital ♀ Female only

♂ Male only A Age ♿ DMEPOS A2-Z3 ASC Payment Indicator A-Y ASC Status Indicator Coding Clinic

⊗ **Q0509** Miscellaneous supply or accessory for use with any implanted ventricular assist device for which payment was not made under Medicare Part A Ⓑ Qp Qh   A

Pharmacy: Supply and Dispensing Fee

⊗ **Q0510** Pharmacy supply fee for initial immunosuppressive drug(s), first month following transplant Ⓑ Qp Qh   B

⊗ **Q0511** Pharmacy supply fee for oral anti-cancer, oral anti-emetic or immunosuppressive drug(s); for the first prescription in a 30-day period Ⓑ Qp Qh   B

⊗ **Q0512** Pharmacy supply fee for oral anti-cancer, oral anti-emetic or immunosuppressive drug(s); for a subsequent prescription in a 30-day period Ⓑ Qp Qh   B

⊗ **Q0513** Pharmacy dispensing fee for inhalation drug(s); per 30 days Ⓑ Qp Qh   B

⊗ **Q0514** Pharmacy dispensing fee for inhalation drug(s); per 90 days Ⓑ Qp Qh   B

Sermorelin Acetate

⊗ **Q0515** Injection, sermorelin acetate, 1 microgram Ⓑ Qp Qh   E2

IOM: 100-02, 15, 50

New Technology: Intraocular Lens

⊗ **Q1004** New technology intraocular lens category 4 as defined in Federal Register notice Ⓑ Qp Qh   E1

⊗ **Q1005** New technology intraocular lens category 5 as defined in Federal Register notice Ⓑ Qp Qh   E1

Solutions and Drugs

⊗ **Q2004** Irrigation solution for treatment of bladder calculi, for example renacidin, per 500 ml Ⓑ Qp Qh   N1 N

IOM: 100-02, 15, 50

Medicare Statute 1861S2B

⊗ **Q2009** Injection, fosphenytoin, 50 mg phenytoin equivalent Ⓑ Qp Qh   K2 K

IOM: 100-02, 15, 50

Medicare Statute 1861S2B

⊗ **Q2017** Injection, teniposide, 50 mg Ⓑ Qp Qh   K2 N

IOM: 100-02, 15, 50

Medicare Statute 1861S2B

⊗ **Q2026** Injection, radiesse, 0.1 ml Ⓑ Qp Qh   E2

Coding Clinic: 2010, Q3, P8

⊗ **Q2028** Injection, sculptra, 0.5 mg Ⓑ Qp Qh   E2

⊗ **Q2034** Influenza virus vaccine, split virus, for intramuscular use (Agriflu) Sipuleucel-t, minimum of 50 million autologous CD54+ cells activated with PAP-GM-CSF, including leukapheresis and all other preparatory procedures, per infusion Ⓑ Qp Qh   L1 L

IOM: 100-02, 15, 50

⊗ **Q2035** Influenza virus vaccine, split virus, when administered to individuals 3 years of age and older, for intramuscular use (Afluria) Ⓑ Qp Qh A   L1 L

Preventive service; no deductible

IOM: 100-02, 15, 50

Coding Clinic: 2011, Q1, P7; 2010, Q4, P8-9

⊗ **Q2036** Influenza virus vaccine, split virus, when administered to individuals 3 years of age and older, for intramuscular use (Flulaval) Ⓑ Qp Qh A   L1 L

Preventive service; no deductible

IOM: 100-02, 15, 50

Coding Clinic: 2011, Q1, P7; 2010, Q4, P8-9

⊗ **Q2037** Influenza virus vaccine, split virus, when administered to individuals3 years of age and older, for intramuscular use (Fluvirin) Ⓑ Qp Qh A   L1 L

Preventive service; no deductible

IOM: 100-02, 15, 50

Coding Clinic: 2011, Q1, P7; 2010, Q4, P8-9

⊗ **Q2038** Influenza virus vaccine, split virus, when administered to individuals 3 years of age or older, for intramuscular use (Fluzone) Ⓑ Qp Qh A   L1 L

Preventive service; no deductible

IOM: 100-02, 15, 50

Coding Clinic: 2011, Q1, P7; 2010, Q4, P8-9

⊗ **Q2039** Influenza virus vaccine, not otherwise specified Ⓑ Qp Qh A   L1 L

Preventive service; no deductible

IOM: 100-02, 15, 50

Coding Clinic: 2011, Q1, P7; 2010, Q4, P8-9

⊗ **Q2041** Axicabtagene ciloleucel, up to 200 million autologous anti-CD 19 CAR-positive viable T cells, including leukapheresis and dose preparation procedures, per therapeutic dose Ⓑ   G

▶ New   ↻ Revised   ✔ Reinstated   ~~deleted~~ Deleted   ⊘ Not covered or valid by Medicare
⊗ Special coverage instructions   ✳ Carrier discretion   Ⓑ Bill Part B MAC   Ⓓ Bill DME MAC

⊙ **Q2042** Tisagenlecleucel, up to 600 million CAR-positive viable T cells, including leukapheresis and dose preparation procedures, per therapeutic dose ⓑ G

⊙ **Q2043** Sipuleucel-T, minimum of 50 million autologous CD54+ cells activated with PAP-GM-CSF, including leukapheresis and all other preparatory procedures, per infusion ⓑ Qp Qh K2 K

Other: Provenge

Coding Clinic: 2012, Q2, P7; Q1, P7, 9; 2011, Q3, P9

✳ **Q2049** Injection, doxorubicin hydrochloride, liposomal, imported lipodox, 10 mg ⓑ ⓓ Qp Qh K2 K

Coding Clinic: 2012, Q3, P10

⊙ **Q2050** Injection, doxorubicin hydrochloride, liposomal, not otherwise specified, 10 mg ⓑ ⓓ Qp Qh K2 K

Other: Doxil

IOM: 100-02, 15, 50

⊙ **Q2052** Services, supplies and accessories used in the home under the Medicare intravenous immune globulin (IVIG) demonstration ⓓ Qp Qh E1

Coding Clinic: 2014, Q2, P6

⊙ **Q2053** Brexucabtagene autoleucel, up to 200 million autologous anti-cd19 car positive viable t cells, including leukapheresis and dose preparation procedures, per therapeutic dose G

⊙ **Q2054** Lisocabtagene maraleucel, up to 110 million autologous anti-cd19 car-positive viable t cells, including leukapheresis and dose preparation procedures, per therapeutic dose G

⊙ **Q2055** Idecabtagene vicleucel, up to 460 million autologous b-cell maturation antigen (bcma) directed car-positive t cells, including leukapheresis and dose preparation procedures, per therapeutic dose G

Q2056 Ciltacabtagene autoleucel, up to 100 million autologous B-cell maturation antigen (bcma) directed car-positive T cells, including leukapheresis and dose preparation procedures, per therapeutic dose G

Brachytherapy Radioelements

⊙ **Q3001** Radioelements for brachytherapy, any type, each ⓑ B

IOM: 100-04, 12, 70; 100-04, 13, 20

Telehealth

✳ **Q3014** Telehealth originating site facility fee ⓑ Qp Qh A

Effective January of each year, the fee for telehealth services is increased by the Medicare Economic Index (MEI). The telehealth originating facility site fee (HCPCS code Q3014) for 2011 was 80 percent of the lesser of the actual charge or $24.10.

Drugs

⊙ **Q3027** Injection, interferon beta-1a, 1 mcg for intramuscular use ⓑ Qp Qh K2 K

Other: Avonex

IOM: 100-02, 15, 50

⊘ **Q3028** Injection, interferon beta-1a, 1 mcg for subcutaneous use ⓑ Qp Qh E1

Skin Test

⊙ **Q3031** Collagen skin test ⓑ Qp Qh N1 N

IOM: 100-03, 4, 280.1

Supplies: Cast

Q4001-Q4051: Payment on a reasonable charge basis is required for splints, casts by regulations contained in 42 CFR 405.501.

✳ **Q4001** Casting supplies, body cast adult, with or without head, plaster ⓑ Qp Qh A ♿ B

✳ **Q4002** Cast supplies, body cast adult, with or without head, fiberglass ⓑ Qp Qh A ♿ B

✳ **Q4003** Cast supplies, shoulder cast, adult (11 years +), plaster ⓑ Qp Qh A ♿ B

✳ **Q4004** Cast supplies, shoulder cast, adult (11 years +), fiberglass ⓑ Qp Qh A ♿ B

✳ **Q4005** Cast supplies, long arm cast, adult (11 years +), plaster ⓑ A ♿ B

✳ **Q4006** Cast supplies, long arm cast, adult (11 years +), fiberglass ⓑ A ♿ B

✳ **Q4007** Cast supplies, long arm cast, pediatric (0-10 years), plaster ⓑ A ♿ B

✳ **Q4008** Cast supplies, long arm cast, pediatric (0-10 years), fiberglass ⓑ A ♿ B

✳ **Q4009** Cast supplies, short arm cast, adult (11 years +), plaster ⓑ A ♿ B

🝐 MIPS	Qp **Quantity Physician**	Qh **Quantity Hospital**	♀ **Female only**
♂ **Male only**	A **Age**	♿ **DMEPOS**	A2-Z3 **ASC Payment Indicator**	A-Y **ASC Status Indicator**	*Coding Clinic*

* **Q4010** Cast supplies, short arm cast, adult (11 years +), fiberglass Ⓟ Ⓐ Ⓖ B

* **Q4011** Cast supplies, short arm cast, pediatric (0-10 years), plaster Ⓟ Ⓐ Ⓖ B

* **Q4012** Cast supplies, short arm cast, pediatric (0-10 years), fiberglass Ⓑ Ⓐ Ⓖ B

* **Q4013** Cast supplies, gauntlet cast (includes lower forearm and hand), adult (11 years +), plaster Ⓑ Ⓐ Ⓖ B

* **Q4014** Cast supplies, gauntlet cast (includes lower forearm and hand), adult (11 years +), fiberglass Ⓑ Ⓐ Ⓖ B

* **Q4015** Cast supplies, gauntlet cast (includes lower forearm and hand), pediatric (0-10 years), plaster Ⓑ Ⓐ Ⓖ B

* **Q4016** Cast supplies, gauntlet cast (includes lower forearm and hand), pediatric (0-10 years), fiberglass Ⓑ Ⓐ Ⓖ B

* **Q4017** Cast supplies, long arm splint, adult (11 years +), plaster Ⓟ Ⓐ Ⓖ B

* **Q4018** Cast supplies, long arm splint, adult (11 years +), fiberglass Ⓑ Ⓐ Ⓖ B

* **Q4019** Cast supplies, long arm splint, pediatric (0-10 years), plaster Ⓟ Ⓐ Ⓖ B

* **Q4020** Cast supplies, long arm splint, pediatric (0-10 years), fiberglass Ⓑ Ⓐ Ⓖ B

* **Q4021** Cast supplies, short arm splint, adult (11 years +), plaster Ⓟ Ⓐ Ⓖ B

* **Q4022** Cast supplies, short arm splint, adult (11 years +), fiberglass Ⓟ Ⓐ Ⓖ B

* **Q4023** Cast supplies, short arm splint, pediatric (0-10 years), plaster Ⓑ Ⓐ Ⓖ B

* **Q4024** Cast supplies, short arm splint, pediatric (0-10 years), fiberglass Ⓑ Ⓐ Ⓖ B

* **Q4025** Cast supplies, hip spica (one or both legs), adult (11 years +), plaster Ⓟ Ⓠp Ⓠh Ⓐ Ⓖ B

* **Q4026** Cast supplies, hip spica (one or both legs), adult (11 years +), fiberglass Ⓟ Ⓠp Ⓠh Ⓐ Ⓖ B

* **Q4027** Cast supplies, hip spica (one or both legs), pediatric (0-10 years), plaster Ⓟ Ⓠp Ⓠh Ⓐ Ⓖ B

* **Q4028** Cast supplies, hip spica (one or both legs), pediatric (0-10 years), fiberglass Ⓑ Ⓠp Ⓠh Ⓐ Ⓖ B

* **Q4029** Cast supplies, long leg cast, adult (11 years +), plaster Ⓑ Ⓐ Ⓖ B

* **Q4030** Cast supplies, long leg cast, adult (11 years +), fiberglass Ⓟ Ⓐ Ⓖ B

* **Q4031** Cast supplies, long leg cast, pediatric (0-10 years), plaster Ⓑ Ⓐ Ⓖ B

* **Q4032** Cast supplies, long leg cast, pediatric (0-10 years), fiberglass Ⓟ Ⓐ Ⓖ B

* **Q4033** Cast supplies, long leg cylinder cast, adult (11 years +), plaster Ⓑ Ⓐ Ⓖ B

* **Q4034** Cast supplies, long leg cylinder cast, adult (11 years +), fiberglass Ⓑ Ⓐ Ⓖ B

* **Q4035** Cast supplies, long leg cylinder cast, pediatric (0-10 years), plaster Ⓑ Ⓐ Ⓖ B

* **Q4036** Cast supplies, long leg cylinder cast, pediatric (0-10 years), fiberglass Ⓑ Ⓐ Ⓖ B

* **Q4037** Cast supplies, short leg cast, adult (11 years +), plaster Ⓟ Ⓐ Ⓖ B

* **Q4038** Cast supplies, short leg cast, adult (11 years +), fiberglass Ⓑ Ⓐ Ⓖ B

* **Q4039** Cast supplies, short leg cast, pediatric (0-10 years), plaster Ⓑ Ⓐ Ⓖ B

* **Q4040** Cast supplies, short leg cast, pediatric (0-10 years), fiberglass Ⓑ Ⓐ Ⓖ B

* **Q4041** Cast supplies, long leg splint, adult (11 years +), plaster Ⓑ Ⓐ Ⓖ B

* **Q4042** Cast supplies, long leg splint, adult (11 years +), fiberglass Ⓟ Ⓐ Ⓖ B

* **Q4043** Cast supplies, long leg splint, pediatric (0-10 years), plaster Ⓑ Ⓐ Ⓖ B

* **Q4044** Cast supplies, long leg splint, pediatric (0-10 years), fiberglass Ⓑ Ⓐ Ⓖ B

* **Q4045** Cast supplies, short leg splint, adult (11 years +), plaster Ⓑ Ⓐ Ⓖ B

* **Q4046** Cast supplies, short leg splint, adult (11 years +), fiberglass Ⓑ Ⓐ Ⓖ B

* **Q4047** Cast supplies, short leg splint, pediatric (0-10 years), plaster Ⓟ Ⓐ Ⓖ B

* **Q4048** Cast supplies, short leg splint, pediatric (0-10 years), fiberglass Ⓑ Ⓐ Ⓖ B

* **Q4049** Finger splint, static Ⓑ Ⓖ B

* **Q4050** Cast supplies, for unlisted types and materials of casts Ⓑ B

* **Q4051** Splint supplies, miscellaneous (includes thermoplastics, strapping, fasteners, padding and other supplies) Ⓑ

Figure 47 Finger splint.

▶ New　　↻ Revised　　✔ Reinstated　　~~deleted~~ Deleted　　⊘ Not covered or valid by Medicare
◎ Special coverage instructions　　✳ Carrier discretion　　Ⓟ Bill Part B MAC　　Ⓑ Bill DME MAC

Drugs

❋ **Q4074** Iloprost, inhalation solution, FDA-approved final product, non-compounded, administered through DME, unit dose form, up to 20 micrograms Ⓠ Ⓑ Ⓠp Ⓠh   Y

    Other: Ventavis

⊙ **Q4081** Injection, epoetin alfa, 100 units (for ESRD on dialysis) Ⓑ Ⓠp Ⓠh   N

    Other: Epogen, Procrit

❋ **Q4082** Drug or biological, not otherwise classified, Part B drug competitive acquisition program (CAP) Ⓑ   B

Skin Substitutes

❋ **Q4100** Skin substitute, not otherwise specified Ⓑ   N1 N

    Coding Clinic: 2018, Q2, P3; 2012, Q2, P7

❋ **Q4101** Apligraf, per square centimeter Ⓑ Ⓠp Ⓠh   N1 N

    Coding Clinic: 2012, Q2, P7; 2011, Q1, P9

❋ **Q4102** Oasis Wound Matrix, per square centimeter Ⓑ Ⓠp Ⓠh   N1 N

    Coding Clinic: 2012, Q3, P8; Q2, P7; 2011, Q1, P9

❋ **Q4103** Oasis Burn Matrix, per square centimeter Ⓑ Ⓠp Ⓠh   N1 N

    Coding Clinic: 2012, Q2, P7; 2011, Q1, P9

❋ **Q4104** Integra Bilayer Matrix Wound Dressing (BMWD), per square centimeter Ⓑ Ⓠp Ⓠh   N1 N

    Coding Clinic: 2012, Q2, P7; 2011, Q1, P9; 2010, Q2, P8

❋ **Q4105** Integra Dermal Regeneration Template (DRT) or integra omnigraft dermal regeneration matrix, per square centimeter Ⓠ Ⓠp Ⓠh   N1 N

    Coding Clinic: 2012, Q2, P7; 2011, Q1, P9; 2010, Q2, P8

❋ **Q4106** Dermagraft, per square centimeter Ⓑ Ⓠp Ⓠh   N1 N

    Coding Clinic: 2012, Q2, P7; 2011, Q1, P9

❋ **Q4107** Graftjacket, per square centimeter Ⓠ Ⓠp Ⓠh   N1 N

    Coding Clinic: 2021, Q1, P9; 2012, Q2, P7; 2011, Q1, P9

❋ **Q4108** Integra Matrix, per square centimeter Ⓑ Ⓠp Ⓠh   N1 N

    Coding Clinic: 2012, Q2, P7; 2011, Q1, P9; 2010, Q2, P8

❋ **Q4110** Primatrix, per square centimeter Ⓑ Ⓠp Ⓠh   N1 N

    Coding Clinic: 2012, Q2, P7; 2011, Q1, P9

❋ **Q4111** GammaGraft, per square centimeter Ⓑ Ⓠp Ⓠh   N1 N

    Coding Clinic: 2012, Q2, P7; 2011, Q1, P9

❋ **Q4112** Cymetra, injectable, 1 cc Ⓑ Ⓠp Ⓠh   N1 N

    Coding Clinic: 2012, Q2, P7; 2011, Q1, P9

❋ **Q4113** GraftJacket Xpress, injectable, 1 cc Ⓠ Ⓠp Ⓠh   N1 N

    Coding Clinic: 2012, Q2, P7; 2011, Q1, P9

❋ **Q4114** Integra Flowable Wound Matrix, injectable, 1 cc Ⓑ Ⓠp Ⓠh   N1 N

    Coding Clinic: 2012, Q2, P7; 2010, Q2, P8

❋ **Q4115** Alloskin, per square centimeter Ⓑ Ⓠp Ⓠh   N1 N

    Coding Clinic: 2012, Q2, P7; 2011, Q1, P9

❋ **Q4116** Alloderm, per square centimeter Ⓑ Ⓠp Ⓠh   N1 N

    Coding Clinic: 2012, Q2, P7; 2011, Q1, P9

❋ **Q4117** Hyalomatrix, per square centimeter Ⓑ Ⓠp Ⓠh   N1 N

    IOM: 100-02, 15, 50

❋ **Q4118** Matristem micromatrix, 1 mg Ⓑ Ⓠp Ⓠh   N1 N

    Coding Clinic: 2013, Q4, P2; 2012, Q2, P7; 2011, Q1, P6

❋ **Q4121** Theraskin, per square centimeter Ⓠ Ⓠp Ⓠh   N1 N

    Coding Clinic: 2012, Q2, P7; 2011, Q1, P6

❋ **Q4122** Dermacell, Dermacell AWM or Dermacell AWM Porous, per square centimeter Ⓑ Ⓠp Ⓠh   N1 N

    Coding Clinic: 2012, Q2, P7; Q1, P8

❋ **Q4123** AlloSkin RT, per square centimeter Ⓑ Ⓠp Ⓠh   N1 N

❋ **Q4124** Oasis Ultra Tri-layer Wound Matrix, per square centimeter Ⓠ Ⓠp Ⓠh   N1 N

    Coding Clinic: 2012, Q2, P7; Q1, P9

❋ **Q4125** Arthroflex, per square centimeter Ⓑ Ⓠp Ⓠh   N1 N

❋ **Q4126** Memoderm, dermaspan, tranzgraft or integuply, per square centimeter Ⓑ Ⓠp Ⓠh   N1 N

❋ **Q4127** Talymed, per square centimeter Ⓑ Ⓠp Ⓠh   N1 N

❋ **Q4128** FlexHD, Allopatch HD, per square centimeter Ⓑ Ⓠp Ⓠh   N1 N

❋ **Q4130** Strattice TM, per square centimeter Ⓑ Ⓠp Ⓠh   N1 N

    Coding Clinic: 2012, Q2, P7

❋ **Q4132** Grafix core and GrafixPL core, per square centimeter Ⓑ Ⓠp Ⓠh   N1 N

---

* **Q4133** Grafix prime, GrafixPL prime, stravix and stravixpl, per square centimeter Ⓑ Qp Qh   N1 N

* **Q4134** Hmatrix, per square centimeter Ⓑ Qp Qh   N1 N

* **Q4135** Mediskin, per square centimeter Ⓑ Qp Qh   N1 N

* **Q4136** Ez-derm, per square centimeter Ⓑ Qp Qh   N1 N

* **Q4137** Amnioexcel, amnioexcel plus or biodexcel, per square centimeter Ⓑ Qp Qh   N1 N

* **Q4138** Biodfence dryflex, per square centimeter Ⓑ Qp Qh   N1 N

* **Q4139** Amniomatrix or biodmatrix, injectable, 1 cc Ⓑ Qp Qh   N1 N

* **Q4140** Biodfence, per square centimeter Ⓑ Qp Qh   N1 N

* **Q4141** Alloskin ac, per square centimeter Ⓑ Qp Qh   N1 N

* **Q4142** XCM biologic tissue matrix, per square centimeter Ⓑ Qp Qh   N1 N

* **Q4143** Repriza, per square centimeter Ⓑ Qp Qh   N1 N

* **Q4145** Epifix, injectable, 1 mg Ⓑ Qp Qh   N1 N

* **Q4146** Tensix, per square centimeter Ⓑ Qp Qh   N1 N

* **Q4147** Architect, architect PX, or architect FX, extracellular matrix, per square centimeter Ⓑ Qp Qh   N1 N

* **Q4148** Neox cord 1K, Neox cord RT, or Clarix cord 1K, per square centimeter Ⓑ Qp Qh   N1 N

* **Q4149** Excellagen, 0.1 cc Ⓑ Qp Qh   N1 N

* **Q4150** AlloWrap DS or dry, per square centimeter Ⓑ Qp Qh   N1 N

* **Q4151** Amnioband or guardian, per square centimeter Ⓑ Qp Qh   N1 N

* **Q4152** DermaPure, per square centimeter Ⓑ Qp Qh   N1 N

* **Q4153** Dermavest and Plurivest, per square centimeter Ⓑ Qp Qh   N1 N

* **Q4154** Biovance, per square centimeter Ⓑ Qp Qh   N1 N

* **Q4155** Neoxflo or clarixflo, 1 mg Ⓑ Qp Qh   N1 N

* **Q4156** Neox 100 or Clarix 100, per square centimeter Ⓑ Qp Qh   N1 N

* **Q4157** Revitalon, per square centimeter Ⓑ Qp Qh   N1 N

* **Q4158** Kerecis Omega3, per square centimeter Ⓑ Qp Qh   N1 N

* **Q4159** Affinity, per square centimeter ⓟ Qp Qh   N1 N

* **Q4160** Nushield, per square centimeter Ⓑ Qp Qh   N1 N

* **Q4161** Bio-ConneKt Wound Matrix, per square centimeter ⓟ Qp Qh   N1 N

* **Q4162** Woundex flow, BioSkin flow 0.5 cc Ⓑ Qp Qh   N1 N

* **Q4163** Woundex, BioSkin per square centimeter Ⓑ Qp Qh   N1 N

* **Q4164** Helicoll, per square centimeter Ⓑ Qp Qh   N1 N

* **Q4165** Keramatrix or kerasorb, per square centimeter Ⓑ Qp Qh   N1 N

* **Q4166** Cytal, per square centimeter Ⓑ Qp Qh   N1 N

    Coding Clinic: 2017, Q1, P10

* **Q4167** TruSkin, per square centimeter Ⓑ Qp Qh   N1 N

    Coding Clinic: 2017, Q1, P10

* **Q4168** AmnioBand, 1 mg ⓟ Qp Qh   N1 N

    Coding Clinic: 2017, Q1, P10

* **Q4169** Artacent wound, per square centimeter Ⓑ Qp Qh   N1 N

    Coding Clinic: 2017, Q1, P10

* **Q4170** Cygnus, per square centimeter Ⓑ Qp Qh   N1 N

    Coding Clinic: 2017, Q1, P10

* **Q4171** Interfyl, 1 mg Ⓑ Qp Qh   N1 N

    Coding Clinic: 2017, Q1, P10

* **Q4173** PalinGen or PalinGen XPlus, per square centimeter Ⓑ Qp Qh   N1 N

    Coding Clinic: 2017, Q1, P10

* **Q4174** PalinGen or ProMatrX, 0.36 mg per 0.25 cc Ⓑ Qp Qh   N1 N

    Coding Clinic: 2017, Q1, P10

* **Q4175** Miroderm, per square centimeter Ⓑ Qp Qh   N1 N

    Coding Clinic: 2017, Q1, P10

* **Q4176** Neopatch or therion, per square centimeter Ⓑ   N1 N

* **Q4177** Floweramnioflo, 0.1 cc Ⓑ   N1 N

* **Q4178** Floweramniopatch, per square centimeter Ⓑ   N1 N

* **Q4179** Flowerderm, per square centimeter Ⓑ   N1 N

* **Q4180** Revita, per square centimeter Ⓑ   N1 N

* **Q4181** Amnio wound, per square centimeter Ⓑ   N1 N

▶ **New**   ⟲ **Revised**   ✓ **Reinstated**   ~~deleted~~ **Deleted**   ⊘ **Not covered or valid by Medicare**
⊛ **Special coverage instructions**   * **Carrier discretion**   Ⓑ **Bill Part B MAC**   ⓟ **Bill DME MAC**

408

* **Q4182** Transcyte, per square centimeter Ⓑ N1 N
* **Q4183** Surgigraft, per square centimeter Ⓑ N
* **Q4184** Cellesta or cellesta duo, per square centimeter Ⓑ N
* **Q4185** Cellesta flowable amnion (25 mg per cc); per 0.5 cc Ⓑ N
* **Q4186** Epifix, per square centimeter Ⓑ N
* **Q4187** Epicord, per square centimeter Ⓑ N
* **Q4188** Amnioarmor, per square centimeter Ⓑ N
* **Q4189** Artacent ac, 1 mg Ⓑ N
* **Q4190** Artacent ac, per square centimeter Ⓑ N
* **Q4191** Restorigin, per square centimeter Ⓑ N
* **Q4192** Restorigin, 1 cc Ⓑ N
* **Q4193** Coll-e-derm, per square centimeter Ⓑ N
* **Q4194** Novachor, per square centimeter Ⓑ N
* **Q4195** Puraply, per square centimeter Ⓑ G
* **Q4196** Puraply am, per square centimeter Ⓑ G
* **Q4197** Puraply xt, per square centimeter Ⓑ N
* **Q4198** Genesis amniotic membrane, per square centimeter Ⓑ N
* **Q4199** Cygnus matrix, per square centimeter N
* **Q4200** Skin te, per square centimeter Ⓑ N
* **Q4201** Matrion, per square centimeter Ⓑ N
* **Q4202** Keroxx (2.5g/cc), 1cc Ⓑ N
* **Q4203** Derma-gide, per square centimeter Ⓑ N
* **Q4204** Xwrap, per square centimeter Ⓑ N
* **Q4205** Membrane graft or membrane wrap, per square centimeter Ⓑ
* **Q4206** Fluid flow or fluid Gf, 1 cc Ⓑ N
* **Q4208** Novafix, per square cenitmeter Ⓑ N
* **Q4209** Surgraft, per square centimeter Ⓑ N
* **Q4210** Axolotl graft or axolotl dualgraft, per square centimeter Ⓑ N
* **Q4211** Amnion bio or axobiomembrane, per square centimeter Ⓑ N
* **Q4212** Allogen, per cc Ⓑ N
* **Q4213** Ascent, 0.5 mg Ⓑ N
* **Q4214** Cellesta cord, per square centimeter Ⓑ N
* **Q4215** Axolotl ambient or axolotl cryo, 0.1 mg Ⓑ N
* **Q4216** Artacent cord, per square centimeter Ⓑ N
* **Q4217** Woundfix, BioWound, Woundfix Plus, BioWound Plus, Woundfix Xplus or BioWound Xplus, per square centimeter Ⓑ N

* **Q4218** Surgicord, per square centimeter Ⓑ N
* **Q4219** Surgigraft-dual, per square centimeter Ⓑ N
* **Q4220** BellaCell HD or Surederm, per square centimeter Ⓑ N
* **Q4221** Amniowrap2, per square centimeter Ⓑ N
* **Q4222** Progenamatrix, per square centimeter Ⓑ N
* **Q4226** MyOwn skin, includes harvesting and preparation procedures, per square centimeter Ⓑ N
* **Q4227** Amniocore, per square centimeter N1 N
* **Q4229** Cogenex amniotic membrane, per square centimeter N1 N
* **Q4230** Cogenex flowable amnion, per 0.5 cc N1 N
* **Q4231** Corplex P, per cc N1 N
* **Q4232** Corplex, per square centimeter N1 N
* **Q4233** Surfactor or Nudyn, per 0.5 cc N1 N
* **Q4234** Xcellerate, per square centimeter N1 N
* **Q4235** Amniorepair or Altiply, per square centimeter N1 N
* **Q4237** Cryo-cord, per square centimeter N1 N
* **Q4238** Derm-maxx, per square centimeter N1 N
* **Q4239** Amnio-maxx or amnio-maxx lite, per square centimeter N1 N
* **Q4240** Corecyte, for topical use only, per 0.5 cc N1 N
* **Q4241** Polycyte, for topical use only, per 0.5 cc N1 N
* **Q4242** Amniocyte plus, per 0.5 cc N1 N
* **Q4244** Procenta, per 200 mg N1 N
* **Q4245** Amniotext, per cc N1 N
* **Q4246** Coretext or Protext, per cc N1 N
* **Q4248** Dermacyte amniotic membrane allograft, per square centimeter N1 N
* **Q4249** Amniply, for topical use only, per square centimeter N
* **Q4950** Amnioamp-MP, per square centimeter N
* **Q4251** Vim, per square centimeter N
* **Q4252** Vendaje, per square centimeter N
* **Q4253** Zenith amniotic membrane, per square centimeter N
* **Q4254** Novafix DL, per square centimeter N
* **Q4255** Reguard, for topical use only, per square centimeter N
* **Q4259** Celera dual layer or celera dual membrane, per square centimeter N

⊚ **Q4260**	Signature apatch, per square centimeter	N	
⊚ **Q4261**	Tag, per square centimeter	N	
⊚ **Q4262**	Dual layer impax membrane, per square centimeter	N	
⊚ **Q4263**	Surgraft tl, per square centimeter	N	
⊚ **Q4264**	Cocoon membrane, per square centimeter	N	
▶ ⊚ **Q4265**	Neostim tl, per square centimeter	N	
▶ ⊚ **Q4266**	Neostim membrane, per square centimeter	N	
▶ ⊚ **Q4267**	Neostim dl, per square centimeter	N	
▶ ⊚ **Q4268**	Surgraft ft, per square centimeter	N	
▶ ⊚ **Q4269**	Surgraft xt, per square centimeter	N	
▶ ⊚ **Q4270**	Complete sl, per square centimeter	N	
▶ ⊚ **Q4271**	Complete ft, per square centimeter	N	
▶ ⊚ **Q4272**	Esano a, per square centimeter	N	
▶ ⊚ **Q4273**	Esano aaa, per square centimeter	N	
▶ ⊚ **Q4274**	Esano ac, per square centimeter	N	
▶ ⊚ **Q4275**	Esano aca, per square centimeter	N	
▶ ⊚ **Q4276**	Orion, per square centimeter	N	
▶ ⊚ **Q4277**	Woundplus membrane or e-graft, per square centimeter	N	
▶ ⊚ **Q4278**	Epieffect, per square centimeter	N	
▶ ⊚ **Q4280**	Xcell amnio matrix, per square centimeter	N	
▶ ⊚ **Q4281**	Barrera sl or barrera dl, per square centimeter	N	
▶ ⊚ **Q4282**	Cygnus dual, per square centimeter	N	
▶ ⊚ **Q4283**	Biovance tri-layer or biovance 3l, per square centimeter	N	
▶ ⊚ **Q4284**	Dermabind sl, per square centimeter	N	
▶ ⊚ **Q4285**	Nudyn dl or nudyn dl mesh, per square centimeter	N	
▶ ⊚ **Q4286**	Nudyn sl or nudyn slw, per square centimeter	N	
⊚ **Q5126**	Injection, bevacizumab-maly, biosimilar, (alymsys), 10 mg	G	
▶ ⊚ **Q5127**	Injection, pegfilgrastim-fpgk (stimufend), biosimilar, 0.5 mg		
▶ ⊚ **Q5128**	Injection, ranibizumab-eqrn (cimerli), biosimilar, 0.1 mg		
▶ ⊚ **Q5129**	Injection, bevacizumab-adcd (vegzelma), biosimilar, 10 mg		
▶ ⊚ **Q5130**	Injection, pegfilgrastim-pbbk (fylnetra), biosimilar, 0.5 mg		
▶ ⊚ **Q5131**	Injection, adalimumab-aacf (idacio), biosimilar, 20 mg		

Hospice Care

⊚ **Q5001**	Hospice or home health care provided in patient's home/residence ⑧	B
⊚ **Q5002**	Hospice or home health care provided in assisted living facility ⑧	B
⊚ **Q5003**	Hospice care provided in nursing long term care facility (LTC) or non-skilled nursing facility (NF) ⑧	B
⊚ **Q5004**	Hospice care provided in skilled nursing facility (SNF) ⑧	B
⊚ **Q5005**	Hospice care provided in inpatient hospital ⑧	B
⊚ **Q5006**	Hospice care provided in inpatient hospice facility ⑧	B

Hospice care provided in an inpatient hospice facility. These are residential facilities, which are places for patients to live while receiving routine home care or continuous home care. These hospice residential facilities are not certified by Medicare or Medicaid for provision of General Inpatient (GIP) or respite care, and regulations at 42 CFR 418.202(e) do not allow provision of GIP or respite care at hospice residential facilities.

⊚ **Q5007**	Hospice care provided in long term care facility ⑧	B
⊚ **Q5008**	Hospice care provided in inpatient psychiatric facility ⑧	B
⊚ **Q5009**	Hospice or home health care provided in place not otherwise specified (NOS) ⑧	B
⊚ **Q5010**	Hospice home care provided in a hospice facility ⑧	B

Biosimilar Drugs

⊚ **Q5101**	Injection, filgrastim-sndz, biosimilar, (zarxio), 1 microgram ⑧ ⑨ **Qp** **Qh**	K2 N
	Other: Zarxio	
⊚ **Q5103**	Injection, infliximab-dyyb, biosimilar, (inflectra), 10 mg ⑧ ⑨	G
	Other: Remicade, Inflectra, Renflexis	
⊚ **Q5104**	Injection, infliximab-abda, biosimilar, (renflexis), 10 mgn ⑧ ⑨	K2 G
	Other: Remicade	
⊚ **Q5105**	Injection, epoetin alfa-epbx, biosimilar, (retacrit) (for ESRD on dialysis), 100 units ⑧ ⑨	K2 G
	Other: Retacrit	

▶ **New**   ↻ **Revised**   ✔ **Reinstated**   ~~deleted~~ **Deleted**   ⊘ **Not covered or valid by Medicare**
⊚ **Special coverage instructions**   ✳ **Carrier discretion**   ⑧ **Bill Part B MAC**   ⑨ **Bill DME MAC**

⊘ **Q5106**   Injection, epoetin alfa-epbx, biosimilar (retacrit) (for non-ESRD use), 1000 units Ⓑ Ⓑ   G

Other: Retacrit

⊘ **Q5107**   Injection, bevacizumab-awwb, biosimilar (mvasi), 10 mg Ⓑ Ⓑ   K

Other: Avastin

↺ ⊘ **Q5108**   Injection, pegfilgrastim-jmdb, (fulphila), biosimilar 0.5 mg Ⓑ Ⓑ   K

Other: Neulasta

⊘ **Q5109**   Injection, infliximab-qbtx, biosimilar (ixifi), 10 mg Ⓑ Ⓑ   E2

Other: Remicade, Inflectra, Renflexis

⊘ **Q5110**   Injection, filgrastim-aafi, biosimilar (nivestym), 1 microgram Ⓑ Ⓑ   K

Other: Nivestym

▶ **Q5111**   Injection, pegfilgrastim-cbqv (udenyca), biosimilar, 0.5 mg   K

✱ **Q5112**   Injection, trastuzumab-dttb, biosimilar (ontruzant), 10 mg Ⓑ Ⓑ   E2

✱ **Q5113**   Injection, trastuzumab-pkrb, biosimilar (herzuma), 10 mg Ⓑ Ⓑ   E2

✱ **Q5114**   Injection, trastuzumab-dkst, biosimilar (ogivri), 10 mg Ⓑ Ⓑ   E2

⊘ **Q5115**   Injection, rituximab-abbs, biosimilar (truxima), 10 mg Ⓑ Ⓑ   E2

✱ **Q5116**   Injection, trastuzumab-qyyp, biosimilar (trazimera), 10 mg Ⓑ Ⓑ   E2

✱ **Q5117**   Injection, trastuzumab-anns, biosimilar (kanjinti), 10 mg Ⓑ Ⓑ   K2 K

✱ **Q5118**   Injection, bevacizumab-bvzr, biosimilar (zirabev), 10 mg Ⓑ Ⓑ   E2

✱ **Q5119**   Injection, rituximab-pvvr, biosimilar (ruxience), 10 mg   G

↺ ✱ **Q5120**   Injection, pegfilgrastim-bmez, (ziextenzo), biosimilar 0.5 mg   K2 G

✱ **Q5121**   Injection, infliximab-axxq, (avsola), biosimilar 10 mg   K2 G

↺ ✱ **Q5122**   Injection, pegfilgrastim-apgf, (nyvepria), biosimilar, 0.5 mg   K5 E1

✱ **Q5123**   Injection, rituximab-arrx, biosimilar, (riabni), 10 mg   K2 G

Q5125   Injection, filgrastim-ayow, biosimilar, (releuko), 1 microgram   K2 G

▶ **Q5126**   Injection, bevacizumab-maly, biosimilar, (alymsys), 10 mg   G

Veteran Services Chaplain

✱ **Q9001**   Assessment by chaplain services   B

✱ **Q9002**   Counseling, individual, by chaplain services   B

✱ **Q9003**   Counseling, group, by chaplain services   B

✱ **Q9004**   Department of veterans affairs whole health partner services   E1

Contrast Agents

✱ **Q9950**   Injection, sulfur hexafluoride lipid microspheres, per ml Ⓑ Qp Qh   N1 N

Other: Lumason

⊘ **Q9951**   Low osmolar contrast material, 400 or greater mg/ml iodine concentration, per ml Ⓑ Qp Qh   N1 N

IOM: 100-04, 12, 70; 100-04, 13, 20; 100-04, 13, 90

Coding Clinic: 2012, Q3, P8

⊘ **Q9953**   Injection, iron-based magnetic resonance contrast agent, per ml Ⓑ Qp Qh   N1 N

IOM: 100-04, 12, 70; 100-04, 13, 20; 100-04, 13, 90

Coding Clinic: 2012, Q3, P8

⊘ **Q9954**   Oral magnetic resonance contrast agent, per 100 ml Ⓑ Qp Qh   N1 N

IOM: 100-04, 12, 70; 100-04, 13, 20; 100-04, 13, 90

Coding Clinic: 2012, Q3, P8

✱ **Q9955**   Injection, perflexane lipid microspheres, per ml Ⓑ Qp Qh   N1 N

Coding Clinic: 2012, Q3, P8

✱ **Q9956**   Injection, octafluoropropane microspheres, per ml Ⓑ Qp Qh   N1 N

Other: Optison

Coding Clinic: 2012, Q3, P8

✱ **Q9957**   Injection, perflutren lipid microspheres, per ml Ⓑ Qp Qh   N1 N

Other: Definity

Coding Clinic: 2012, Q3, P8

⊘ **Q9958**   High osmolar contrast material, up to 149 mg/ml iodine concentration, per ml Ⓑ Qp Qh   N1 N

Other: Conray 30, Cysto-Conray II, Cystografin

IOM: 100-04, 12, 70; 100-04, 13, 20; 100-04, 13, 90

Coding Clinic: 2012, Q3, P8; 2007, Q1, P6

🔖 MIPS   Qp Quantity Physician   Qh Quantity Hospital   ♀ Female only

♂ Male only   Ⓐ Age   🦽 DMEPOS   A2-Z3 ASC Payment Indicator   A-Y ASC Status Indicator   Coding Clinic

⊛ **Q9959** High osmolar contrast material, 150-199 mg/ml iodine concentration, per ml Ⓑ Qp Qh   N1 N

IOM: 100-04, 12, 70; 100-04, 13, 20; 100-04, 13, 90

Coding Clinic: 2012, Q3, P8; 2007, Q1, P6

⊛ **Q9960** High osmolar contrast material, 200-249 mg/ml iodine concentration, per ml Ⓑ Qp Qh   N1 N

Other: Conray 43

IOM: 100-04, 12, 70; 100-04, 13, 20; 100-04, 13, 90

Coding Clinic: 2012, Q3, P8; 2007, Q1, P6

⊛ **Q9961** High osmolar contrast material, 250-299 mg/ml iodine concentration, per ml Ⓑ Qp Qh   N1 N

Other: Conray, Cholografin Meglumine

IOM: 100-04, 12, 70; 100-04, 13, 20; 100-04, 13, 90

Coding Clinic: 2012, Q3, P8; 2007, Q1, P6

⊛ **Q9962** High osmolar contrast material, 300-349 mg/ml iodine concentration, per ml Ⓑ Qp Qh   N1 N

IOM: 100-04, 12, 70; 100-04, 13, 20; 100-04, 13, 90

Coding Clinic: 2012, Q3, P8; 2007, Q1, P6

⊛ **Q9963** High osmolar contrast material, 350-399 mg/ml iodine concentration, per ml Ⓑ Qp Qh   N1 N

Other: Gastrografin, MD-76R, MD Gastroview, Sinografin

IOM: 100-04, 12, 70; 100-04, 13, 20; 100-04, 13, 90

Coding Clinic: 2012, Q3, P8; 2007, Q1, P6

⊛ **Q9964** High osmolar contrast material, 400 or greater mg/ml iodine concentration, per ml Ⓑ Qp Qh   N1 N

IOM: 100-04, 12, 70; 100-04, 13, 20; 100-04, 13, 90

Coding Clinic: 2012, Q3, P8; 2007, Q1, P6

⊛ **Q9965** Low osmolar contrast material, 100-199 mg/ml iodine concentration, per ml Ⓑ   N1 N

Other: Omnipaque

IOM: 100-04, 12, 70; 100-04, 13, 20; 100-04, 13, 90

Coding Clinic: 2012, Q3, P8

⊛ **Q9966** Low osmolar contrast material, 200-299 mg/ml iodine concentration, per ml Ⓑ Qp Qh   N1 N

Other: Isovue, Omnipaque, Optiray, Ultravist 240, Visipaque

IOM: 100-04, 12, 70; 100-04, 13, 20; 100-04, 13, 90

Coding Clinic: 2012, Q3, P8

⊛ **Q9967** Low osmolar contrast material, 300-399 mg/ml iodine concentration, per ml Ⓑ Qp Qh   N1 N

Other: Hexabrix 320, Isovue, Omnipaque, Optiray, Oxilan, Ultravist, Vispaque

IOM: 100-04, 12, 70; 100-04, 13, 20; 100-04, 13, 90

Coding Clinic: 2012, Q3, P8

❋ **Q9968** Injection, non-radioactive, non-contrast, visualization adjunct (e.g., Methylene Blue, Isosulfan Blue), 1 mg Ⓑ   K2 K

⊛ **Q9969** Tc-99m from non-highly enriched uranium source, full cost recovery add-on, per study dose Ⓥ Qp Qh   K

Radiopharmaceuticals

⊛ **Q9982** Flutemetamol F18, diagnostic, per study dose, up to 5 millicuries Ⓑ Qp Qh   K2 G

Other: Vizamyl

⊛ **Q9983** Florbetaben F18, diagnostic, per study dose, up to 8.1 millicuries Ⓑ Qp Qh   K2 G

Other: Neuraceq

❋ **Q9991** Injection, buprenorphine extended-release (sublocade), less than or equal to 100 mg Ⓑ Ⓥ   G

Other: Subutex, Buprenex, Belbuca, Probuphine, Butrans

❋ **Q9992** Injection, buprenorphine extended-release (sublocade), greater than 100 mg Ⓑ Ⓥ   G

Other: Subutex, Buprenex, Belbuca, Probuphine, Butrans

▶ New   ↻ Revised   ✔ Reinstated   ~~deleted~~ Deleted   ⊘ Not covered or valid by Medicare   ⊛ Special coverage instructions   ❋ Carrier discretion   Ⓑ Bill Part B MAC   Ⓥ Bill DME MAC

DIAGNOSTIC RADIOLOGY SERVICES
(R0000-R9999)

Transportation/Setup of Portable Equipment

⚙ **R0070** Transportation of portable x-ray equipment and personnel to home or nursing home, per trip to facility or location, one patient seen Ⓑ **Qp** **Qh** B

CMS Transmittal B03-049; specific instructions to contractors on pricing

IOM: 100-04, 13, 90; 100-04, 13, 90.3

⚙ **R0075** Transportation of portable x-ray equipment and personnel to home or nursing home, per trip to facility or location, more than one patient seen Ⓑ **Qp** **Qh** B

This code would not apply to the x-ray equipment if stored at the location where the x-ray was performed (e.g., a nursing home).

IOM: 100-04, 13, 90; 100-04, 13, 90.3

⚙ **R0076** Transportation of portable ECG to facility or location, per patient Ⓑ **Qp** **Qh** B

EKG procedure code 93000 or 93005 must be submitted on same claim as transportation code. Bundled status on physician fee schedule

IOM: 100-01, 5, 90.2; 100-02, 15, 80; 100-03, 1, 20.15; 100-04, 13, 90; 100-04, 16, 10; 100-04, 16, 110.4

⚙ MIPS	**Qp** Quantity Physician	**Qh** Quantity Hospital	♀ Female only
♂ Male only Ⓐ Age ♿ DMEPOS	A2-Z3 ASC Payment Indicator	A-Y ASC Status Indicator	Coding Clinic

TEMPORARY NATIONAL CODES ESTABLISHED BY PRIVATE PAYERS (S0000–S9999)

NOTE: Medicare and other federal payers do not recognize "S" codes; however, S codes may be useful for claims to some private insurers.

Non-Medicare Drugs

⊘ **S0012** Butorphanol tartrate, nasal spray, 25 mg

⊘ **S0013** Esketamine, nasal spray, 1 mg

⊘ **S0014** Tacrine hydrochloride, 10 mg

⊘ **S0017** Injection, aminocaproic acid, 5 grams

~~S0020~~ ~~Injection, bupivacaine hydrochloride, 30 ml~~

⊘ **S0021** Injection, cefoperazone sodium, 1 gram

⊘ **S0023** Injection, cimetidine hydrochloride, 300 mg

⊘ **S0028** Injection, famotidine, 20 mg

~~S0030~~ ~~Injection, metronidazole, 500 mg~~

⊘ **S0032** Injection, nafcillin sodium, 2 grams

⊘ **S0034** Injection, ofloxacin, 400 mg

⊘ **S0039** Injection, sulfamethoxazole and trimethoprim, 10 ml

⊘ **S0040** Injection, ticarcillin disodium and clavulanate potassium, 3.1 grams

~~S0073~~ ~~Injection, aztreonam, 500 mg~~

⊘ **S0074** Injection, cefotetan disodium, 500 mg

⊘ **S0077** Injection, clindamycin phosphate, 300 mg

⊘ **S0078** Injection, fosphenytoin sodium, 750 mg

⊘ **S0080** Injection, pentamidine isethionate, 300 mg

⊘ **S0081** Injection, piperacillin sodium, 500 mg

⊘ **S0088** Imatinib, 100 mg

⊘ **S0090** Sildenafil citrate, 25 mg Ⓐ

⊘ **S0091** Granisetron hydrochloride, 1 mg (for circumstances falling under the Medicare Statute, use Q0166)

⊘ **S0092** Injection, hydromorphone hydrochloride, 250 mg (loading dose for infusion pump)

⊘ **S0093** Injection, morphine sulfate, 500 mg (loading dose for infusion pump)

⊘ **S0104** Zidovudine, oral, 100 mg

⊘ **S0106** Bupropion HCl sustained release tablet, 150 mg, per bottle of 60 tablets

⊘ **S0108** Mercaptopurine, oral, 50 mg

⊘ **S0109** Methadone, oral, 5 mg

⊘ **S0117** Tretinoin, topical, 5 grams

⊘ **S0119** Ondansetron, oral, 4 mg (for circumstances falling under the Medicare statute, use HCPCS Q code)

⊘ **S0122** Injection, menotropins, 75 IU

⊘ **S0126** Injection, follitropin alfa, 75 IU

⊘ **S0128** Injection, follitropin beta, 75 IU

⊘ **S0132** Injection, ganirelix acetate, 250 mcg

⊘ **S0136** Clozapine, 25 mg

⊘ **S0137** Didanosine (DDI), 25 mg

⊘ **S0138** Finasteride, 5 mg

⊘ **S0139** Minoxidil, 10 mg

⊘ **S0140** Saquinavir, 200 mg

⊘ **S0142** Colistimethate sodium, inhalation solution administered through DME, concentrated form, per mg

⊘ **S0145** Injection, pegylated interferon alfa-2a, 180 mcg per ml

⊘ **S0148** Injection, pegylated interferon ALFA-2b, 10 mcg

⊘ **S0155** Sterile dilutant for epoprostenol, 50 ml

⊘ **S0156** Exemestane, 25 mg

⊘ **S0157** Becaplermin gel 0.01%, 0.5 gm

⊘ **S0160** Dextroamphetamine sulfate, 5 mg

⊘ **S0164** Injection, pantoprazole sodium, 40 mg

⊘ **S0166** Injection, olanzapine, 2.5 mg

⊘ **S0169** Calcitrol, 0.25 microgram

⊘ **S0170** Anastrozole, oral, 1 mg

⊘ **S0171** Injection, bumetanide, 0.5 mg

⊘ **S0172** Chlorambucil, oral, 2 mg

⊘ **S0174** Dolasetron mesylate, oral 50 mg (for circumstances falling under the Medicare Statute, use Q0180)

⊘ **S0175** Flutamide, oral, 125 mg

⊘ **S0176** Hydroxyurea, oral, 500 mg

~~S0177~~ ~~Levamisole hydrochloride, oral, 50 mg~~

⊘ **S0178** Lomustine, oral, 10 mg

⊘ **S0179** Megestrol acetate, oral, 20 mg

⊘ **S0182** Procarbazine hydrochloride, oral, 50 mg

⊘ **S0183** Prochlorperazine maleate, oral, 5 mg (for circumstances falling under the Medicare Statute, use Q0164)

▶ New   ↻ Revised   ✔ Reinstated   ~~deleted~~ Deleted   ⊘ Not covered or valid by Medicare
Ⓢ Special coverage instructions   ✳ Carrier discretion   Ⓑ Bill Part B MAC   Ⓓ Bill DME MAC

⊘ **S0187** Tamoxifen citrate, oral, 10 mg

⊘ **S0189** Testosterone pellet, 75 mg

⊘ **S0190** Mifepristone, oral, 200 mg

⊘ **S0191** Misoprostol, oral 200 mcg

⊘ **S0194** Dialysis/stress vitamin supplement, oral, 100 capsules

⊘ **S0197** Prenatal vitamins, 30-day supply ♀

Provider Services

⊘ **S0199** Medically induced abortion by oral ingestion of medication including all associated services and supplies (e.g., patient counseling, office visits, confirmation of pregnancy by HCG, ultrasound to confirm duration of pregnancy, ultrasound to confirm completion of abortion) except drugs ♀

⊘ **S0201** Partial hospitalization services, less than 24 hours, per diem

⊘ **S0207** Paramedic intercept, non-hospital-based ALS service (non-voluntary), non-transport

⊘ **S0208** Paramedic intercept, hospital-based ALS service (non-voluntary), non-transport

⊘ **S0209** Wheelchair van, mileage, per mile

⊘ **S0215** Non-emergency transportation; mileage per mile

⊘ **S0220** Medical conference by a physician with interdisciplinary team of health professionals or representatives of community agencies to coordinate activities of patient care (patient is present); approximately 30 minutes

⊘ **S0221** Medical conference by a physician with interdisciplinary team of health professionals or representatives of community agencies to coordinate activities of patient care (patient is present); approximately 60 minutes

⊘ **S0250** Comprehensive geriatric assessment and treatment planning performed by assessment team [A]

⊘ **S0255** Hospice referral visit (advising patient and family of care options) performed by nurse, social worker, or other designated staff

⊘ **S0257** Counseling and discussion regarding advance directives or end of life care planning and decisions, with patient and/or surrogate (list separately in addition to code for appropriate evaluation and management service)

⊘ **S0260** History and physical (outpatient or office) related to surgical procedure (list separately in addition to code for appropriate evaluation and management service)

⊘ **S0265** Genetic counseling, under physician supervision, each 15 minutes

⊘ **S0270** Physician management of patient home care, standard monthly case rate (per 30 days)

⊘ **S0271** Physician management of patient home care, hospice monthly case rate (per 30 days)

⊘ **S0272** Physician management of patient home care, episodic care monthly case rate (per 30 days)

⊘ **S0273** Physician visit at member's home, outside of a capitation arrangement

⊘ **S0274** Nurse practitioner visit at member's home, outside of a capitation arrangement

⊘ **S0280** Medical home program, comprehensive care coordination and planning, initial plan

⊘ **S0281** Medical home program, comprehensive care coordination and planning, maintenance of plan

⊘ **S0285** Colonoscopy consultation performed prior to a screening colonoscopy procedure

⊘ **S0302** Completed Early Periodic Screening Diagnosis and Treatment (EPSDT) service (list in addition to code for appropriate evaluation and management service) [A]

⊘ **S0310** Hospitalist services (list separately in addition to code for appropriate evaluation and management service)

⊘ **S0311** Comprehensive management and care coordination for advanced illness, per calendar month

⊘ **S0315** Disease management program; initial assessment and initiation of the program

⊘ **S0316** Disease management program; follow-up/reassessment

⊘ **S0317** Disease management program; per diem

⊘ **S0320** Telephone calls by a registered nurse to a disease management program member for monitoring purposes; per month

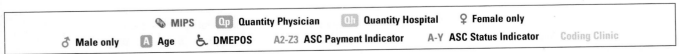

⊘ **S0340** Lifestyle modification program for management of coronary artery disease, including all supportive services; first quarter/stage

⊘ **S0341** Lifestyle modification program for management of coronary artery disease, including all supportive services; second or third quarter/stage

⊘ **S0342** Lifestyle modification program for management of coronary artery disease, including all supportive services; fourth quarter/stage

⊘ **S0353** Treatment planning and care coordination management for cancer, initial treatment

⊘ **S0354** Treatment planning and care coordination management for cancer, established patient with a change of regimen

⊘ **S0390** Routine foot care; removal and/or trimming of corns, calluses and/or nails and preventive maintenance in specific medical conditions (e.g., diabetes), per visit

⊘ **S0395** Impression casting of a foot performed by a practitioner other than the manufacturer of the orthotic

⊘ **S0400** Global fee for extracorporeal shock wave lithotripsy treatment of kidney stone(s)

Vision Supplies

⊘ **S0500** Disposable contact lens, per lens

⊘ **S0504** Single vision prescription lens (safety, athletic, or sunglass), per lens

⊘ **S0506** Bifocal vision prescription lens (safety, athletic, or sunglass), per lens

⊘ **S0508** Trifocal vision prescription lens (safety, athletic, or sunglass), per lens

⊘ **S0510** Non-prescription lens (safety, athletic, or sunglass), per lens

⊘ **S0512** Daily wear specialty contact lens, per lens

⊘ **S0514** Color contact lens, per lens

⊘ **S0515** Scleral lens, liquid bandage device, per lens

⊘ **S0516** Safety eyeglass frames

⊘ **S0518** Sunglasses frames

⊘ **S0580** Polycarbonate lens (list this code in addition to the basic code for the lens)

⊘ **S0581** Nonstandard lens (list this code in addition to the basic code for the lens)

⊘ **S0590** Integral lens service, miscellaneous services reported separately

⊘ **S0592** Comprehensive contact lens evaluation

⊘ **S0595** Dispensing new spectacle lenses for patient supplied frame

⊘ **S0596** Phakic intraocular lens for correction of refractive error

Screening and Examinations

⊘ **S0601** Screening proctoscopy

⊘ **S0610** Annual gynecological examination, new patient ♀

⊘ **S0612** Annual gynecological examination, established patient ♀

⊘ **S0613** Annual gynecological examination; clinical breast examination without pelvic evaluation ♀

⊘ **S0618** Audiometry for hearing aid evaluation to determine the level and degree of hearing loss

⊘ **S0620** Routine ophthalmological examination including refraction; new patient

Many non-Medicare vision plans may require code for routine encounter, no complaints

⊘ **S0621** Routine ophthalmological examination including refraction; established patient

Many non-Medicare vision plans may require code for routine encounter, no complaints

⊘ **S0622** Physical exam for college, new or established patient (list separately) in addition to appropriate evaluation and management code Ⓐ

Provider Services and Supplies

⊘ **S0630** Removal of sutures; by a physician other than the physician who originally closed the wound

⊘ **S0800** Laser in situ keratomileusis (LASIK)

▶ New   ↻ Revised   ✔ Reinstated   ~~deleted~~ Deleted   ⊘ Not covered or valid by Medicare

⊙ Special coverage instructions   ✳ Carrier discretion   Ⓑ Bill Part B MAC   Ⓑ Bill DME MAC

Figure 48
Phototherapeutic keratectomy (PRK).

⊘ **S0810** Photorefractive keratectomy (PRK)

⊘ **S0812** Phototherapeutic keratectomy (PTK)

⊘ **S1001** Deluxe item, patient aware (list in addition to code for basic item)

⊘ **S1002** Customized item (list in addition to code for basic item)

⊘ **S1015** IV tubing extension set

⊘ **S1016** Non-PVC (polyvinyl chloride) intravenous administration set, for use with drugs that are not stable in PVC (e.g., paclitaxel)

⊘ **S1030** Continuous noninvasive glucose monitoring device, purchase (for physician interpretation of data, use CPT code)

⊘ **S1031** Continuous noninvasive glucose monitoring device, rental, including sensor, sensor replacement, and download to monitor (for physician interpretation of data, use CPT code)

⊘ **S1034** Artificial pancreas device system (e.g., low glucose suspend (LGS) feature) including continuous glucose monitor, blood glucose device, insulin pump and computer algorithm that communicates with all of the devices

⊘ **S1035** Sensor; invasive (e.g., subcutaneous), disposable, for use with artificial pancreas device system

⊘ **S1036** Transmitter; external, for use with artificial pancreas device system

⊘ **S1037** Receiver (monitor); external, for use with artificial pancreas device system

⊘ **S1040** Cranial remolding orthosis, pediatric, rigid, with soft interface material, custom fabricated, includes fitting and adjustment(s) **A**

⊘ **S1091** Stent, non-coronary, temporary, with delivery system (propel)

⊘ **S2053** Transplantation of small intestine and liver allografts

⊘ **S2054** Transplantation of multivisceral organs

⊘ **S2055** Harvesting of donor multivisceral organs, with preparation and maintenance of allografts; from cadaver donor

⊘ **S2060** Lobar lung transplantation

⊘ **S2061** Donor lobectomy (lung) for transplantation, living donor

⊘ **S2065** Simultaneous pancreas kidney transplantation

⊘ **S2066** Breast reconstruction with gluteal artery perforator (GAP) flap, including harvesting of the flap, microvascular transfer, closure of donor site and shaping the flap into a breast, unilateral ♀

⊘ **S2067** Breast reconstruction of a single breast with "stacked" deep inferior epigastric perforator (DIEP) flap(s) and/or gluteal artery perforator (GAP) flap(s), including harvesting of the flap(s), microvascular transfer, closure of donor site(s) and shaping the flap into a breast, unilateral ♀

⊘ **S2068** Breast reconstruction with deep inferior epigastric perforator (DIEP) flap, or superficial inferior epigastric artery (SIEA) flap, including harvesting of the flap, microvascular transfer, closure of donor site and shaping the flap into a breast, unilateral ♀

⊘ **S2070** Cystourethroscopy, with ureteroscopy and/or pyeloscopy; with endoscopic laser treatment of ureteral calculi (includes ureteral catheterization)

⊘ **S2079** Laparoscopic esophagomyotomy (Heller type)

⊘ **S2080** Laser-assisted uvulopalatoplasty (LAUP)

⊘ **S2083** Adjustment of gastric band diameter via subcutaneous port by injection or aspiration of saline

Figure 49 Gastric band.

⊘ **S2095** Transcatheter occlusion or embolization for tumor destruction, percutaneous, any method, using yttrium-90 microspheres

⊘ **S2102** Islet cell tissue transplant from pancreas; allogeneic

⊘ **S2103** Adrenal tissue transplant to brain

⊘ **S2107** Adoptive immunotherapy i.e. development of specific anti-tumor reactivity (e.g., tumor-infiltrating lymphocyte therapy) per course of treatment

⊘ **S2112** Arthroscopy, knee, surgical for harvesting of cartilage (chondrocyte cells)

⊘ **S2115** Osteotomy, periacetabular, with internal fixation

⊘ **S2117** Arthroereisis, subtalar

⊘ **S2118** Metal-on-metal total hip resurfacing, including acetabular and femoral components

⊘ **S2120** Low density lipoprotein (LDL) apheresis using heparin-induced extracorporeal LDL precipitation

⊘ **S2140** Cord blood harvesting for transplantation, allogeneic

⊘ **S2142** Cord blood-derived stem cell transplantation, allogeneic

⊘ **S2150** Bone marrow or blood-derived stem cells (peripheral or umbilical), allogeneic or autologous, harvesting, transplantation, and related complications; including: pheresis and cell preparation/storage; marrow ablative therapy; drugs, supplies, hospitalization with outpatient follow-up; medical/surgical, diagnostic, emergency, and rehabilitative services; and the number of days of pre- and post-transplant care in the global definition

⊘ **S2152** Solid organ(s), complete or segmental, single organ or combination of organs; deceased or living donor(s), procurement, transplantation, and related complications; including: drugs; supplies; hospitalization with outpatient follow-up; medical/surgical, diagnostic, emergency, and rehabilitative services, and the number of days of pre- and post-transplant care in the global definition

⊘ **S2202** Echosclerotherapy

⊘ **S2205** Minimally invasive direct coronary artery bypass surgery involving mini-thoracotomy or mini-sternotomy surgery, performed under direct vision; using arterial graft(s), single coronary arterial graft

⊘ **S2206** Minimally invasive direct coronary artery bypass surgery involving mini-thoracotomy or mini-sternotomy surgery, performed under direct vision; using arterial graft(s), two coronary arterial grafts

⊘ **S2207** Minimally invasive direct coronary artery bypass surgery involving mini-thoracotomy or mini-sternotomy surgery, performed under direct vision; using venous graft only, single coronary venous graft

⊘ **S2208** Minimally invasive direct coronary artery bypass surgery involving mini-thoracotomy or mini-sternotomy surgery, performed under direct vision; using single arterial and venous graft(s), single venous graft

⊘ **S2209** Minimally invasive direct coronary artery bypass surgery involving mini-thoracotomy or mini-sternotomy surgery, performed under direct vision; using two arterial grafts and single venous graft

⊘ **S2225** Myringotomy, laser-assisted

⊘ **S2230** Implantation of magnetic component of semi-implantable hearing device on ossicles in middle ear

⊘ **S2235** Implantation of auditory brain stem implant

⊘ **S2260** Induced abortion, 17 to 24 weeks ♀

⊘ **S2265** Induced abortion, 25 to 28 weeks ♀

⊘ **S2266** Induced abortion, 29 to 31 weeks ♀

⊘ **S2267** Induced abortion, 32 weeks or greater ♀

⊘ **S2300** Arthroscopy, shoulder, surgical; with thermally-induced capsulorrhaphy

⊘ **S2325** Hip core decompression

Coding Clinic: 2017, Q3, P1

⊘ **S2340** Chemodenervation of abductor muscle(s) of vocal cord

⊘ **S2341** Chemodenervation of adductor muscle(s) of vocal cord

⊘ **S2342** Nasal endoscopy for post-operative debridement following functional endoscopic sinus surgery, nasal and/or sinus cavity(s), unilateral or bilateral

▶ New   ↻ Revised   ✔ Reinstated   ~~deleted~~ Deleted   ⊘ Not covered or valid by Medicare   ✲ Special coverage instructions   ✳ Carrier discretion   Ⓑ Bill Part B MAC   Ⓓ Bill DME MAC

418

⊘ **S2348** Decompression procedure, percutaneous, of nucleus pulpous of intervertebral disc, using radiofrequency energy, single or multiple levels, lumbar

⊘ **S2350** Diskectomy, anterior, with decompression of spinal cord and/or nerve root(s), including osteophytectomy; lumbar, single interspace

⊘ **S2351** Diskectomy, anterior, with decompression of spinal cord and/or nerve root(s) including osteophytectomy; lumbar, each additional interspace (list separately in addition to code for primary procedure)

⊘ **S2400** Repair, congenital diaphragmatic hernia in the fetus using temporary tracheal occlusion, procedure performed in utero ♀ A

⊘ **S2401** Repair, urinary tract obstruction in the fetus, procedure performed in utero ♀ A

⊘ **S2402** Repair, congenital cystic adenomatoid malformation in the fetus, procedure performed in utero ♀ A

⊘ **S2403** Repair, extralobar pulmonary sequestration in the fetus, procedure performed in utero ♀ A

⊘ **S2404** Repair, myelomeningocele in the fetus, procedure performed in utero ♀ A

⊘ **S2405** Repair of sacrococcygeal teratoma in the fetus, procedure performed in utero ♀ A

⊘ **S2409** Repair, congenital malformation of fetus, procedure performed in utero, not otherwise classified ♀ A

⊘ **S2411** Fetoscopic laser therapy for treatment of twin-to-twin transfusion syndrome A

⊘ **S2900** Surgical techniques requiring use of robotic surgical system (list separately in addition to code for primary procedure)

Coding Clinic: 2010, Q2, P6

⊘ **S3000** Diabetic indicator; retinal eye exam, dilated, bilateral

⊘ **S3005** Performance measurement, evaluation of patient self assessment, depression

⊘ **S3600** STAT laboratory request (situations other than S3601)

⊘ **S3601** Emergency STAT laboratory charge for patient who is homebound or residing in a nursing facility

⊘ **S3620** Newborn metabolic screening panel, includes test kit, postage and the laboratory tests specified by the state for inclusion in this panel (e.g., galactose; hemoglobin, electrophoresis; hydroxyprogesterone, 17-D; phenylalanine (PKU); and thyroxine, total) A

⊘ **S3630** Eosinophil count, blood, direct

⊘ **S3645** HIV-1 antibody testing of oral mucosal transudate

⊘ **S3650** Saliva test, hormone level; during menopause ♀

⊘ **S3652** Saliva test, hormone level; to assess preterm labor risk ♀

⊘ **S3655** Antisperm antibodies test (immunobead) ♀

⊘ **S3708** Gastrointestinal fat absorption study

⊘ **S3722** Dose optimization by area under the curve (AUC) analysis, for infusional 5-fluorouracil

Genetic Testing

⊘ **S3800** Genetic testing for amyotrophic lateral sclerosis (ALS)

⊘ **S3840** DNA analysis for germline mutations of the RET proto-oncogene for susceptibility to multiple endocrine neoplasia type 2

⊘ **S3841** Genetic testing for retinoblastoma

⊘ **S3842** Genetic testing for von Hippel-Lindau disease

⊘ **S3844** DNA analysis of the connexin 26 gene (GJB2) for susceptibility to congenital, profound deafness

⊘ **S3845** Genetic testing for alpha-thalassemia

⊘ **S3846** Genetic testing for hemoglobin E beta-thalassemia

⊘ **S3849** Genetic testing for Niemann-Pick disease

⊘ **S3850** Genetic testing for sickle cell anemia

⊘ **S3852** DNA analysis for APOE epilson 4 allele for susceptibility to Alzheimer's disease

⊘ **S3853** Genetic testing for myotonic muscular dystrophy

⊘ **S3854** Gene expression profiling panel for use in the management of breast cancer treatment ♀

⊘ **S3861** Genetic testing, sodium channel, voltage-gated, type V, alpha subunit (SCN5A) and variants for suspected Brugada syndrome

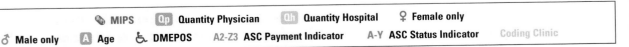

⊘ **S3865** Comprehensive gene sequence analysis for hypertrophic cardiomyopathy

⊘ **S3866** Genetic analysis for a specific gene mutation for hypertrophic cardiomyopathy (HCM) in an individual with a known HCM mutation in the family

⊘ **S3870** Comparative genomic hybridization (CGH) microarray testing for developmental delay, autism spectrum disorder and/or intellectual disability

Other Tests

⊘ **S3900** Surface electromyography (EMG)

⊘ **S3902** Ballistrocardiogram

⊘ **S3904** Masters two step

Bill on paper. Requires a report.

Obstetric and Fertility Services

⊘ **S4005** Interim labor facility global (labor occurring but not resulting in delivery) ♀

⊘ **S4011** In vitro fertilization; including but not limited to identification and incubation of mature oocytes, fertilization with sperm, incubation of embryo(s), and subsequent visualization for determination of development ♀

⊘ **S4013** Complete cycle, gamete intrafallopian transfer (GIFT), case rate ♀

⊘ **S4014** Complete cycle, zygote intrafallopian transfer (ZIFT), case rate ♀

⊘ **S4015** Complete in vitro fertilization cycle, not otherwise specified, case rate ♀

⊘ **S4016** Frozen in vitro fertilization cycle, case rate ♀

⊘ **S4017** Incomplete cycle, treatment cancelled prior to stimulation, case rate ♀

⊘ **S4018** Frozen embryo transfer procedure cancelled before transfer, case rate ♀

⊘ **S4020** In vitro fertilization procedure cancelled before aspiration, case rate ♀

⊘ **S4021** In vitro fertilization procedure cancelled after aspiration, case rate ♀

⊘ **S4022** Assisted oocyte fertilization, case rate ♀

⊘ **S4023** Donor egg cycle, incomplete, case rate ♀

⊘ **S4025** Donor services for in vitro fertilization (sperm or embryo), case rate

⊘ **S4026** Procurement of donor sperm from sperm bank ♂

⊘ **S4027** Storage of previously frozen embryos ♀

⊘ **S4028** Microsurgical epididymal sperm aspiration (MESA) ♂

⊘ **S4030** Sperm procurement and cryopreservation services; initial visit ♂

⊘ **S4031** Sperm procurement and cryopreservation services; subsequent visit ♂

⊘ **S4035** Stimulated intrauterine insemination (IUI), case rate ♀

⊘ **S4037** Cryopreserved embryo transfer, case rate ♀

⊘ **S4040** Monitoring and storage of cryopreserved embryos, per 30 days ♀

⊘ **S4042** Management of ovulation induction (interpretation of diagnostic tests and studies, non-face-to-face medical management of the patient), per cycle ♀

⊘ **S4981** Insertion of levonorgestrel-releasing intrauterine system ♀

⊘ **S4989** Contraceptive intrauterine device (e.g., Progestasert IUD), including implants and supplies ♀

Therapeutic Substances and Medications

⊘ **S4990** Nicotine patches, legend

⊘ **S4991** Nicotine patches, non-legend

⊘ **S4993** Contraceptive pills for birth control ♀

Only billed by Family Planning Clinics

⊘ **S4995** Smoking cessation gum

⊘ **S5000** Prescription drug, generic

⊘ **S5001** Prescription drug, brand name

Figure 50 IUD.

⊘ **S5010** 5% dextrose and 0.45% normal saline, 1000 ml

⊘ **S5012** 5% dextrose with potassium chloride, 1000 ml

⊘ **S5013** 5% dextrose/0.45% normal saline with potassium chloride and magnesium sulfate, 1000 ml

⊘ **S5014** 5% dextrose/0.45% normal saline with potassium chloride and magnesium sulfate, 1500 ml

Home Care Services

⊘ **S5035** Home infusion therapy, routine service of infusion device (e.g., pump maintenance)

⊘ **S5036** Home infusion therapy, repair of infusion device (e.g., pump repair)

⊘ **S5100** Day care services, adult; per 15 minutes [A]

⊘ **S5101** Day care services, adult; per half day [A]

⊘ **S5102** Day care services, adult; per diem [A]

⊘ **S5105** Day care services, center-based; services not included in program fee, per diem

⊘ **S5108** Home care training to home care client, per 15 minutes

⊘ **S5109** Home care training to home care client, per session

⊘ **S5110** Home care training, family; per 15 minutes

⊘ **S5111** Home care training, family; per session

⊘ **S5115** Home care training, non-family; per 15 minutes

⊘ **S5116** Home care training, non-family; per session

⊘ **S5120** Chore services; per 15 minutes

⊘ **S5121** Chore services; per diem

⊘ **S5125** Attendant care services; per 15 minutes

⊘ **S5126** Attendant care services; per diem

⊘ **S5130** Homemaker service, NOS; per 15 minutes

⊘ **S5131** Homemaker service, NOS; per diem

⊘ **S5135** Companion care, adult (e.g., IADL/ADL); per 15 minutes [A]

⊘ **S5136** Companion care, adult (e.g., IADL/ADL); per diem [A]

⊘ **S5140** Foster care, adult; per diem [A]

⊘ **S5141** Foster care, adult; per month [A]

⊘ **S5145** Foster care, therapeutic, child; per diem [A]

⊘ **S5146** Foster care, therapeutic, child; per month [A]

⊘ **S5150** Unskilled respite care, not hospice; per 15 minutes

⊘ **S5151** Unskilled respite care, not hospice; per diem

⊘ **S5160** Emergency response system; installation and testing

⊘ **S5161** Emergency response system; service fee, per month (excludes installation and testing)

⊘ **S5162** Emergency response system; purchase only

⊘ **S5165** Home modifications; per service

⊘ **S5170** Home delivered meals, including preparation; per meal

⊘ **S5175** Laundry service, external, professional; per order

⊘ **S5180** Home health respiratory therapy, initial evaluation

⊘ **S5181** Home health respiratory therapy, NOS, per diem

⊘ **S5185** Medication reminder service, non-face-to-face; per month

⊘ **S5190** Wellness assessment, performed by non-physician

⊘ **S5199** Personal care item, NOS, each

Home Infusion Therapy

⊘ **S5497** Home infusion therapy, catheter care/maintenance, not otherwise classified; includes administrative services, professional pharmacy services, care coordination, and all necessary supplies and equipment (drugs and nursing visits coded separately), per diem

⊘ **S5498** Home infusion therapy, catheter care/maintenance, simple (single lumen), includes administrative services, professional pharmacy services, care coordination and all necessary supplies and equipment, (drugs and nursing visits coded separately), per diem

⊘ **S5501** Home infusion therapy, catheter care/maintenance, complex (more than one lumen), includes administrative services, professional pharmacy services, care coordination, and all necessary supplies and equipment (drugs and nursing visits coded separately), per diem

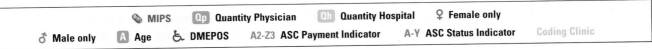

🪶 MIPS   [Qp] **Quantity Physician**   [Qh] **Quantity Hospital**   ♀ **Female only**   ♂ **Male only**   [A] **Age**   ♿ **DMEPOS**   A2-Z3 **ASC Payment Indicator**   A-Y **ASC Status Indicator**   Coding Clinic

⊘ **S5502** Home infusion therapy, catheter care/maintenance, implanted access device, includes administrative services, professional pharmacy services, care coordination, and all necessary supplies and equipment, (drugs and nursing visits coded separately), per diem (use this code for interim maintenance of vascular access not currently in use)

⊘ **S5517** Home infusion therapy, all supplies necessary for restoration of catheter patency or declotting

⊘ **S5518** Home infusion therapy, all supplies necessary for catheter repair

⊘ **S5520** Home infusion therapy, all supplies (including catheter) necessary for a peripherally inserted central venous catheter (PICC) line insertion

Bill on paper. Requires a report.

⊘ **S5521** Home infusion therapy, all supplies (including catheter) necessary for a midline catheter insertion

⊘ **S5522** Home infusion therapy, insertion of peripherally inserted central venous catheter (PICC), nursing services only (no supplies or catheter included)

⊘ **S5523** Home infusion therapy, insertion of midline central venous catheter, nursing services only (no supplies or catheter included)

Insulin Services

⊘ **S5550** Insulin, rapid onset, 5 units

⊘ **S5551** Insulin, most rapid onset (Lispro or Aspart); 5 units

⊘ **S5552** Insulin, intermediate acting (NPH or Lente); 5 units

⊘ **S5553** Insulin, long acting; 5 units

⊘ **S5560** Insulin delivery device, reusable pen; 1.5 ml size

⊘ **S5561** Insulin delivery device, reusable pen; 3 ml size

⊘ **S5565** Insulin cartridge for use in insulin delivery device other than pump; 150 units

⊘ **S5566** Insulin cartridge for use in insulin delivery device other than pump; 300 units

Figure 51 Nova pen.

⊘ **S5570** Insulin delivery device, disposable pen (including insulin); 1.5 ml size

⊘ **S5571** Insulin delivery device, disposable pen (including insulin); 3 ml size

Imaging

⊘ **S8030** Scleral application of tantalum ring(s) for localization of lesions for proton beam therapy

⊘ **S8035** Magnetic source imaging

⊘ **S8037** Magnetic resonance cholangiopancreatography (MRCP)

⊘ **S8040** Topographic brain mapping

⊘ **S8042** Magnetic resonance imaging (MRI), low-field

⊘ **S8055** Ultrasound guidance for multifetal pregnancy reduction(s), technical component (only to be used when the physician doing the reduction procedure does not perform the ultrasound, guidance is included in the CPT code for multifetal pregnancy reduction - 59866) ♀

⊘ **S8080** Scintimammography (radioimmunoscintigraphy of the breast), unilateral, including supply of radiopharmaceutical ♀

⊘ **S8085** Fluorine-18 fluorodeoxyglucose (F-18 FDG) imaging using dual-head coincidence detection system (non-dedicated PET scan)

⊘ **S8092** Electron beam computed tomography (also known as ultrafast CT, cine CT)

Assistive Breathing Supplies

⊘ **S8096** Portable peak flow meter

⊘ **S8097** Asthma kit (including but not limited to portable peak expiratory flow meter, instructional video, brochure, and/or spacer)

⊘ **S8100** Holding chamber or spacer for use with an inhaler or nebulizer; without mask

⊘ **S8101** Holding chamber or spacer for use with an inhaler or nebulizer; with mask

⊘ **S8110** Peak expiratory flow rate (physician services)

⊘ **S8120** Oxygen contents, gaseous, 1 unit equals 1 cubic foot

⊘ **S8121** Oxygen contents, liquid, 1 unit equals 1 pound

▶ New   ↻ Revised   ✔ Reinstated   ~~deleted~~ Deleted   ⊘ Not covered or valid by Medicare
✿ Special coverage instructions   ✳ Carrier discretion   Ⓑ Bill Part B MAC   Ⓓ Bill DME MAC

⊘ **S8130** Interferential current stimulator, 2 channel

⊘ **S8131** Interferential current stimulator, 4 channel

⊘ **S8185** Flutter device

⊘ **S8186** Swivel adapter

⊘ **S8189** Tracheostomy supply, not otherwise classified

⊘ **S8210** Mucus trap

Miscellaneous Supplies and Services

⊘ **S8265** Haberman feeder for cleft lip/palate

⊘ **S8270** Enuresis alarm, using auditory buzzer and/or vibration device

⊘ **S8301** Infection control supplies, not otherwise specified

⊘ **S8415** Supplies for home delivery of infant Ⓐ

⊘ **S8420** Gradient pressure aid (sleeve and glove combination), custom made

⊘ **S8421** Gradient pressure aid (sleeve and glove combination), ready made

⊘ **S8422** Gradient pressure aid (sleeve), custom made, medium weight

⊘ **S8423** Gradient pressure aid (sleeve), custom made, heavy weight

⊘ **S8424** Gradient pressure aid (sleeve), ready made

⊘ **S8425** Gradient pressure aid (glove), custom made, medium weight

⊘ **S8426** Gradient pressure aid (glove), custom made, heavy weight

⊘ **S8427** Gradient pressure aid (glove), ready made

⊘ **S8428** Gradient pressure aid (gauntlet), ready made

⊘ **S8429** Gradient pressure exterior wrap

⊘ **S8430** Padding for compression bandage, roll

⊘ **S8431** Compression bandage, roll

⊘ **S8450** Splint, prefabricated, digit (specify digit by use of modifier)

⊘ **S8451** Splint, prefabricated, wrist or ankle

⊘ **S8452** Splint, prefabricated, elbow

⊘ **S8460** Camisole, post-mastectomy

⊘ **S8490** Insulin syringes (100 syringes, any size)

⊘ **S8930** Electrical stimulation of auricular acupuncture points; each 15 minutes of personal one-on-one contact with the patient

⊘ **S8940** Equestrian/Hippotherapy, per session

⊘ **S8948** Application of a modality (requiring constant provider attendance) to one or more areas; low-level laser; each 15 minutes

⊘ **S8950** Complex lymphedema therapy, each 15 minutes

⊘ **S8990** Physical or manipulative therapy performed for maintenance rather than restoration

⊘ **S8999** Resuscitation bag (for use by patient on artificial respiration during power failure or other catastrophic event)

⊘ **S9001** Home uterine monitor with or without associated nursing services ♀

⊘ **S9007** Ultrafiltration monitor

⊘ **S9024** Paranasal sinus ultrasound

⊘ **S9025** Omnicardiogram/cardiointegram

⊘ **S9034** Extracorporeal shockwave lithotripsy for gall stones (if performed with ERCP, use 43265)

⊘ **S9055** Procuren or other growth factor preparation to promote wound healing

⊘ **S9056** Coma stimulation per diem

⊘ **S9061** Home administration of aerosolized drug therapy (e.g., pentamidine); administrative services, professional pharmacy services, care coordination, all necessary supplies and equipment (drugs and nursing visits coded separately), per diem

⊘ **S9083** Global fee urgent care centers

⊘ **S9088** Services provided in an urgent care center (list in addition to code for service)

⊘ **S9090** Vertebral axial decompression, per session

⊘ **S9097** Home visit for wound care

⊘ **S9098** Home visit, phototherapy services (e.g., Bili-Lite), including equipment rental, nursing services, blood draw, supplies, and other services, per diem

⊘ **S9110** Telemonitoring of patient in their home, including all necessary equipment; computer system, connections, and software; maintenance; patient education and support; per month

⊘ **S9117** Back school, per visit

⊘ **S9122** Home health aide or certified nurse assistant, providing care in the home; per hour

---

🅜 MIPS	Ⓠp Quantity Physician	Ⓠh Quantity Hospital	♀ Female only
♂ Male only	Ⓐ Age	♿ DMEPOS	A2-Z3 ASC Payment Indicator	A-Y ASC Status Indicator	Coding Clinic

⊘ **S9123** Nursing care, in the home; by registered nurse, per hour (use for general nursing care only, not to be used when CPT codes 99500-99602 can be used)

⊘ **S9124** Nursing care, in the home; by licensed practical nurse, per hour

⊘ **S9125** Respite care, in the home, per diem

⊘ **S9126** Hospice care, in the home, per diem

⊘ **S9127** Social work visit, in the home, per diem

⊘ **S9128** Speech therapy, in the home, per diem

⊘ **S9129** Occupational therapy, in the home, per diem

⊘ **S9131** Physical therapy; in the home, per diem

⊘ **S9140** Diabetic management program, follow-up visit to non-MD provider

⊘ **S9141** Diabetic management program, follow-up visit to MD provider

⊘ **S9145** Insulin pump initiation, instruction in initial use of pump (pump not included)

⊘ **S9150** Evaluation by ocularist

⊘ **S9152** Speech therapy, re-evaluation

Home Management of Pregnancy

⊘ **S9208** Home management of preterm labor, including administrative services, professional pharmacy services, care coordination, and all necessary supplies or equipment (drugs and nursing visits coded separately), per diem (do not use this code with any home infusion per diem code) ♀

⊘ **S9209** Home management of preterm premature rupture of membranes (PPROM), including administrative services, professional pharmacy services, care coordination, and all necessary supplies or equipment (drugs and nursing visits coded separately), per diem (do not use this code with any home infusion per diem code) ♀

⊘ **S9211** Home management of gestational hypertension, includes administrative services, professional pharmacy services, care coordination, and all necessary supplies and equipment (drugs and nursing visits coded separately); per diem (do not use this code with any home infusion per diem code) ♀

⊘ **S9212** Home management of postpartum hypertension, includes administrative services, professional pharmacy services, care coordination, and all necessary supplies and equipment (drugs and nursing visits coded separately), per diem (do not use this code with any home infusion per diem code) ♀

⊘ **S9213** Home management of preeclampsia, includes administrative services, professional pharmacy services, care coordination, and all necessary supplies and equipment (drugs and nursing services coded separately); per diem (do not use this code with any home infusion per diem code) ♀

⊘ **S9214** Home management of gestational diabetes, includes administrative services, professional pharmacy services, care coordination, and all necessary supplies and equipment (drugs and nursing visits coded separately); per diem (do not use this code with any home infusion per diem code) ♀

Home Infusion Therapy

⊘ **S9325** Home infusion therapy, pain management infusion; administrative services, professional pharmacy services, care coordination, and all necessary supplies and equipment, (drugs and nursing visits coded separately), per diem (do not use this code with S9326, S9327 or S9328)

⊘ **S9326** Home infusion therapy, continuous (twenty-four hours or more) pain management infusion; administrative services, professional pharmacy services, care coordination, and all necessary supplies and equipment (drugs and nursing visits coded separately), per diem

⊘ **S9327** Home infusion therapy, intermittent (less than twenty-four hours) pain management infusion; administrative services, professional pharmacy services, care coordination, and all necessary supplies and equipment (drugs and nursing visits coded separately), per diem

▶ New   ↻ Revised   ✔ Reinstated   ~~deleted~~ Deleted   ⊘ Not covered or valid by Medicare
✧ Special coverage instructions   ✳ Carrier discretion   Ⓟ Bill Part B MAC   Ⓓ Bill DME MAC

⊘ **S9328** Home infusion therapy, implanted pump pain management infusion; administrative services, professional pharmacy services, care coordination, and all necessary supplies and equipment (drugs and nursing visits coded separately), per diem

⊘ **S9329** Home infusion therapy, chemotherapy infusion; administrative services, professional pharmacy services, care coordination, and all necessary supplies and equipment (drugs and nursing visits coded separately), per diem (do not use this code with S9330 or S9331)

⊘ **S9330** Home infusion therapy, continuous (twenty-four hours or more) chemotherapy infusion; administrative services, professional pharmacy services, care coordination, and all necessary supplies and equipment (drugs and nursing visits coded separately), per diem

⊘ **S9331** Home infusion therapy, intermittent (less than twenty-four hours) chemotherapy infusion; administrative services, professional pharmacy services, care coordination, and all necessary supplies and equipment (drugs and nursing visits coded separately), per diem

⊘ **S9335** Home therapy, hemodialysis; administrative services, professional pharmacy services, care coordination, and all necessary supplies and equipment (drugs and nursing services coded separately), per diem

⊘ **S9336** Home infusion therapy, continuous anticoagulant infusion therapy (e.g., heparin), administrative services, professional pharmacy services, care coordination, and all necessary supplies and equipment (drugs and nursing visits coded separately), per diem

⊘ **S9338** Home infusion therapy, immunotherapy, administrative services, professional pharmacy services, care coordination, and all necessary supplies and equipment (drug and nursing visits coded separately), per diem

⊘ **S9339** Home therapy; peritoneal dialysis, administrative services, professional pharmacy services, care coordination and all necessary supplies and equipment (drugs and nursing visits coded separately), per diem

⊘ **S9340** Home therapy; enteral nutrition; administrative services, professional pharmacy services, care coordination, and all necessary supplies and equipment (enteral formula and nursing visits coded separately), per diem

⊘ **S9341** Home therapy; enteral nutrition via gravity; administrative services, professional pharmacy services, care coordination, and all necessary supplies and equipment (enteral formula and nursing visits coded separately), per diem

⊘ **S9342** Home therapy; enteral nutrition via pump; administrative services, professional pharmacy services, care coordination, and all necessary supplies and equipment (enteral formula and nursing visits coded separately), per diem

⊘ **S9343** Home therapy; enteral nutrition via bolus; administrative services, professional pharmacy services, care coordination, and all necessary supplies and equipment (enteral formula and nursing visits coded separately), per diem

⊘ **S9345** Home infusion therapy, anti-hemophilic agent infusion therapy (e.g., Factor VIII); administrative services, professional pharmacy services, care coordination, and all necessary supplies and equipment (drugs and nursing visits coded separately), per diem

⊘ **S9346** Home infusion therapy, alpha-1-proteinase inhibitor (e.g., Prolastin); administrative services, professional pharmacy services, care coordination, and all necessary supplies and equipment (drugs and nursing visits coded separately), per diem

⊘ **S9347** Home infusion therapy, uninterrupted, long-term, controlled rate intravenous or subcutaneous infusion therapy (e.g., Epoprostenol); administrative services, professional pharmacy services, care coordination, and all necessary supplies and equipment (drugs and nursing visits coded separately), per diem

⊘ **S9348** Home infusion therapy, sympathomimetic/inotropic agent infusion therapy (e.g., Dobutamine); administrative services, professional pharmacy services, care coordination, all necessary supplies and equipment (drugs and nursing visits coded separately), per diem

⊘ **S9349** Home infusion therapy, tocolytic infusion therapy; administrative services, professional pharmacy services, care coordination, and all necessary supplies and equipment (drugs and nursing visits coded separately), per diem

⊘ **S9351** Home infusion therapy, continuous or intermittent anti-emetic infusion therapy; administrative services, professional pharmacy services, care coordination, and all necessary supplies and equipment (drugs and visits coded separately), per diem

⊘ **S9353** Home infusion therapy, continuous insulin infusion therapy; administrative services, professional pharmacy services, care coordination, and all necessary supplies and equipment (drugs and nursing visits coded separately), per diem

⊘ **S9355** Home infusion therapy, chelation therapy; administrative services, professional pharmacy services, care coordination, and all necessary supplies and equipment (drugs and nursing visits coded separately), per diem

⊘ **S9357** Home infusion therapy, enzyme replacement intravenous therapy (e.g., Imiglucerase); administrative services, professional pharmacy services, care coordination, and all necessary supplies and equipment (drugs and nursing visits coded separately), per diem

⊘ **S9359** Home infusion therapy, anti-tumor necrosis factor intravenous therapy (e.g., Infliximab); administrative services, professional pharmacy services, care coordination, and all necessary supplies and equipment (drugs and nursing visits coded separately), per diem

⊘ **S9361** Home infusion therapy, diuretic intravenous therapy; administrative services, professional pharmacy services, care coordination, and all necessary supplies and equipment (drugs and nursing visits coded separately), per diem

⊘ **S9363** Home infusion therapy, anti-spasmotic therapy; administrative services, professional pharmacy services, care coordination, and all necessary supplies and equipment (drugs and nursing visits coded separately), per diem

⊘ **S9364** Home infusion therapy, total parenteral nutrition (TPN); administrative services, professional pharmacy services, care coordination, and all necessary supplies and equipment including standard TPN formula (lipids, specialty amino acid formulas, drugs other than in standard formula, and nursing visits coded separately) per diem (do not use with home infusion codes S9365-S9368 using daily volume scales)

⊘ **S9365** Home infusion therapy, total parenteral nutrition (TPN); one liter per day, administrative services, professional pharmacy services, care coordination, and all necessary supplies and equipment including standard TPN formula (lipids, specialty amino acid formulas, drugs other than in standard formula and nursing visits coded separately), per diem

⊘ **S9366** Home infusion therapy, total parenteral nutrition (TPN); more than one liter but no more than two liters per day, administrative services, professional pharmacy services, care coordination, and all necessary supplies and equipment including standard TPN formula (lipids, specialty amino acid formulas, drugs other than in standard formula and nursing visits coded separately), per diem

⊘ **S9367** Home infusion therapy, total parenteral nutrition (TPN); more than two liters but no more than three liters per day, administrative services, professional pharmacy services, care coordination, and all necessary supplies and equipment including standard TPN formula (lipids, specialty amino acid formulas, drugs other than in standard formula and nursing visits coded separately), per diem

⊘ **S9368** Home infusion therapy, total parenteral nutrition (TPN); more than three liters per day, administrative services, professional pharmacy services, care coordination, and all necessary supplies and equipment (including standard TPN formula; lipids, specialty amino acid formulas, drugs other than in standard formula and nursing visits coded separately), per diem

▶ New   ↻ Revised   ✔ Reinstated   deleted Deleted   ⊘ Not covered or valid by Medicare
⊚ Special coverage instructions   ✳ Carrier discretion   Ⓑ Bill Part B MAC   Ⓑ Bill DME MAC

⊘ **S9370** Home therapy, intermittent anti-emetic injection therapy; administrative services, professional pharmacy services, care coordination, and all necessary supplies and equipment (drugs and nursing visits coded separately), per diem

⊘ **S9372** Home therapy; intermittent anticoagulant injection therapy (e.g., heparin); administrative services, professional pharmacy services, care coordination, and all necessary supplies and equipment (drugs and nursing visits coded separately), per diem (do not use this code for flushing of infusion devices with heparin to maintain patency)

⊘ **S9373** Home infusion therapy, hydration therapy; administrative services, professional pharmacy services, care coordination, and all necessary supplies and equipment (drugs and nursing visits coded separately), per diem (do not use with hydration therapy codes S9374-S9377 using daily volume scales)

⊘ **S9374** Home infusion therapy, hydration therapy; one liter per day, administrative services, professional pharmacy services, care coordination, and all necessary supplies and equipment (drugs and nursing visits coded separately), per diem

⊘ **S9375** Home infusion therapy, hydration therapy; more than one liter but no more than two liters per day, administrative services, professional pharmacy services, care coordination, and all necessary supplies and equipment (drugs and nursing visits coded separately), per diem

⊘ **S9376** Home infusion therapy, hydration therapy; more than two liters but no more than three liters per day, administrative services, professional pharmacy services, care coordination, and all necessary supplies and equipment (drugs and nursing visits coded separately), per diem

⊘ **S9377** Home infusion therapy, hydration therapy; more than three liters per day, administrative services, professional pharmacy services, care coordination, and all necessary supplies (drugs and nursing visits coded separately), per diem

⊘ **S9379** Home infusion therapy, infusion therapy, not otherwise classified; administrative services, professional pharmacy services, care coordination, and all necessary supplies and equipment (drugs and nursing visits coded separately), per diem

Miscellaneous Supplies and Services

⊘ **S9381** Delivery or service to high risk areas requiring escort or extra protection, per visit

⊘ **S9401** Anticoagulation clinic, inclusive of all services except laboratory tests, per session

⊘ **S9430** Pharmacy compounding and dispensing services

⊘ **S9432** Medical foods for non-inborn errors of metabolism

⊘ **S9433** Medical food nutritionally complete, administered orally, providing 100% of nutritional intake

⊘ **S9434** Modified solid food supplements for inborn errors of metabolism

⊘ **S9435** Medical foods for inborn errors of metabolism

⊘ **S9436** Childbirth preparation/Lamaze classes, non-physician provider, per session ♀

⊘ **S9437** Childbirth refresher classes, non-physician provider, per session ♀

⊘ **S9438** Cesarean birth classes, non-physician provider, per session ♀

⊘ **S9439** VBAC (vaginal birth after cesarean) classes, non-physician provider, per session ♀

⊘ **S9441** Asthma education, non-physician provider, per session

⊘ **S9442** Birthing classes, non-physician provider, per session ♀

⊘ **S9443** Lactation classes, non-physician provider, per session ♀

⊘ **S9444** Parenting classes, non-physician provider, per session

⊘ **S9445** Patient education, not otherwise classified, non-physician provider, individual, per session

⊘ **S9446** Patient education, not otherwise classified, non-physician provider, group, per session

⊘ **S9447** Infant safety (including CPR) classes, non-physician provider, per session

⊘ **S9449** Weight management classes, non-physician provider, per session

---

🏷 MIPS   **Qp** Quantity Physician   **Qh** Quantity Hospital   ♀ Female only

♂ Male only   **A** Age   DMEPOS   A2-Z3 ASC Payment Indicator   A-Y ASC Status Indicator   Coding Clinic

⊘ **S9451** Exercise classes, non-physician provider, per session

⊘ **S9452** Nutrition classes, non-physician provider, per session

⊘ **S9453** Smoking cessation classes, non-physician provider, per session

⊘ **S9454** Stress management classes, non-physician provider, per session

⊘ **S9455** Diabetic management program, group session

⊘ **S9460** Diabetic management program, nurse visit

⊘ **S9465** Diabetic management program, dietitian visit

⊘ **S9470** Nutritional counseling, dietitian visit

⊘ **S9472** Cardiac rehabilitation program, non-physician provider, per diem

⊘ **S9473** Pulmonary rehabilitation program, non-physician provider, per diem

⊘ **S9474** Enterostomal therapy by a registered nurse certified in enterostomal therapy, per diem

⊘ **S9475** Ambulatory setting substance abuse treatment or detoxification services, per diem

⊘ **S9476** Vestibular rehabilitation program, non-physician provider, per diem

⊘ **S9480** Intensive outpatient psychiatric services, per diem

⊘ **S9482** Family stabilization services, per 15 minutes

⊘ **S9484** Crisis intervention mental health services, per hour

⊘ **S9485** Crisis intervention mental health services, per diem

Home Therapy Services

⊘ **S9490** Home infusion therapy, corticosteroid infusion; administrative services, professional pharmacy services, care coordination, and all necessary supplies and equipment (drugs and nursing visits coded separately), per diem

⊘ **S9494** Home infusion therapy, antibiotic, antiviral, or antifungal therapy; administrative services, professional pharmacy services, care coordination, and all necessary supplies and equipment (drugs and nursing visits coded separately) per diem (do not use this code with home infusion codes for hourly dosing schedules S9497-S9504)

⊘ **S9497** Home infusion therapy, antibiotic, antiviral, or antifungal therapy; once every 3 hours; administrative services, professional pharmacy services, care coordination, and all necessary supplies and equipment (drugs and nursing visits coded separately), per diem

⊘ **S9500** Home infusion therapy, antibiotic, antiviral, or antifungal therapy; once every 24 hours; administrative services, professional pharmacy services, care coordination, and all necessary supplies and equipment (drugs and nursing visits coded separately), per diem

⊘ **S9501** Home infusion therapy, antibiotic, antiviral, or antifungal therapy; once every 12 hours; administrative services, professional pharmacy services, care coordination, and all necessary supplies and equipment (drugs and nursing visits coded separately), per diem

⊘ **S9502** Home infusion therapy, antibiotic, antiviral, or antifungal therapy; once every 8 hours, administrative services, professional pharmacy services, care coordination, and all necessary supplies and equipment (drugs and nursing visits coded separately), per diem

⊘ **S9503** Home infusion therapy, antibiotic, antiviral, or antifungal; once every 6 hours; administrative services, professional pharmacy services, care coordination, and all necessary supplies and equipment (drugs and nursing visits coded separately), per diem

⊘ **S9504** Home infusion therapy, antibiotic, antiviral, or antifungal; once every 4 hours; administrative services, professional pharmacy services, care coordination, and all necessary supplies and equipment (drugs and nursing visits coded separately), per diem

⊘ **S9529** Routine venipuncture for collection of specimen(s), single home bound, nursing home, or skilled nursing facility patient

⊘ **S9537** Home therapy; hematopoietic hormone injection therapy (e.g., erythropoietin, G-CSF, GM-CSF); administrative services, professional pharmacy services, care coordination, and all necessary supplies and equipment (drugs and nursing visits coded separately), per diem

▶ New   ⟳ Revised   ✔ Reinstated   ~~deleted~~ Deleted   ⊘ Not covered or valid by Medicare   ⊙ Special coverage instructions   ✳ Carrier discretion   Ⓑ Bill Part B MAC   Ⓓ Bill DME MAC

⊘ **S9538** Home transfusion of blood product(s); administrative services, professional pharmacy services, care coordination, and all necessary supplies and equipment (blood products, drugs, and nursing visits coded separately), per diem

⊘ **S9542** Home injectable therapy; not otherwise classified, including administrative services, professional pharmacy services, care coordination, and all necessary supplies and equipment (drugs and nursing visits coded separately), per diem

⊘ **S9558** Home injectable therapy; growth hormone, including administrative services, professional pharmacy services, care coordination, and all necessary supplies and equipment (drugs and nursing visits coded separately), per diem

⊘ **S9559** Home injectable therapy; interferon, including administrative services, professional pharmacy services, care coordination, and all necessary supplies and equipment (drugs and nursing visits coded separately), per diem

⊘ **S9560** Home injectable therapy; hormonal therapy (e.g., Leuprolide, Goserelin), including administrative services, professional pharmacy services, care coordination, and all necessary supplies and equipment (drugs and nursing visits coded separately), per diem

⟲⊘ **S9562** Home injectable therapy, palivizumab, or other monoclonal antibody for rsv, including administrative services, professional pharmacy services, care coordination, and all necessary supplies and equipment (drugs and nursing visits coded separately), per diem

▶⊘ **S9563** Home injectable therapy, immunotherapy, including administrative services, professional pharmacy services, care coordination, and all necessary supplies and equipment (drugs and nursing visits coded separately), per diem

⊘ **S9590** Home therapy, irrigation therapy (e.g., sterile irrigation of an organ or anatomical cavity); including administrative services, professional pharmacy services, care coordination, and all necessary supplies and equipment (drugs and nursing visits coded separately), per diem

⊘ **S9810** Home therapy; professional pharmacy services for provision of infusion, specialty drug administration, and/or disease state management, not otherwise classified, per hour (do not use this code with any per diem code)

Other Services and Fees

⊘ **S9900** Services by journal-listed Christian Science Practitioner for the purpose of healing, per diem

⊘ **S9901** Services by a journal-listed Christian Science nurse, per hour

⊘ **S9960** Ambulance service, conventional air service, nonemergency transport, one way (fixed wing)

⊘ **S9961** Ambulance service, conventional air service, nonemergency transport, one way (rotary wing)

⊘ **S9970** Health club membership, annual

⊘ **S9975** Transplant related lodging, meals and transportation, per diem

⊘ **S9976** Lodging, per diem, not otherwise classified

⊘ **S9977** Meals, per diem, not otherwise specified

⊘ **S9981** Medical records copying fee, administrative

⊘ **S9982** Medical records copying fee, per page

⊘ **S9986** Not medically necessary service (patient is aware that service not medically necessary)

⊘ **S9988** Services provided as part of a Phase I clinical trial

⊘ **S9989** Services provided outside of the United States of America (list in addition to code(s) for services(s))

⊘ **S9990** Services provided as part of a Phase II clinical trial

⊘ **S9991** Services provided as part of a Phase III clinical trial

⊘ **S9992** Transportation costs to and from trial location and local transportation costs (e.g., fares for taxicab or bus) for clinical trial participant and one caregiver/companion

⊘ **S9994** Lodging costs (e.g., hotel charges) for clinical trial participant and one caregiver/companion

⊘ **S9996** Meals for clinical trial participant and one caregiver/companion

⊘ **S9999** Sales tax

🐾 MIPS	**Qp** Quantity Physician	**Qh** Quantity Hospital	♀ Female only
♂ Male only	**A** Age	👤 DMEPOS	A2-Z3 **ASC Payment Indicator**	A-Y **ASC Status Indicator**	Coding Clinic

TEMPORARY NATIONAL CODES ESTABLISHED BY MEDICAID (T1000-T9999)

Not Valid For Medicare

⊘ **T1000** Private duty/independent nursing service(s) - licensed, up to 15 minutes

⊘ **T1001** Nursing assessment/evaluation

⊘ **T1002** RN services, up to 15 minutes

⊘ **T1003** LPN/LVN services, up to 15 minutes

⊘ **T1004** Services of a qualified nursing aide, up to 15 minutes

⊘ **T1005** Respite care services, up to 15 minutes

⊘ **T1006** Alcohol and/or substance abuse services, family/couple counseling

⊘ **T1007** Alcohol and/or substance abuse services, treatment plan development and/or modification

⊘ **T1009** Child sitting services for children of the individual receiving alcohol and/or substance abuse services A

⊘ **T1010** Meals for individuals receiving alcohol and/or substance abuse services (when meals not included in the program)

⊘ **T1012** Alcohol and/or substance abuse services, skills development

⊘ **T1013** Sign language or oral interpretive services, per 15 minutes

⊘ **T1014** Telehealth transmission, per minute, professional services bill separately

⊘ **T1015** Clinic visit/encounter, all-inclusive

⊘ **T1016** Case Management, each 15 minutes

⊘ **T1017** Targeted Case Management, each 15 minutes

⊘ **T1018** School-based individualized education program (IEP) services, bundled

⊘ **T1019** Personal care services, per 15 minutes, not for an inpatient or resident of a hospital, nursing facility, ICF/MR or IMD, part of the individualized plan of treatment (code may not be used to identify services provided by home health aide or certified nurse assistant)

⊘ **T1020** Personal care services, per diem, not for an inpatient or resident of a hospital, nursing facility, ICF/MR or IMD, part of the individualized plan of treatment (code may not be used to identify services provided by home health aide or certified nurse assistant)

⊘ **T1021** Home health aide or certified nurse assistant, per visit

⊘ **T1022** Contracted home health agency services, all services provided under contract, per day

⊘ **T1023** Screening to determine the appropriateness of consideration of an individual for participation in a specified program, project or treatment protocol, per encounter

⊘ **T1024** Evaluation and treatment by an integrated, specialty team contracted to provide coordinated care to multiple or severely handicapped children, per encounter A

⊘ **T1025** Intensive, extended multidisciplinary services provided in a clinic setting to children with complex medical, physical, mental and psychosocial impairments, per diem A

⊘ **T1026** Intensive, extended multidisciplinary services provided in a clinic setting to children with complex medical, physical, medical and psychosocial impairments, per hour A

⊘ **T1027** Family training and counseling for child development, per 15 minutes A

⊘ **T1028** Assessment of home, physical and family environment, to determine suitability to meet patient's medical needs

⊘ **T1029** Comprehensive environmental lead investigation, not including laboratory analysis, per dwelling

⊘ **T1030** Nursing care, in the home, by registered nurse, per diem

⊘ **T1031** Nursing care, in the home, by licensed practical nurse, per diem

⊘ **T1032** Services performed by a doula birth worker, per 15 minutes

⊘ **T1033** Services performed by a doula birth worker, per diem

⊘ **T1040** Medicaid certified community behavioral health clinic services, per diem

⊘ **T1041** Medicaid certified community behavioral health clinic services, per month

⊘ **T1502** Administration of oral, intramuscular and/or subcutaneous medication by health care agency/professional, per visit

⊘ **T1503** Administration of medication, other than oral and/or injectable, by a health care agency/professional, per visit

▶ New ↻ Revised ✔ Reinstated ~~deleted~~ Deleted ⊘ Not covered or valid by Medicare 🔵 Special coverage instructions ✱ Carrier discretion Ⓑ Bill Part B MAC Ⓑ Bill DME MAC

⊘ **T1505** Electronic medication compliance management device, includes all components and accessories, not otherwise classified

⊘ **T1999** Miscellaneous therapeutic items and supplies, retail purchases, not otherwise classified; identify product in "remarks"

⊘ **T2001** Non-emergency transportation; patient attendant/escort

⊘ **T2002** Non-emergency transportation; per diem

⊘ **T2003** Non-emergency transportation; encounter/trip

⊘ **T2004** Non-emergency transport; commercial carrier, multi-pass

⊘ **T2005** Non-emergency transportation: stretcher van

⊘ **T2007** Transportation waiting time, air ambulance and non-emergency vehicle, one-half (1/2) hour increments

⊘ **T2010** Preadmission screening and resident review (PASRR) level I identification screening, per screen

⊘ **T2011** Preadmission screening and resident review (PASRR) level II evaluation, per evaluation

⊘ **T2012** Habilitation, educational, waiver; per diem

⊘ **T2013** Habilitation, educational, waiver; per hour

⊘ **T2014** Habilitation, prevocational, waiver; per diem

⊘ **T2015** Habilitation, prevocational, waiver; per hour

⊘ **T2016** Habilitation, residential, waiver; per diem

⊘ **T2017** Habilitation, residential, waiver; 15 minutes

⊘ **T2018** Habilitation, supported employment, waiver; per diem

⊘ **T2019** Habilitation, supported employment, waiver; per 15 minutes

⊘ **T2020** Day habilitation, waiver; per diem

⊘ **T2021** Day habilitation, waiver; per 15 minutes

⊘ **T2022** Case management, per month

⊘ **T2023** Targeted case management; per month

⊘ **T2024** Service assessment/plan of care development, waiver

⊘ **T2025** Waiver services; not otherwise specified (NOS)

⊘ **T2026** Specialized childcare, waiver; per diem

⊘ **T2027** Specialized childcare, waiver; per 15 minutes

⊘ **T2028** Specialized supply, not otherwise specified, waiver

⊘ **T2029** Specialized medical equipment, not otherwise specified, waiver

⊘ **T2030** Assisted living, waiver; per month

⊘ **T2031** Assisted living; waiver, per diem

⊘ **T2032** Residential care, not otherwise specified (NOS), waiver; per month

⊘ **T2033** Residential care, not otherwise specified (NOS), waiver; per diem

⊘ **T2034** Crisis intervention, waiver; per diem

⊘ **T2035** Utility services to support medical equipment and assistive technology/devices, waiver

⊘ **T2036** Therapeutic camping, overnight, waiver; each session

⊘ **T2037** Therapeutic camping, day, waiver; each session

⊘ **T2038** Community transition, waiver; per service

⊘ **T2039** Vehicle modifications, waiver; per service

⊘ **T2040** Financial management, self-directed, waiver; per 15 minutes

⊘ **T2041** Supports brokerage, self-directed, waiver; per 15 minutes

⊘ **T2042** Hospice routine home care; per diem

⊘ **T2043** Hospice continuous home care; per hour

⊘ **T2044** Hospice inpatient respite care; per diem

⊘ **T2045** Hospice general inpatient care; per diem

⊘ **T2046** Hospice long term care, room and board only; per diem

⊘ **T2047** Habilitation, prevocational, waiver; per 15 minutes

⊘ **T2048** Behavioral health; long-term care residential (non-acute care in a residential treatment program where stay is typically longer than 30 days), with room and board, per diem

⊘ **T2049** Non-emergency transportation; stretcher van, mileage; per mile

⊘ **T2101** Human breast milk processing, storage and distribution only ♀

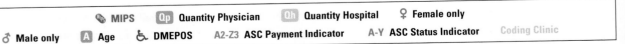

⊘ **T4521** Adult sized disposable incontinence product, brief/diaper, small, each Ⓐ
IOM: 100-03, 4, 280.1

⊘ **T4522** Adult sized disposable incontinence product, brief/diaper, medium, each Ⓐ
IOM: 100-03, 4, 280.1

⊘ **T4523** Adult sized disposable incontinence product, brief/diaper, large, each Ⓐ
IOM: 100-03, 4, 280.1

⊘ **T4524** Adult sized disposable incontinence product, brief/diaper, extra large, each Ⓐ
IOM: 100-03, 4, 280.1

⊘ **T4525** Adult sized disposable incontinence product, protective underwear/pull-on, small size, each Ⓐ
IOM: 100-03, 4, 280.1

⊘ **T4526** Adult sized disposable incontinence product, protective underwear/pull-on, medium size, each Ⓐ
IOM: 100-03, 4, 280.1

⊘ **T4527** Adult sized disposable incontinence product, protective underwear/pull-on, large size, each Ⓐ
IOM: 100-03, 4, 280.1

⊘ **T4528** Adult sized disposable incontinence product, protective underwear/pull-on, extra large size, each Ⓐ
IOM: 100-03, 4, 280.1

⊘ **T4529** Pediatric sized disposable incontinence product, brief/diaper, small/medium size, each Ⓐ
IOM: 100-03, 4, 280.1

⊘ **T4530** Pediatric sized disposable incontinence product, brief/diaper, large size, each Ⓐ
IOM: 100-03, 4, 280.1

⊘ **T4531** Pediatric sized disposable incontinence product, protective underwear/pull-on, small/medium size, each Ⓐ
IOM: 100-03, 4, 280.1

⊘ **T4532** Pediatric sized disposable incontinence product, protective underwear/pull-on, large size, each Ⓐ
IOM: 100-03, 4, 280.1

⊘ **T4533** Youth sized disposable incontinence product, brief/diaper, each Ⓐ
IOM: 100-03, 4, 280.1

⊘ **T4534** Youth sized disposable incontinence product, protective underwear/pull-on, each Ⓐ
IOM: 100-03, 4, 280.1

⊘ **T4535** Disposable liner/shield/guard/pad/undergarment, for incontinence, each
IOM: 100-03, 4, 280.1

⊘ **T4536** Incontinence product, protective underwear/pull-on, reusable, any size, each
IOM: 100-03, 4, 280.1

⊘ **T4537** Incontinence product, protective underpad, reusable, bed size, each
IOM: 100-03, 4, 280.1

⊘ **T4538** Diaper service, reusable diaper, each diaper
IOM: 100-03, 4, 280.1

⊘ **T4539** Incontinence product, diaper/brief, reusable, any size, each
IOM: 100-03, 4, 280.1

⊘ **T4540** Incontinence product, protective underpad, reusable, chair size, each
IOM: 100-03, 4, 280.1

⊘ **T4541** Incontinence product, disposable underpad, large, each

⊘ **T4542** Incontinence product, disposable underpad, small size, each

⊘ **T4543** Adult sized disposable incontinence product, protective brief/diaper, above extra large, each Ⓐ
IOM: 100-03, 4, 280.1

⊘ **T4544** Adult sized disposable incontinence product, protective underwear/pull-on, above extra large, each Ⓐ
IOM: 100-03, 4, 280.1

⊘ **T4545** Incontinence product, disposable, penile wrap, each ♂

⊘ **T5001** Positioning seat for persons with special orthopedic needs, supply, not otherwise specified

⊘ **T5999** Supply, not otherwise specified

▶ **New**   ↻ **Revised**   ✔ **Reinstated**   ~~deleted~~ **Deleted**   ⊘ **Not covered or valid by Medicare**   ✦ **Special coverage instructions**   ✳ **Carrier discretion**   Ⓑ **Bill Part B MAC**   Ⓑ **Bill DME MAC**

CORONAVIRUS DIAGNOSTIC PANEL
(U0001–U0002)

U0001 CDC 2019 novel coronavirus (2019-nCoV) real-time RT-PCR diagnostic panel **A**

U0002 2019-nCoV coronavirus, SARS-CoV-2/2019-nCoV (COVID-19), any technique, multiple types or subtypes (includes all targets), non-CDC **A**

~~U0003 Infectious agent detection by nucleic acid (DNA or RNA); severe acute respiratory syndrome coronavirus 2 (SARS-CoV-2) (Coronavirus disease [COVID-19]), amplified probe technique, making use of high throughput technologies as described by CMS-2020-01-R~~ **A**

~~U0004 2019-nCoV Coronavirus, SARS-CoV-2/2019-nCoV (COVID-19), any technique, multiple types or subtypes (includes all targets), non-CDC, making use of high throughput technologies as described by CMS-2020-01-R~~ **A**

~~U0005 Infectious agent detection by nucleic acid (DNA or RNA); severe acute respiratory syndrome coronavirus 2 (SARS-CoV-2) (Coronavirus disease [COVID-19]), amplified probe technique, CDC or non-CDC, making use of high throughput technologies, completed within 2 calendar days from date of specimen collection (list separately in addition to either HCPCS code U0003 or U0004) as described by CMS-2020-01-R2~~ **A**

VISION SERVICES (V0000–V2999)

Frames

⊛ **V2020** Frames, purchases Ⓑ Qp Qh ♿ A

Includes cost of frame/replacement and dispensing fee. One unit of service represents one pair of eyeglass frames.

IOM: 100-02, 15, 120

⊘ **V2025** Deluxe frame Ⓑ Qp Qh E1

Not a benefit. Billing deluxe frames- submit V2020 on one line; V2025 on second line.

IOM: 100-04, 1, 30.3.5

If a CPT procedure code for supply of spectacles or a permanent prosthesis is reported, recode with the specific lens type listed below.

Single Vision Lenses

✻ **V2100** Sphere, single vision, plano to plus or minus 4.00, per lens Ⓑ Qp Qh ♿ A

✻ **V2101** Sphere, single vision, plus or minus 4.12 to plus or minus 7.00d, per lens Ⓑ Qp Qh ♿ A

✻ **V2102** Sphere, single vision, plus or minus 7.12 to plus or minus 20.00d, per lens Ⓑ Qp Qh ♿ A

✻ **V2103** Spherocylinder, single vision, plano to plus or minus 4.00d sphere, .12 to 2.00d cylinder, per lens Ⓑ Qp Qh ♿ A

✻ **V2104** Spherocylinder, single vision, plano to plus or minus 4.00d sphere, 2.12 to 4.00d cylinder, per lens Ⓑ Qp Qh ♿ A

✻ **V2105** Spherocylinder, single vision, plano to plus or minus 4.00d sphere, 4.25 to 6.00d cylinder, per lens Ⓑ Qp Qh ♿ A

✻ **V2106** Spherocylinder, single vision, plano to plus or minus 4.00d sphere, over 6.00d cylinder, per lens Ⓑ Qp Qh ♿ A

✻ **V2107** Spherocylinder, single vision, plus or minus 4.25 to plus or minus 7.00 sphere, .12 to 2.00d cylinder, per lens Ⓑ Qp Qh ♿ A

✻ **V2108** Spherocylinder, single vision, plus or minus 4.25d to plus or minus 7.00d sphere, 2.12 to 4.00d cylinder, per lens Ⓑ Qp Qh ♿ A

✻ **V2109** Spherocylinder, single vision, plus or minus 4.25 to plus or minus 7.00d sphere, 4.25 to 6.00d cylinder, per lens Ⓑ Qp Qh ♿ A

✻ **V2110** Sperocylinder, single vision, plus or minus 4.25 to 7.00d sphere, over 6.00d cylinder, per lens Ⓑ Qp Qh ♿ A

✻ **V2111** Spherocylinder, single vision, plus or minus 7.25 to plus or minus 12.00d sphere, .25 to 2.25d cylinder, per lens Ⓑ Qp Qh ♿ A

✻ **V2112** Spherocylinder, single vision, plus or minus 7.25 to plus or minus 12.00d sphere, 2.25d to 4.00d cylinder, per lens Ⓑ Qp Qh ♿ A

✻ **V2113** Spherocylinder, single vision, plus or minus 7.25 to plus or minus 12.00d sphere, 4.25 to 6.00d cylinder, per lens Ⓑ Qp Qh ♿ A

✻ **V2114** Spherocylinder, single vision, sphere over plus or minus 12.00d, per lens Ⓑ Qp Qh ♿ A

✻ **V2115** Lenticular, (myodisc), per lens, single vision Ⓑ Qp Qh ♿ A

✻ **V2118** Aniseikonic lens, single vision Ⓑ Qp Qh ♿ A

⊛ **V2121** Lenticular lens, per lens, single Ⓑ Qp Qh ♿ A

IOM: 100-02, 15, 120; 100-04, 3, 10.4

✻ **V2199** Not otherwise classified, single vision lens Ⓑ Qp Qh A

Bill on paper. Requires report of type of single vision lens and optical lab invoice.

Bifocal Lenses

✻ **V2200** Sphere, bifocal, plano to plus or minus 4.00d, per lens Ⓑ Qp Qh ♿ A

✻ **V2201** Sphere, bifocal, plus or minus 4.12 to plus or minus 7.00d, per lens Ⓑ Qp Qh ♿ A

✻ **V2202** Sphere, bifocal, plus or minus 7.12 to plus or minus 20.00d, per lens Ⓑ Qp Qh ♿ A

✻ **V2203** Spherocylinder, bifocal, plano to plus or minus 4.00d sphere, .12 to 2.00d cylinder, per lens Ⓑ Qp Qh ♿ A

✻ **V2204** Spherocylinder, bifocal, plano to plus or minus 4.00d sphere, 2.12 to 4.00d cylinder, per lens Ⓑ Qp Qh ♿ A

✻ **V2205** Spherocylinder, bifocal, plano to plus or minus 4.00d sphere, 4.25 to 6.00d cylinder, per lens Ⓑ Qp Qh ♿ A

✻ **V2206** Spherocylinder, bifocal, plano to plus or minus 4.00d sphere, over 6.00d cylinder, per lens Ⓑ Qp Qh ♿ A

▶ New   ↻ Revised   ✔ Reinstated   ~~deleted~~ Deleted   ⊘ Not covered or valid by Medicare
⊛ Special coverage instructions   ✻ Carrier discretion   Ⓑ Bill Part B MAC   Ⓑ Bill DME MAC

* **V2207** Spherocylinder, bifocal, plus or minus 4.25 to plus or minus 7.00d sphere, .12 to 2.00d cylinder, per lens Ⓑ Qp Qh ♿   A

* **V2208** Spherocylinder, bifocal, plus or minus 4.25 to plus or minus 7.00d sphere, 2.12 to 4.00d cylinder, per lens Ⓑ Qp Qh ♿   A

* **V2209** Spherocylinder, bifocal, plus or minus 4.25 to plus or minus 7.00d sphere, 4.25 to 6.00d cylinder, per lens Ⓑ Qp Qh ♿   A

* **V2210** Spherocylinder, bifocal, plus or minus 4.25 to plus or minus 7.00d sphere, over 6.00d cylinder, per lens Ⓑ Qp Qh ♿   A

* **V2211** Spherocylinder, bifocal, plus or minus 7.25 to plus or minus 12.00d sphere, .25 to 2.25d cylinder, per lens Ⓑ Qp Qh ♿   A

* **V2212** Spherocylinder, bifocal, plus or minus 7.25 to plus or minus 12.00d sphere, 2.25 to 4.00d cylinder, per lens Ⓑ Qp Qh ♿   A

* **V2213** Spherocylinder, bifocal, plus or minus 7.25 to plus or minus 12.00d sphere, 4.25 to 6.00d cylinder, per lens Ⓑ Qp Qh ♿   A

* **V2214** Spherocylinder, bifocal, sphere over plus or minus 12.00d, per lens Ⓑ Qp Qh ♿   A

* **V2215** Lenticular (myodisc), per lens, bifocal Ⓑ Qp Qh ♿   A

* **V2218** Aniseikonic, per lens, bifocal Ⓑ Qp Qh ♿   A

* **V2219** Bifocal seg width over 28 mm Ⓑ Qp Qh ♿   A

* **V2220** Bifocal add over 3.25d Ⓑ Qp Qh ♿ A

⊛ **V2221** Lenticular lens, per lens, bifocal Ⓑ Qp Qh ♿   A

    IOM: 100-02, 15, 120; 100-04, 3, 10.4

* **V2299** Specialty bifocal (by report) Ⓑ Qp Qh   A

    Bill on paper. Requires report of type of specialty bifocal lens and optical lab invoice.

Trifocal Lenses

* **V2300** Sphere, trifocal, plano to plus or minus 4.00d, per lens Ⓑ Qp Qh ♿   A

* **V2301** Sphere, trifocal, plus or minus 4.12 to plus or minus 7.00d per lens Ⓑ Qp Qh ♿   A

* **V2302** Sphere, trifocal, plus or minus 7.12 to plus or minus 20.00, per lens Ⓑ Qp Qh ♿   A

* **V2303** Spherocylinder, trifocal, plano to plus or minus 4.00d sphere, .12 to 2.00d cylinder, per lens Ⓑ Qp Qh ♿ A

* **V2304** Spherocylinder, trifocal, plano to plus or minus 4.00d sphere, 2.25-4.00d cylinder, per lens Ⓑ Qp Qh ♿ A

* **V2305** Spherocylinder, trifocal, plano to plus or minus 4.00d sphere, 4.25 to 6.00 cylinder, per lens Ⓑ Qp Qh ♿   A

* **V2306** Spherocylinder, trifocal, plano to plus or minus 4.00d sphere, over 6.00d cylinder, per lens Ⓑ Qp Qh ♿   A

* **V2307** Spherocylinder, trifocal, plus or minus 4.25 to plus or minus 7.00d sphere, .12 to 2.00d cylinder, per lens Ⓑ Qp Qh ♿   A

* **V2308** Spherocylinder, trifocal, plus or minus 4.25 to plus or minus 7.00d sphere, 2.12 to 4.00d cylinder, per lens Ⓑ Qp Qh ♿   A

* **V2309** Spherocylinder, trifocal, plus or minus 4.25 to plus or minus 7.00d sphere, 4.25 to 6.00d cylinder, per lens Ⓑ Qp Qh ♿   A

* **V2310** Spherocylinder, trifocal, plus or minus 4.25 to plus or minus 7.00d sphere, over 6.00d cylinder, per lens Ⓑ Qp Qh ♿   A

* **V2311** Spherocylinder, trifocal, plus or minus 7.25 to plus or minus 12.00d sphere, .25 to 2.25d cylinder, per lens Ⓑ Qp Qh ♿   A

* **V2312** Spherocylinder, trifocal, plus or minus 7.25 to plus or minus 12.00d sphere, 2.25 to 4.00d cylinder, per lens Ⓑ Qp Qh ♿   A

* **V2313** Spherocylinder, trifocal, plus or minus 7.25 to plus or minus 12.00d sphere, 4.25 to 6.00d cylinder, per lens Ⓑ Qp Qh ♿   A

* **V2314** Spherocylinder, trifocal, sphere over plus or minus 12.00d, per lens Ⓑ Qp Qh ♿   A

* **V2315** Lenticular, (myodisc), per lens, trifocal Ⓑ Qp Qh ♿   A

* **V2318** Aniseikonic lens, trifocal Ⓑ Qp Qh ♿   A

* **V2319** Trifocal seg width over 28 mm Ⓑ Qp Qh ♿   A

* **V2320** Trifocal add over 3.25d Ⓑ Qp Qh ♿ A

🄼 MIPS	Qp Quantity Physician	Qh Quantity Hospital	♀ Female only
♂ Male only	A Age	♿ DMEPOS	A2-Z3 ASC Payment Indicator A-Y ASC Status Indicator Coding Clinic

○ **V2321** Lenticular lens, per lens, trifocal ⑥ Qp Qh ♿   A

IOM: 100-02, 15, 120; 100-04, 3, 10.4

✳ **V2399** Specialty trifocal (by report) ⑥ Qp Qh   A

Bill on paper. Requires report of type of trifocal lens and optical lab invoice.

Variable Asphericity/Sphericity Lenses

✳ **V2410** Variable asphericity lens, single vision, full field, glass or plastic, per lens ⑥ Qp Qh ♿   A

✳ **V2430** Variable asphericity lens, bifocal, full field, glass or plastic, per lens ⑥ Qp Qh ♿   A

✳ **V2499** Variable sphericity lens, other type ⑥ Qp Qh   A

Bill on paper. Requires report of other ptical lab invoice.

Contact Lenses

If a CPT procedure code for supply of contact lens is reported, recode with specific lens type listed below (per lens).

✳ **V2500** Contact lens, PMMA, spherical, per lens ⑧ Qp Qh ♿   A

Requires prior authorization for patients under age 21.

✳ **V2501** Contact lens, PMMA, toric or prism ballast, per lens ⑧ Qp Qh ♿   A

Requires prior authorization for clients under age 21.

✳ **V2502** Contact lens, PMMA, bifocal, per lens ⑥ Qp Qh ♿   A

Requires prior authorization for clients under age 21. Bill on paper. Requires optical lab invoice.

✳ **V2503** Contact lens PMMA, color vision deficiency, per lens ⑧ Qp Qh ♿   A

Requires prior authorization for clients under age 21. Bill on paper. Requires optical lab invoice.

✳ **V2510** Contact lens, gas permeable, spherical, per lens ⑥ Qp Qh ♿   A

Requires prior authorization for clients under age 21.

✳ **V2511** Contact lens, gas permeable, toric, prism ballast, per lens ⑧ Qp Qh ♿   A

Requires prior authorization for clients under age 21.

✳ **V2512** Contact lens, gas permeable, bifocal, per lens ⑧ Qp Qh ♿   A

Requires prior authorization for clients under age 21.

✳ **V2513** Contact lens, gas permeable, extended wear, per lens ⑥ Qp Qh ♿   A

Requires prior authorization for clients under age 21.

○ **V2520** Contact lens, hydrophilic, spherical, per lens ⑨ ⑧ Qp Qh ♿   A

Requires prior authorization for clients under age 21.

IOM: 100-03, 1, 80.1; 100-03, 1, 80.4

○ **V2521** Contact lens, hydrophilic, toric, or prism ballast, per lens ⑨ ⑥ Qp Qh ♿   A

Requires prior authorization for clients under age 21.

IOM: 100-03, 1, 80.1; 100-03, 1, 80.4

○ **V2522** Contact lens, hydrophilic, bifocal, per lens ⑧ ⑥ Qp Qh ♿   A

Requires prior authorization for clients under age 21.

IOM: 100-03, 1, 80.1; 100-03, 1, 80.4

○ **V2523** Contact lens, hydrophilic, extended wear, per lens ⑥ ⑧ Qp Qh ♿   A

Requires prior authorization for clients under age 21.

IOM: 100-03, 1, 80.1; 100-03, 1, 80.4

○ **V2524** Contact lens, hydrophilic, spherical, photochromic additive, per lens ♿   A

▶ **V2526** Contact lens, hydrophilic, with blue-violet filter, per lens   E1

✳ **V2530** Contact lens, scleral, gas impermeable, per lens (for contact lens modification, see 92325) ⑥ Qp Qh ♿   A

Requires prior authorization for clients under age 21.

○ **V2531** Contact lens, scleral, gas permeable, per lens (for contact lens modification, see 92325) ⑥ Qp Qh ♿   A

Requires prior authorization for clients under age 21. Bill on paper. Requires optical lab invoice.

IOM: 100-03, 1, 80.5

▶ New   ↻ Revised   ✔ Reinstated   ~~deleted~~ Deleted   ⊘ Not covered or valid by Medicare
○ Special coverage instructions   ✳ Carrier discretion   ⑧ Bill Part B MAC   ⑥ Bill DME MAC

✳ **V2599** Contact lens, other type ⒷⒷ ⓆⓅ Ⓠⓗ A

Requires prior authorization for clients under age 21. Bill on paper. Requires report of other type of contact lens and optical invoice.

Low Vision Aids

If a CPT procedure code for supply of low vision aid is reported, recode with specific systems listed below.

✳ **V2600** Hand held low vision aids and other nonspectacle mounted aids Ⓖ ⓆⓅ Ⓠⓗ   A

Requires prior authorization.

✳ **V2610** Single lens spectacle mounted low vision aids Ⓖ ⓆⓅ Ⓠⓗ   A

Requires prior authorization.

✳ **V2615** Telescopic and other compound lens system, including distance vision telescopic, near vision telescopes and compound microscopic lens system Ⓖ ⓆⓅ Ⓠⓗ   A

Requires prior authorization. Bill on paper. Requires optical lab invoice.

Prosthetic Eye

⊘ **V2623** Prosthetic eye, plastic, custom Ⓑ ⓆⓅ Ⓠⓗ ♿   A

DME regional carrier. Requires prior authorization. Bill on paper. Requires optical lab invoice.

✳ **V2624** Polishing/resurfacing of ocular prosthesis Ⓖ ⓆⓅ Ⓠⓗ ♿   A

Requires prior authorization. Bill on paper. Requires optical lab invoice.

✳ **V2625** Enlargement of ocular prosthesis Ⓖ ⓆⓅ Ⓠⓗ ♿   A

Requires prior authorization. Bill on paper. Requires optical lab invoice.

✳ **V2626** Reduction of ocular prosthesis Ⓖ ⓆⓅ Ⓠⓗ ♿   A

Requires prior authorization. Bill on paper. Requires optical lab invoice.

⊘ **V2627** Scleral cover shell Ⓖ ⓆⓅ Ⓠⓗ ♿   A

DME regional carrier

Requires prior authorization. Bill on paper. Requires optical lab invoice.

IOM: 100-03, 4, 280.2

✳ **V2628** Fabrication and fitting of ocular conformer Ⓖ ⓆⓅ Ⓠⓗ ♿   A

Requires prior authorization. Bill on paper. Requires optical lab invoice.

✳ **V2629** Prosthetic eye, other type Ⓖ ⓆⓅ Ⓠⓗ   A

Requires prior authorization. Bill on paper. Requires optical lab invoice.

Intraocular Lenses

⊘ **V2630** Anterior chamber intraocular lens Ⓑ ⓆⓅ Ⓠⓗ ♿   N1 N

IOM: 100-02, 15, 120

⊘ **V2631** Iris supported intraocular lens Ⓑ ⓆⓅ Ⓠⓗ ♿   N1 N

IOM: 100-02, 15, 120

⊘ **V2632** Posterior chamber intraocular lens Ⓑ ⓆⓅ Ⓠⓗ ♿   N1 N

IOM: 100-02, 15, 120

Figure 52 Posterior intraocular lens.

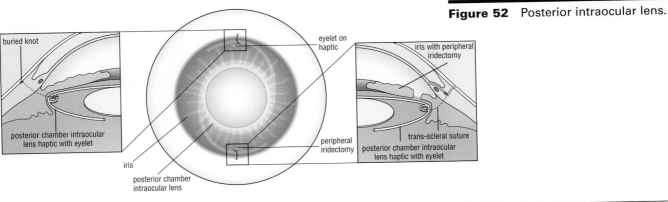

buried knot

posterior chamber intraocular lens haptic with eyelet

iris

posterior chamber intraocular lens

eyelet on haptic

peripheral iridectomy

iris with peripheral iridectomy

trans-scleral suture

posterior chamber intraocular lens haptic with eyelet

🝆 **MIPS**   ⓆⓅ **Quantity Physician**   Ⓠⓗ **Quantity Hospital**   ♀ **Female only**

♂ **Male only**   A **Age**   ♿ **DMEPOS**   A2-Z3 **ASC Payment Indicator**   A-Y **ASC Status Indicator**   *Coding Clinic*

Miscellaneous Vision Services

✳ **V2700** Balance lens, per lens Ⓑ Qp Qh ♿ A

⊘ **V2702** Deluxe lens feature Ⓑ Qp Qh E1

IOM: 100-02, 15, 120; 100-04, 3, 10.4

✳ **V2710** Slab off prism, glass or plastic, per lens Ⓓ Qp Qh ♿ A

✳ **V2715** Prism, per lens Ⓑ Qp Qh ♿ A

✳ **V2718** Press-on lens, Fresnel prism, per lens Ⓓ Qp Qh ♿ A

✳ **V2730** Special base curve, glass or plastic, per lens Ⓓ Qp Qh ♿ A

⊛ **V2744** Tint, photochromatic, per lens Ⓑ Qp Qh ♿ A

Requires prior authorization.

IOM: 100-02, 15, 120; 100-04, 3, 10.4

⊛ **V2745** Addition to lens, tint, any color, solid, gradient or equal, excludes photochroatic, any lens material, per lens Ⓑ Qp Qh ♿ A

Includes photochromatic lenses (V2744) used as sunglasses, which are prescribed in addition to regular prosthetic lenses for aphakic patient will be denied as not medically necessary.

IOM: 100-02, 15, 120; 100-04, 3, 10.4

⊛ **V2750** Anti-reflective coating, per lens Ⓓ Qp Qh ♿ A

Requires prior authorization.

IOM: 100-02, 15, 120; 100-04, 3, 10.4

⊛ **V2755** U-V lens, per lens Ⓓ Qp Qh ♿ A

IOM: 100-02, 15, 120; 100-04, 3, 10.4

✳ **V2756** Eye glass case Ⓓ Qp Qh E1

✳ **V2760** Scratch resistant coating, per lens Ⓓ Qp Qh ♿ E1

⊛ **V2761** Mirror coating, any type, solid, gradient or equal, any lens material, per lens Ⓓ Qp Qh B

IOM: 100-02, 15, 120; 100-04, 3, 10.4

⊛ **V2762** Polarization, any lens material, per lens Ⓑ Qp Qh ♿ E1

IOM: 100-02, 15, 120; 100-04, 3, 10.4

✳ **V2770** Occluder lens, per lens Ⓑ Qp Qh ♿ A

Requires prior authorization.

✳ **V2780** Oversize lens, per lens Ⓓ Qp Qh ♿ A

Requires prior authorization.

✳ **V2781** Progressive lens, per lens Ⓑ Qp Qh B

Requires prior authorization.

⊛ **V2782** Lens, index 1.54 to 1.65 plastic or 1.60 to 1.79 glass, excludes polycarbonate, per lens Ⓑ Qp Qh ♿ A

Do not bill in addition to V2784

IOM: 100-02, 15, 120; 100-04, 3, 10.4

⊛ **V2783** Lens, index greater than or equal to 1.66 plastic or greater than or equal to 1.80 glass, excludes polycarbonate, per lens Ⓓ Qp Qh ♿ A

Do not bill in addition to V2784

IOM: 100-02, 15, 120; 100-04, 3, 10.4

⊛ **V2784** Lens, polycarbonate or equal, any index, per lens Ⓑ Qp Qh ♿ A

Covered only for patients with functional vision in one eye-in this situation, an impact-resistant material is covered for both lenses if eyeglasses are covered. Claims with V2784 that do not meet this coverage criterion will be denied as not medically necessary.

IOM: 100-02, 15, 120; 100-04, 3, 10.4

✳ **V2785** Processing, preserving and transporting corneal tissue Ⓑ Qp Qh F4 F

For ASC, bill on paper. Must attach eye bank invoice to claim.

For Hospitals, bill charges for corneal tissue to receive cost based reimbursement.

IOM: 100-⊠4, 4, 200.1

⊛ **V2786** Specialty occupational multifocal lens, per lens Ⓑ Qp Qh ♿ E1

IOM: 100-02, 15, 120; 100-04, 3, 10.4

⊘ **V2787** Astigmatism correcting function of intraocular lens Ⓑ E1

Medicare Statute 1862(a)(7)

⊘ **V2788** Presbyopia correcting function of intraocular lens Ⓑ E1

Medicare Statute 1862a7

✳ **V2790** Amniotic membrane for surgical reconstruction, per procedure Ⓑ Qp Qh N1 N

✳ **V2797** Vision supply, accessory and/or service component of another HCPCS vision code Ⓑ Qp Qh E1

✳ **V2799** Vision item or service, miscellaneous Ⓑ A

Bill on paper. Requires report of miscellaneous service and optical lab invoice.

▶ New ⟲ Revised ✔ Reinstated ~~deleted~~ Deleted ⊘ Not covered or valid by Medicare
⊛ Special coverage instructions ✳ Carrier discretion Ⓑ Bill Part B MAC Ⓓ Bill DME MAC

HEARING SERVICES (V5000-V5999)

These codes are for non-physician services.

Assessments and Evaluations

⊘ **V5008** Hearing screening Ⓑ Qp Qh   E1
IOM: 100-02, 16, 90

⊘ **V5010** Assessment for hearing aid Ⓑ Qp Qh   E1
Medicare Statute 1862a7

⊘ **V5011** Fitting/orientation/checking of hearing aid Ⓑ Qp Qh   E1
Medicare Statute 1862a7

⊘ **V5014** Repair/modification of a hearing aid Ⓑ   E1
Medicare Statute 1862a7

⊘ **V5020** Conformity evaluation Ⓑ   E1
Medicare Statute 1862a7

Monaural Hearing Aid

⊘ **V5030** Hearing aid, monaural, body worn, air conduction Ⓑ   E1
Medicare Statute 1862a7

⊘ **V5040** Hearing aid, monaural, body worn, bone conduction Ⓑ   E1
Medicare Statute 1862a7

⊘ **V5050** Hearing aid, monaural, in the ear Ⓑ E1
Medicare Statute 1862a7

⊘ **V5060** Hearing aid, monaural, behind the ear Ⓑ   E1
Medicare Statute 1862a7

Miscellaneous Services and Supplies

⊘ **V5070** Glasses, air conduction Ⓑ   E1
Medicare Statute 1862a7

⊘ **V5080** Glasses, bone conduction Ⓑ   E1
Medicare Statute 1862a7

⊘ **V5090** Dispensing fee, unspecified hearing aid Ⓑ   E1
Medicare Statute 1862a7

⊘ **V5095** Semi-implantable middle ear hearing prosthesis Ⓑ   E1
Medicare Statute 1862a7

⊘ **V5100** Hearing aid, bilateral, body worn Ⓑ   E1
Medicare Statute 1862a7

⊘ **V5110** Dispensing fee, bilateral Ⓑ   E1
Medicare Statute 1862a7

Hearing Aids

⊘ **V5120** Binaural, body Ⓑ   E1
Medicare Statute 1862a7

⊘ **V5130** Binaural, in the ear Ⓑ   E1
Medicare Statute 1862a7

⊘ **V5140** Binaural, behind the ear Ⓑ   E1
Medicare Statute 1862a7

⊘ **V5150** Binaural, glasses Ⓑ   E1
Medicare Statute 1862a7

⊘ **V5160** Dispensing fee, binaural Ⓟ   E1
Medicare Statute 1862a7

⊘ **V5171** Hearing aid, contralateral routing device, monaural, in the ear (ITE)   E1
Medicare Statute 1862a7

⊘ **V5172** Hearing aid, contralateral routing device, monaural, in the canal (ITC)   E1
Medicare Statute 1862a7

⊘ **V5181** Hearing aid, contralateral routing device, monaural, behind the ear (BTE)   E1
Medicare Statute 1862a7

⊘ **V5190** Hearing aid, contralateral routing, monaural, glasses Ⓑ   E1
Medicare Statute 1862a7

⊘ **V5200** Dispensing fee, contralateral, monaural Ⓑ   E1
Medicare Statute 1862a7

⊘ **V5211** Hearing aid, contralateral routing system, binaural, ITE/ITE   E1
Medicare Statute 1862a7

⊘ **V5212** Hearing aid, contralateral routing system, binaural, ITE/ITC   E1
Medicare Statute 1862a7

⊘ **V5213** Hearing aid, contralateral routing system, binaural, ITE/BTE   E1
Medicare Statute 1862a7

🐾 **MIPS**   Qp **Quantity Physician**   Qh **Quantity Hospital**   ♀ **Female only**

♂ **Male only**   Ⓐ **Age**   ♿ **DMEPOS**   A2-Z3 **ASC Payment Indicator**   A-Y **ASC Status Indicator**   Coding Clinic

⊘ **V5214** Hearing aid, contralateral routing system, binaural, ITC/ITC   E1

Medicare Statute 1862a7

⊘ **V5215** Hearing aid, contralateral routing system, binaural, ITC/BTE   E1

Medicare Statute 1862a7

⊘ **V5221** Hearing aid, contralateral routing system, binaural, BTE/BTE   E1

Medicare Statute 1862a7

⊘ **V5230** Hearing aid, contralateral routing system, binaural, glasses ⑧   E1

Medicare Statute 1862a7

⊘ **V5240** Dispensing fee, contralateral routing system, binaural ⑧   E1

Medicare Statute 1862a7

⊘ **V5241** Dispensing fee, monaural hearing aid, any type ⑧   E1

Medicare Statute 1862a7

⊘ **V5242** Hearing aid, analog, monaural, CIC (completely in the ear canal) ⑧   E1

Medicare Statute 1862a7

⊘ **V5243** Hearing aid, analog, monaural, ITC (in the canal) ⑧   E1

Medicare Statute 1862a9

⊘ **V5244** Hearing aid, digitally programmable analog, monaural, CIC ⑧   E1

Medicare Statute 1862a7

⊘ **V5245** Hearing aid, digitally programmable, analog, monaural, ITC ⑧   E1

Medicare Statute 1862a7

⊘ **V5246** Hearing aid, digitally programmable analog, monaural, ITE (in the ear) ⑧ E1

Medicare Statute 1862a7

⊘ **V5247** Hearing aid, digitally programmable analog, monaural, BTE (behind the ear) ⑧   E1

Medicare Statute 1862a7

⊘ **V5248** Hearing aid, analog, binaural, CIC ⑧ E1

Medicare Statute 1862a7

⊘ **V5249** Hearing aid, analog, binaural, ITC ⑧ E1

Medicare Statute 1862a7

⊘ **V5250** Hearing aid, digitally programmable analog, binaural, CIC ⑧   E1

Medicare Statute 1862a7

⊘ **V5251** Hearing aid, digitally programmable analog, binaural, ITC ⑧   E1

Medicare Statute 1862a7

⊘ **V5252** Hearing aid, digitally programmable, binaural, ITE ⑧   E1

Medicare Statute 1862a7

⊘ **V5253** Hearing aid, digitally programmable, binaural, BTE ⑧   E1

Medicare Statute 1862a7

⊘ **V5254** Hearing aid, digital, monaural, CIC ⑧E1

Medicare Statute 1862a7

⊘ **V5255** Hearing aid, digital, monaural, ITC ⑧E1

Medicare Statute 1862a7

⊘ **V5256** Hearing aid, digital, monaural, ITE ⑧E1

Medicare Statute 1862a7

⊘ **V5257** Hearing aid, digital, monaural, BTE ⑧   E1

Medicare Statute 1862a7

⊘ **V5258** Hearing aid, digital, binaural, CIC ⑧ E1

Medicare Statute 1862a7

⊘ **V5259** Hearing aid, digital, binaural, ITC ⑧ E1

Medicare Statute 1862a7

⊘ **V5260** Hearing aid, digital, binaural, ITE ⑧ E1

Medicare Statute 1862a7

⊘ **V5261** Hearing aid, digital, binaural, BTE ⑧E1

Medicare Statute 1862a7

⊘ **V5262** Hearing aid, disposable, any type, monaural ⑧   E1

Medicare Statute 1862a7

⊘ **V5263** Hearing aid, disposable, any type, binaural ⑧   E1

Medicare Statute 1862a7

⊘ **V5264** Ear mold/insert, not disposable, any type ⑧   E1

Medicare Statute 1862a7

⊘ **V5265** Ear mold/insert, disposable, any type ⑧   E1

Medicare Statute 1862a7

⊘ **V5266** Battery for use in hearing device ⑧ E1

Medicare Statute 1862a7

⊘ **V5267** Hearing aid or assistive listening device/supplies/accessories, not otherwise specified ⑧   E1

Medicare Statute 1862a7

▶ **New**   ↻ **Revised**   ✔ **Reinstated**   ~~deleted~~ **Deleted**   ⊘ **Not covered or valid by Medicare**

⊛ **Special coverage instructions**   ✳ **Carrier discretion**   ⑧ **Bill Part B MAC**   ⑧ **Bill DME MAC**

Assistive Listening Devices

⊘ **V5268** Assistive listening device, telephone amplifier, any type ⑧   E1

Medicare Statute 1862a7

⊘ **V5269** Assistive listening device, alerting, any type ⑧   E1

Medicare Statute 1862a7

⊘ **V5270** Assistive listening device, television amplifier, any type ⑧   E1

Medicare Statute 1862a7

⊘ **V5271** Assistive listening device, television caption decoder ⑧   E1

Medicare Statute 1862a7

⊘ **V5272** Assistive listening device, TDD ⑧   E1

Medicare Statute 1862a7

⊘ **V5273** Assistive listening device, for use with cochlear implant ⑧   E1

Medicare Statute 1862a7

⊘ **V5274** Assistive listening device, not otherwise specified ⑧ Qp Qh   E1

Medicare Statute 1862a7

⊘ **V5275** Ear impression, each ⑧   E1

Medicare Statute 1862a7

⊘ **V5281** Assistive listening device, personal FM/DM system, monaural (1 receiver, transmitter, microphone), any type ⑧ Qp Qh   E1

Medicare Statute 1862a7

⊘ **V5282** Assistive listening device, personal FM/DM system, binaural (2 receivers, transmitter, microphone), any type ⑧ Qp Qh   E1

Medicare Statute 1862a7

⊘ **V5283** Assistive listening device, personal FM/DM neck, loop induction receiver ⑧ Qp Qh   E1

Medicare Statute 1862a7

⊘ **V5284** Assistive listening device, personal FM/DM, ear level receiver ⑧ Qp Qh E1

Medicare Statute 1862a7

⊘ **V5285** Assistive listening device, personal FM/DM, direct audio input receiver ⑧ Qp Qh   E1

Medicare Statute 1862a7

⊘ **V5286** Assistive listening device, personal Bluetooth FM/DM receiver ⑧ Qp Qh E1

Medicare Statute 1862a7

⊘ **V5287** Assistive listening device, personal FM/DM receiver, not otherwise specified ⑧ Qp Qh   E1

Medicare Statute 1862a7

⊘ **V5288** Assistive listening device, personal FM/DM transmitter assistive listening device ⑧ Qp Qh   E1

Medicare Statute 1862a7

⊘ **V5289** Assistive listening device, personal FM/DM adapter/boot coupling device for receiver, any type ⑧ Qp Qh   E1

Medicare Statute 1862a7

⊘ **V5290** Assistive listening device, transmitter microphone, any type ⑧ Qp Qh   E1

Medicare Statute 1862a7

Other Supllies and Miscellaneous Services

⊘ **V5298** Hearing aid, not otherwise classified ⑧   E1

Medicare Statute 1862a7

⊛ **V5299** Hearing service, miscellaneous ⑧   B

IOM: 100-02, 16, 90

Repair/Modification

⊘ **V5336** Repair/modification of augmentative communicative system or device (excludes adaptive hearing aid) ⑧   E1

Medicare Statute 1862a7

Speech, Language, and Pathology Screening

These codes are for non-physician services.

⊘ **V5362** Speech screening ⑧   E1

Medicare Statute 1862a7

⊘ **V5363** Language screening ⑧   E1

Medicare Statute 1862a7

⊘ **V5364** Dysphagia screening ⑧   E1

Medicare Statute 1862a7

⚒ MIPS	Qp Quantity Physician	Qh Quantity Hospital	♀ Female only	
♂ Male only	A Age	♿ DMEPOS	A2-Z3 ASC Payment Indicator	A-Y ASC Status Indicator Coding Clinic

APPENDIX A

Jurisdiction List for DMEPOS HCPCS Codes

Deleted codes are valid for dates of service on or before the date of deletion. The jurisdiction list includes codes that are not payable by Medicare. Please consult the Medicare contractor in whose jurisdiction a claim would be filed in order to determine coverage under Medicare.

NOTE: All Local Carrier language has been changed to Part B MAC

HCPCS	DESCRIPTION	JURISDICTION
A4206 - A4209	Medical, Surgical, and Self-Administered Injection, Supplies	Part B MAC if incident to a physician's service (not separately payable). If other, DME MAC.
A4210	Needle Free Injection Device	DME MAC
A4211	Medical, Surgical, and Self-Administered Injection, Supplies	Part B MAC if incident to a physician's service (not separately payable). If other, DME MAC.
A4213 - A4215	Medical, Surgical, and Self-Administered Injection, Supplies	Part B MAC if incident to a physician's service (not separately payable). If other, DME MAC.
A4216 - A4218	Saline	Part B MAC if incident to a physician's service (not separately payable). If other, DME MAC.
A4221 - A4239	Self-Administered Injection and Diabetic Supplies	DME MAC
A4244 - A4250	Medical, Surgical, and Self-Administered Injection, Supplies	Part B MAC if incident to a physician's service (not separately payable). If other, DME MAC.
A4252 - A4259	Diabetic Supplies	DME MAC
A4265	Paraffin	Part B MAC if incident to a physician's service (not separately payable). If other, DME MAC.
A4280	Accessory for Breast Prosthesis	DME MAC
A4281 - A4286	Accessory for Breast Pump	DME MAC
A4305 - A4306	Disposable Drug Delivery System	Part B MAC if incident to a physician's service (not separately payable). If other, DME MAC.
A4310 - A4358	Incontinence Supplies/ Urinary Supplies	If provided in the physician's office for a temporary condition, the item is incident to the physician's service & billed to the Part B MAC. If provided in the physician's office or other place of service for a permanent condition, the item is a prosthetic device & billed to the DME MAC.
A4360 - A4437	Urinary Supplies	If provided in the physician's office for a temporary condition, the item is incident to the physician's service & billed to the Part B MAC. If provided in the physician's office or other place of service for a permanent condition, the item is a prosthetic device & billed to the DME MAC.

HCPCS	DESCRIPTION	JURISDICTION
A4450 - A4452	Tape; Adhesive Remover	Part B MAC if incident to a physician's service (not separately payable), or if supply for implanted prosthetic device. If other, DME MAC.
A4453	Enema Catheter	DME MAC
A4455 - A4456	Tape; Adhesive Remover	Part B MAC if incident to a physician's service (not separately payable), or if supply for implanted prosthetic device. If other, DME MAC.
A4458 - A4459	Enema Bag/System	DME MAC
A4461 - A4463	Surgical Dressing Holders	Part B MAC if incident to a physician's service (not separately payable). If other, DME MAC.
A4465 - A4467	Non-elastic Binder and Garment, Strap, Covering	DME MAC
A4481	Tracheostomy Supply	Part B MAC if incident to a physician's service (not separately payable). If other, DME MAC.
A4483	Moisture Exchanger	DME MAC
A4490 - A4510	Surgical Stockings	DME MAC
A4520	Diapers	DME MAC
A4553 - A4554	Underpads	DME MAC
A4555 - A4558	Electrodes; Lead Wires; Conductive Paste	**Part B MAC** if incident to a physician's service (not separately payable). If other, **DME MAC.**
A4559	Coupling Gel	**Part B MAC** if incident to a physician's service (not separately payable). If other, **DME MAC.**
A4575	Topical Hyperbaric Oxygen Chamber, Disposable	DME MAC
A4595	TENS Supplies	Part B MAC if incident to a physician's service (not separately payable). If other, DME MAC.
A4596	Electrical Stimulator Supplies	**DME MAC**
A4600	Sleeve for Intermittent Limb Compression Device	DME MAC
A4601 - A4602	Lithium Replacement Batteries	DME MAC
A4604	Tubing for Positive Airway Pressure Device	DME MAC

HCPCS	DESCRIPTION	JURISDICTION
A4605	Tracheal Suction Catheter	DME MAC
A4606	Oxygen Probe for Oximeter	DME MAC
A4608	Transtracheal Oxygen Catheter	DME MAC
A4611 - A4613	Oxygen Equipment Batteries and Supplies	DME MAC
A4614	Peak Flow Rate Meter	Part B MAC if incident to a physician's service (not separately payable). If other, DME MAC.
A4615 - A4629	Oxygen & Tracheostomy Supplies	Part B MAC if incident to a physician's service (not separately payable). If other, DME MAC.
A4630 - A4640	DME Supplies	DME MAC
A4649	Miscellaneous Surgical Supplies	Part B MAC if incident to a physician's service (not separately payable), or if supply for implanted prosthetic device or implanted DME. If other, DME MAC.
A4651 - A4932	Supplies for ESRD	DME MAC (not separately payable)
A5051 - A5093	Additional Ostomy Supplies	If provided in the physician's office for a temporary condition, the item is incident to the physician's service & billed to the Part B MAC. If provided in the physician's office or other place of service for a permanent condition, the item is a prosthetic device & billed to the DME MAC.
A5102 - A5200	Additional Incontinence and Ostomy Supplies	If provided in the physician's office for a temporary condition, the item is incident to the physician's service & billed to the Part B MAC. If provided in the physician's office or other place of service for a permanent condition, the item is a prosthetic device & billed to the DME MAC.
A5500 - A5514	Therapeutic Shoes	DME MAC
A6000	Non-Contact Wound Warming Cover	DME MAC
A6010-A6024	Surgical Dressing	Part B MAC if incident to a physician's service (not separately payable) or if supply for implanted prosthetic device or implanted DME. If other, DME MAC.
A6025	Silicone Gel Sheet	Part B MAC if incident to a physician's service (not separately payable) or if supply for implanted prosthetic device or implanted DME. If other, DME MAC.
A6154 - A6411	Surgical Dressing	Part B MAC if incident to a physician's service (not separately payable) or if supply for implanted prosthetic device or implanted DME. If other, DME MAC.

HCPCS	DESCRIPTION	JURISDICTION
A6412	Eye Patch	Part B MAC if incident to a physician's service (not separately payable) or if supply for implanted prosthetic device or implanted DME. If other, DME MAC.
A6413	Adhesive Bandage	Part B MAC if incident to a physician's service (not separately payable) or if supply for implanted prosthetic device or implanted DME. If other, DME MAC.
A6441 - A6457	Surgical Dressing	Part B MAC if incident to a physician's service (not separately payable) or if supply for implanted prosthetic device or implanted DME. If other, DME MAC.
A6501 - A6512	Surgical Dressing	Part B MAC if incident to a physician's service (not separately payable) or if supply for implanted prosthetic device or implanted DME. If other, DME MAC.
A6513	Compression Burn Mask	DME MAC
A6530 - A6549	Compression Gradient Stockings	DME MAC
A6550	Supplies for Negative Pressure Wound Therapy Electrical Pump	DME MAC
A7000 - A7002	Accessories for Suction Pumps	DME MAC
A7003 - A7039	Accessories for Nebulizers, Aspirators and Ventilators	DME MAC
A7044 - A7047	Respiratory Accessories	DME MAC
A7501-A7527	Tracheostomy Supplies	DME MAC
A8000-A8004	Protective Helmets	DME MAC
A9270	Noncovered Items or Services	DME MAC
A9272	Disposable Wound Suction Pump	DME MAC
A9273	Hot Water Bottles, Ice Caps or Collars, and Heat and/or Cold Wraps	DME MAC
A9274 - A9278	Glucose Monitoring	DME MAC
A9279	Monitoring Feature/ Device	DME MAC
A9280	Alarm Device	DME MAC
A9281	Reaching/Grabbing Device	DME MAC
A9282	Wig	DME MAC
A9283	Foot Off Loading Device	DME MAC
A9284- A9286	Non-electric Spirometer, Inversion Devices and Hygienic Items	DME MAC
A9300	Exercise Equipment	DME MAC
A9900	Miscellaneous DME Supply or Accessory	Part B MAC if used with implanted DME. If other, DME MAC.
A9901	Delivery	DME MAC

HCPCS	DESCRIPTION	JURISDICTION
A9999	Miscellaneous DME Supply or Accessory	Part B MAC if used with implanted DME. If other, DME MAC.
B4034 - B9999	Enteral and Parenteral Therapy	DME MAC
E0100 - E0105	Canes	DME MAC
E0110 - E0118	Crutches	DME MAC
E0130 - E0159	Walkers	DME MAC
E0160 - E0175	Commodes	DME MAC
E0181 - E0199	Decubitus Care Equipment	DME MAC
E0200 - E0239	Heat/Cold Applications	DME MAC
E0240 - E0248	Bath and Toilet Aids	DME MAC
E0249	Pad for Heating Unit	DME MAC
E0250 - E0304	Hospital Beds	DME MAC
E0305 - E0326	Hospital Bed Accessories	DME MAC
E0328 - E0329	Pediatric Hospital Beds	DME MAC
E0350 - E0352	Electronic Bowel Irrigation System	DME MAC
E0370	Heel Pad	DME MAC
E0371 - E0373	Decubitus Care Equipment	DME MAC
E0424 - E0484	Oxygen and Related Respiratory Equipment	DME MAC
E0485 - E0486	Oral Device to Reduce Airway Collapsibility	DME MAC
E0487	Electric Spirometer	DME MAC
E0500	IPPB Machine	DME MAC
E0550 - E0585	Compressors/Nebulizers	DME MAC
E0600	Suction Pump	DME MAC
E0601	CPAP Device	DME MAC
E0602 - E0604	Breast Pump	DME MAC
E0605	Vaporizer	DME MAC
E0606	Drainage Board	DME MAC
E0607	Home Blood Glucose Monitor	DME MAC
E0610 - E0615	Pacemaker Monitor	DME MAC
E0617	External Defibrillator	DME MAC
E0618 - E0619	Apnea Monitor	DME MAC
E0620	Skin Piercing Device	DME MAC
E0621 - E0636	Patient Lifts	DME MAC
E0637 - E0642	Standing Devices/Lifts	DME MAC
E0650 - E0676	Pneumatic Compressor and Appliances	DME MAC
E0691 - E0694	Ultraviolet Light Therapy Systems	DME MAC
E0700	Safety Equipment	DME MAC
E0705	Transfer Board	DME MAC
E0710	Restraints	DME MAC

HCPCS	DESCRIPTION	JURISDICTION
E0720 - E0745	Electrical Nerve Stimulators	DME MAC
E0747 - E0748	Osteogenic Stimulators	DME MAC
E0755- E0770	Stimulation Devices	DME MAC
E0776	IV Pole	DME MAC
E0779 - E0780	External Infusion Pumps	DME MAC
E0781	Ambulatory Infusion Pump	DME MAC
E0784	Infusion Pumps, insulin	DME MAC
E0791	Parenteral Infusion Pump	DME MAC
E0830	Ambulatory Traction Device	DME MAC
E0840 - E0900	Traction Equipment	DME MAC
E0910 - E0930	Trapeze/Fracture Frame	DME MAC
E0935 - E0936	Passive Motion Exercise Device	DME MAC
E0940	Trapeze Equipment	DME MAC
E0941	Traction Equipment	DME MAC
E0942 - E0945	Orthopedic Devices	DME MAC
E0946 - E0948	Fracture Frame	DME MAC
E0950 - E1298	Wheelchairs	DME MAC
E1300 - E1310	Whirlpool Equipment	DME MAC
E1352 - E1392	Additional Oxygen Related Equipment	DME MAC
E1399	Miscellaneous DME	Part B MAC if implanted DME. If other, DME MAC.
E1405 - E1406	Additional Oxygen Equipment	DME MAC
E1500 - E1625	Artificial Kidney Machines and Accessories	DME MAC (not separately payable)
E1630 - E1699	Artifical Kidney Machines and Accessories	DME MAC (not separately payable)
E1700 - E1702	TMJ Device and Supplies	DME MAC
E1800 - E1841	Dynamic Flexion Devices	DME MAC
E1902	Communication Board	DME MAC
E2000	Gastric Suction Pump	DME MAC
E2100 - E2103	Blood Glucose Monitors with Special Features	DME MAC
E2120	Pulse Generator for Tympanic Treatment of Inner Ear	DME MAC
E2201 - E2398	Wheelchair Accessories	DME MAC
E2402	Negative Pressure Wound Therapy Pump	DME MAC
E2500 - E2599	Speech Generating Device	DME MAC

HCPCS	DESCRIPTION	JURISDICTION
E2601 - E2633	Wheelchair Cushions and Accessories	DME MAC
E8000 - E8002	Gait Trainers	DME MAC
G0333	Dispensing Fee	DME MAC
J0120 - J1094	Injection	Part B MAC if incident to a physician's service or used in an implanted infusion pump. If other, DME MAC.
J1100 - J2786	Injection	Part B MAC if incident to a physician's service or used in an implanted infusion pump. If other, DME MAC.
J2788 - J3570	Injection	Part B MAC if incident to a physician's service or used in an implanted infusion pump. If other, DME MAC.
J7030 - J7131	Miscellaneous Drugs and Solutions	Part B MAC if incident to a physician's service or used in an implanted infusion pump. If other, DME MAC.
J7340	Carbidopa/Levodopa	Part B MAC if incident to a physician's service or used in an implanted infusion pump. If other, DME MAC.
J7500 - J7599	Immunosuppressive Drugs	Part B MAC if incident to a physician's service or used in an implanted infusion pump. If other, DME MAC.
J7604 - J7699	Inhalation Solutions	Part B MAC if incident to a physician's service. If other, DME MAC.
J7799 - J7999	NOC Drugs, Other than Inhalation Drugs	Part B MAC if incident to a physician's service or used in an implanted infusion pump. If other, DME MAC.
J8498	Anti-emetic Drug	DME MAC
J8499	Prescription Drug, Oral, Non Chemotherapeutic	Part B MAC if incident to a physician's service. If other, DME MAC.
J8501 - J8999	Oral Anti-Cancer Drugs	DME MAC
J9000 - J9999	Chemotherapy Drugs	Part B MAC if incident to a physician's service or used in an implanted infusion pump. If other, DME MAC.
K0001 - K0108	Wheelchairs	DME MAC
K0195	Elevating Leg Rests	DME MAC
K0455	Infusion Pump used for Uninterrupted Administration of Epoprostenal	DME MAC
K0462	Loaner Equipment	DME MAC
K0552 - K0605	External Infusion Pump Supplies	DME MAC
K0606 - K0609	Defibrillator Accessories	DME MAC
K0669	Wheelchair Cushion	DME MAC
K0672	Soft Interface for Orthosis	DME MAC
K0730	Inhalation Drug Delivery System	DME MAC

HCPCS	DESCRIPTION	JURISDICTION
K0733	Power Wheelchair Accessory	DME MAC
K0738	Oxygen Equipment	DME MAC
K0739	Repair or Nonroutine Service for DME	Part B MAC if implanted DME. If other, DME MAC.
K0740	Repair or Nonroutine Service for Oxygen Equipment	DME MAC
K0743 - K0746	Suction Pump and Dressings	DME MAC
K0800 - K0899	Power Mobility Devices	DME MAC
K0900	Custom DME, other than Wheelchair	DME MAC
K1001 - K1003	Devices	DME MAC
K1004	Devices	DME MAC when the supplier considers the item DMEPOS. Part B MAC if the supplier considers the item something other than DMEPOS (e.g., supplies furnished incident to the professional service of physician).
K1005 - K1006	Devices	DME MAC
K1007	Devices	DME MAC when the supplier considers the item DMEPOS. Part B MAC if the supplier considers the item something other than DMEPOS (e.g., supplies furnished incident to the professional service of a physician).
K1009	Devices	DME MAC
K1013	Devices	Part B MAC if supply for or inserted by a licensed healthcare provider. If other, DME MAC.
K1014 - K1026	Devices	DME MAC
K1027	Devices	DME MAC when the supplier considers the item DMEPOS. Part B MAC if the supplier considers the item something other than DMEPOS (e.g., supplies furnished incident to the professional service of a physician).
K1028 - K1029	Devices	DME MAC
K1031 - K1033	Devices	DME MAC
L0112 - L4631	Orthotics & Devices	DME MAC
L5000 - L5999	Lower Limb Prosthetics	DME MAC
L6000 - L7499	Upper Limb Prosthetics	DME MAC
L7510 - L7520	Repair of Prosthetic Device	Part B MAC if repair of implanted prosthetic device. If other, DME MAC.
L7600 - L8485	Prosthetics	DME MAC
L8499	Unlisted Procedure for Miscellaneous Prosthetic Services	Part B MAC if implanted prosthetic device. If other, DME MAC.
L8500 - L8501	Artificial Larynx; Tracheostomy Speaking Valve	DME MAC
L8505	Artificial Larynx Accessory	DME MAC

HCPCS	DESCRIPTION	JURISDICTION
L8507	Voice Prosthesis, Patient Inserted	DME MAC
L8509	Voice Prosthesis, Inserted by a Licensed Health Care Provider	Part B MAC for dates of service on or after 10/01/2010. DME MAC for dates of service prior to 10/01/2010
L8510	Voice Prosthesis	DME MAC
L8511 - L8515	Voice Prosthesis	Part B MAC if used with tracheoesophageal voice prostheses inserted by a licensed health care provider. If other, DME MAC
L8701 - L8702	Assist Device	DME MAC
L9900	Miscellaneous Orthotic or Prosthetic Component or Accessory	Part B MAC if used with implanted prosthetic device. If other, DME MAC.
Q0144	Azithromycin Dihydrate	Part B MAC if incident to a physician's service. If other, DME MAC.
Q0161 - Q0181	Anti-emetic	DME MAC
Q0510 - Q0514	Drug Dispensing Fees	DME MAC
Q2049 -Q2050	Doxorubicin	Part B MAC if incident to a physician's service or used in an implanted infusion pump. If other, DME MAC.
Q2052	IVIG Demonstration	DME MAC
Q4074	Inhalation Drug	Part B MAC if incident to a physician's service. If other, DME MAC.
Q5101 - Q5121	Injection	Part B MAC if incident to a physician's service. If other, DME MAC.

HCPCS	DESCRIPTION	JURISDICTION
Q9991 - Q9992	Injection	Part B MAC if incident to a physician's service or used in an implanted infusion pump. If other, DME MAC.
V2020 - V2025	Frames	DME MAC
V2100 - V2513	Lenses	DME MAC
V2520 - V2523	Hydrophilic Contact Lenses	Part B MAC if incident to a physician's service. If other, DME MAC.
V2524 - V2525	Hydrophilic Contact Lenses	DME MAC
V2530 - V2531	Contact Lenses, Scleral	DME MAC
V2599	Contact Lens, Other Type	Part B MAC if incident to a physician's service. If other, DME MAC.
V2600 - V2615	Low Vision Aids	DME MAC
V2623 - V2629	Prosthetic Eyes	DME MAC
V2700 - V2780	Miscellaneous Vision Service	DME MAC
V2781	Progressive Lens	DME MAC
V2782 - V2784	Lenses	DME MAC
V2786	Lens	DME MAC
V2797	Vision Supply	DME MAC
V2799	Miscellaneous Vision Service	Part B MAC if supply for an implanted prosthetic device. If other, DME MAC
V5336	Repair/Modification of Augmentative Communicative System or Device	DME MAC

APPENDIX B

CHAPTER I
GENERAL CORRECT CODING POLICIES
MEDICARE NATIONAL CORRECT CODING INITIATIVE POLICY MANUAL
Revised January *31, 2023*

Current Procedural Terminology (CPT) codes, descriptions and other data only are copyright *2022* American Medical Association. All rights reserved.

CPT® is a registered trademark of the American Medical Association.

Applicable FARS\DFARS Restrictions Apply to Government Use.

Fee schedules, relative value units, conversion factors and/or related components *aren't* assigned by the AMA, *aren't* part of CPT, and the AMA *isn't* recommending their use. The AMA *doesn't* directly or indirectly practice medicine or dispense medical services. The AMA assumes no liability for the data contained or not contained herein.

CMS issues the Hospital Outpatient Prospective Payment System (OPPS) and Ambulatory Surgical Center (ASC) Payment System.

Chapter I
Revision Date 1/*31/2023*
GENERAL CORRECT CODING POLICIES

A. Introduction

Healthcare providers/suppliers use Healthcare Common Procedure Coding System/Current Procedural Terminology (HCPCS/CPT) codes to report medical services performed on patients to Medicare Administrative Contractors (MACs). Healthcare Common Procedure Coding System (HCPCS) consists of Level I CPT (Current Procedural Terminology) codes and Level II codes. CPT codes are defined in the American Medical Association's (AMA's) "CPT Manual," which is updated and published annually. HCPCS Level II codes are defined by the Centers for Medicare & Medicaid Services (CMS) and are updated throughout the year as necessary. Changes in CPT codes are approved by the AMA CPT Editorial Panel, which meets 3 times per year.

CPT and HCPCS Level II codes define medical and surgical procedures performed on patients. Some procedure codes are very specific in defining a single service (e.g., CPT code 93000 (electrocardiogram)), while other codes define procedures consisting of many services (e.g., CPT code 58263 (Vaginal hysterectomy, for uterus 250 g or less; with removal of tube(s) and/*or* ovary(s), *with* repair of enterocele)). Because many procedures can be performed via different approaches, different methods, or in combination with other procedures, there are often multiple HCPCS/CPT codes defining similar or related procedures.

CPT and HCPCS Level II code descriptors usually do not define all services included in a procedure. There are often services inherent in a procedure or group of procedures. For example, anesthesia services include certain preparation and monitoring services.

The CMS developed the National Correct Coding Initiative (NCCI) program to prevent inappropriate payment of services that should not be reported together. Prior to April 1, 2012, NCCI Procedure-to-Procedure (PTP) edits were placed into either the "Column One/Column Two Correct Coding Edit Table" or the "Mutually Exclusive Edit Table." However, on April 1, 2012, the edits in the "Mutually Exclusive Edit Table" were moved to the "Column One/Column Two Correct Coding Edit Table"

so that all NCCI PTP edits are currently contained in this single table. Combining the 2 tables simplifies researching NCCI PTP edits and online use of the NCCI tables.

Each edit table contains edits which are pairs of HCPCS/CPT codes that in general should not be reported together. Each edit has a Column One and Column Two HCPCS/CPT code. If a provider/supplier reports the 2 codes of an edit pair, the Column Two code is denied, and the Column One code is eligible for payment. However, if it is clinically appropriate to use an NCCI PTP-associated modifier, both the Column One and Column Two codes are eligible for payment. (NCCI PTP-associated modifiers and their appropriate use are discussed elsewhere in this chapter.)

When the NCCI program was first established and during its early years, the "Column One/Column Two Correct Coding Edit Table" was termed the "Comprehensive/Component Edit Table." This latter terminology was a misnomer. Although the Column Two code is often a component of a more comprehensive Column One code, this relationship is not true for many edits. In the latter type of edit, the code pair edit simply represents 2 codes that should not be reported together. For example, a provider/supplier shall not report a vaginal hysterectomy code and total abdominal hysterectomy code together.

In this chapter, Sections B–Q address various issues relating to NCCI PTP edits.

Medically Unlikely Edits (MUEs) prevent payment for a potentially inappropriate number/quantity of the same service on a single day. An MUE *is the maximum units of service (UOS) reported for a HCPCS/CPT code on the vast majority of appropriately reported claims by the same provider/ supplier for the same beneficiary on the same date of service.* For more information concerning MUEs, see Section V of this chapter.

In this Manual, many policies are described using the term "physician." Unless otherwise indicated, the use of this term does not restrict the application of policies to physicians only. Rather, the policies apply to all practitioners, hospitals, providers, or suppliers eligible to bill the relevant HCPCS/ CPT codes pursuant to applicable portions of the Social Security Act (SSA) of 1965, the Code of Federal Regulations (CFR), and Medicare rules. In some sections of this Manual, the term "physician" would not include some of these entities because specific rules do not apply to them. For example,

Anesthesia Rules [e.g., CMS "Internet-only Manual (IOM)," Publication 100-04 ("Medicare Claims Processing Manual"), Chapter 12 (Physician/Nonphysician Practitioners), Section 50 (Payment for Anesthesiology Services)] and Global Surgery Rules [e.g., CMS "Internet-only Manual (IOM)," Publication 100-04 ("Medicare Claims Processing Manual"), Chapter 12 (Physician/Nonphysician Practitioners), Section 40 (Surgeons and Global Surgery)] do not apply to hospitals.

Providers/suppliers reporting services under Medicare's hospital Outpatient Prospective Payment System (OPPS) shall report all services in accordance with appropriate Medicare "IOM" instructions.

Providers/suppliers must report services correctly. This manual discusses general coding principles in Chapter I, and principles more relevant to other specific groups of HCPCS/CPT codes in the other chapters. There are certain types of improper coding that providers/suppliers must avoid.

Procedures shall be reported with the most comprehensive CPT code that describes the services performed. Providers/suppliers must not unbundle the services described by a HCPCS/CPT code. Some examples follow:

- A provider/supplier shall not report multiple HCPCS/CPT codes when a single comprehensive HCPCS/CPT code describes these services. For example, if a physician performs a vaginal hysterectomy on a uterus weighing less than 250 grams with bilateral salpingo-oophorectomy, the provider/supplier shall report CPT code 58262 (Vaginal hysterectomy, for uterus 250 g or less; with removal of tube(s), and/or ovary(s)). The provider/supplier shall not report CPT code 58260 (Vaginal hysterectomy, for uterus 250 g or less;) plus CPT code 58720 (Salpingo-oophorectomy, complete or partial, unilateral, or bilateral (separate procedure)).
- A physician shall not fragment a procedure into component parts. For example, if a physician performs an anal endoscopy with biopsy, the provider/supplier shall report CPT code 46606 (Anoscopy; with biopsy, single or multiple). It is improper to unbundle this procedure and report CPT code 46600 (Anoscopy; diagnostic...) plus CPT code 45100 (Biopsy of anorectal wall, anal approach...). The latter code is not intended to be used with an endoscopic procedure code.
- A provider/supplier shall not unbundle a bilateral procedure code into 2 unilateral procedure codes. For example, if a physician performs bilateral mammography, the provider/supplier shall report CPT code 77066 (Diagnostic mammography... bilateral). The provider/supplier shall not report CPT code 77065 (Diagnostic mammography...unilateral) with 2 UOS or 77065 LT plus 77065 RT.
- A provider/supplier shall not unbundle services that are integral to a more comprehensive procedure. For example, surgical access is integral to a surgical procedure. A provider/supplier shall not report CPT code 49000 (Exploratory laparotomy...) when performing an open abdominal procedure such as a total abdominal colectomy (e.g., CPT code 44150).
- Providers/suppliers shall only report a biopsy separately when pathologic examination results in a decision to immediately proceed with a more extensive procedure (e.g., excision, destruction, removal) on the same lesion; or when performed on a separate lesion.
- Providers/suppliers shall not report a biopsy separately when it is to assess resection margins or to verify resectability; or when performed and submitted for pathologic evaluation completed after performing the more extensive procedure.

Providers/suppliers must avoid downcoding. If a HCPCS/CPT code exists that describes the services performed, the providers/suppliers must report this code rather than report a less comprehensive code with other codes describing the services not included in the less comprehensive code. For example, if a physician performs a unilateral partial mastectomy with axillary lymphadenectomy, the provider/supplier shall report CPT code 19302 (Mastectomy, partial...; with axillary lymphadenectomy). A provider/supplier shall not report CPT code 19301 (Mastectomy, partial...) plus CPT code 38745 (Axillary lymphadenectomy; complete).

Providers/suppliers must avoid upcoding. A HCPCS/CPT code may be reported only if all services described by that code have been performed. For example, if a physician performs a superficial axillary lymphadenectomy (CPT code 38740), the provider/supplier shall not report CPT code 38745 (Axillary lymphadenectomy; complete).

Providers/suppliers must report UOS correctly. Each HCPCS/CPT code has a defined unit of service for reporting purposes. A provider/supplier shall not report UOS for a HCPCS/CPT code using a criterion that differs from the code's defined unit of service. For example, some therapy codes are reported in fifteen-minute increments (e.g., CPT codes 97110-97124). Others are reported per session (e.g., CPT codes 92507, 92508). A provider/supplier shall not report a per session code using fifteen-minute increments. CPT code 92507 or 92508 should be reported with one unit of service on a single date of service.

The MUE values and NCCI PTP edits are based on services provided by the same physician to the same beneficiary on the same date of service. Physicians shall not inconvenience beneficiaries nor increase risks to beneficiaries by performing services on different dates of service to avoid MUE or NCCI PTP edits.

In 2010, the "CPT Manual" modified the numbering of codes so that the sequence of codes as they appear in the "CPT Manual" does not necessarily correspond to a sequential numbering of codes. In the "National Correct Coding Initiative Policy Manual for Medicare Services", use of a numerical range of codes reflects all codes that numerically fall within the range regardless of their sequential order in the "CPT Manual".

This chapter addresses general coding principles, issues, and policies. Many of these principles, issues, and policies are addressed further in subsequent chapters dealing with specific groups of HCPCS/CPT codes. In this chapter, examples are often used to clarify principles, issues, or policies. The examples do not represent the only codes to which the principles, issues, or policies apply.

B. Coding Based on Standards of Medical/Surgical Practice

Most HCPCS/CPT code defined procedures include services that are integral to them. Some of these integral services have specific CPT codes for reporting the service when not performed as an integral part of another procedure. (For example, CPT code 36000 (Introduction of needle or intracatheter, vein) is integral to all nuclear medicine procedures requiring injection of a radiopharmaceutical into a vein. CPT code 36000 is not separately reportable with these types of nuclear medicine procedures. However, CPT code 36000 may be reported alone if the only service provided is the introduction of a needle into a vein. Other integral services do not have specific CPT codes. (For example, wound irrigation is integral to the treatment of all wounds and does not have a HCPCS/CPT code.) Services integral to HCPCS/CPT code defined procedures are included in those procedures based upon the standards of medical/surgical practice. It is inappropriate to separately report services that are integral to another procedure with that procedure.

Many NCCI PTP edits are based upon the standards of medical/surgical practice. Services that are integral to another service are component parts of the more comprehensive service. When integral component services have their own HCPCS/CPT codes, NCCI PTP edits place the comprehensive service in Column One and the component service in Column Two. Since a component service integral to a comprehensive service is not separately reportable, the Column Two code is not separately reportable with the Column One code.

Some services are integral to large numbers of procedures. Other services are integral to a more limited number of procedures. Examples of services integral to a large number of procedures include:

- Cleansing, shaving and prepping of skin
- Draping and positioning of patient
- Insertion of intravenous access for medication administration;
- Insertion of urinary catheter
- Sedative administration by the physician performing a procedure (see Chapter II, Anesthesia Services)
- Local, topical or regional anesthesia administered by the physician performing the procedure
- Surgical approach including identification of anatomical landmarks, incision, evaluation of the surgical field, debridement of traumatized tissue, lysis of adhesions, and isolation of structures limiting access to the surgical field such as bone, blood vessels, nerve, and muscles including stimulation for identification or monitoring - Surgical cultures
- Wound irrigation
- Insertion and removal of drains, suction devices, and pumps into same site
- Surgical closure and dressings
- Application, management, and removal of postoperative dressings and analgesic devices (peri-incisional)
- Application of TENS unit
- Institution of Patient Controlled Anesthesia
- Preoperative, intraoperative and postoperative documentation, including photographs, drawings, dictation, or transcription as necessary to document the services provided
- Imaging and/or ultrasound guidance
- Surgical supplies, except for specific situations where CMS policy permits separate payment.

Although other chapters in this Manual further address issues related to the standards of medical/surgical practice for the procedures covered by that chapter, it is not possible to discuss all NCCI PTP edits based upon the principle of the standards of medical/surgical practice due to space limitations. However, there are several general principles that can be applied to the edits, as follows:

1. The component service is an accepted standard of care when performing the comprehensive service.
2. The component service is usually necessary to complete the comprehensive service.
3. The component service is not a separately distinguishable procedure when performed with the comprehensive service.

Specific examples of services that are not separately reportable because they are components of more comprehensive services follow:

Medical Examples

1. Because interpretation of cardiac rhythm is an integral component of the interpretation of an electrocardiogram, a rhythm strip is not separately reportable.
2. Because determination of ankle/brachial indices requires both upper and lower extremity Doppler studies, an upper extremity Doppler study is not separately reportable.
3. Because a cardiac stress test includes multiple electrocardiograms, an electrocardiogram is not separately reportable.

Surgical Examples

1. Because a myringotomy requires access to the tympanic membrane through the external auditory canal, removal of impacted cerumen from the external auditory canal is not separately reportable.
2. A "scout" bronchoscopy to assess the surgical field, anatomic landmarks, extent of disease, etc., is not separately reportable with an open pulmonary procedure such as a pulmonary lobectomy. By contrast, an initial diagnostic bronchoscopy is separately reportable. If the diagnostic bronchoscopy is performed at the same patient encounter as the open pulmonary procedure and does not duplicate an earlier diagnostic bronchoscopy by the same or another physician, the diagnostic bronchoscopy may be reported with modifier 58 appended to the open pulmonary procedure code to indicate a staged procedure. A cursory examination of the upper airway during a bronchoscopy with the bronchoscope shall not be reported separately as a laryngoscopy. However, separate endoscopies of anatomically distinct areas with different endoscopes may be reported separately (e.g., thoracoscopy and mediastinoscopy).
3. If an endoscopic procedure is performed at the same patient encounter as a nonendoscopic procedure to ensure no intraoperative injury occurred or verify the procedure was performed correctly, the endoscopic procedure is not separately reportable with the nonendoscopic procedure.
4. Because a colectomy requires exposure of the colon, the laparotomy and adhesiolysis to expose the colon are not separately reportable.

Medical/Surgical Package

Most medical and surgical procedures include pre-procedure, intra-procedure, and postprocedure work. When multiple procedures are performed at the same patient encounter, there is often overlap of the pre-procedure and post-procedure work. Payment methodologies for surgical procedures account for the overlap of the pre-procedure and post-procedure work.

The component elements of the pre-procedure and post-procedure work for each procedure are included component services of that procedure as a standard of medical/surgical practice. Some general guidelines follow:

1. Many invasive procedures require vascular and/or airway access. The work associated with obtaining the required access is included in the pre-procedure or intra-procedure work. The work associated with returning a patient to the appropriate post-procedure state is included in the post-procedure work.

Airway access is necessary for general anesthesia and is not separately reportable. There is no CPT code for elective endotracheal intubation. CPT code 31500 describes an emergency endotracheal intubation and shall not be reported for elective endotracheal intubation. Visualization of the airway is a component part of an endotracheal intubation, and CPT codes describing procedures that visualize the airway (e.g., nasal endoscopy, laryngoscopy, bronchoscopy) shall not be reported with an endotracheal intubation. These CPT codes describe diagnostic and therapeutic endoscopies, and it is a misuse of these codes to report visualization of the airway for endotracheal intubation.

Intravenous access (e.g., CPT codes 36000, 36400, 36410) is not separately reportable when performed with many types of procedures (e.g., surgical procedures, anesthesia procedures, radiological procedures requiring intravenous contrast, nuclear medicine procedures requiring intravenous radiopharmaceutical).

After vascular access is achieved, the access must be maintained by a slow infusion (e.g., saline) or injection of heparin or saline into a "lock." Since these services are necessary for maintenance of the vascular access, they are not separately reportable with the vascular access CPT codes or procedures requiring vascular access as a standard of medical/surgical practice. CPT codes 37211-37214 (Transcatheter therapy with infusion for thrombolysis) shall not be reported for use of an anticoagulant to maintain vascular access.

The global surgical package includes the administration of fluids and drugs during the operative procedure. CPT codes 96360-*96379* shall not be reported separately for that operative procedure. Under OPPS, the administration of fluids and drugs during or for an operative procedure are included services and are not separately reportable (e.g., CPT codes 96360-*96379*).

When a procedure requires more invasive vascular access services (e.g., central venous access, pulmonary artery access), the more invasive vascular service is separately reportable if it is not typical of the procedure and the work of the more invasive vascular service has not been included in the valuation of the procedure.

Insertion of a central venous access device (e.g., central venous catheter, pulmonary artery catheter) requires passage of a catheter through central venous vessels and, in the case of a pulmonary artery catheter, through the right atrium and ventricle. These services often require the use of fluoroscopic guidance. Separate reporting of CPT codes for right heart catheterization, selective venous catheterization, or pulmonary artery catheterization is not appropriate when reporting a CPT code for insertion of a central venous access device. Since CPT code 77001 describes fluoroscopic guidance for central venous access device procedures, CPT codes for more general fluoroscopy (e.g., 76000, 77002) shall not be reported separately. (CPT code 76001 was deleted January 1, 2019.)

2. Medicare Anesthesia Rules prevent separate payment for anesthesia services by the same physician performing a surgical or medical procedure. The physician performing a surgical or medical procedure shall not report CPT codes 96360-*96379* for the administration of anesthetic agents during the procedure. If it is medically reasonable and necessary that a separate provider/supplier (anesthesia practitioner) perform anesthesia services (e.g., monitored anesthesia care) for a surgical or medical procedure, a separate anesthesia service may be reported by the second provider/supplier.

Under the OPPS, anesthesia for a surgical procedure is an included service and is not separately reportable. For example, a provider/supplier shall not report CPT codes 96360-*96379* for anesthesia services.

When anesthesia services are not separately reportable, providers/suppliers shall not unbundle components of anesthesia and report them in lieu of an anesthesia code.

3. If an endoscopic procedure is performed at the same patient encounter as a nonendoscopic procedure to ensure that no intraoperative injury occurred or to verify that the procedure was performed correctly, the endoscopic procedure is not separately reportable with the non-endoscopic procedure.
4. Many procedures require cardiopulmonary monitoring, either by the physician performing the procedure or an anesthesia practitioner. Since these services are integral to the procedure, they are not separately reportable. Examples of these services include cardiac monitoring, pulse oximetry, and ventilation management (e.g., 93000-93010, 93040-93042, 94760, 94761).
5. *For more information regarding biopsies, see Section A, Introduction.*
6. Exposure and exploration of the surgical field is integral to an operative procedure and is not separately reportable. For example, an exploratory laparotomy (CPT code 49000) is not separately reportable with an intra-abdominal procedure. If exploration of the surgical field results in additional procedures other than the primary procedure, the additional procedures may generally be reported separately. However, a procedure designated by the CPT code descriptor as a "separate procedure" is not separately reportable if performed in a region anatomically related to the other procedure(s) through the same skin incision, orifice, or surgical approach.
7. If a definitive surgical procedure requires access through diseased tissue (e.g., necrotic skin, abscess, hematoma, seroma), a separate service for this access (e.g., debridement, incision, and drainage) is not separately reportable. Types of procedures to which this principle applies include, but are not limited to, -ectomy, -otomy, excision, resection, -plasty, insertion, revision, replacement, relocation, removal, or closure. For example, debridement of skin and subcutaneous tissue at the site of an abdominal incision made to perform an intra-abdominal procedure is not separately reportable. (See Chapter IV, Section I (General Policy Statements), Subsection 11 for guidance on reporting debridement with open fractures and dislocations.)
8. If removal, destruction, or other form of elimination of a lesion requires coincidental elimination of other pathology, only the primary procedure may be reported. For example, if an area of pilonidal disease contains an abscess, incision, and drainage of the abscess during the procedure to excise the area of pilonidal disease is not separately reportable.
9. An excision and removal (-ectomy) includes the incision and opening (-otomy) of the organ. A HCPCS/CPT code for an –otomy procedure shall not be reported with an –ectomy code for the same organ.
10. Multiple approaches to the same procedure are mutually exclusive of one another and shall not be reported sepa-

rately. For example, both a vaginal hysterectomy and abdominal hysterectomy shall not be reported separately.

11. If a procedure using one approach fails and is converted to a procedure using a different approach, only the completed procedure may be reported. For example, if a laparoscopic hysterectomy is converted to an open hysterectomy, only the open hysterectomy procedure code may be reported.

12. If a laparoscopic procedure fails and is converted to an open procedure, the physician shall not report a diagnostic laparoscopy in lieu of the failed laparoscopic procedure. For example, if a laparoscopic cholecystectomy is converted to an open cholecystectomy, the physician shall not report the failed laparoscopic cholecystectomy nor a diagnostic laparoscopy.

13. If a diagnostic endoscopy is the basis for and precedes an open procedure, the diagnostic endoscopy may be reported with modifier 58 appended to the open procedure code. However, the medical record must document the medical reasonableness and necessity for the diagnostic endoscopy. A scout endoscopy to assess anatomic landmarks and extent of disease is not separately reportable with an open procedure. When an endoscopic procedure fails and is converted to another surgical procedure, only the completed surgical procedure may be reported. The endoscopic procedure is not separately reportable with the completed surgical procedure.

14. Treatment of complications of primary surgical procedures is separately reportable with some limitations. The global surgical package for an operative procedure includes all intra-operative services that are normally a usual and necessary part of the procedure. Additionally, the global surgical package includes all medical and surgical services required of the surgeon during the postoperative period of the surgery to treat complications that do not require return to the operating room. Thus, treatment of a complication of a primary surgical procedure is not separately reportable:

    (1) if it represents usual and necessary care in the operating room during the procedure; or

    (2) if it occurs postoperatively and does not require return to the operating room. For example, control of hemorrhage is a usual and necessary component of a surgical procedure in the operating room and is not separately reportable. Control of postoperative hemorrhage is also not separately reportable unless the patient must be returned to the operating room for treatment. In the latter case, the control of hemorrhage may be separately reportable with modifier 78.

D. Evaluation & Management (E&M) Services

Medicare Global Surgery Rules define the rules for reporting Evaluation & Management (E&M) services with procedures covered by these rules. This section summarizes some of the rules.

All procedures on the Medicare Physician Fee Schedule are assigned a global period of 000, 010, 090, XXX, YYY, ZZZ, or MMM. The global concept does not apply to XXX procedures. The global period for YYY procedures is defined by the MAC. All procedures with a global period of ZZZ are related to another procedure, and the applicable global period for the ZZZ code is determined by the related procedure. Procedures with a global period of MMM are maternity procedures.

Since NCCI PTP edits are applied to same-day services by the same provider/supplier to the same beneficiary, certain Global Surgery Rules are applicable to the NCCI program. An E&M service is separately reportable on the same date of service as a procedure with a global period of 000, 010, or 090 under limited circumstances.

If a procedure has a global period of 090 days, it is defined as a major surgical procedure. If an E&M service is performed on the same date of service as a major surgical procedure to decide whether to perform this surgical procedure, the E&M service is separately reportable with modifier 57. Other preoperative E&M services on the same date of service as a major surgical procedure are included in the global payment for the procedure and are not separately reportable. NCCI does not contain edits based on this rule because MACs have separate edits.

If a procedure has a global period of 000 or 010 days, it is defined as a minor surgical procedure. In general, E&M services performed on the same date of service as a minor surgical procedure are included in the payment for the procedure. The decision to perform a minor surgical procedure is included in the payment for the minor surgical procedure and shall not be reported separately as an E&M service. However, a significant and separately identifiable E&M service unrelated to the decision to perform the minor surgical procedure is separately reportable with modifier 25. The E&M service and minor surgical procedure do not require different diagnoses. If a minor surgical procedure is performed on a new patient, the same rules for reporting E&M services apply. The fact that the patient is "new" to the provider/supplier is not sufficient alone to justify reporting an E&M service on the same date of service as a minor surgical procedure. NCCI contains many, but not all, possible edits based on these principles.

For major and minor surgical procedures, postoperative E&M services related to recovery from the surgical procedure during the postoperative period are included in the global surgical package as are E&M services related to complications of the surgery. Postoperative visits unrelated to the diagnosis for which the surgical procedure was performed, unless related to a complication of surgery, may be reported separately on the same day as a surgical procedure with modifier 24 ("Unrelated Evaluation and Management Service by the Same Physician or Other Qualified Health Care Professional During a Postoperative Period").

Procedures with a global surgery indicator of "XXX" are not covered by these rules. Many of these "XXX" procedures are performed by physicians and have inherent pre-procedure, intraprocedure, and post-procedure work usually performed each time the procedure is completed. This work shall **not** be reported as a separate E&M code. Other "XXX" procedures are not usually performed by a physician and have no physician work relative value units associated with them. A physician shall **not** report a separate E&M code with these procedures for the supervision of others performing the procedure or for the interpretation of the procedure. With most "XXX" procedures, the physician may, however, perform a significant and separately identifiable E&M service on the same date of service which may be reported by appending modifier 25 to the E&M code. This E&M service may be related to the same diagnosis necessitating performance of the "XXX" procedure but cannot include any work inherent in the "XXX" procedure, supervision of others performing the "XXX" procedure, or time for interpreting the result of the "XXX" procedure. Appending modifier 25 to a significant, separately identifiable E&M service when performed on the same date of service as an "XXX" procedure is correct coding.

E. Modifiers and Modifier Indicators

1. The AMA "CPT Manual" and the CMS define modifiers that may be appended to HCPCS/CPT codes to provide additional information about the services rendered. Modifiers consist of 2 alphanumeric characters.

Modifiers may be appended to HCPCS/CPT codes only if the clinical circumstances justify the use of the modifier. A modifier shall not be appended to a HCPCS/CPT code solely to bypass an NCCI PTP edit if the clinical circumstances do not justify its use. If the Medicare program imposes restrictions on the use of a modifier, the modifier may only be used to bypass an NCCI PTP edit if the Medicare restrictions are fulfilled. Modifiers that may be used under appropriate clinical circumstances to bypass an NCCI PTP edit include:

Anatomic modifiers: E1-E4, FA, F1-F9, TA, T1-T9, LT, RT, LC, LD, RC, LM, RI

Global surgery modifiers: 24, 25, 57, 58, 78, 79

Other modifiers: 27, 59, 91, XE, XS, XP, XU

Modifiers 76 ("Repeat Procedure or Service by Same Physician") and 77 ("Repeat Procedure by Another Physician") are not NCCI PTP-associated modifiers. Use of either of these modifiers does not bypass an NCCI PTP edit.

Each NCCI PTP edit has an assigned modifier indicator. A modifier indicator of "0" indicates that NCCI PTP-associated modifiers cannot be used to bypass the edit. A modifier indicator of "1" indicates that NCCI PTP-associated modifiers may be used to bypass an edit under appropriate circumstances. A modifier indicator of "9" indicates that the edit has been deleted, and the modifier indicator is not relevant.

It is very important that NCCI PTP-associated modifiers only be used when appropriate. In general, these circumstances relate to separate patient encounters, separate anatomic sites, or separate specimens. (See subsequent discussion of modifiers in this section.) Most edits involving paired organs or structures (e.g., eyes, ears, extremities, lungs, kidneys) have NCCI PTP modifier indicators of "1" because the 2 codes of the code pair edit may be reported if performed on the contralateral organs or structures. Most of these code pairs should not be reported with NCCI PTPassociated modifiers when performed on the ipsilateral organ or structure unless there is a specific coding rationale to bypass the edit. The existence of the NCCI PTP edit indicates that the 2 codes generally cannot be reported together unless the 2 corresponding procedures are performed at 2 separate patient encounters or 2 separate anatomic locations. However, if the 2 corresponding procedures are performed at the same patient encounter and in contiguous structures in the same organ or anatomic region, NCCI PTP-associated modifiers generally should not be used.

The appropriate use of most of these modifiers is straightforward. However, further explanation is provided regarding modifiers 25, 58, and 59. Although modifier 22 is not a modifier that bypasses an NCCI PTP edit, its use is occasionally relevant to an NCCI PTP edit and is discussed below.

a) **Modifier 22**: Modifier 22 is defined by the "CPT Manual" as "Increased Procedural Services." This modifier shall not be reported unless the service(s) performed is (are) substantially more extensive than the usual service(s) included in the procedure described by the HCPCS/CPT code reported.

When an NCCI PTP edit allows use of NCCI PTP-associated modifiers to bypass *the edit* and the clinical circumstances justify use of one of these modifiers, both services may be reported with the NCCI PTP-associated modifier. However, if the NCCI PTP edit does not allow use of NCCI PTP-associated modifiers to bypass it and the procedure qualifies as an unusual procedural service, the physician may report the Column One HCPCS/CPT code of the NCCI PTP edit with modifier 22. The MAC may then evaluate the unusual procedural service to determine whether additional payment is justified.

For example, CMS limits payment for CPT code 69990 (Microsurgical techniques, requiring use of operating microscope...) to procedures listed in the "IOM" ("Claims Processing Manual", Publication 100-04, 12-§20.4.5). If a physician reports CPT code 69990 with 2 other CPT codes and 1 of the codes is not on this list, an NCCI PTP edit with the code not on the list will prevent payment for CPT code 69990. Claims processing systems do not determine which procedure is linked with CPT code 69990. In situations such as this, the physician may submit their claim to the local MAC for readjudication appending modifier 22 to the CPT code. Although MAC cannot override an NCCI PTP edit that does not allow use of NCCI PTP-associated modifiers, the MAC has discretion to adjust payment to include use of the operating microscope based on modifier 22.

b) **Modifier 25**: The "CPT Manual" defines modifier 25 as a "Significant, Separately Identifiable Evaluation and Management Service by the Same Physician or Other Qualified Health Care Professional on the Same Day of the Procedure or Other Service." Modifier 25 may be appended to an evaluation and management (E&M) CPT code to indicate that the E&M service is significant and separately identifiable from other services reported on the same date of service. The E&M service may be related to the same or different diagnosis as the other procedure(s).

Modifier 25 may be appended to E&M services reported with minor surgical procedures (with global periods of 000 or 010 days) or procedures not covered by Global Surgery Rules (with a global indicator of XXX). Since minor surgical procedures and XXX procedures include preprocedure, intra-procedure, and post-procedure work inherent in the procedure, the provider/supplier shall not report an E&M service for this work. Furthermore, Medicare Global Surgery Rules prevent the reporting of a separate E&M service for the work associated with the decision to perform a minor surgical procedure regardless of whether the patient is a new or established patient.

c) **Modifier 58**: Modifier 58 is defined by the "CPT Manual" as a "Staged or Related Procedure or Service by the Same Physician or Other Qualified Health Care Professional During the Postoperative Period." It may be used to indicate that a procedure was followed by a second procedure during the post-operative period of the first procedure. This situation may occur because the second procedure was planned prospectively, was more extensive than the first procedure, or was therapy after a diagnostic surgical service. Use of modifier 58 will bypass NCCI PTP edits that allow use of NCCI PTP-associated modifiers.

If a diagnostic endoscopic procedure results in the decision to perform an open procedure, both procedures may be reported with modifier 58 appended to the HCPCS/CPT code for the open procedure. However, if the endoscopic procedure preceding an open procedure is a "scout" procedure to assess anatomic landmarks and/or extent of disease, it is not separately reportable.

Diagnostic endoscopy is never separately reportable with another endoscopic procedure of the same organ(s)or anatomic region when performed at the same patient encounter. Similarly, diagnostic laparoscopy is never separately reportable with a surgical laparoscopic procedure of the same body cavity when performed at the same patient encounter.

If a planned laparoscopic procedure fails and is converted to an open procedure, only the open procedure may be reported. The failed laparoscopic procedure is not separately reportable. The NCCI program contains many, but not all, edits bundling laparoscopic procedures into open procedures. Since the number of possible code combinations bundling a laparoscopic procedure into an open procedure is much greater than the number of such edits in the NCCI program, the principle stated in this paragraph is applicable regardless of whether the selected code pair combination is included in the NCCI tables. A provider/supplier shall not select laparoscopic and open HCPCS/CPT codes to report because the combination is not included in the NCCI tables.

d) **Modifier 59:** Modifier 59 is an important NCCI PTP-associated modifier that is often used incorrectly. For the NCCI program, its primary purpose is to indicate that 2 or more procedures are performed at different anatomic sites or different patient encounters. One function of NCCI PTP edits is to prevent payment for codes that report overlapping services, except in those instances where the services are "separate and distinct." Modifier 59 shall only be used if no other modifier more appropriately describes the relationships of the 2 or more procedure codes (see Section E for modifiers -X{EPSU}). The "CPT Manual" defines modifier 59 as follows:

Modifier 59: Distinct Procedural Service: Under certain circumstances, it may be necessary to indicate that a procedure or service was distinct or independent from other non-E/M services performed on the same day. Modifier 59 is used to identify procedures/services, other than E/M services, that are not normally reported together, but are appropriate under the circumstances. Documentation must support a different session, different procedure or surgery, different site or organ system, separate incision/excision, separate lesion, or separate injury (or area of injury in extensive injuries) not ordinarily encountered or performed on the same day by the same individual. However, when another already established modifier is appropriate, it should be used rather than modifier 59. Only if no more descriptive modifier is available, and the use of modifier 59 best explains the circumstances, should modifier 59 be used. Note: Modifier 59 should not be appended to an E/M service. To report a separate and distinct E/M service with a nonE/M service performed on the same date, see modifier 25."

Modifier 59 and other NCCI-associated modifiers should **NOT** be used to bypass a PTP edit unless the proper criteria for use of the modifier are met. Documentation in the medical record

must satisfy the criteria required by any NCCI-associated modifier that is used. Modifier "-59" shall not be used with code 77427 Radiation treatment management, 5 treatments.

NCCI PTP edits define when 2 procedure HCPCS/CPT codes may not be reported together, except under special circumstances. If an edit allows use of NCCI PTP-associated modifiers, the 2 procedure codes may be reported together when the 2 procedures are performed at different anatomic sites or different patient encounters. MAC processing systems use NCCI PTP associated modifiers to allow payment of both codes of an edit. Modifiers 59 or -X{EPSU} and other NCCI PTP-associated modifiers shall NOT be used to bypass an NCCI PTP edit unless the proper criteria for use of the modifier are met. Documentation in the medical record must satisfy the criteria required by any NCCI PTP-associated modifier used. Some examples of the appropriate use of modifiers 59 or -X{EPSU} are contained in the individual chapter policies.

One of the common misuses of modifier 59 is related to the portion of the definition of modifier 59 allowing its use to describe "different procedure or surgery." The code descriptors of the 2 codes of a code pair edit usually represent different procedures or surgeries. The edit indicates that the 2 procedures/surgeries cannot be reported together if performed at the same anatomic site and same patient encounter. The provider/supplier cannot use modifier 59 for such an edit based on the 2 codes being different procedures/surgeries. However, if the 2 procedures/surgeries are performed at separate anatomic sites or at separate patient encounters on the same date of service, modifiers 59 or -X{ES} may be appended to indicate that they are different procedures/surgeries on that date of service.

Modifier 59 or XS is used appropriately for different anatomic sites during the same encounter only when procedures which are not ordinarily performed or encountered on the same day are performed on different organs, or different anatomic regions, or in limited situations on different, non-contiguous lesions in different anatomic regions of the same organ.

There are several exceptions to this general principle about misuse of modifiers 59 or X{EPSU} that apply to some code pair edits for procedures performed at the same patient encounter.

(1) When a diagnostic procedure precedes a surgical or non-surgical therapeutic procedure and is the basis on which the decision to perform the surgical or non-surgical therapeutic procedure is made, that diagnostic procedure may be considered to be a separate and distinct procedure as long as (a) it occurs before the therapeutic procedure and is not interspersed with services that are required for the therapeutic intervention; (b) it clearly provides the information needed to decide whether to proceed with the therapeutic procedure; and (c) it does not constitute a service that would have otherwise been required during the therapeutic intervention. If the diagnostic procedure is an inherent component of the surgical or non-surgical therapeutic procedure, it shall not be reported separately.

(2) When a diagnostic procedure follows a surgical procedure or non-surgical therapeutic procedure, that diagnostic procedure may be considered to be a separate and distinct procedure as long as (a) it occurs after the completion of the therapeutic procedure and is not interspersed with or otherwise commingled with services that are only required for the therapeutic intervention, and (b) it does not constitute a service that

would have otherwise been required during the therapeutic intervention. If the postprocedure diagnostic procedure is an inherent component or otherwise included (or not separately payable) post-procedure service of the surgical procedure or non-surgical therapeutic procedure, it shall not be reported separately.

(3) There is an appropriate use for modifiers 59 or -X[ES] that is applicable only to codes for which the unit of service is a measure of time (e.g., per 15 minutes, per hour). If 2 separate and distinct timed services are provided in separate and distinct time blocks, modifier 59 may be used to identify the services. The separate and distinct time blocks for the 2 services may be sequential to one another or split. When the 2 services are split, the time block for 1 service may be followed by a time block for the second service followed by another time block for the first service. All Medicare rules for reporting timed services are applicable. For example, the total time is calculated for all related timed services performed. The number of reportable UOS is based on the total time, and these UOS are allocated between the HCPCS/CPT codes for the individual services performed. The practitioner is not permitted to perform multiple services, each for the minimal reportable time, and report each of these as separate UOS.

Use of modifiers 59 or -X[ES] to indicate different procedures/surgeries does not require a different diagnosis for each HCPCS/CPT coded procedure/surgery. Additionally, different diagnoses are not adequate criteria for use of modifiers 59 or -X[EPSU]. The HCPCS/CPT codes remain bundled unless the procedures/surgeries are performed at different anatomic sites or separate patient encounters.

From an NCCI program perspective, the definition of different anatomic sites includes different organs, different anatomic regions, or different lesions in the same organ. It does not include treatment of contiguous structures in the same organ or anatomic region. For example, treatment of the nail, nail bed, and adjacent soft tissue constitutes treatment of a single anatomic site. Treatment of posterior segment structures in the ipsilateral eye constitutes treatment of a single anatomic site.

If the same procedure is performed at different anatomic sites, it does not necessarily imply that a HCPCS/CPT code may be reported with more than one unit of service for the procedure. Determining whether additional UOS may be reported depends in part upon the HCPCS/CPT code descriptor including the definition of the code's unit of service when present.

Example 1

The Column One/Column Two code edit with Column One CPT code 38221 (Diagnostic bone marrow biopsy(ies)) and Column Two CPT code 38220 (Diagnostic bone marrow, aspiration) includes two distinct procedures when performed at separate anatomic sites (e.g., contralateral iliac bones) or separate patient encounters. In these circumstances, it would be acceptable to use modifier 59. However, if both 38221 and 38220 are performed on the same iliac bone at the same patient encounter which is the usual practice, modifier 59 shall NOT be used. Although CMS does not allow separate payment for CPT code 38220 with CPT code 38221 when bone marrow aspiration and biopsy are performed on the same iliac bone at a single patient encounter, a physician may report CPT code 38222 (Diagnostic bone marrow; biopsy(ies) and aspiration(s)).

Example 2

The Column One/Column Two code edit with Column One CPT code 11055 (Paring or cutting of benign hyperkeratotic lesion (eg, corn or callus); single lesion) and Column Two CPT code 11720 (Debridement of nail(s) by any method(s); 1 to 5) should not be reported together for services performed on skin distal to and including the skin overlying the distal interphalangeal joint of the same toe. Modifiers 59 or –X[EPSU] should not be used if a nail is debrided on the same toe on which a hyperkeratotic lesion of the skin on or distal to the distal interphalangeal joint is pared. Modifiers 59 or –XS may be reported with code 11720 if 1 to 5 nails are debrided, and a hyperkeratotic lesion is pared on a toe other than 1 with a debrided toenail or the hyperkeratotic lesion is proximal to the skin overlying the distal interphalangeal joint of a toe on which a nail is debrided.

e) **Modifiers XE, XS, XP, XU:** These modifiers were effective January 1, 2015. These modifiers were developed to provide greater reporting specificity in situations where modifier 59 was previously reported and may be used in lieu of modifier 59 whenever possible. The modifiers are defined as follows:

XE – "Separate Encounter, A service that is distinct because it occurred during a separate encounter." This modifier shall only be used to describe separate encounters on the same date of service.

XS – "Separate Structure, A service that is distinct because it was performed on a separate organ/structure"

XP – "Separate Practitioner, A service that is distinct because it was performed by a different practitioner"

XU – "Unusual Non-Overlapping Service, the use of a service that is distinct because it does not overlap usual components of the main service"

F. Standard Preparation/Monitoring Services for Anesthesia

With few exceptions, anesthesia HCPCS/CPT codes do not specify the mode of anesthesia for a particular procedure. Regardless of the mode of anesthesia, preparation and monitoring services are not separately reportable with anesthesia service HCPCS/CPT codes when performed in association with the anesthesia service. However, if the provider/*supplier* of the anesthesia service performs 1 or more of these services prior to and unrelated to the anticipated anesthesia service or after the patient is released from the anesthesia practitioner's postoperative care, the service may be separately reportable with modifiers 59 or -X[EU].

G. Anesthesia Service Included in the Surgical Procedure

Under the CMS Anesthesia Rules, with limited exceptions, Medicare does not allow separate payment for anesthesia services performed by the physician who also furnishes the medical or surgical service. In this case, payment for the anesthesia service is included in the payment for the medical or surgical procedure. Likewise, under OPPS, payment for the anesthesia service is generally included in the payment for the medical or surgical procedure. For example, separate payment is not allowed for the physician's performance of local, regional, or most other anesthesia including nerve blocks if the physician also performs the medical or surgical procedure. Medicare generally allows separate reporting for moderate conscious sedation services (CPT codes 99151-99153) when provided by the same physician performing a medical or surgical procedure except when the anesthesia service is bundled into the procedure, e.g., radiation treatment management.

CPT codes describing anesthesia services (00100-01999) or services that are bundled into anesthesia shall not be reported in addition to the surgical or medical procedure requiring the anesthesia services if performed by the same physician. Examples of improperly reported services that are bundled into the anesthesia service when anesthesia is provided by the physician performing the medical or surgical procedure include introduction of needle or intracatheter into a vein (CPT code 36000), venipuncture (CPT code 36410), intravenous infusion/injection (CPT codes 96360-96368, 96374-96377) or cardiac assessment (e.g., CPT codes 93000-93010, 9304093042). However, if these services are not related to the delivery of an anesthetic agent or are not an inherent component of the procedure or global service, they may be reported separately.

The physician performing a surgical or medical procedure shall not report an epidural/subarachnoid injection (CPT codes 62320-62327) or nerve block (CPT codes 6440064530) for anesthesia for that procedure.

H. HCPCS/CPT Procedure Code Definition

The HCPCS/CPT code descriptors of 2 codes are often the basis of an NCCI PTP edit. If 2 HCPCS/CPT codes describe redundant services, they shall not be reported separately. Several general principles follow:

1. A family of CPT codes may include a CPT code followed by one or more indented CPT codes. The first CPT code descriptor includes a semicolon. The portion of the descriptor of the first code in the family preceding the semicolon is a common part of the descriptor for each subsequent code of the family. For example:

CPT code 70120 Radiologic examination, mastoids; less than 3 views per side

CPT code 70130 complete, minimum of 3 views per side

The portion of the descriptor preceding the semicolon ("Radiologic examination, mastoids") is common to both CPT codes 70120 and 70130. The difference between the 2 codes is the portion of the descriptors following the semicolon. Often, as in this case, 2 codes from a family may not be reported separately. A physician cannot report CPT codes 70120 and 70130 for a procedure performed on ipsilateral mastoids at the same patient encounter. It is important to recognize, however, that there are numerous circumstances when it may be appropriate to report more than one code from a family of codes. For example, CPT codes 70120 and 70130 may be reported separately if the 2 procedures are performed on contralateral mastoids or at 2 separate patient encounters on the same date of service.

2. If a HCPCS/CPT code is reported, it includes all components of the procedure defined by the descriptor. For example, CPT code 58291 includes a vaginal hysterectomy with "removal of tube(s) and/or ovary(s)." A physician cannot report a salpingo-oophorectomy (CPT code 58720) separately with CPT code 58291.

3. CPT code descriptors often define correct coding relationships where 2 codes may not be reported separately with one another at the same anatomic site and/or same patient encounter. A few examples follow:
   a) A "partial" procedure is not separately reportable with a "complete" procedure.
   b) A "partial" procedure is not separately reportable with a "total" procedure.
   c) A "unilateral" procedure is not separately reportable with a "bilateral" procedure.
   d) A "single" procedure is not separately reportable with a "multiple" procedure.
   e) A "with" procedure is not separately reportable with a "without" procedure.
   f) An "initial" procedure is not separately reportable with a "subsequent" procedure.

I. CPT Manual and CMS Coding Manual Instructions

The CMS often publishes coding instructions in its rules, manuals, and notices. Physicians must use these instructions when reporting services rendered to Medicare patients.

The "CPT Manual" also includes coding instructions which may be found in the "Introduction," individual chapters, and appendices. In individual chapters, the instructions may appear at the beginning of a chapter, at the beginning of a subsection of the chapter, or after specific CPT codes. Physicians should follow "CPT Manual" instructions unless the CMS has provided different coding or reporting instructions.

The American Medical Association publishes "CPT Assistant" which contains coding guidelines. The CMS does not review nor approve the information in this publication. In the development of NCCI PTP edits, the CMS occasionally disagrees with the information in this publication. If a physician uses information from "CPT Assistant" to report services rendered to Medicare patients, it is possible that MACs may use different criteria to process claims.

J. CPT "Separate Procedure" Definition

If a CPT code descriptor includes the term "separate procedure," the CPT code may not be reported separately with a related procedure. The CMS interprets this designation to prohibit the separate reporting of a "separate procedure" when performed with another procedure in an anatomically related region often through the same skin incision, orifice, or surgical approach.

A CPT code with the "separate procedure" designation may be reported with another procedure if it is performed at a separate patient encounter on the same date of service or at the same patient encounter in an anatomically unrelated area often through a separate skin incision, orifice, or surgical approach. Modifiers 59 or -X[ES] (or a more specific modifier, e.g., anatomic modifier) may be appended to the "separate procedure" CPT code to indicate that it qualifies as a separately reportable service.

K. Family of Codes

The "CPT Manual" often contains a group of codes that describe related procedures that may be performed in various combinations. Some codes describe limited component services, and other codes describe various combinations of component services. Physicians must use several principles in selecting the correct code to report:

1. A HCPCS/CPT code may be reported if and only if all services described by the code are performed.
2. The HCPCS/CPT code describing the services performed shall be reported. A physician shall not report multiple codes corresponding to component services if a single comprehensive code describes the services performed. There are limited exceptions to this rule which are specifically identified in this Manual.
3. HCPCS/CPT code(s) corresponding to component service(s) of other more comprehensive HCPCS/CPT code(s) shall not be reported separately with the more comprehensive HCPCS/CPT code(s) that include the component service(s).
4. If the HCPCS/CPT codes do not correctly describe the procedure(s) performed, the physician shall report a "not otherwise specified" CPT code rather than a HCPCS/CPT code that most closely describes the procedure(s) performed.

L. More Extensive Procedure

The "CPT Manual" often describes groups of similar codes differing in the complexity of the service. Unless services are performed at separate patient encounters or at separate anatomic sites, the less complex service is included in the more complex service and is not separately reportable. Several examples of this principle follow:

1. If 2 procedures only differ in that 1 is described as a "simple" procedure and the other as a "complex" procedure, the "simple" procedure is included in the "complex" procedure and is not separately reportable unless the 2 procedures are performed at separate patient encounters or at separate anatomic sites.
2. If 2 procedures only differ in that 1 is described as a "simple" procedure and the other as a "complicated" procedure, the "simple" procedure is included in the "complicated" procedure and is not separately reportable unless the 2 procedures are performed at separate patient encounters or at separate anatomic sites.
3. If 2 procedures only differ in that 1 is described as a "limited" procedure and the other as a "complete" procedure, the "limited" procedure is included in the "complete" procedure and is not separately reportable unless the 2 procedures are performed at separate patient encounters or at separate anatomic sites.
4. If 2 procedures only differ in that 1 is described as an "intermediate" procedure and the other as a "comprehensive" procedure, the "intermediate" procedure is included in the "comprehensive" procedure and is not separately reportable unless the 2 procedures are performed at separate patient encounters or at separate anatomic sites.
5. If 2 procedures only differ in that 1 is described as a "superficial" procedure and the other as a "deep" procedure, the "superficial" procedure is included in the "deep" procedure and is not separately reportable unless the 2 procedures are

performed at separate patient encounters or at separate anatomic sites.
6. If 2 procedures only differ in that 1 is described as an "incomplete" procedure and the other as a "complete" procedure, the "incomplete" procedure is included in the "complete" procedure and is not separately reportable unless the 2 procedures are performed at separate patient encounters or at separate anatomic sites.
7. If 2 procedures only differ in that 1 is described as an "external" procedure and the other as an "internal" procedure, the "external" procedure is included in the "internal" procedure and is not separately reportable unless the 2 procedures are performed at separate patient encounters or at separate anatomic sites.

M. Sequential Procedure

Some surgical procedures may be performed by different surgical approaches. If an initial surgical approach to a procedure fails and a second surgical approach is used at the same patient encounter, only the HCPCS/CPT code corresponding to the second surgical approach may be reported. If there are different HCPCS/CPT codes for the 2 different surgical approaches, the 2 procedures are considered "sequential," and only the HCPCS/CPT code corresponding to the second surgical approach may be reported. For example, a physician may begin a cholecystectomy procedure using a laparoscopic approach and have to convert the procedure to an open abdominal approach. Only the CPT code for the open cholecystectomy may be reported. The CPT code for the failed laparoscopic cholecystectomy is not separately reportable.

N. Laboratory Panel

The "CPT Manual" defines organ and disease specific panels of laboratory tests. If a laboratory performs all tests included in one of these panels, the laboratory shall report the CPT code for the panel. If the laboratory repeats 1 of these component tests as a medically reasonable and necessary service on the same date of service, the CPT code corresponding to the repeat laboratory test may be reported with modifier 91 appended (See Chapter X, Section C (Organ or Disease Oriented Panels).

O. Misuse of Column Two Column Code with Column One Code (Misuse of Code Edit Rationale)

The CMS manuals and instructions often describe groups of HCPCS/CPT codes that should not be reported together for the Medicare program. Edits based on these instructions are often included as misuse of a Column Two code with a Column One code.

A HCPCS/CPT code descriptor does not include exhaustive information about the code. Physicians who are not familiar with a HCPCS/CPT code may incorrectly report the code in a context different than intended. The NCCI program has identified HCPCS/CPT codes that are incorrectly reported with other HCPCS/CPT codes as a result of the misuse of the Column

Two code with the Column One code. If these edits allow use of NCCI PTP-associated modifiers (modifier indicator of "1"), there are limited circumstances when the Column Two code may be reported on the same date of service as the Column One code. Two examples follow:

1. Three or more HCPCS/CPT codes may be reported on the same date of service. Although the Column Two code is misused if reported as a service associated with the Column One code, the Column Two code may be appropriately reported with a third HCPCS/CPT code reported on the same date of service. For example, the CMS limits separate payment for use of the operating microscope for microsurgical techniques (CPT code 69990) to a group of procedures listed in the online "Claims Processing Manual" (Chapter 12, Section 20.4.5 (Allowable Adjustments)). The NCCI program has edits with Column One codes of surgical procedures not listed in this section of the manual and Column Two CPT code of 69990. Some of these edits allow use of NCCI PTP-associated modifiers because the 2 services listed in the edit may be performed at the same patient encounter as a third procedure for which CPT code 69990 is separately reportable.
2. There may be limited circumstances when the Column Two code is separately reportable with the Column One code. For example, the NCCI program has an edit with Column One CPT code of 47600 (Cholecystectomy) and Column Two CPT code of 12035 (Repair, intermediate, wounds of scalp, axillae, trunk and/or extremities (excluding hands and feet); 12.6 cm to 20.0 cm). If the patient has an abdominal wound in addition to and separate from the cholecystectomy surgical incision, then it may be separately reportable with CPT code 12035 using an NCCI PTP-associated modifier to bypass the edit. 47600 includes repair of the cholecystectomy surgical incision.

Misuse of code as an edit rationale may be applied to PTP edits where the Column Two code is not separately reportable with the Column One code based on the nature of the Column One coded procedure. This edit rationale may also be applied to code pairs where use of the Column Two code with the Column One code is deemed to be a coding error.

P. Mutually Exclusive Procedures

Many procedure codes cannot be reported together because they are mutually exclusive of each other. Mutually exclusive procedures cannot reasonably be performed at the same anatomic site or same patient encounter. An example of a mutually exclusive situation is the repair of an organ that can be performed by 2 different methods. Only one method can be chosen to repair the organ. A second example is a service that can be reported as an "initial" service or a "subsequent" service.

Q. Gender-Specific Procedures

The descriptor of some HCPCS/CPT codes includes a gender-specific restriction on the use of the code. HCPCS/CPT codes specific for one gender should not be reported with HCPCS/CPT codes for the opposite gender. For example, CPT code 53210 describes a total urethrectomy including cystostomy in a female, and CPT code 53215 describes the same procedure in a male. Since the patient cannot have both the male and female procedures performed, the 2 CPT codes cannot be reported together.

R. Add-on Codes

Some codes in the "CPT Manual" are identified as "Add-on" Codes (AOCs), which describe a service that can only be reported in addition to a primary procedure. "CPT Manual" instructions specify the primary procedure code(s) for most AOCs. For other AOCs, the primary procedure code(s) is (are) not specified. When the "CPT Manual" identifies specific primary codes, the AOCs shall not be reported as a supplemental service for other HCPCS/CPT codes not listed as a primary code.

AOCs permit the reporting of significant supplemental services commonly performed in addition to the primary procedure. By contrast, incidental services that are necessary to accomplish the primary procedure (e.g., lysis of adhesions in the course of an open cholecystectomy) are not separately reportable with an AOC. Similarly, complications inherent in an invasive procedure occurring during the procedure are not separately reportable. For example, control of bleeding during an invasive procedure is considered part of the procedure and is not separately reportable.

In general, NCCI PTP edits do not include edits with most AOCs because edits related to the primary procedure(s) are adequate to prevent inappropriate payment for an add-on coded procedure (i.e., if an edit prevents payment of the primary procedure code, the AOC shall not be paid). However, the NCCI program does include edits for some AOCs when coding edits related to the primary procedures must be supplemented. Examples include edits with add-on HCPCS/CPT codes 69990 (Microsurgical techniques requiring use of operating microscope) and 95940/95941/G0453 (Intraoperative neurophysiology testing).

HCPCS/CPT codes that are not designated as AOCs shall not be misused as an AOC to report a supplemental service. A HCPCS/CPT code may be reported if and only if all services described by the CPT code are performed. A HCPCS/CPT code shall not be reported with another service because a portion of the service described by the HCPCS/CPT code was performed with the other procedure. For example, if an ejection fraction is estimated from an echocardiogram study, it would be inappropriate to additionally report CPT code 78472 (Cardiac blood pool imaging gated equilibrium; planar, single study at rest or stress (exercise and/or pharmacologic), wall motion study plus ejection fraction, with or without additional quantitative processing) with the echocardiography (e.g., CPT code 93307). Although the procedure described by CPT code 78472 includes an ejection fraction, it is measured by gated equilibrium with a radionuclide which is not used in echocardiography.

S. Excluded Service

The NCCI program does not generally address issues related to HCPCS/CPT codes describing services that are excluded from Medicare coverage or are not otherwise recognized for payment under the Medicare program.

T. Unlisted Procedure Codes

The "CPT Manual" includes codes to identify services or procedures not described by other HCPCS/CPT codes. These unlisted procedure codes are generally identified as XXX99 or XXXX9 codes and are located at the end of each section or subsection of the Manual. If a physician provides a service that is not accurately described by other HCPCS/CPT codes, the service shall be reported using an unlisted procedure code. A physician shall not report a CPT code for a specific procedure if it does not accurately describe the service performed. It is inappropriate to report the best fit HCPCS/CPT code unless it accurately describes the service performed, and all components of the HCPCS/CPT code were performed. Since unlisted procedure codes may be reported for a very diverse group of services, the NCCI program generally does not include edits with these codes.

U. Modified, Deleted, and Added Code Pairs/Edits — Information moved to Introduction chapter, Section (Purpose), Page Intro-5 of this Manual

V. Medically Unlikely Edits (MUEs)

To lower the Medicare Fee-For-Service Paid Claims Error Rate, the CMS has established units of service edits referred to as Medically Unlikely Edit(s)(MUEs).

An MUE is the maximum units of service (UOS) reported for a HCPCS/CPT code on the vast majority of appropriately reported claims by the same provider/supplier for the same beneficiary on the same date of service.

All claims submitted to MACs and Durable Medical Equipment (DME) MACs, and outpatient facility services claims (Type of Bill 13X, 14X, 85X, *87X*) are tested against MUEs.

Prior to April 1, 2013, each line of a claim was adjudicated separately against the MUE value for the HCPCS/CPT code reported on that claim line. If the UOS on that claim line exceeded the MUE value, the entire claim line was denied.

In the April 1, 2013, version of MUEs, the CMS began introducing date of service (DOS) MUEs. Over time the CMS will convert many, but not all, MUEs to DOS MUEs. Since April 1, 2013, MUEs are adjudicated either as claim line edits or DOS edits. If the MUE is adjudicated as a claim line edit, the UOS on each claim line are compared to the MUE value for the HCPCS/CPT code on that claim line. If the UOS exceed the MUE value, all UOS on that claim line are denied. If the MUE is adjudicated as a DOS MUE, all UOS on each claim line for the same date of service for the same HCPCS/CPT code are summed, and the sum is compared to the MUE value. If the summed UOS exceed the MUE value, all UOS for the HCPCS/CPT code for that date of service are denied. Denials due to claim line MUEs or DOS MUEs may be appealed to the local claims processing contractor. DOS MUEs are used for HCPCS/CPT codes where it would be extremely unlikely that more UOS than the MUE value would ever be performed on the same date of service for the same patient.

The MUE files on the CMS NCCI website display an "MUE Adjudication Indicator" (MAI) for each HCPCS/CPT code. An MAI of "1" indicates that the edit is a claim line MUE. An MAI of "2" or "3" indicates that the edit is a DOS MUE.

If a HCPCS/CPT code has an MUE that is adjudicated as a claim line edit, (i.e., MAI equal to "1") appropriate use of CPT modifiers (i.e., 59 or -X{EPSU}, 76, 77, 91, anatomic) may be used to report the same HCPCS/CPT code on separate lines of a claim. Each line of the claim with that HCPCS/CPT code will be separately adjudicated against the MUE value for that HCPCS/CPT code. Claims processing contractors have rules limiting use of these modifiers with some HCPCS/CPT codes.

MUEs for HCPCS codes with an MAI of "2" are absolute date of service edits. These are "per day edits based on policy." HCPCS codes with an MAI of "2" have been rigorously reviewed and vetted within CMS and obtain this MAI designation because UOS on the same date of service (DOS) in excess of the MUE value would be considered impossible because it was contrary to statute, regulation, or subregulatory guidance. This subregulatory guidance includes clear correct coding policy that is binding on both providers/suppliers and CMS claims processing contractors. Limitations created by anatomical, or coding limitations are incorporated in correct coding policy, both in the HIPAA mandated coding descriptors and CMS-approved coding guidance as well as specific guidance in the CMS and NCCI manuals. For example, it would be contrary to correct coding policy to report more than one unit of service for CPT 94002 (Ventilation assist and management . . . initial day) because such use could not accurately describe 2 initial days of management occurring on the same date of service as would be required by the code descriptor. As a result, claims processing contractors are instructed that an MAI of "2" denotes a claims processing restriction for which override during processing, reopening, or redetermination would be contrary to CMS policy.

MUEs for HCPCS codes with an MAI of "3" are "per day edits based on clinical benchmarks." MUEs assigned an MAI of "3" are based on criteria (e.g., nature of service, prescribing information) combined with data such that it would be possible but medically highly unlikely that higher values would represent correctly reported medically necessary services. If contractors have evidence (e.g., medical review) that UOS in excess of the MUE value were actually provided, were correctly coded and were medically necessary, the contractor may bypass the MUE for a HCPCS code with an MAI of "3" during claim processing, reopening, or redetermination, or in response to effectuation instructions from a reconsideration or higher-level appeal.

Both the MAI and MUE value for each HCPCS/CPT code are based on one or more of the following criteria:

(1) Anatomic considerations may limit UOS based on anatomic structures. For example:
   a) The MUE value for an appendectomy is "1" since there is only 1 appendix.
   b) The MUE for a knee brace is "2" because there are 2 knees and Medicare policy does not cover back-up equipment.
   c) The MUE value for a lumbar spine procedure reported per lumbar vertebra or per lumbar interspace cannot exceed "5" since there are only 5 lumbar vertebrae or interspaces.
   d) The MUE value for a procedure reported per lung lobe cannot exceed "5" since there are only 5 lung lobes (3 in right lung and 2 in left lung).
(2) CPT code descriptors/CPT coding instructions in the "CPT Manual" may limit UOS. For example:

a) A procedure described as the "initial 30 minutes" would have an MUE value of "1" because of the use of the term "initial." A different code may be reported for additional time.

b) If a code descriptor uses the plural form of the procedure, it must not be reported with multiple UOS. For example, if the code descriptor states "biopsies," the code is reported with "1" unit of service regardless of the number of biopsies performed.

c) The MUE value for a procedure with "per day," "per week," or "per month" in its code descriptor is "1" because MUEs are based on number of services per day of service.

d) The MUE value of a code for a procedure described as "unilateral" is "1" if there is a different code for the procedure described as "bilateral."

e) The code descriptors of a family of codes may define different levels of service, each having an MUE of "1." For example, CPT codes 78102-78104 describe bone marrow imaging. CPT code 78102 is reported for imaging a "limited area." CPT code 78103 is reported for imaging "multiple areas." CPT code 78104 is reported for imaging the "whole body."

f) The MUE value for CPT code 86021 (Antibody identification; leukocyte antibodies) is "1" because the code descriptor is plural including testing for any and all leukocyte antibodies. On a single date of service only one specimen from a patient would be tested for leukocyte antibodies.

g) When reporting codes, it is important to assure the accuracy of coding and the correct UOS by selecting a code that accurately identifies the service performed based on factors including but not limited to, the route of administration. For example, for intravitreal injection of bevacizumab, select an intravitreal code (e.g., C9257) rather than an intravenous code (e.g., J9035).

(3) Edits based on established CMS policies may limit UOS. For example:

a) The MUE value for a surgical or diagnostic procedure may be based on the bilateral surgery indicator on the Medicare Physician Fee Schedule Database (MPFSDB).

i. If the bilateral surgery indicator is "0," a bilateral procedure must be reported with "1" unit of service. There is no additional payment for the code if reported as a unilateral or bilateral procedure because of anatomy or physiology. Alternatively, the code descriptor may specifically state that the procedure is a unilateral procedure, and there is a separate code for a bilateral procedure.

ii. If the bilateral surgery indicator is "1," a bilateral surgical procedure must be reported with "1" unit of service and modifier 50 (bilateral modifier). A bilateral diagnostic procedure may be reported with "1" unit of service and modifier 50 on 1 claim line, or "1" unit of service with modifier RT on 1 claim line plus "1" unit of service and modifier LT on a second claim line.

iii. If the bilateral surgery indicator is "2," a bilateral procedure must be reported with "1" unit of service. The procedure is priced as a bilateral procedure because (1) the code descriptor defines the procedure as bilateral; (2) the code descriptor states that the procedure is performed unilaterally or bilaterally; or (3) the procedure is usually performed as a bilateral procedure.

iv. If the bilateral surgery indicator is "3," a bilateral surgical procedure must be reported with "1" unit of service and modifier 50 (bilateral modifier). A bilateral diagnostic procedure may be reported with "2" UOS on 1 claim line, "1" unit of service and modifier 50 on 1 claim line, or 1 unit of service with modifier RT on 1 claim line plus "1" unit of service and modifier LT on a second claim line.

b) The MUE value for a code may be "1" where the code descriptor does not specify a unit of service and the CMS considers the default UOS to be "per day." c) The MUE value for a code may be "0" because the code is listed as invalid, not covered, bundled, not separately payable, statutorily excluded, not reasonable and necessary, etc. based on:
i. The Medicare Physician Fee Schedule Database
ii. OPPS Addendum B
iii. Alpha-Numeric HCPCS Code File
iv. DMEPOS Jurisdiction List
v. Medicare "Internet-Only Manual ("IOM")

(4) The nature of an analyte may limit UOS and is in general determined by:

a) The nature of the specimen may limit the UOS. For example, CPT code 82575 describes a creatinine clearance test and has an MUE of "1" because the test requires a twenty-four-hour urine collection; or

b) The physiology, pathophysiology, or clinical application of the analyte is such that a maximum unit of service for a single date of service can be determined. For example, the MUE for CPT code 82747 (RBC folic acid) is "1" because the test result would not be expected to change during a single day, and thus it is not necessary to perform the test more than once on a single date of service.

(5) The nature of a procedure/service may limit UOS and is in general determined by the amount of time required to perform a procedure/service (e.g., overnight sleep studies) or clinical application of a procedure/service (e.g., motion analysis tests).

a) The MUE for many surgical or medical procedures is "1" because the procedure is rarely, if ever, performed more than 1 time per day (e.g., colonoscopy, motion analysis tests).

b) The MUE value for a procedure is "1" because of the amount of time required to perform the procedure (e.g., overnight sleep study).

(6) The nature of equipment may limit UOS and is in general determined by the number of items of equipment that would be used. For example, the MUE value for a wheelchair code is "1" because only 1 wheelchair is used at 1 time and Medicare policy does not cover back-up equipment.

(7) Although clinical judgment considerations and determinations based on input from numerous physicians and certified coders are sometimes initially used to establish some MUE values, these values are subsequently validated or changed based on submitted and/or paid claims data.

(8) Prescribing information is based on FDA labeling as well as off-label information published in CMS-approved drug compendia. See below for additional information about how prescribing information is used in determining the MUE values.

(9) Submitted and paid claims data (100%) from a six-month period is used to ascertain the distribution pattern of UOS typically reported for a given HCPCS/CPT code.

(10) Published policies of the Durable Medical Equipment (DME) Medicare Administrative Contractors (MACs) may

limit UOS for some durable medical equipment, prosthetics, orthotics, and supplies (DMEPOS). For example:

a) The MUE values for many ostomy and urological supply codes, nebulizer codes, and CPAP accessory codes are typically based on a three-month supply of items.

b) The MUE values for surgical dressings, parenteral and enteral nutrition, immunosuppressive drugs, and oral anti-cancer drugs are typically based on a one-month supply.

c) The MUE values take into account the requirement for reporting certain codes with date spans.

d) The MUE value of a code may be "0" if the item is noncovered, not medically necessary, or not separately payable.

e) The MUE value of a code may be "0" if the code is invalid for claim submission to the DME MAC.

UOS denied based on an MUE may be appealed. Because a denial of services due to an MUE is a coding denial, not a medical necessity denial, the presence of an Advanced Beneficiary Notice of Noncoverage (ABN) shall not shift liability to the beneficiary for UOS denied based on an MUE. If during reopening or redetermination medical records are provided with respect to an MUE denial for an edit with an MAI of "3," contractors will review the records to determine if the provider actually furnished units in excess of the MUE, if the codes were used correctly, and whether the services were medically reasonable and necessary. If the units were actually provided but one of the other conditions is not met, a change in denial reason may be warranted (for example, a change from the MUE denial based on incorrect coding to a determination that the item/service is not reasonable and necessary under section 1862(a)(1)). This may also be true for certain edits with an MAI of "1." The CMS interprets the notice delivery requirements under §1879 of the Social Security Act (the Act) as applying to situations in which a provider expects the initial claim determination to be a reasonable and necessary denial. Consistent with NCCI guidance, denials resulting from MUEs are not based on any of the statutory provisions that give liability protection to beneficiaries under Section 1879 of the Act. Thus, ABN issuance based on an MUE is NOT appropriate. A provider/supplier may not issue an ABN in connection with services denied due to an MUE and cannot bill the beneficiary for UOS denied based on an MUE.

HCPCS J-code and drug related C and Q-code MUEs are based on prescribing information and 100% claims data for a six-month period of time. Using the prescribing information, the highest total daily dose for each drug was determined. This dose and its corresponding UOS were evaluated against paid and submitted claims data. Some of the guiding principles used in developing these edits are as follows:

(1) If the prescribing information defined a maximum daily dose, this value was used to determine the MUE value. For some drugs there is an absolute maximum daily dose. For others there is a maximum "recommended" or "usual" dose. In the latter 2 cases, the daily dose calculation was evaluated against claims data.

(2) If the maximum daily dose calculation is based on actual body weight, a dose based on a weight range of 110-150 kg was evaluated against the claims data. If the maximum daily dose calculation is based on ideal body weight, a dose based on a weight range of 90-110 kg was evaluated against claims data. If the maximum daily dose calculation is based on body surface area (BSA), a dose based on a BSA range of 2.4-3.0 square meters was evaluated against claims data.

(3) For drugs where the maximum daily dose is based on patient response or need, prescribing information and claims data were used to establish the MUE values.

(4) Published off-label use of a drug was considered for the maximum daily dose calculation.

(5) The MUE values for some drug codes are set to "0." The rationale for such values include but are not limited to: discontinued manufacture of drug, non-FDA-approved compounded drug, practitioner MUE values for oral antineoplastic, oral anti-emetic, and oral immune suppressive drugs which should be billed to the DME MACs, outpatient hospital MUE values for inhalation drugs which should be billed to the DME MACs, and Practitioner/ASC MUE values for HCPCS C codes describing medications that would not be related to a procedure performed in an ASC.

Non-drug-related HCPCS/CPT codes may be assigned an MUE of "0" for a variety of reasons including, but not limited to, outpatient hospital MUE value for a surgical procedure only performed as an inpatient procedure, noncovered service, bundled service, DME MUE value for implanted devices and items related to implanted devices which should not be billed to the DME MACs, or packaged service.

The MUE files on the CMS NCCI website display an "Edit Rationale" for each HCPCS/CPT code. Although an MUE may be based on several rationales, only one is displayed on the website. One of the listed rationales is "Data." This rationale indicates that 100% claims data from a six-month period of time was the major factor in determining the MUE value. If a physician appeals an MUE denial for a HCPCS/CPT code where the MUE is based on "Data," the reviewer will usually confirm that (1) the correct code is reported; (2) the correct UOS are used; (3) the number of reported UOS were performed; and (4) all UOS were medically reasonable and necessary.

The first MUEs were implemented January 1, 2007. Additional MUEs are added on a quarterly basis on the same schedule as NCCI PTP updates. Prior to implementation proposed MUEs are sent to numerous national healthcare organizations for a 60-day review and comment period.

Many surgical procedures may be performed bilaterally. Instructions in the CMS "IOM" (Publication 100-04 "Medicare Claims Processing Manual," Chapter 12 (Physicians/Nonphysician Practitioners), Section 40.7.B. and Chapter 4 (Part B Hospital (Including Inpatient Hospital Part B and OPPS)), Section 20.6.2 require that bilateral surgical procedures be reported using modifier 50 with one unit of service unless the code descriptor defines the procedure as "bilateral." If the code descriptor defines the procedure as a "bilateral" procedure, it shall be reported with one unit of service without modifier 50. If a bilateral surgical procedure is performed at different sites bilaterally, one unit of service may be reported for each site. That is, the HCPCS/CPT code may be reported with modifier 50 and one unit of service for each site at which it was performed bilaterally.

Some A/B MACs allow providers/*suppliers* to report repetitive services performed over a range of dates on a single line of a claim with multiple UOS. If a provider/*supplier* reports services in this fashion, the provider/*supplier* should report the "from date" and "to date" on the claim line. Contractors are instructed to divide the UOS reported on the claim line by the number of days in the date span and round to the nearest whole number. This number is compared to the MUE value for the code on the claim line.

Providers/Suppliers billing services to the DME MACs typically report some HCPCS codes for supply items for a period exceeding a single day. The DME MACs have billing rules for these codes. For some codes the DME MACs require that the "from date" and "to date" be reported. The MUEs for these codes are based on the maximum number of UOS that may be reported for a single date of service. For other codes the DME MACs permit multiple days' supply items to be reported on a single claim line where the "from date" and "to date" are the same. The DME MACs have rules allowing supply items for a maximum number of days to be reported at one time for each of these types of codes. The MUE values for these codes are based on the maximum number of days that may be reported at one time. As with all MUEs, the MUE value does not represent a utilization guideline. Providers/suppliers shall not assume that they may report UOS up to the MUE value on each date of service. Providers/suppliers may only report supply items that are medically reasonable and necessary.

Most MUE values are set so that a provider or supplier would only very occasionally have a claim line denied. If a provider/*supplier* encounters a code with frequent denials due to the MUE or frequent use of a CPT modifier to bypass the MUE, the provider or supplier should consider the following: (1) Is the HCPCS/CPT code being used correctly? (2) Is the unit of service being counted correctly? (3) Are all reported services medically reasonable and necessary? and (4) Why does the provider's or supplier's practice differ from national patterns? A provider or supplier may choose to discuss these questions with the local Medicare contractor or a national healthcare organization whose members frequently perform the procedure.

Most MUE values are published on the CMS MUE webpage. However, some MUE values are not published and are confidential. These values shall not be published in oral or written form by any party that acquires one or more of them.

MUEs are not utilization edits. Although the MUE value for some codes may represent the commonly reported UOS (e.g., MUE of "1" for appendectomy), the usual UOS for many HCPCS/CPT codes is less than the MUE value. Claims reporting UOS less than the MUE value may be subject to review by claims processing contractors, Unified Program Integrity Contractor (UPICS), Recovery Audit Contractors (RACs), and Department of Justice (DOJ).

Since MUEs are coding edits, rather than medical necessity edits, claims processing contractors may have UOS edits that are more restrictive than MUEs. In such cases, the more restrictive claims processing contractor edit would be applied to the claim. Similarly, if the MUE is more restrictive than a claims processing contractor edit, the more restrictive MUE would apply.

W. Add-on Code Edit Tables

Add-on Codes (AOCs) are discussed in Chapter I, Section R (Add-on Codes). The CMS publishes a list of AOCs and their primary codes annually prior to January 1. The list is updated quarterly based on the AMA's "CPT Errata" documents or implementation of new HCPCS/CPT add-on codes. The CMS identifies AOCs and their primary codes based on "CPT Manual" instructions, CMS interpretation of HCPCS/CPT codes, and CMS coding instructions.

The NCCI program includes 3 AOC Edit Tables, 1 table for each of 3 "Types" of AOC. Each table lists the AOC with its primary codes. An AOC is a HCPCS/CPT code that describes a service that, with rare exception, is performed in conjunction with another primary service by the same practitioner. An AOC is rarely eligible for payment if it is the only procedure reported by a practitioner.

The "Type *1* AOC Edit Table" lists AOCs for which the "CPT Manual" or HCPCS tables define all acceptable primary codes. Claims processing contractors should not allow other primary codes with Type I AOCs. CPT code 99292 (Critical care, evaluation, and management of the critically ill or critically injured patient; each additional 30 minutes (List separately in addition to code for primary service)) is included as a Type I AOC since its only primary code is CPT code 99291 (Critical care, evaluation, and management of the critically ill or critically injured patient; first 30-74 minutes). For Medicare purposes, CPT code 99292 may be eligible for payment to a physician without CPT code 99291 if another physician of the same specialty and physician group reports and is paid for CPT code 99291.

The "Type *2* AOC Edit Table" lists AOC for which the "CPT Manual" and HCPCS tables do not define any primary codes. Claims processing contractors should develop their own lists of acceptable primary codes.

The "Type *3* AOC Edit Table" lists AOCs for which the "CPT Manual" or HCPCS tables define some, but not all, acceptable primary codes. Claims processing contractors should allow the listed primary codes for these AOCs but may develop their own lists of additional acceptable primary codes.

Although the AOC and primary code are normally reported for the same date of service, there are unusual circumstances where the 2 services may be reported for different dates of service (e.g., CPT codes 99291 and 99292).

CMS will update the complete list of AOC edits with their primary procedure codes on an annual basis on or by January 1 every year based on changes to the CPT Manual or HCPCS Level II Manual. Quarterly updates will be posted as a complete list of AOC edits, if necessary, on April 1, July 1, and October 1 of each year. If no changes occur in the AOC edits, no quarterly update will be posted.

FIGURE CREDITS

1. From Little J, et al: *Dental Management of the Medically Compromised Patient*, ed 9, St. Louis, 2017, Mosby. *(Courtesy Medtronic, Minneapolis)*
2. From Franklin I, Dawson P, Rodway A: *Essentials of Clinical Surgery*, ed 2, St. Louis, 2012, Saunders.
3. Modified from Grosfeld J, et al: *Pediatric Surgery*, ed 7, Philadelphia, 2012, Mosby.
4. Modified from Hsu J, Michael J, Fisk J: *AAOS Atlas of Orthoses and Assistive Devices*, ed 4, Philadelphia, 2008, Mosby.
5. From Wold G: *Basic Geriatric Nursing*, ed 5, St. Louis, 2011, Mosby.
6. Modified from Roberts J, Hedges J: *Clinical Procedures in Emergency Medicine*, ed 6, St. Louis, 2013, Saunders.
7. From Auerbach P: *Wilderness Medicine*, ed 7, Philadelphia, 2016, Mosby. (Courtesy Black Diamond Equipment, Ltd.)
8. *(Original to book)*.
9. Modified from Abeloff M, et al: *Clinical Oncology*, ed 5, Philadelphia, 2013, Churchill Livingstone.
10. *(Original to book)*.
11. Modified from Duthie E, Katz P, Malone M: *Practice of Geriatrics*, ed 4, Philadelphia, 2007, Saunders.
12. Modified from Roberts J, Hedges J: *Clinical Procedures in Emergency Medicine*, ed 6, St. Louis, 2013, Saunders.
13. From Young A, Proctor D: *Kinn's The Medical Assistant*, ed 13, St. Louis, 2016, Saunders.
14. From Bonewit-West K: *Clinical Procedures for Medical Assistants*, ed 9, Philadelphia, 2015, WB Saunders.
15. From Roberts J, Hedges J: *Clinical Procedures in Emergency Medicine*, ed 6, St. Louis, 2013, Saunders.
16. From Yeo: *Shackelford's Surgery of the Alimentary Tract*, ed 7, Philadelphia, 2012, Saunders.
17. Redrawn from Bragg D, Rubin P, Hricak H: *Oncologic Imaging*, ed 2, 2002, Saunders.
18. From Roberts J, Hedges J: *Clinical Procedures in Emergency Medicine*, ed 6, St. Louis, 2013, Saunders. *(Courtesy Atrium Medical Corp., Hudson, NH 03051)*
19. **A** From Auerbach P: *Wilderness Medicine*, ed 7, Philadelphia, 2016, Mosby. **B** Modified from Hsu J, Michael J, Fisk J: *AAOS Atlas of Orthoses and Assistive Devices*, ed 4, Philadelphia, 2008, Mosby.
20. Modified from Lusardi M, Nielsen C: *Orthotics and Prosthetics in Rehabilitation*, ed 3, St. Louis, 2013, Butterworth-Heinemann.
21. Modified from Lusardi M, Nielsen C: *Orthotics and Prosthetics in Rehabilitation*, ed 3, St. Louis, 2013, Butterworth-Heinemann.
22. Modified from Lusardi M, Nielsen C: *Orthotics and Prosthetics in Rehabilitation*, ed 3, St. Louis, 2013, Butterworth-Heinemann.
23. From Buck C: *The Next Step, Advanced Medical Coding 2023/2024 edition*, St. Louis, 2023, Elsevier.
24. From Jardins T: *Clinical Manifestations and Assessment of Respiratory Disease*, ed 7, St. Louis, 2015, Elsevier.
25. From Hsu J, Michael J, Fisk J: *AAOS Atlas of Orthoses and Assistive Devices*, ed 4, Philadelphia, 2008, Mosby.
26. Modified from Hsu J, Michael J, Fisk J: *AAOS Atlas of Orthoses and Assistive Devices*, ed 4, Philadelphia, 2008, Mosby.
27. Modified from Hsu J, Michael J, Fisk J: *AAOS Atlas of Orthoses and Assistive Devices*, ed 4, Philadelphia, 2008, Mosby.
28. From Didomenico L, Gatlyak N: "End-Stage Ankle Arthritis." *Clinics in Podiatric Medicine and Surgery* 29.3 (2012): 391-412.
29. Cameron M, Monroe L: *Physical Rehabilitation for the Physical Therapist Assistant*, ed 1, St. Louis, 2011, Saunders.
30. From Rowe D, Jadhav A: "Care of the Adolescent with Spina Bifida." *Pediatric Clinics of North America* 55.6 (2008): 1359-374.
31. Modified from Lusardi M, Nielsen C: *Orthotics and Prosthetics in Rehabilitation*, ed 3, St. Louis, 2013, Butterworth-Heinemann.
32. From Hsu J, Michael J, Fisk J: *AAOS Atlas of Orthoses and Assistive Devices*, ed 4, Philadelphia, 2008, Mosby.
33. *(Original to book.)*
34. From Hochberg M: *Rheumatology*, ed 5, Philadelphia, 2011, Mosby.
35. Modified from Hsu J, Michael J, Fisk J: *AAOS Atlas of Orthoses and Assistive Devices*, ed 4, Philadelphia, 2008, Mosby.
36. From Coughlin M, Mann R, Saltzman C: *Surgery of the Foot and Ankle*, ed 9, Philadelphia, 2013, Mosby.
37. From Canale S: *Campbell's Operative Orthopaedics*, ed 12, St. Louis, 2012, Mosby.
38. From Sorrentino S, Gorek B: *Mosby's Textbook for Long-term Care Nursing Assistants*, ed 7, St. Louis, 2014, Mosby.
39. From Pedretti L, Pendleton H, Schultz-Krohn W: *Pedretti's Occupational Therapy: Practice Skills for Physical Dysfunction*, ed 7, St. Louis, 2013, Elsevier.
40. From Skirven T: *Rehabilitation of the Hand and Upper Extremity*, ed 6, Philadelphia, 2010, Mosby.
41. From Lusardi M, Nielsen C: *Orthotics and Prosthetics in Rehabilitation*, ed 3, St. Louis, 2013, Butterworth-Heinemann. *(Courtesy Michael Curtain)*
42. Schickendantz M: "Diagnosis and Treatment of Elbow Disorders in the Overhead Athlete." *Hand Clinics* 18.1 (2002): 65-75.
43. Modified from Bland K, Copeland E: *The Breast: Comprehensive Management of Benign and Malignant Disorders*, ed 4, St. Louis, 2009, Saunders.
44. From Shah J, Patel S, Singh B, Shah J: *Jatin Shah's Head and Neck Surgery and Oncology*, ed 4, Philadelphia, 2012, Mosby, 2012. From Subburaj K, Nair C, Rajesh S, Ravi B: "Rapid Development of Auricular Prosthesis Using CAD and Rapid Prototyping Technologies." *International Journal of Oral and Maxillofacial Surgery* 36.10 (2007): 938-43.
45. From Weinzweig J: *Plastic Surgery Secrets*, ed 2, Philadelphia, 2010, Hanley & Belfus, p 543.
46. Modified from Mann D: *Heart Failure: A Companion to Braunwald's Heart Disease*, ed 3, Philadelphia, 2015, Saunders.
47. Modified from Roberts J, Hedges J: *Clinical Procedures in Emergency Medicine*, ed 6, Philadelphia, 2013, Saunders.
48. From Yanoff M, Duker J: *Ophthalmology*, ed 4, St. Louis, 2014, Mosby.
49. From Feldman M, Friedman L, Brandt L: *Sleisenger and Fordtran's Gastrointestinal and Liver Disease*, ed 10, Philadelphia, 2015, Saunders.
50. From Katz V, et al: *Comprehensive Gynecology*, ed 7, Philadelphia, 2016, Mosby.
51. From Young A, Proctor D: *Kinn's The Medical Assistant*, ed 13, St. Louis, 2016, Saunders.
52. From Yanoff M, Duker J: *Ophthalmology*, ed 4, St. Louis, 2014, Mosby.